T0206123

The GLYCEMIC INDEX

Applications in Practice

The GLYCEMIC INDEX

Applications in Practice

Edited by

Elena Philippou

Assistant Professor in Nutrition and Dietetics
Department of Life and Health Sciences
University of Nicosia
Nicosia, Cyprus

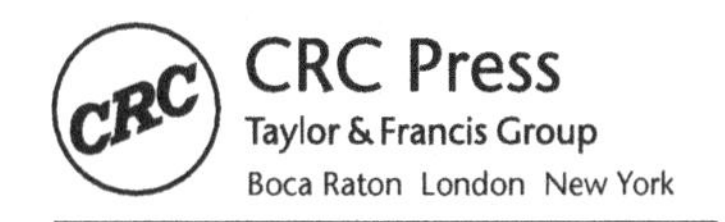

CRC Press is an imprint of the
Taylor & Francis Group, an **informa** business

CRC Press
Taylor & Francis Group
6000 Broken Sound Parkway NW, Suite 300
Boca Raton, FL 33487-2742

First issued in paperback 2021

ISBN 13: 978-1-03-209769-5 (pbk)
ISBN 13: 978-1-4987-0366-6 (hbk)

Publisher's Note
The publisher has gone to great lengths to ensure the quality of this reprint but points out that some imperfections in the original copies may be apparent.

Visit the Taylor & Francis Web site at
http://www.taylorandfrancis.com

and the CRC Press Web site at
http://www.crcpress.com

Contents

Foreword

By 1981, the United States was in the grip of the low-fat diet craze. Based upon tenuous evidence, nutrition authorities began to recommend that everyone consume as little fat as possible to avoid obesity, diabetes, heart disease, and possibly cancer. Instead, the public was advised to base their diet on carbohydrates. Natural high-fat foods such as nuts, avocado, and whole milk yoghurt acquired a bad reputation, whereas highly processed carbohydrates inundated the food supply. Amazingly, these products—including prepared breakfast, crackers, baked chips, breads, reduced fat cookies and cakes, and sugary beverages—were marketed as healthful or at least innocuous, even though they were composed primarily of refined grains and concentrated sugar. Very soon, this low-fat message spread throughout the world.

The year 1981 also witnessed the introduction of the glycemic index (GI) by David Jenkins, Thomas Wolever, and colleagues at the University of Toronto. At that time, the concept of the GI represented a radical departure from conventional thinking, by proposing that the health effects of carbohydrates differ according to how they affect blood glucose in the postprandial state. On account of the brain's critical dependence on this metabolic fuel under most conditions, the concentration of glucose in the blood is ordinarily tightly controlled. However, most highly processed carbohydrates digest rapidly, raising blood glucose and insulin levels much more than traditionally consumed carbohydrates such as legumes, fruits, and minimally processed grains. Early investigators in the field recognized that a high-GI diet stressed the body's energy homeostasis mechanisms, with major implications not only to diabetes management but also to the prevention of type 2 diabetes, heart disease, obesity, and other modern chronic degenerative conditions. Indeed, the science surrounding the GI helped explain why the conventional low-fat diet loaded with processed carbohydrates had actually contributed to many of the diseases it was intended to prevent.

Fortunately, the concept of the GI has also spread around the globe and is poised to outlast and supersede the low-fat diet craze. A new scientific study on the topic is now being published at a rate of almost one a day, providing a wealth of new information about how diet affects hormones, metabolism, and health. All fats are not the same, and neither are carbohydrates. Thus, the GI leads us away from simplistic debates about nutrient "quantity," to a critically important focus on food "quality."

Almost from its inception, the GI elicited controversy, perhaps precisely because it challenged an entrenched paradigm that implicitly considers all carbohydrates alike. Some critics dismissed the GI, arguing that ostensibly unhealthful foods such as ice cream rate low on this scale. But such arguments miss the point: No one dietary factor can ever define a healthful diet. Others point to the existence of negative studies, neglecting the inherent complexity and heterogeneity of nutritional research and the large body of mechanistic, translational, interventional, and observational research supporting a critical role for the GI in human health. In addition, the field is relatively young—many methodological issues have just recently been resolved.

The Glycemic Index: Applications in Practice is a wonderful birthday gift, 36 years after Jenkins, Wolever, and other visionaries brought the GI into the world. In it, the reader will find chapters ranging from state-of-the-art science to clinical application, written by luminaries in the field. I recommend this book with enthusiasm to everyone interested in improving public health through diet.

David S. Ludwig
Boston Children's Hospital
Harvard Medical School
Harvard School of Public Health

Foreword

Preface

It is already been 36 years since 1981 when David Jenkins, Thomas Wolever, and colleagues introduced the concept of glycemic index (GI) to differentiate carbohydrates based on the rate of blood glucose rise following their consumption. Although GI was first used in the diet therapy of diabetes, since then, research evidence has accumulated to thousands of publications from all over the world with applications for prevention and/or management of metabolic syndrome, cardiovascular disease, obesity, polycystic ovary syndrome, certain types of cancer, effects on pregnancy outcomes, sports performance, eye health, and cognitive functioning.

As eloquently put by Professor David S. Ludwig in his Foreword to this book, the GI concept has faced much controversy and criticism arising mainly from misconceptions on its use and application; nevertheless, it has led the way into understanding the importance of macronutrient *quality* rather than just *quantity* on metabolic pathways and diet–disease relationships.

The Glycemic Index: Applications in Practice has gathered in a systematic way all the up-to-date research in the field of GI. It also provides a detailed explanation of how to correctly measure a food's GI, how the GI of food products can be altered, and the use and misuse of GI labeling around the globe. Additionally, it provides practical recommendations on how the GI concept can be applied in the dietary management of certain disease conditions. It is a valuable source of information for healthcare professionals of various disciplines, such as nutritionists, dietitians, food scientists, medical doctors, sports scientists, psychologists, public health (nutrition) policy makers, and students in these fields, as well as an important addition to university libraries for reference purposes.

This book is a result of the combined effort of many experts, including pioneers in the area of GI research, and I wish to express my sincere gratitude to each one of them for making it such a valuable addition to the literature. I also thank CRC Press and especially Dr. Ira Wolinsky, who invited me to edit this book, Randy Brehm, senior editor of the nutrition program, and Kathryn Everett, production coordinator.

I hope you find this book stimulating and useful in your studies and practice.

Elena Philippou
University of Nicosia

Preface

Editor

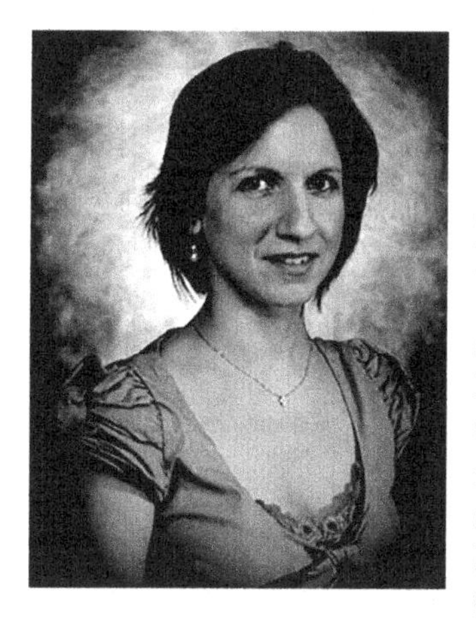

Dr. Elena Philippou is an Assistant Professor in Nutrition and Dietetics at the University of Nicosia, Cyprus, and a Visiting Lecturer in Nutrition and Dietetics at King's College London, United Kingdom. As a registered dietitian, she also holds private consultations on diet-related issues, including obesity, cardiovascular disease, and diabetes.

She obtained a BSc degree in Nutrition and a postgraduate diploma in Dietetics from King's College London, London, England, in 2001 and 2002, respectively. She worked as a dietitian for the National Health Service in the United Kingdom and in parallel completed a postgraduate certificate in behavioral management of adult obesity awarded by the University of Central Lancashire, Preston, England. In 2008, she completed her PhD studies at Imperial College London, focusing on the role of dietary carbohydrates and specifically dietary GI in weight maintenance and cardiovascular disease prevention. Her research has been published in international peer-reviewed scientific journals and presented in scientific conferences.

In 2012, Dr. Philippou obtained a postgraduate certificate in continuing professional academic development program in learning and teaching in higher education awarded by the University of Hertfordshire, Hatfield, England, and became a member of U.K.'s Higher Education Academy. She lectures on various topics, including public health nutrition, nutritional assessment, and medical nutrition therapy of various diseases.

Dr. Philippou's current research interest is in the role of dietary GI manipulation and the Mediterranean diet on cognitive function including investigation of the potential underlying mechanisms.

Editor

Contributors

Ayesha Salem Al Dhaheri
Department of Nutrition and Health
United Arab Emirates University
Al Ain, United Arab Emirates

Fiona S. Atkinson
School of Life and Environmental Sciences
Charles Perkins Centre
The University of Sydney
Sydney, New South Wales, Australia

Livia S.A. Augustin
Clinical Nutrition and Risk Factor Modification Centre
St. Michael's Hospital
Toronto, Ontario, Canada

and

National Cancer Institute "Fondazione G. Pascale"
Naples, Italy

Alan W. Barclay
The Glycemic Index Symbol Foundation
Sydney, New South Wales, Australia

David Bentley
School of Medicine
Department of Social and Health Sciences
Flinders University
Adelaide, South Australia, Australia

Jennie C. Brand-Miller
School of Life and Environmental Sciences
Charles Perkins Centre
The University of Sydney
Sydney, New South Wales, Australia

Gautier Cesbron-Lavau
Mondelez International R&D, Nutrition Research
Saclay, France

Min-Lee Chang
Jean Mayer United States Department of Agriculture Human Nutrition Research Center on Aging
Department of Ophthalmology School of Medicine
Tufts University
Boston, Massachusetts

Laura Chiavaroli
Faculty of Medicine
Department of Nutritional Sciences
University of Toronto
and
Clinical Nutrition and Risk Factor Modification Centre
St. Michael's Hospital
Toronto, Ontario, Canada

Chung-Jung Chiu
Jean Mayer United States Department of Agriculture Human Nutrition Research Center on Aging
Department of Ophthalmology School of Medicine
and
School of Medicine
Department of Ophthalmology
Tufts University
Boston, Massachusetts

Marios Constantinou
School of Humanities, Social Sciences and Law
Department of Social Sciences
University of Nicosia
Nicosia, Cyprus

Russell J. de Souza
Faculty of Medicine
Department of Nutritional Sciences
University of Toronto
and
Clinical Nutrition and Risk Factor Modification Centre
St. Michael's Hospital
Toronto, Ontario, Canada

Kai Lin Ek
Human Nutrition Asia Pacific
BASF South East Asia Pte Ltd
Singapore

Martí Juanola-Falgarona
Department of Neurology
Columbia University Medical Centre
New York, New York

Aurélie Goux
Mondelez International R&D, Nutrition Research
Saclay, France

Vanessa Ha
Faculty of Health Sciences
Department of Clinical Epidemiology and Biostatistics
McMaster University
Hamilton, Ontario, Canada

and

Faculty of Medicine
Department of Nutritional Sciences
University of Toronto
and
Clinical Nutrition and Risk Factor Modification Centre
St. Michael's Hospital
Toronto, Ontario, Canada

Viranda H. Jayalath
Clinical Nutrition and Risk Factor Modification Centre
St. Michael's Hospital
and
Princess Margaret Cancer Center
Department of Surgical Oncology-Urology
University Health Network
and
Faculty of Medicine
Department of Medicine
University of Toronto
Toronto, Ontario, Canada

David J.A. Jenkins
Faculty of Medicine
Department of Nutritional Sciences
University of Toronto
and
Clinical Nutrition and Risk Factor Modification Centre
St. Michael's Hospital
and
Faculty of Medicine
Department of Medicine
University of Toronto
and
Li Ka Shing Knowledge Institute
St. Michael's Hospital
Toronto, Ontario, Canada

Cyril W.C. Kendall
Faculty of Medicine
Department of Nutritional Sciences
University of Toronto
and
Clinical Nutrition and Risk Factor Modification Centre
St. Michael's Hospital
Toronto, Ontario, Canada

and

College of Pharmacy and Nutrition
Division of Nutrition and Dietetics
University of Saskatchewan
Saskatoon, Saskatchewan, Canada

Aurélie Lesdéma
Mondelez International R&D, Nutrition Research
Saclay, France

Kate Marsh
Northside Nutrition & Dietetics
and
The PCOS Health & Nutrition Centre
Sydney, New South Wales, Australia

Lars McNaughton
Department of Sport and Physical Activity
Edge Hill University
Ormskirk, United Kingdom

Alexandra Meynier
Mondelez International R&D, Nutrition Research
Saclay, France

Arash Mirrahimi
School of Medicine
Department of Medicine, Faculty of Health Sciences
Queen's University
Kingston, Ontario, Canada

and

Clinical Nutrition and Risk Factor Modification Centre
St. Michael's Hospital
Toronto, Ontario, Canada

Stephanie Nishi
Faculty of Medicine
Department of Nutritional Sciences
University of Toronto
and
Clinical Nutrition and Risk Factor Modification Centre
St. Michael's Hospital
Toronto, Ontario, Canada

Signe Nyby
Faculty of Science
Department of Nutrition, Exercise and Sports
University of Copenhagen
Copenhagen, Denmark

Elena Philippou
School of Sciences and Engineering
Department of Life and Health Sciences
University of Nicosia
Nicosia, Cyprus

and

Department of Nutrition and Dietetics
King's College London
London, United Kingdom

Anne Raben
Faculty of Science
Department of Nutrition, Exercise and Sports
University of Copenhagen
Copenhagen, Denmark

John L. Sievenpiper
Faculty of Medicine
Department of Nutritional Sciences
University of Toronto
and
Clinical Nutrition and Risk Factor Modification Centre
and
Division of Endocrinology & Metabolism
and
Li Ka Shing Knowledge Institute
and
Toronto 3D Knowledge Synthesis and Clinical Trials Unit
St. Michael's Hospital
Toronto, Ontario, Canada

S. Andy Sparks
Department of Sport and Physical Activity
Edge Hill University
Ormskirk, United Kingdom

Allen Taylor
Jean Mayer United States Department of Agriculture Human Nutrition Research Center on Aging
Department of Ophthalmology School of Medicine
Tufts University
Boston, Massachusetts

Effie Viguiliouk
Faculty of Medicine
Department of Nutritional Sciences
University of Toronto
and
Clinical Nutrition and Risk Factor Modification Centre
and
Toronto 3D Knowledge Synthesis and Clinical Trials Unit
St. Michael's Hospital
Toronto, Ontario, Canada

Sophie Vinoy
Mondelez International R&D, Nutrition Research
Saclay, France

Thomas M.S. Wolever
Faculty of Medicine
Department of Nutritional Sciences
University of Toronto
and
Clinical Nutrition and Risk Factor Modification Centre
St. Michael's Hospital
Toronto, Ontario, Canada

1 Introduction to Dietary Carbohydrates and the Glycemic Index

Elena Philippou and Ayesha Salem Al Dhaheri

CONTENTS

1.1 DIETARY CARBOHYDRATES

Dietary carbohydrates or "hydrates of carbon" are the chemical compounds of carbon, hydrogen, and oxygen, in the ratio of $C_n(H_2O)_n$, the basic unit of which is monosaccharide (a single sugar unit) (Bender 1997). Carbohydrates are the main energy-providing macronutrient in the diet. They are diverse in their characteristics and have a range of chemical, physical, and physiological properties (Cummings and Stephen 2007). Apart from their principal role in energy metabolism, they also affect satiety, blood glucose, and insulin, as well as lipid metabolism. Additionally, they have a central role in colonic function through fermentation and subsequently affect transit time, bowel habit, intestinal flora, and epithelial cell health of the large bowel. Less-known influences of carbohydrates are those on immune function and calcium absorption (Mann et al. 2007). It is thus commonly acknowledged that carbohydrates play many diverse roles, ranging from overall well-being to contributing to the regulation of body weight, cognition, dental health, exercise endurance, gut health and resistance to gut infection, bone mineral density, as well as in the prevention and management of diseases such as cardiovascular disease (CVD), diabetes and cancer of the large bowel (Mann et al. 2007).

This introductory chapter on carbohydrates and the glycemic index (GI) will provide an overview of dietary carbohydrates, including their classification, dietary intake recommendations, roles in the diet and the risks associated with the intake of simple sugars. The concepts of GI and glycemic load (GL) will be introduced and factors affecting the GI of foods will be explained. This chapter will end with a very brief overview of the role of GI in different physiologic conditions and disease states.

1.2 CARBOHYDRATE CLASSIFICATION AND TERMINOLOGY

Carbohydrates are classified based on their molecular size (determined by the degree of polymerization [DP]) into sugars (DP 1–2), oligosaccharides (DP 3–9), and polysaccharides (DP >10); type of linkage (α and non-α); and characteristic of the individual monomers, as shown in Table 1.1 (Cummings and Stephen 2007). Sugars can be monosaccharides, disaccharides, or sugar alcohols, whereas oligosaccharides can either be α-glucans, mainly resulting from the hydrolysis of starch, or non-α-glucans. Polysaccharides are divided into starch and nonstarch polysaccharides (NSPs), mainly composed of plant cell wall polysaccharides, but also including plant gums, mucilages, and hydrocolloids (Cummings and Stephen 2007). However, not all carbohydrates fit into this scheme, an example being inulin from plants, which may have between 2 and 200 fructose units and thus crosses the boundary between oligosaccharides and polysaccharides (Roberfroid et al. 1993). The 2007 scientific update of the Food and Agriculture Organization/World Health Organization (FAO/WHO) on carbohydrates in human nutrition endorsed the primary classification, recommended by the 1997 expert consultation based on chemical form, as explained above, but acknowledging that this classification should also have dimensions of physical effects, functional and/or physiologic effects, and health outcomes (Cummings and Stephen 2007). The explanation of carbohydrate terminology and classification that follows is based on the 2007 scientific update of FAO/WHO on carbohydrates.

1.2.1 TOTAL CARBOHYDRATE

"Total carbohydrate" reported in food tables may be derived by using either the "by difference" approach or the direct measurement of the individual components, which are then added to give a total (Cummings and Stephen 2007). Determination is done by measuring all other components of a food, including moisture, protein, fat, ash, and alcohol, and then subtracting the sum of these from the total weight of the food, thus considering the remainder or "difference" to be the carbohydrate. Although the calculation of carbohydrate by difference for the determination of the nutrient content of foods is used by the U.S. Department of Agriculture (U.S. Department of Agriculture 2015), it is limited by the fact that the derived figure includes noncarbohydrate components such as lignin,

TABLE 1.1
Carbohydrate Classification

Class (DP)	Subgroup	Examples
Sugars (1–2)	Monosaccharides	Glucose, galactose, and fructose
	Disaccharides	Sucrose, lactose, maltose, and trehalose
	Polyols (sugar alcohol)	Sorbitol, mannitol, lactitol, xylitol, erythritol, isomalt, and maltitol
Oligosaccharides (3–9)	Maltooligosaccharides (α-glucans)	Maltodextrins
	Non-α-glucan oligosaccharides	Raffinose, stachyose, fructo- and galactooligosaccharides, polydextrose, and inulin
Polysaccharides (≥10)	Starch (α-glucans)	Amylose, amylopectin, and modified starches
	Nonstarch polysaccharides	Cellulose, hemicellulose, pectin, arabinoxylans, β-glucan, glucomannans, plant gums and mucilages, and hydrocolloids

Source: Cummings, J.H. and Stephen, A.M. 2007. Eur. J. Clin. Nutr., 61, Suppl 1, S5–S18. With permission.
Note: DP = degree of polymerization or number of single-sugar units.

organic acids, tannins, waxes, and some Maillard products and obviously combines all the analytical errors from other analyses (Cummings and Stephen 2007). In addition, knowing only the total carbohydrate content of a food without breakdown into the different types does not provide enough information on the potential health effects. Alternatively, direct analysis to determine the carbohydrate content can be used, and the United Kingdom's McCance and Widdowson's composition of foods expresses carbohydrate content in this approach (Food Standard Agency and Public Health England 2014). The "available carbohydrate" obtained by the direct method does not include the plant cell wall polysaccharide, fiber, and is not limited by the errors that occur during analysis of other food components. Perhaps more importantly, direct analysis of total carbohydrate and its components allows diet-disease risks to be explored. The 2007 scientific update of FAO/WHO on carbohydrates recommends that the direct measurement of total carbohydrate should be preferred and that simplified methods to do this should be developed (Cummings and Stephen 2007). Here, it should be noted that the determination of carbohydrate by the above two methods will result in apparently different carbohydrate content and total energy of certain foods such as pasta (Stephen 2006). Thus, the comparison of carbohydrate intake or carbohydrate content of foods between countries should be viewed with caution, especially if the method of determination differs.

1.2.2 Sugars and Terms Used to Define Sugars

The term "sugars" refers to mono- and disaccharides, which either naturally occur in foods or are added for sweetness. The three monosaccharides, glucose, fructose, and galactose, are the building blocks of the bigger di-, oligo-, or polysaccharides. As free sugars, glucose and fructose occur in small amounts in honey and cooked or dried fruits and in larger amounts in fruit and berries (Holland et al. 1992). A nonnatural form of these sugars is the one used by the food industry as corn syrup and high-fructose corn syrup (HFCS) (Cummings and Stephen 2007). In addition to sweetening foods, sugars have a number of functions such as food preservation and conferring functional characteristics to foods such as viscosity, texture, body, and browning capacity (Institute of Medicine 2006). Sugar alcohols, for example, sorbitol, may be used to replace sugar and are both found naturally in some fruits and made commercially (Cummings and Stephen 2007).

The main disaccharides are sucrose, made of glucose and fructose (α-Glc(1→2)β-Fru), and lactose, made of galactose and glucose (β-Gal(1→4)Glc). Sucrose is extracted from sugar cane or beet and is found widely in fruits, berries, and vegetables, whereas lactose is the main sugar found in milk. In addition, there are other less-abundant disaccharides such as maltose (α-Glc(1→4)α-Glc), which consists of two glucose molecules and occur in sprouted wheat and barley, and trehalose (α-Glc(1→1)α-Glc), which also consists of two glucose molecules and is found abundantly in yeast and fungi and in small amounts in bread and honey (Cummings and Stephen 2007). Sugars are categorized on food labels by using a number of different terms, as outlined below; this mainly aims to differentiate their origin and thus perceived health impact.

1.2.2.1 Total Sugars

Used on labels and accepted by the European Union, Australia, and New Zealand, the term "all sugars" includes all sugars from whatever source in a food and is defined as "all monosaccharides and disaccharides other than polyols" (European Union 2011). The "Carbohydrate Terminology and Classification" paper of the 2007 updated scientific report of FAO/WHO on carbohydrates describes "total sugars" as "probably the most useful way to describe, measure and label sugars" (Cummings and Stephen 2007).

1.2.2.2 Free Sugars

Free sugars are traditionally referred to "any sugars in a food that are free and not bound" (Holland et al. 1992) and thus include all mono- and disaccharides and lactose (Southgate et al. 1978). The same term was used to describe the carbohydrate components of a hydrolyzed food detected by chromatography or calorimetric methods (Southgate et al. 1978). The term has now changed to refer to "monosaccharides and disaccharides added to foods by the manufacturer, cook, and consumer, plus sugars naturally present in honey, syrups, and fruit juices" (WHO/FAO 2003), and thus, care needs to be taken to avoid confusion between the two terms (Cummings and Stephen 2007).

1.2.2.3 Added Sugars

The U.S. Institute of Medicine defines "added sugars" as "sugars and syrups that are added to foods during processing or preparation" (Institute of Medicine 2006). Naturally occurring sugars, for example, lactose (in milk) or fructose (in fruit), are not included in this definition. Examples of added sugars include white, brown, or raw sugar; syrups such as corn syrup, HFCS, and malt syrup; liquid fructose; honey; molasses; and dextrose (Institute of Medicine 2006). The Institute of Medicine notes that foods and beverages that are major sources of added sugars have lower micronutrient densities compared with those that contain these sugars naturally. However, there is no difference in the chemical composition of the two (Institute of Medicine 2006). (See also Section 1.4.1 that discusses the possible health risks posed by the consumption of free sugars.)

1.2.2.4 Extrinsic and Intrinsic Sugars

The terms "extrinsic" and "intrinsic" sugars originated from the U.K. Department of Health Committee report in 1989 in order to "distinguish sugars naturally intergraded into the cellular structure of a food (intrinsic) from those that are free in the food or added to it (extrinsic)" (Department of Health 1989). Examples of intrinsic sugars include whole fruits and vegetables that contain mainly fructose, glucose, and sucrose, whereas examples of extrinsic sugars include fruit juice and sugars added to processed foods (Cummings and Stephen 2007). The term "nonmilk extrinsic sugar" was also introduced to differentiate the sugar present in milk, lactose, which is nutritionally beneficial despite being extrinsic (Department of Health 1989). In practical terms, analysis of sugars in this way or the use of these terms on food labels is problematic, and although the terminology is used in scientific reports, it is not well understood or used by the public (Cummings and Stephen 2007).

The "Carbohydrate Terminology and Classification" paper of the 2007 updated scientific report of FAO/WHO on carbohydrates notes that apart from the terms "total sugars" and the subdivision into mono- and disaccharides, the use of most of the other terms, including "refined sugars," "natural sugars," and "discretionary sugar," is not really justified. In addition, a uniform terminology is important in order to be able to make direct comparisons between foods and intakes in different populations (Cummings and Stephen 2007).

1.2.3 Oligosaccharides

Oligosaccharides are defined as "compounds in which monosaccharide units are joined by glycosidic linkages," but their DP definition may vary from 2 to 19 monosaccharide units (Cummings and Stephen 2007). As shown in Table 1.1, food oligosaccharides can be either maltodextrins, which are used in the food industry as sweeteners and fat substitutes and for texture modification, or non-α-glucan oligosaccharides, which are found in peas, beans, and lentils. The latter group also includes inulin and fructooligosaccharides, which are storage carbohydrates in artichokes and chicory and are also found in smaller amounts in wheat, rye, asparagus, onion, leek, and garlic. The above-mentioned oligosaccharides are also used by the industry and are referred to as "nondigestible oligosaccharides" because they are not susceptible to pancreatic or brush border enzyme breakdown. Some members of this group such as fructans and galactans are also known for their prebiotic properties, discussed in Section 1.3.1 (Cummings and Stephen 2007).

1.2.4 Starch

Starch consists of only glucose molecules and is the storage carbohydrate of plants such as cereals, root vegetables, and legumes. It is mainly composed of two polymers: the nonbranched helical chain of glucose linked by α-1,4 glucosidic bonds, called "amylose," which has a DP of about 10^3, shown in Figure 1.1, and the highly branched polymer containing both α-1,4 and α-1,6 bonds, called amylopectin, which has a DP of 10^4–10^5, shown in Figure 1.2. Although most starches contain 10%–30% amylose, "waxy" varieties of starches from maize, rice, barley, and sorghum contain

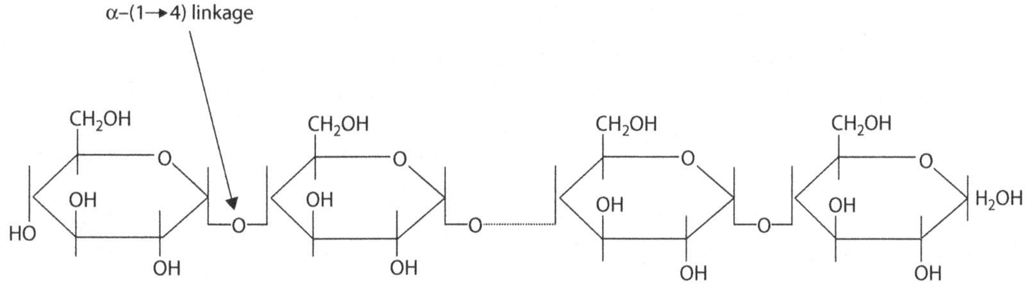

FIGURE 1.1 Amylose molecule.

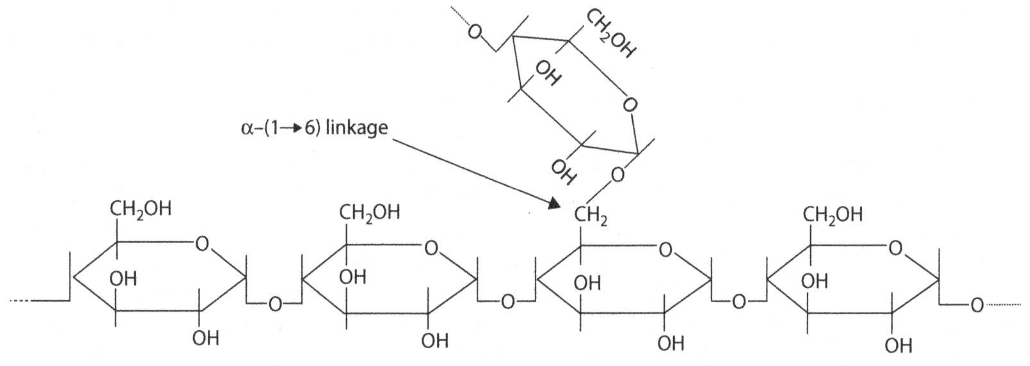

FIGURE 1.2 Amylopectin molecule.

largely amylopectin. Different varieties of cereals such as rice have different proportions of amylose and amylopectin (Kennedy and Burlingame 2003), which, as discussed in detail under Section 1.7.1, affect their GI.

Heating starch in water results in the loss of its crystalline structure, which is referred to as gelatinization, whereas recrystallization or retrogradation results when cooked starch is cooled down, such as that found in cold potato salad (Cummings and Stephen 2007). Gelatinization occurs at higher temperatures in higher-amylose starches, which are also more prone to retrograde and form amylose-lipid complexes. Thus, these types of starches can be used to form foods with high-resistant starch (high-RS) content, the definition and properties of which are explained in Section 1.3.2.

Starches can also be modified chemically (modified starch) to change their properties, resulting in qualities such as gel stability; decrease in viscosity; changes in mouth feel, appearance, and texture; and resistance to heat treatment, which are important in the food industry (Cummings and Stephen 2007). The applications are so diverse that some of these modifications are classed as additives and others as ingredients (Coultate 2009). The two most important processes to modify starch are substitution and cross-linking. Substitution involves esterification of a small proportion (<1%) of glucose units with organic acids or phosphates to produce "stabilized" starches (Coultate 2009). Depending on which groups are attached, the resulting modified starch may have properties such as freeze stability in gels, resistance to retrogradation, which is involved in bread staling, and increase in viscosity (Coultate 2009). Cross-linking is a process in which a limited number of linkages between the chains of amylose and amylopectin are introduced (Cummings and Stephen 2007). In fact, fewer than one cross-linkage per 1000 glucose units is enough to produce significant changes in starch properties, which result in strengthening the starch granule (Coultate 2009). The resulting properties include resilience to low pH and extended cooking, control of viscosity during processing, and also resistance to digestion (Coultate 2009; Cummings and Stephen 2007). The use of starch modification to alter GI is discussed extensively in Chapter 13.

1.2.5 Nonstarch Polysaccharides

Nonstarch polysaccharides are non-α-glucan polysaccharides, principally found in the plant cell wall and are defined as "macromolecules consisting of a large number of monosaccharide residues joined to each other by glycosidic linkages" (IUB-IUPAC Joint Commission on Biochemical Nomenclature 1982). Cellulose, a straight-chain β1–4-linked glucan (DP 10^3–10^6), comprises 10%–30% of NSP in foods and gives the plant cell wall its structure by its close packing to form microfibrils. The hemicelluloses (DP 150–200) are highly branched chains containing a mixture of hexose (6C) and pentose (5C) sugars, mostly comprising a backbone of xylose sugars with branches of arabinose, mannose, galactose, and glucose. An example of NSP is arabinoxylans, found in cereals containing uronic acids—the carboxylated derivatives of glucose and galactose; they are able to form salts with calcium and zinc, an important determinant of their properties (Cummings and Stephen 2007). Another NSP is pectin, a 1–4β-D galacturonic acid polymer, with possible side chains of other sugars such as rhamnose, galactose, and arabinose, known for its gel-forming properties. Other NSPs include plant gums and mucilages (Cummings and Stephen 2007). Plant gums, mostly highly branched, complex uronic-acid-containing polymers, are sticky exudates formed at the sites of injuries to plants. The most well-known plant gum is gum arabic, used as a thickener (Cummings and Stephen 2007). Plant mucilages, the most well known of them being guar gum and carob gums, are mixed with the endosperm of storage carbohydrates of seeds and have water-retaining and desiccation-preventing properties (Cummings and Stephen 2007). These are also used by the food and pharmaceutical industries as thickeners and stabilizers. Finally, another NSP category is algal polysaccharides, such as carageenan, which is used in dairy products and chocolate because of its ability to react with milk protein. Other examples include agar and alginate, which are the NSPs extracted from seaweed or algae, and have gel-forming properties (Cummings and Stephen 2007).

1.3 CARBOHYDRATE TERMINOLOGY BASED ON PHYSIOLOGY

The "Carbohydrate Terminology and Classification" paper of the 2007 updated scientific report of FAO/WHO on carbohydrates explains that the classification of carbohydrates based on their chemistry does not allow a simple translation into nutritional benefits because their physiologic effects are varied and overlapping (Cummings and Stephen 2007). It is thus preferable to classify them based on their physiologic properties, which focuses more on the potential health benefits of carbohydrates. An example of physiologic grouping is that based on the effect of carbohydrates on stool weight, where some carbohydrates such as polyols (except erythritol), some starches, NSP, lactose (in lactose-intolerant populations), and fructose (in large amounts) increase stool weight, whereas others such as glucose, galactose, sucrose, maltose, trehalose, maltodextrins, oligosaccharides, and most starches have no effect on stool weight (Cummings and Stephen 2007). However, it should be noted that the physiology of carbohydrates can vary among individuals and populations, with examples including lactose, which is poorly hydrolyzed by most adults, except Caucasians, and polyols and starch, whose digestion and absorption are variable (Cummings and Stephen 2007). Table 1.2 shows the preferred terminology of dietary carbohydrates suggested by the 2007 scientific update of FAO/WHO on dietary carbohydrates and also lists the less useful terms. In the following sections, the physiologic or botanical terminology will be discussed.

1.3.1 Prebiotics

The first definition of prebiotics, just more than 20 years ago, was "nondigestible food ingredients that beneficially affect the host by selectively stimulating the growth and/or activity of one or a limited number of bacteria in the colon, thus improving host health" (Gibson and Roberfroid 1995). This was later refined to include other areas that may benefit from selective targeting of particular microorganisms to: "a selectively fermented ingredient that allows specific changes, both in the composition and/or activity in the gastrointestinal microbiota that confers benefits" (Gibson et al. 2004). For an ingredient to be characterized as prebiotic, it has to abide to the following criteria:

TABLE 1.2
Preferred Terminology of Dietary Carbohydrates

	Chemical	Physiologic or Botanical
Useful	Monosaccharides	Prebiotic
	Disaccharides	Resistant starch
	Polyols	Dietary fiber[a]
	Short-chain carbohydrates	Glycemic
	Oligosaccharides	
	Polysaccharides	
	Starch	
	Nonstarch polysaccharides	
	Total carbohydrate	
Less useful	Sugars	Nondigestible oligosaccharides
	Sugar	Soluble and insoluble fiber
	Free sugars	Available and unavailable carbohydrate
	Refined sugars	Complex carbohydrate
	Added sugars	
	Extrinsic and intrinsic sugars	

Source: Cummings, J.H. and Stephen, A.M. 2007. *Eur. J. Clin. Nutr.*, 61, Suppl 1, S5–S18. With permission.
[a] Intrinsic plant cell wall polysaccharides.

(1) resist gastric acidity, hydrolysis by mammalian enzymes, and absorption in the upper GI tract; (2) be fermented by the intestinal microbiota; and (3) selectively stimulate the growth and/or activity of intestinal bacteria potentially associated with health and well-being (Gibson and Roberfroid 1995; Gibson et al. 2004;). The latter of these criteria is what separates prebiotics from traditional fibers (Brownawell et al. 2012). The benefits of prebiotics are many and diverse; however, their discussion is outside the scope of this chapter.

1.3.2 Resistant Starch

Resistant starch, an example of a nonglycemic carbohydrate, is defined as "starch and starch degradation products not absorbed in the small intestine of healthy humans" (Englyst and Cummings 1990). A range of physical and chemical properties alter the rate and extent to which starch is broken down (Cummings and Stephen 2007), leading to a suggested classification of RS as follows: physically enclosed starch, for example, within intact cell structures (RS_1), in foods such as bulgur wheat, legumes, and pumpernickel bread (whole grains); (RS_2), which is the starch resistant to amylolytic digestion because of its compact unbranched nature such as amylose; retrograded amylose (RS_3) formed by the cooling of gelatinized high-amylose starch; and modified starches (RS_4) (Englyst et al. 1992; Englyst and Cummings 1990).

The fact that the rate and extent of starch digestion varies formed the basis of GI, and the 2007 scientific update of FAO/WHO on carbohydrates reports this as "one of the most important developments in the understanding of carbohydrates in the past 30 years" (Cummings and Stephen 2007).

Trowell defined dietary fiber as "the cellular walls of plants that are resistant to hydrolysis by the enzymes of man" (Trowell 2006). This term, however, does not refer precisely to a chemical component of the diet, and the nondigestibility of plant cell walls varies from person to person and is affected by food storage, cooking, chewing, ripeness, and the presence of other foods (Cummings and Stephen 2007). Cummings and Stephen (2007) explain that apart from the plant cell wall, it includes many dietary components such as lactose in some populations, some polyols, and some RS, and there is no enforceable method that can be used to measure this physiologic fraction of the diet. Based on this and on the fact that dietary fiber has been linked to many health benefits, the FAO/WHO in its scientific update meeting on carbohydrates in human nutrition (July 2006) agreed that the definition of dietary fiber should be more clearly linked to health. Thus, the following definition was proposed: "dietary fiber consists of intrinsic plant cell wall polysaccharides" (Cummings and Stephen 2007). As described previously, NSPs comprise a mixture of many molecular forms, of which cellulose is the most widely distributed. The plant cell wall polysaccharides can be determined using the enzymatic-chemical method. This method is designed to remove all starch, and thus, it measures NSP as the sum of chemically identified NSP constituent sugars (Englyst et al. 1994). The advantage of measuring NSP is that it is not in itself created or destroyed by normal food preparation or storage techniques, and thus, it is a consistent indicator of plant cell wall material. Any added preparations of NSP will also be measured (Englyst et al. 2007). Dietary fiber may also be measured using the enzymatic-gravimetric method, which is based on the "indigestibility" approach (AOAC 2007; Englyst et al. 2007). This aims to measure the sum of indigestible polysaccharides and lignin, and in practice, it includes RS, the amount of which may be affected by food processing and the addition of RS preparations; noncarbohydrate materials such as lignin; and food-processing artifacts such as Maillard reaction products (Englyst et al. 2007; Tuohy et al. 2006).

1.3.2.1 Soluble and Insoluble Fiber

The terms "soluble fiber" and "insoluble fiber" are based on the fractional extraction of NSP, which can be controlled under laboratory conditions by changing the pH of solutions (Joint FAO/WHO Expert Consultation 1998). In the initial understanding of the properties of dietary fiber, these terms proved very useful, allowing a simple division of NSPs into those that were soluble and had effects on glucose and lipid absorption in the small intestine (Lairon 1994) and those that were insoluble and thus fermented more slowly and incompletely and had more pronounced effects on bowel habit (Cummings 1997). However, their physiologic differences are not always so distinct; for example, much insoluble fiber is completely fermented and not all soluble fiber has an effect on glucose and lipid absorption. Moreover, their separation is dependent on the conditions of extraction (Asp et al. 1992; Cummings and Stephen 2007). It should be noted that a lot of the earlier work was done on isolated gums or extracts of cell walls; however, fiber exists together mostly in intact plant cell walls (Cummings and Stephen 2007).

1.3.3 Available and Unavailable Carbohydrates

McCance and Lawrence in 1929 introduced the terms "available" and "unavailable" carbohydrates in their attempt to prepare food tables for diabetic diets and the realization that not all carbohydrates could be "utilized and metabolized," to the same extend. This definition referred to available carbohydrate as "starch and soluble sugars" and unavailable carbohydrate as "mainly hemicelluloses and fiber (cellulose)" (McCance and Laurence 1929). The concept drew attention to the fact that some carbohydrates are not digested and absorbed in the small intestine but reach the large bowel, where they are fermented and excreted in feces (Cummings and Stephen 2007). A later definition of available carbohydrate given by an FAO technical workshop was: "that fraction of carbohydrate that can be digested by human enzymes, is absorbed and enters into intermediary metabolism" (FAO 2003).

The "Carbohydrate Terminology and Classification" paper of the 2007 updated scientific report of FAO/WHO on carbohydrates argues that the use of the term "unavailable" for carbohydrates is misleading because carbohydrates that reach the colon would still provide energy through fermentation and absorption of short-chain fatty acids (Cummings and Stephen 2007). Alternatively, the terms "glycemic," which means providing carbohydrate for metabolism, and "non-glycemic" were recommended and referred to as more precise and measurable fractions (Cummings and Stephen 2007). These terms are discussed in more detail below.

1.3.3.1 Glycemic Carbohydrate

Depending on their gastrointestinal handling, carbohydrates can be referred to as "glycemic carbohydrates," which refer to the carbohydrates that are digested and absorbed in the small intestine and cause a rise in blood glucose (e.g., free sugars, maltodextrins, and starch [even if it is slowly digested]), and "non-glycemic," which refer to the carbohydrates (or their components) that are not absorbed in the small intestine and move down to become fermented in the colon, with the production of short-chain fatty acids, methane, and hydrogen gas. Examples of the latter are RS, NSPs, and sugar alcohols (Englyst and Englyst 2005). Most unprocessed foods containing carbohydrates include both glycemic and nonglycemic types. From the categorization of glycemic carbohydrates stems the term "glycemic index," which refers to the extent to which carbohydrate in foods raises the blood glucose concentration compared with an equivalent amount of reference carbohydrate (glucose or white bread) (Jenkins et al. 1981).

1.3.4 Complex Carbohydrates

The term "complex carbohydrates" is mostly used in the United States and was first introduced in 1977 in the McGovern report "Dietary Goals for the United States," in which it was denoted to include "fruit, vegetables, and whole grains." Although the idea behind its use was to encourage the consumption of healthy foods, it is limited by the fact that fruits and vegetables are low in starch. The "Carbohydrate Terminology and Classification" paper of the 2007 updated scientific report of FAO/WHO on carbohydrates recommends discussing carbohydrates by using their common chemical names rather than by using this term (Cummings and Stephen 2007).

1.3.5 Whole Grain

Intake of whole grains has been associated with lower risks of CVD, type 2 diabetes, and weight gain (Ferruzzi et al. 2014) and is embodied in many dietary recommendations, including the WHO/FAO report on "Diet, Nutrition, and the Prevention of Chronic Diseases" (WHO/FAO 2003). However, the definition of whole grains may vary from country to country. In 1999, the definition of a wholegrain ingredient was developed by the Whole Grains Working Group of the American Association of Cereal Chemists International, which stated that whole grains are "intact, ground, cracked or flaked fruit of the grain whose principal components, the starchy endosperm, germ and bran, are present in the same relative proportions as they exist in the intact grain" (American Association of Cereal Chemists International 1999). The United States adopted this definition in its Whole Grain Label Guidance (U.S. Food and Drug Administration 2006). Another definition of whole grains published by the European HEALTHGRAIN Forum is "consisting of the intact, ground, cracked or flaked kernel after the removal of inedible parts such as the hull and husk. The principle anatomic components—the endosperm, germ and bran—are to be present in the same relative proportions as they exist in the intact kernel. Small losses of components, that is, <2% of the germ or <10% of the bran, which may occur through processing methods consistent with safety and quality, are allowed" (Bjorck et al. 2012). The difference between the two definitions is that the latter allows for small losses during the initial processing and/or cleaning of the grain (Ferruzzi et al. 2014). A wholegrain "food" had not been defined up until 2012, when a group of experts held a Whole Grain Roundtable in Chicago, Illinois, to discuss this. After examining the scientific evidence, the expert panel recommended that 8 g of whole grain/30 g serving (27 g/100 g), without a fiber requirement, be considered the minimum content of whole grains that is nutritionally meaningful and that a food providing at least 8 g of whole grains/30 g serving be defined as a wholegrain food (Ferruzzi et al. 2014). However, Cumming and Stephen rightly pointed out that because the type of grain contributing to whole grains varies from country to country, with most of the wholegrain intake being wheat in the United Kingdom and oats in the United States, the differences in their physical and physiologic properties, including, we could add, GI, need to be considered when examining the health impacts of wholegrain consumption (Cummings and Stephen 2007).

1.4 CARBOHYDRATE INTAKE RECOMMENDATIONS AND DIETARY ROLES

Dietary recommendations across the world point to the essential and central role of carbohydrates in the diet. The 1998 FAO/WHO Expert Consultation on carbohydrates in human nutrition recommends that carbohydrates provide 55%–75% of the total energy intake from a variety of sources and that excessive intake of sugars, which compromise micronutrient density, should be avoided (Joint FAO/WHO Expert Consultation 1998). The consultation endorses that the bulk of carbohydrate-containing foods consumed should be rich in NSP and should have low GI (Joint FAO/WHO Expert Consultation 1998). However, the 2007 scientific update of FAO/WHO on carbohydrates identified the need to review the recommended lower limit because of insufficient justification and suggested a possible revision of 50% of total energy (Cummings and Stephen 2007).

The dietary recommendations of countries around the globe for carbohydrates are similar. The U.S. Institute of Medicine recommends the acceptable macronutrient distribution range (AMDR) for carbohydrates to be between 45% and 65% of total energy and suggests a tolerable upper intake level of 25% of total energy from added sugars. For all ages, starting from 1 to more than 70 years, the Dietary Reference Intakes for carbohydrates are set as: Estimated Average Requirement, 100 g/day, and Recommended Dietary Allowance, 130 g/day (Institute of Medicine 2006). (The Estimated Average Requirement refers to "the average daily nutrient intake level estimated to meet the requirements of half of the healthy individuals in a group" whereas the Recommended Dietary Allowance is the "average daily dietary intake level sufficient to meet the nutrient requirements of 97%–98% of the health individuals in a group" [Institute of Medicine 2006].) The Dietary Guidelines of

Americans 2010 recommend that at least half of all grains consumed should be whole grains and also recommend to achieve this by replacing refined grains with whole grains (U.S. Department of Agriculture and U.S. Department of Health and Human Services 2010). Similarly, Canada's Food Guide recommends that at least half of the grain products each day should be whole grain and also recommends to choose grain products that are low in fat, sugar, or salt (Health Canada 2015).

The European Food Safety Authority (EFSA) Scientific Panel's recommended reference intake for carbohydrates is 45%–60% of energy, with an adequate fiber intake considered as 25 g/day (EFSA 2010). The U.K.'s recommendations refer to 50% of total food energy consumed as carbohydrates and this to be broken down to not more than 11% nonmilk extrinsic sugars and 39% intrinsic and milk sugars and starch. The individual Dietary Reference Intakes (minimum to maximum) for NSPs are 12–24 g/day, with 18 g/day being the recommended population average intake. With regard to public health messages, the U.K. Government recommends consuming "plenty of starchy foods such as rice, bread, pasta, and potatoes (using wholegrain varieties when possible)." Australia's dietary guidelines also recommend daily consumption of "grain (cereal) foods, mostly wholegrain and/or high-cereal-fiber varieties, such as breads, cereals, rice, pasta, noodles, polenta, couscous, oats, quinoa, and barley" (National Health and Medical Research Council 2013).

The dietary roles of carbohydrates are shown in Table 1.3. Carbohydrate-containing foods are the staple foods in most countries, because their most important role is to provide energy (Joint FAO/WHO Expert Consultation 1998), with significant effects on satiety (Blundell et al. 1994). In addition, they are an important vehicle for protein intake and a source of vitamin B complex and minerals (calcium, magnesium, potassium, phosphorus, selenium, manganese, zinc, and iron) (Joint FAO/WHO Expert Consultation 1998). In particular, wholegrain carbohydrate foods are important sources of fiber, vitamin E, antioxidants, and phytoestrogens, found in their bran and germ components (Anderson et al. 2000).

1.4.1 Possible Health Risks Posed by Consumption of Free Sugars

Consumption of free sugars, being, as defined by WHO "monosaccharides and disaccharides added to foods and beverages by the manufacturer, cook or consumer, and sugars naturally present in honey, syrups, fruit juices, and fruit juice concentrates" (WHO 2015), has been implicated in the development of dental caries and overweight and obesity.

With regard to dental caries, sugars are reported to be "cariogenic," which refers to "foods/drinks containing fermentable carbohydrates that can cause a decrease in salivary pH to <5.5 and demineralization when in contact with microorganisms in the mouth" (American Dietetic Association 2003), but not all sugars have the same potency. The most cariogenic sugar is sucrose, followed by fructose, glucose, and maltose, whereas lactose, galactose, maltodextrins, and polysaccharides

TABLE 1.3
Roles of Dietary Carbohydrates

Roles
Energy provision
Enhancement of satiety
Blood glucose and insulin control
Protein glycosylation
Bile acid dehydroxylation
Laxative
Through fermentation:
Hydrogen and/or methane production
Increase in microbial biomass
Control of colonic epithelial cell function
Selective stimulation of microbial growth (e.g., bifidobacteria)

have very little effect and sorbitol and xylitol are noncariogenic and are used in products such as sugar-free chewing gums. Those carbohydrate-containing foods that are chewy and/or sticky are particularly detrimental to teeth. A WHO-commissioned meta-analysis of the effect of sugar on dental caries found a strong positive association between consumption of free sugars and dental caries in children, with higher rates of dental caries when consumption of free sugar was more than 10% of total energy. In three national population studies, per-capita sugar intake below 10 kg/person/year (approximately 5% of total energy intake) was associated with lower levels of dental caries development (Moynihan and Kelly 2014).

The question of whether sugar-sweetened foods and beverages (SSB) are implicated in weight gain, and in particular whether reducing consumption of SSB will also reduce the prevalence of obesity and obesity-related diseases, has been a matter of heated debate (Hu 2013; Kaiser et al. 2013). It is true that in the past few decades, there has been a huge increase in the intake of SSB, especially in the United States (Bray 2010), which are most commonly sweetened using HFCS but also using sucrose or fruit juice concentrates. This increase in consumption parallels the increase in obesity prevalence (Malik et al. 2013). Of course, this by itself does not prove a cause-and-effect relationship; indeed, there has also been an increase in water consumption during the same time period (Earth Policy Institute 2007). Nevertheless, well-powered prospective cohort studies have shown a significant dose–response relationship between SSB consumption and long-term weight gain and risk of type 2 diabetes (Odegaard et al. 2010; Palmer et al. 2008; Schulze et al. 2004). Consumption of 1–2 servings of SSB per day was associated with a 26% (95% confidence interval [CI] 12%–41%) greater risk of developing type 2 diabetes compared with just occasional intake (Malik et al. 2010), whereas a meta-analysis of randomized controlled trials (RCTs) commissioned by WHO found that decreased intake of added sugars significantly reduced body weight (0.80 kg, 95% CI 0.39–1.21; $P < .001$), whereas increased sugar intake led to a comparable weight increase (0.75 kg, CI 0.30–1.19; $P = .001$) (Te et al. 2013). Similarly, in children, it has been shown that a higher intake of SSB is associated with a 55% (95% CI 32%–82%) higher risk of overweight or obesity compared with a lower intake (Te et al. 2013). Moreover, considerable epidemiologic evidence also suggests that increased intake of added sugars, sucrose, and/or HFCS, or SSB is associated with dyslipidemia, CVD, and metabolic syndrome (Richelsen 2013), whereas the higher the intake of added sugar, the greater the risk (Yang et al. 2014).

With regard to the effect of reduction of intake, two large long-term RCTs in children and adolescents showed that reduction in the consumption of SSB leads to significant reduction in weight gain and adiposity (de Ruyter et al. 2012; Ebbeling et al. 2012). Furthermore, in a study lasting 6 months, sugar-sweetened cola was shown to significantly increase visceral, liver, and muscle fat; triglycerides; total cholesterol; and systolic blood pressure in comparison with milk, diet cola, or water, which did not affect body weight or total body fat, showing that SSB can mimic many features of the metabolic syndrome (Maersk et al. 2012). Even so, Kaiser et al. (2013) in an updated meta-analysis of RCTs attempting to reduce SSB consumption concluded that the evidence is equivocal on whether reducing SSB will reduce the prevalence of obesity. To this, Hu (2013) answered that prospective cohort studies that address dietary determinants of long-term weight gain and chronic diseases are as critical as RCTs in evaluating causality and thus cannot be ignored.

Another issue of debate is where the metabolism of HFCS, typically composed of 55% fructose and 45% glucose (for beverages) or 42% fructose and 58% glucose (for baked goods) (White et al. 2010), is different to that of sucrose, composed of 50% fructose and 50% glucose. It has been demonstrated that acute responses to HFCS and sucrose are identical with regard to glucose, insulin, leptin, ghrelin, triglycerides, and appetite (Melanson et al. 2007; Soenen and Westerterp-Plantenga 2007). Whether research comparing fructose with glucose is relevant to human nutrition has also been questioned, because these sugars are rarely consumed in isolation in the human diet (Rippe and Angelopoulos 2013). The same researchers reported that 10-week consumption of added sugar (sugar and HFCS at 8%, 18%, or 30% of calories) up to the 90th percentile population consumption for fructose did not affect blood pressure and had modest effects on blood lipids (Lowndes et al. 2014), whereas a meta-analysis of controlled feeding studies on the effect of fructose on blood pressure also reported no effect (Ha et al. 2012). However, yet another study produced conflicting results by finding that consumption of beverages containing 10%, 17.5%, or 25% of estimated energy requirements from HFCS resulted in dose-dependent increases of circulating lipid and/or lipoprotein risk factors for CVD and uric acid within 2 weeks, prompting the authors to suggest that these results provide mechanistic support for the epidemiologic evidence, linking the increasing consumption of added sugar with cardiovascular mortality (Stanhope et al. 2015).

Based on the available evidence on body weight and dental caries, WHO issued a guideline in 2015 recommending that adults and children reduce their daily intake of free sugars to less than 10% of total energy intake. A further reduction to less than 5% or roughly 25 g (6 teaspoons) per day would provide additional health benefits (WHO 2015). Finally, there is no doubt that sugar-sweetened beverages and sucrose provide only empty calories and they have never been shown to provide any benefit that would support their intake.

1.5 INSULIN

Central to the health effects of carbohydrates is insulin, a hormone produced by the β (beta) cells of the pancreas, which was isolated by Frederic Banting and Charles Best in 1921 in Canada and which is required for the proper use of glucose by the body. Insulin appears to activate a process that helps glucose molecules enter the cells of striated muscle and adipose tissue. In addition, it stimulates the production of glycogen by the liver. Insulin also promotes protein synthesis and helps the body store fat by preventing its breakdown for energy.

1.5.1 Insulin and the Metabolic Syndrome

Metabolic syndrome is a cluster of disorders linked with obesity and hyperinsulinemia and is associated with a markedly increased risk of type 2 diabetes and CVD (Soderberg et al. 2005). The metabolic syndrome is characterized by impaired insulin sensitivity (insulin resistance), hyperglycemia, dyslipidemia, and hypertension. Insulin resistance is the most approved and unifying hypothesis to explain the pathophysiology of the metabolic syndrome (Eckel et al. 2005), and it is strongly associated with obesity, especially its central or visceral component. A number of mechanisms

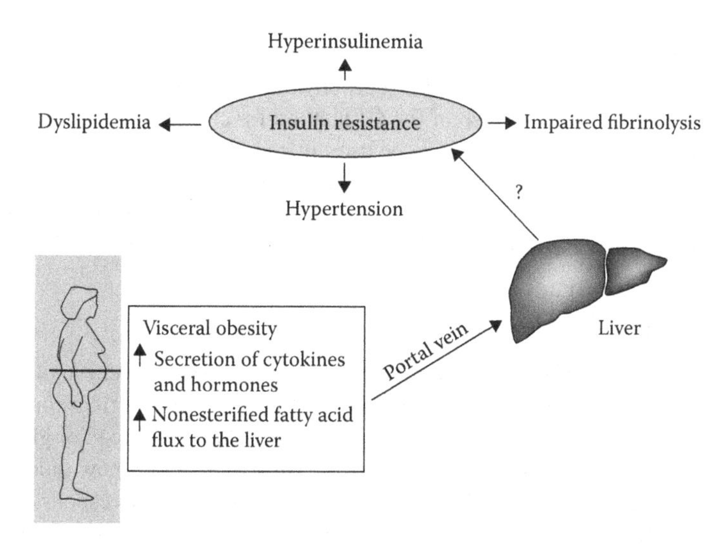

FIGURE 1.3 The metabolic syndrome. (From Davy, B.M. and Melby, C.L. 2003. *J. Am. Diet Assoc.*, 103, 1, 86–96. With permission.)

have been suggested regarding the development of insulin resistance and the metabolic syndrome, which may be caused by visceral obesity (Frayn 2000). First, as illustrated in Figure 1.3, visceral adipose tissue secretes cytokines and hormones that drain into the portal vein and may alter hepatic metabolism. Second, the visceral adipose depot releases nonesterified fatty acids more rapidly that subcutaneous adipose tissue, consequently increasing fatty acid flux to the liver. The increased hepatic uptake of nonesterified fatty acids could increase hepatic glucose production while decreasing glucose oxidation, thus resulting in glucose intolerance (Belfiore and Iannello 1998; Ferrannini et al. 1983); increase hepatic very-low-density lipoprotein-triglyceride secretion, which causes hypertriglyceridemia (Frayn 2000); and decrease hepatic insulin removal, thus leading to hyperinsulinemia (Wiesenthal et al. 1999). Thus, increased accumulation of visceral fat may be the main factor that leads to the development of the metabolic syndrome. It is apparent that healthy subjects show marked variability in the location and size of fat depots, and this may contribute to differences in disease risk.

The dietary influences on metabolic syndrome are many and complex, with potentially synergistic effects both in protective and detrimental dietary patterns. A recently conducted review identified three dietary patterns that have potentially beneficial effects on the prevalence of the metabolic syndrome: the Mediterranean diet, the Dietary Approaches to Stop Hypertension (DASH) diet, and the Nordic diet. On the contrary, the Western dietary pattern characterized by high intakes of total and saturated fats and simple and added sugars has been associated with higher risk of the metabolic syndrome. Although it is outside the scope of this book to discuss them in detail, these dietary patterns include increased consumption of fruits, vegetables, whole grains, and (low-fat) dairy, and their relatively low GI, among others (such as calcium, vitamin D, and omega-3 fatty acids), has been suggested as one of the likely mechanisms in which they may exert their protective effects (Calton et al. 2014).

1.6 GLYCEMIC INDEX: A HISTORY

The GI was conceived in 1981 by David Jenkins and his colleagues at the University of Toronto, Canada, as a tool for classifying carbohydrates according to their effect on blood glucose concentrations (Jenkins et al. 1981). At that time, it was thought that all simple sugars caused a more rapid rise in blood sugar than complex carbohydrates, but some studies were beginning to emerge that challenged this conventional wisdom about sugars. The GI was developed to predict postprandial (after a meal) increases in blood glucose concentration, originally in diabetic patients.

In 1997, a committee of experts was brought together by FAO and WHO to review the available research evidence regarding the importance of carbohydrate in human nutrition and health (FAO 1998). The committee authorized the use of the GI method for classifying carbohydrate-rich foods and recommended that the GI values of foods be used in combination with information about food composition to guide food choices. Tables on the measured GIs of various carbohydrate-rich foods have been published, aiming to bring together all the published data on the GI values of individual foods for the convenience of users (Atkinson et al. 2008; Foster-Powell et al. 2002).

1.6.1 Definition of the Glycemic Index

GI is defined as "the incremental area under the blood glucose response curve of a 50 g carbohydrate portion of a test food, expressed as a percentage of the response to the same amount of carbohydrate from a standard food taken by the same subject (either white bread or glucose)" (Jenkins et al. 1981). In effect, GI ranks carbohydrate-containing foods based on how quickly they elevate blood sugar concentration. By comparing the area under the blood glucose response curve of the test food with that of the standard food, which is given a relative value of 100, foods receive a numeric value and are then generally classified as having a low, moderate, or high GI (Jenkins et al. 1984). Foods containing carbohydrates that are quickly digested have the highest GI, because the blood sugar response is fast and high. Slowly digested carbohydrates have a low GI, because they release glucose gradually into the bloodstream (Brand-Miller et al. 2002; 2003a). In general, most refined carbohydrate-rich foods have a high GI, whereas nonstarchy vegetables, fruits, and legumes tend to have a low GI (Ludwig 2002). However, there are many factors that determine the GI of a food, and these are discussed in Section 1.7.

The GI of a food is measured by comparing the increase in blood glucose concentration after eating 50 g of available carbohydrate (i.e., the total carbohydrate content of foods completely hydrolyzed and absorbed in the small intestine and used in metabolism, i.e., total carbohydrate minus dietary fiber) from a test food with the same quantity of available carbohydrate from a standard food, which is either pure glucose or white bread. The average change in blood sugar concentration over the next 2 h, compared with the change in blood sugar concentration after consuming the standard food is the GI value of that particular food. The blood sugar response of the standard food, usually glucose or white bread, is given a value of 100, and all other foods are compared with this value. A detailed explanation of how GI is calculated, including example calculations, can be found in Chapter 2.

The GI is defined as: (Joint FAO/WHO Expert Consultation 1998)

$$\begin{aligned} GI = & \left(\text{iAUC for test food containing 50g available carbohydrate}\right)/ \\ & \left(\text{iAUC 50g standard food}\right) \times 100 \end{aligned}$$

where iAUC = incremental area under the curve (i.e., area above fasting concentrations).

There is a direct correlation between a food's glycemic response and insulinemic response, also referred to as insulin index, calculated in the same way as the GI by using the 2-h postprandial insulin iAUC rather than the glucose iAUC (Bornet et al. 1987).

Carbohydrate-containing foods can be ranked according to their glucose response as low, medium, or high GI; however, the cutoff values are arbitrary. The most widely acceptable classification is shown in Table 1.4 (Brand-Miller et al. 2003a).

1.6.2 Glycemic Load

The GL is a measure of the overall glycemic impact of the food and is the product of the food's GI and the amount of carbohydrate it provides. It incorporates both the quantity and quality of the dietary carbohydrate consumed, as opposed to GI, which measures only the quality of carbohydrate intake (Wolever 2003). Each unit of GL is equal to the glycemic effect produced after the ingestion of 1 g of glucose (used as a reference food), and the higher the GL, the greater the expected elevation in blood glucose and insulin.

The GL is defined as: (Salmeron et al. 1997)

$$GL = (GI \times \text{amount of carbohydrate})/100$$

The question of whether the GI or the carbohydrate content of a food is the greatest determinant of GL was addressed by Brand-Miller and colleagues in 2003, and it was shown that the carbohydrate

TABLE 1.4
Glycemic Index Classification

Glycemic Index (GI) Category	Values
Low GI	55 or less
Medium GI	56–69 inclusive
High GI	70 or higher

content of foods alone explained 68% of the variance in GL values, whereas the GI value alone explained 49% of the variance, concluding that carbohydrate content (rather than GI) is the greatest determinant of GL (Brand-Miller et al. 2003b). Foods with a GL $\leq$ 10 are classified as low GL and those with a GL $\geq$ 20 are classified as high GL (Brand-Miller et al. 2003b), but this classification is mainly used for research purposes.

1.7 FACTORS INFLUENCING THE BLOOD GLUCOSE RESPONSES OF FOODS

It is inaccurate to predict the glycemic response or GI of food from food composition tables, because the glycemic response to foods is influenced by many factors, including the type of carbohydrate, the nature of the starch (amylose or amylopectin), cooking and food processing (degree of starch gelatinization, particle size, cellular form, etc.), the food form, and other food components (fat, protein, and natural or added substances that reduce digestion, such as viscous fiber and acidity). Furthermore, the GI of a food is determined by a complex interaction of factors, including but not limited to the physical and chemical properties of foods, the rate of carbohydrate digestion, the rate of gastric emptying, the presence of other nutrients or antinutrients, and the insulin response elicited by the food. Therefore, the GI reflects the combined effect of all the properties of a food or meal that influence the rate of influx and removal of glucose from the circulation (Englyst and Englyst 2005; Wolever 2006). Hence, a GI value is an *in vivo* measurement and does not always correlate with *in vitro* measurements of glycemic response, because the latter cannot fully account for all the factors that determine a GI value (Brand-Miller and Holt 2004). It should also be noted that not all the food factors or mechanisms that determine the glycemic response to a food or meal are equally beneficial to health. A brief overview of the factors that affect a food's GI is provided below, but further details can be found in Chapter 13.

1.7.1 Starch Type

Different kinds of a specific food, for example, rice, have different GI values, because the type of starch determines the rate of digestion. As explained in Section 1.2.4, there are two types of starch: amylose and amylopectin; amylose is a linear molecule and amylopectin is highly branched. In most starchy foods, 70%–80% of the total starch consists of amylopectin, with the remaining being amylose (Cummings and Englyst 1995). As a result of its linear structure, amylose has more extensive hydrogen bonding and is easier to retrograde than amylopectin. Thus, amylose is more resistant to hydrolytic enzymes, with resultant lower glycemic and insulinemic responses than amylopectin. There are also various genotypes of cereals such as barley, corn, and rice with different amylose-to-amylopectin ratios. Individuals consuming high amylose-containing rice (Juliano and Goddard 1986) and corn (Behall et al. 1988; 1989; Granfeldt et al. 1995) were reported to have significantly lower postprandial serum glucose and insulin responses. However, rice varieties with similar high-amylose contents can also differ in physicochemical properties, and this, in turn, may influence starch digestibility. Examples of rice with different GIs are basmati rice, a high-amylose rice, which has a GI of 58, and instant rice, which has a higher proportion of amylopectin and a GI of 87 (Foster-Powell et al. 2002).

1.7.2 Processing

The method of processing a single food can greatly change its GI. Grinding, rolling, or milling starchy foods reduces particle size and makes it easier for water to be absorbed and digestive enzymes to attack the food. Processing can also remove the fibrous outer coat of the grain that slows down the access of digestive enzymes to the starch inside and at the same time increases the GI value (Asp 1987). Chemically modifying a food also affects its GI. For instance, 1%–2% acetylated potato starch results in a decrease in GI (Raben et al. 1997), as does the addition of β-cyclodextrin to stabilize the carbohydrate (Raben et al. 1997).

1.7.3 Preparation

The applications of heat and moisture and cooking time, all have a significant effect on GI (Vaaler et al. 1984). During cooking, water and heat expand the starch granules to varying degrees. Foods containing starch that has gelatinized to bursting point, such as boiled or baked potatoes, are more easily digested and therefore have higher GI values compared with foods containing starch granules that are less gelatinized, such as oatmeal or brown rice. For illustration, the GI of a baked potato is 85, whereas that of brown rice is 50 (Englyst and Cummings 1987; Foster-Powell et al. 2002).

1.7.4 Protein, Fat, and Carbohydrate

Numerous studies have shown that protein and fat decrease the blood glucose response and enhance insulin secretion when added to a carbohydrate meal (Estrich et al. 1967; Gulliford et al. 1989). Eating protein-rich food in the same meal stimulates insulin secretion and thus reduces the blood glucose response of that meal (Nuttall et al. 1984). Protein foods delay stomach emptying, which in effect delays digestion of starches. In addition, foods or meals with a higher fat content will have a lower GI than those with a lower fat content because of the property of fat to delay gastric emptying (Thompson et al. 1982). However, foods with a high fat content have also been shown to enhance postprandial insulin secretion because of the large increase in gastric inhibitory polypeptide concentration (Collier and Odea 1983). Gastric inhibitory polypeptide potentiates glucose-induced insulin secretion (Sarson et al. 1984). To demonstrate the effect of protein and fat, the GI of potato chips is 57, that of French fries is 75, and that of baked potato is 85 (Foster-Powell et al. 2002).

1.7.5 Fiber

Viscous, soluble fiber thickens the mixture of food in the digestive tract, which slows down enzymes from digesting the starch (Jenkins et al. 1986). This results in a lower blood sugar response and a lower GI. Foods containing viscous fiber such as barley (Wolever et al. 1988) and legumes (Jenkins et al. 1983) have a low GI. However, it is not possible to differentiate the effects of the type of fiber from those of the food form, particle size, starch type, antinutrients, and the starch-protein interaction.

1.7.6 Sugar

Different sugars have different GI values. For example, sucrose (table sugar), which is made up of glucose and fructose, has a lower GI than glucose because half of the sucrose molecule is made up of fructose, a type of sugar that results in lower blood glucose spikes after consumption. Using glucose as a standard (i.e., GI of glucose: 100), the GI of sucrose is 68 and that of fructose is 19. Therefore, it is expected that adding sugar to a food would lower the GI, however, both Jenkins et al. (1981) and Brand-Miller (1994) found no relation between the sugar content in foods and GI in 62 commonly eaten foods.

1.7.7 Acidity

An increase in the acidity of a meal can significantly lower its GI and the blood sugar response. Organic acid in food slows down stomach emptying, which slows down the rate of carbohydrate digestion. Increasing the amount of vinegar and lemon juice in a meal leads to this effect. Moreover, the addition of sourdough bread to a meal can result in different GIs, depending on its organic acid content (Liljeberg and Bjorck 1996).

1.8 ROLE OF GLYCEMIC INDEX IN HEALTH AND DISEASE

Since the concept of diet GI was first introduced, there has been a lot of research interest in its role in certain disease states, both in terms of prevention and management. Diseases in which GI has been shown to play a role include diabetes and prediabetic states, CVD, obesity and general weight management, cancer, polycystic ovary syndrome, and eye disease. Moreover, there is a lot of research interest in the manipulation of dietary GI and its effect on pregnancy outcome, exercise performance, endurance and recovery, and cognitive function. These diseases and physiologic states or conditions will be discussed in detail in the following chapters, which will provide the research evidence, as it currently stands, and where appropriate, provide recommendations for future research and applications in practice. In addition, Chapter 2 will discuss the common criticisms of the GI; Chapter 3, the methodology used to measure the GI of foods, Chapter 12 will discuss the controversy with regard to using GI on food labels and Chapter 13 will deal with how to create foods with a lower GI.

REFERENCES

American Association of Cereal Chemists International 1999. Whole grain definition. *Cereal Foods World*, 45, 79.

American Dietetic Association 2003. Position of the American Dietetic Association: Oral health and nutrition. *J. Am. Diet. Assoc.*, 103, 615–625.

Anderson, J.W., Hanna, T.J., Peng, X., and Kryscio, R.J. 2000. Whole grain foods and heart disease risk. *J. Am. Coll. Nutr.*, 19(3 Suppl), 291S–299S.

AOAC 2007. *Official Methods of Analysis*, 18th ed., Revision 2 ed. Gaithersburg, MD: AOAC International.

Asp, N.G. 1987. Definition and analysis of dietary fibre. *Scand. J Gastroenterol.,* 129, 16–20.

Asp, N.G., Schweizer, T.F., Southgate, D.A.T., and Theander, O. 1992, Dietary fibre analysis. In *Dietary Fibre: A Component of Food: Nutritional Function in Health and Disease*, T.F. Schweizer and C.A. Edwards, eds., London: Springer, pp. 57–102.

Atkinson, F.S., Foster-Powell, K., and Brand-Miller, J.C. 2008. International tables of glycemic index and glycemic load values: 2008. *Diabetes Care*, 31(12), 2281–2283.

Behall, K.M., Scholfield, D.J., and Canary, J. 1988. Effect of starch structure on glucose and insulin responses in adults. *Am. J. Clin. Nutr.*, 47(3), 428–432.

Behall, K.M., Scholfield, D.J., Yuhaniak, I., and Canary, J. 1989. Diets containing high amylose vs amylopectin starch: Effects on metabolic variables in human subjects. *Am. J. Clin. Nutr.*, 49(2), 337–344.

Belfiore, F. and Iannello, S. 1998. Insulin resistance in obesity: Metabolic mechanisms and measurement methods. *Mol. Genet. Metab.*, 65(2), 121–128.

Bender, D.A. 1997, Digestion and absorption. In *Introduction to Nutrition and Metabolism*, 2nd ed. London: Taylor & Francis Group, pp. 111–140.

Bjorck, I., Ostman, E., Kristensen, M., Anson, N.M., Price, R., Haenen, G.R.M.M., Havenaar, R. et al. 2012. Cereal grains for nutrition and health benefits: Overview of results from in vitro, animal and human studies in the HEALTHGRAIN project. *Trends Food Sci. Tech.*, 25, 87–100.

Blundell, J.E., Green, S., and Burley, V. 1994. Carbohydrates and human appetite. *Am. J. Clin. Nutr.*, 59(3 Suppl), 728S–734S.

Bornet, F.R., Costagliola, D., Rizkalla, S.W., Blayo, A., Fontvieille, A.M., Haardt, M.J., Letanoux, M., Tchobroutsky, G., and Slama, G. 1987. Insulinemic and glycemic indexes of six starch-rich foods taken alone and in a mixed meal by type 2 diabetics. *Am. J. Clin. Nutr.*, 45(3), 588–595.

Brand-Miller, J. and Holt, S. 2004. Testing the glycaemic index of foods: In vivo, not in vitro. *Eur. J. Clin. Nutr.*, 58(4), 700–701.

Brand-Miller, J., Wolever, T.M.S., Foster-Powell, K., and Colagiuri, S. 2003a. *The New Glucose Revolution*, 2nd ed. New Work: Marlowe & Company.

Brand-Miller, J.C. 1994. Importance of glycemic index in diabetes. *Am. J. Clin. Nutr.*, 59(3), S747–S752.

Brand-Miller, J.C., Holt, S.H., Pawlak, D.B., and McMillan, J. 2002. Glycemic index and obesity. *Am. J. Clin. Nutr.*, 76(1), 281S–285S.

Brand-Miller, J.C., Holt, S.H.A., and Petocz, P. 2003b. Reply to R. Mendosa. *Am. J. Clin. Nutr.*, 77, 994–995.

Bray, G.A. 2010. Fructose: Pure, white, and deadly? Fructose, by any other name, is a health hazard. *J. Diabetes Sci. Tech.*, 4, 1003–1007.

Brownawell, A.M., Caers, W., Gibson, G.R., Kendall, C.W., Lewis, K.D., Ringel, Y., and Slavin, J.L. 2012. Prebiotics and the health benefits of fiber: Current regulatory status, future research, and goals. *J. Nutr.*, 142(5), 962–974.

Calton, E.K., James, A.P., Pannu, P.K., and Soares, M.J. 2014. Certain dietary patterns are beneficial for the metabolic syndrome: Reviewing the evidence. *Nutr. Res.*, 34(7), 559–568.

Collier, G. and Odea, K. 1983. The effect of coingestion of fat on the glucose, insulin, and gastric-inhibitory polypeptide responses to carbohydrate and protein. *Am. J. Clin. Nutr.*, 37(6), 941–944.

Coultate, T. P. 2009, Polysaccharides. In *Food: The Chemistry of Its Components*, 5th ed. T. P. Coultate, ed., Cambridge: The Royal Society of Chemistry, pp. 51–96.

Cummings, J.H. 1997, The large intestine in nutrition and disease. In *Danome Chair Monograph*, Brussels, Belgium: Institute Danome.

Cummings, J.H. and Englyst, H.N. 1995. Gastrointestinal effects of food carbohydrate. *Am. J. Clin. Nutr.*, 61(4 Suppl), 938S–945S.

Cummings, J.H. and Stephen, A.M. 2007. Carbohydrate terminology and classification. *Eur. J. Clin. Nutr.*, 61(Suppl 1), S5–S18.

Davy, B.M. and Melby, C.L. 2003. The effect of fiber-rich carbohydrates on features of syndrome X. *J. Am. Diet Assoc.*, 103(1), 86–96.

de Ruyter, J.C., Olthof, M.R., Seidell, J.C., and Katan, M.B. 2012. A trial of sugar-free or sugar-sweetened beverages and body weight in children. *N. Engl. J. Med.*, 367(15), 1397–1406.

Department of Health 1989. *Dietary Sugars and Human Disease.* London: Her Majesty's Stationery Office.

Earth Policy Institute 2007. Bottled Water Consumption Per Person in the United States, 1976–2007. http://www.earth-policy.org/index.php?/data_center/C21/. (Accessed June 16, 2016.)

Ebbeling, C.B., Feldman, H.A., Chomitz, V.R., Antonelli, T.A., Gortmaker, S.L., Osganian, S.K., and Ludwig, D.S. 2012. A randomized trial of sugar-sweetened beverages and adolescent body weight. *N. Engl. J. Med.*, 367(15), 1407–1416.

Eckel, R.H., Grundy, S.M., and Zimmet, P.Z. 2005. The metabolic syndrome. *Lancet*, 365(9468), 1415–1428.

EFSA 2010. Scientific opinion on dietary reference values for carbohydrates and dietary fibre. *EFSA J.*, 8(3), 1462–1539.

Englyst, H.N. and Cummings, J.H. 1987. Digestion of polysaccharides of potato in the small intestine of man. *Am. J. Clin. Nutr.*, 45(2), 423–431.

Englyst, H.N. and Cummings, J.H. 1990, Non-starch polysaccharides (dietary fiber) and resistant starch. In *New Developments in Dietary Fiber. Physiological, Physicochemical, and Analytical Aspects*, I. Furda and C.J. Brine, eds., New York and London: Plenum Press, pp. 205–225.

Englyst, H.N., Kingman, S.M., and Cummings, J.H. 1992. Classification and measurement of nutritionally important starch fractions. *Eur. J. Clin. Nutr.*, 46, S33–S50.

Englyst, H.N., Quigley, M.E., and Hudson, G.J. 1994. Determination of dietary fibre as non-starch polysaccharides with gas-liquid chromatographic, high-performance liquid chromatographic or spectrophotometric measurement of constituent sugars. *Analyst*, 119(7), 1497–1509.

Englyst, K.N. and Englyst, H.N. 2005. Carbohydrate bioavailability. *Brit. J. Nutr.*, 94(1), 1–11.

Englyst, K.N., Liu, S., and Englyst, H.N. 2007. Nutritional characterization and measurement of dietary carbohydrates. *Eur. J. Clin. Nutr.*, 61(Suppl 1), S19–S39.

Estrich, D., Ravnik, A., Schlierf, G., Fukayama, G., and Kinsell, L. 1967. Effects of Co-ingestion of fat and protein upon carbohydrate-induced hyperglycemia. *Diabetes*, 16(4), 232–237.

European Union 2011. Regulation (EU) No 1169/2011 of the European parliament and of the council of 25 October 2011 on the provision of food information to consumers, amending Regulations (EC) No 1924/2006 and (EC) No 1925/2006 of the European parliament and of the council, and repealing commission directive 87/250/EEC, council directive 90/496/EEC, commission directive 1999/10/EC, directive 2000/13/EC of the European parliament and of the council, commission directives 2002/67/EC and 2008/5/EC and commission regulation (EC) No 608/2004. *OJEU*, L 304, 18–63.

FAO 1998, *FAO Food and Nutrition Paper 66: Carbohydrates in Human Nutrition.* Rome, Italy: *FAO.*

FAO 2003, *Food Energy—Methods of Analysis and Conversion Factors.* Rome, Italy: Food and Agriculture Organisation of the United Nations, FAO Food and Nutrition Paper no 77.

Ferrannini, E., Barrett, E.J., Bevilacqua, S., and DeFronzo, R.A. 1983. Effect of fatty acids on glucose production and utilization in man. *J. Clin. Invest.*, 72(5), 1737–1747.

Ferruzzi, M.G., Jonnalagadda, S.S., Liu, S., Marquart, L., McKeown, N., Reicks, M., Riccardi, G.et al. 2014. Developing a standard definition of whole-grain foods for dietary recommendations: Summary report of a multidisciplinary expert roundtable discussion. *Adv. Nutr.*, 5(2), 164–176.

Food Standard Agency and Public Health England 2014. *The Composition of Foods: 7th Summary Edition.* Cambridge: Royal Society of Chemisty.

Foster-Powell, K., Holt, S.H., and Brand-Miller, J.C. 2002. International table of glycemic index and glycemic load values: 2002. *Am. J. Clin. Nutr.*, 76(1), 5–56.

Frayn, K.N. 2000. Visceral fat and insulin resistance—causative or correlative? *Br. J. Nutr.*, 83(Suppl 1), S71–S77.
Gibson, G.R., Probert, H.M., Loo, J.V., Rastall, R.A., and Roberfroid, M.B. 2004. Dietary modulation of the human colonic microbiota: Updating the concept of prebiotics. *Nutr. Res. Rev.*, 17(2), 259–275.
Gibson, G.R. and Roberfroid, M.B. 1995. Dietary modulation of the human colonic microbiota: Introducing the concept of prebiotics. *J. Nutr.*, 125(6), 1401–1412.
Granfeldt, Y., Drews, A., and Bjorck, I. 1995. Arepas made from high amylose corn flour produce favorably low glucose and insulin responses in healthy humans. *J. Nutr.*, 125(3), 459–465.
Gulliford, M.C., Bicknell, E.J., and Scarpello, J.H. 1989. Differential effect of protein and fat ingestion on blood glucose responses to high- and low-glycemic-index carbohydrates in noninsulin-dependent diabetic subjects. *Am. J. Clin. Nutr.*, 50(4), 773–777.
Ha, V., Sievenpiper, J.L., de Souza, R.J., Chiavaroli, L., Wang, D.D., Cozma, A.I., Mirrahimi, A. et al. 2012. Effect of fructose on blood pressure: A systematic review and meta-analysis of controlled feeding trials. *Hypertension*, 59(4), 787–795.
Health Canada 2015. Canada's Food Guide. http://www.hc-sc.gc.ca/fn-an/food-guide-aliment/index-eng.php. (Accessed April 7, 2016.)
Holland, B., Unwin, I.D., and Buss, D.H. 1992. *Fruit and Nuts. First Supplement to 5th Edition of McCance and Widdowson's The Composition of Foods.* London: Her Majesty's Stationary Office.
Hu, F.B. 2013. Resolved: There is sufficient scientific evidence that decreasing sugar-sweetened beverage consumption will reduce the prevalence of obesity and obesity-related diseases. *Obes. Rev.*, 14(8), 606–619.
Institute of Medicine 2006. *Dietary Reference Intakes: The Essential Guide to Nutrient Requirements.* Washington, DC: The National Academies Press.
IUB-IUPAC Joint Commission on Biochemical Nomenclature 1982. Abbreviated terminology of oligosaccharide chains. *J. Biol. Chem.*, 257, 3347–3351.
Jenkins, D.J., Wolever, T.M., Jenkins, A.L., Josse, R.G., and Wong, G.S. 1984. The glycaemic response to carbohydrate foods. *Lancet*, 2(8399), 388–391.
Jenkins, D.J., Wolever, T.M., Jenkins, A.L., Thorne, M.J., Lee, R., Kalmusky, J., Reichert, R., and Wong, G.S. 1983. The glycaemic index of foods tested in diabetic patients: A new basis for carbohydrate exchange favouring the use of legumes. *Diabetologia*, 24(4), 257–264.
Jenkins, D.J., Wolever, T.M., Taylor, R.H., Barker, H., Fielden, H., Baldwin, J.M., Bowling, A.C., Newman, H.C., Jenkins, A.L., and Goff, D.V. 1981. Glycemic index of foods: A physiological basis for carbohydrate exchange. *Am. J. Clin. Nutr.*, 34(3), 362–366.
Jenkins, D.J.A., Jenkins, M.J.A., Wolever, T.M.S., Taylor, R.H., and Ghafari, H. 1986. Slow release carbohydrate: mechanism of action of viscous fibers. *J. Clin. Nutr.*, 1, 237–241.
Joint FAO/WHO Expert Consultation 1998, *Carbohydrates in Human Nutrition.* Rome, Italy: *FAO Food and Nutrition Paper 66*, FAO.
Juliano, B.O. and Goddard, M.S. 1986. Cause of varietal difference in insulin and glucose responses to ingested rice. *Qual. Plant.*, 36, 35–41.
Kaiser, K.A., Shikany, J.M., Keating, K.D., and Allison, D.B. 2013. Will reducing sugar-sweetened beverage consumption reduce obesity? Evidence supporting conjecture is strong, but evidence when testing effect is weak. *Obes. Rev.*, 14(8), 620–633.
Kennedy, G. and Burlingame, B. 2003. Analysis of food composition data on rice from a plant genetic resources perspective. *Food Chem.*, 80, 589–596.
Lairon, D. 1994, *Mechanisms of Action of Dietary Fibre on Lipid and Cholesterol Metabolism.* Luxembourg: Commission of the European Communities.
Liljeberg, H.G. and Bjorck, I.M. 1996. Delayed gastric emptying rate as a potential mechanism for lowered glycemia after eating sourdough bread: Studies in humans and rats using test products with added organic acids or an organic salt. *Am. J. Clin. Nutr.*, 64(6), 886–893.
Lowndes, J., Sinnett, S., Yu, Z., and Rippe, J. 2014. The effects of fructose-containing sugars on weight, body composition and cardiometabolic risk factors when consumed at up to the 90th percentile population consumption level for fructose. *Nutrients*, 6(8), 3153–3168.
Ludwig, D.S. 2002. The glycemic index: Physiological mechanisms relating to obesity, diabetes, and cardiovascular disease. *JAMA*, 287(18), 2414–2423.
Maersk, M., Belza, A., Stodkilde-Jorgensen, H., Ringgaard, S., Chabanova, E., Thomsen, H., Pedersen, S.B., Astrup, A., and Richelsen, B. 2012. Sucrose-sweetened beverages increase fat storage in the liver, muscle, and visceral fat depot: A 6-mo randomized intervention study. *Am. J. Clin. Nutr.*, 95(2), 283–289.
Malik, V.S., Popkin, B.M., Bray, G.A., Despres, J.P., Willett, W.C., and Hu, F.B. 2010. Sugar-sweetened beverages and risk of metabolic syndrome and type 2 diabetes: A meta-analysis. *Diabetes Care*, 33(11), 2477–2483.

Malik, V.S., Willett, W.C., and Hu, F.B. 2013. Global obesity: Trends, risk factors and policy implications. *Nat. Rev. Endocrinol.*, 9, 13–27.
Mann, J., Cummings, J.H., Englyst, H.N., Key, T., Liu, S., Riccardi, G. et al. 2007. FAO/WHO scientific update on carbohydrates in human nutrition: Conclusions. *Eur. J. Clin. Nutr.*, 61(Suppl 1), S132–S137.
McCance, R.A. and Laurence, R.D. 1929. *The Carbohydrate Content of Foods.* London: Her Majesty's Stationery Office.
Melanson, K.J., Zukley, L., Lowndes, J., Nguyen, V., Angelopoulos, T.J., and Rippe, J.M. 2007. Effects of high-fructose corn syrup and sucrose consumption on circulating glucose, insulin, leptin, and ghrelin and on appetite in normal-weight women. *Nutrition*, 23(2), 103–112.
Moynihan, P.J. and Kelly, S.A. 2014. Effect on caries of restricting sugars intake: Systematic review to inform WHO guidelines. *J. Dent. Res.*, 93(1), 8–18.
National Health and Medical Research Council 2013. *Australian Dietary Guidelines.* Canberra, Australia: National Health and Medical Research Council.
Nuttall, F.Q., Mooradian, A.D., Gannon, M.C., Billington, C., and Krezowski, P. 1984. Effect of protein ingestion on the glucose and insulin response to a standardized oral glucose load. *Diabetes Care*, 7(5), 465–470.
Odegaard, A.O., Koh, W.P., Arakawa, K., Yu, M.C., and Pereira, M.A. 2010. Soft drink and juice consumption and risk of physician-diagnosed incident type 2 diabetes: The Singapore Chinese Health Study. *Am. J. Epidemiol.*, 171(6), 701–708.
Palmer, J.R., Boggs, D.A., Krishnan, S., Hu, F.B., Singer, M., and Rosenberg, L. 2008. Sugar-sweetened beverages and incidence of type 2 diabetes mellitus in African American women. *Arch. Intern. Med.*, 168(14), 1487–1492.
Raben, A., Andersen, K., Karberg, M.A., Holst, J.J., and Astrup, A. 1997. Acetylation of or beta-cyclodextrin addition to potato beneficial effect on glucose metabolism and appetite sensations. *Am. J. Clin. Nutr.*, 66(2), 304–314.
Richelsen, B. 2013. Sugar-sweetened beverages and cardio-metabolic disease risks. *Curr. Opin. Clin. Nutr. Metab. Care*, 16(4), 478–484.
Rippe, J.M. and Angelopoulos, T.J. 2013. Sucrose, high-fructose corn syrup, and fructose, their metabolism and potential health effects: What do we really know? *Adv. Nutr.*, 4(2), 236–245.
Roberfroid, M., Gibson, G.R., and Delzenne, N. 1993. The biochemistry of oligofructose, a nondigestible fiber: An approach to calculate its caloric value. *Nutr. Rev.*, 51(5), 137–146.
Salmeron, J., Manson, J.E., Stampfer, M.J., Colditz, G.A., Wing, A.L., and Willett, W.C. 1997. Dietary fiber, glycemic load, and risk of non-insulin-dependent diabetes mellitus in women. *J. Am. Med. Assoc.*, 277(6), 472–477.
Sarson, D.L., Wood, S.M., Kansal, P.C., and Bloom, S.R. 1984. Glucose-dependent insulinotropic polypeptide augmentation of insulin. Physiology or pharmacology? *Diabetes*, 33(4), 389–393.
Schulze, M.B., Manson, J.E., Ludwig, D.S., Colditz, G.A., Stampfer, M.J., Willett, W.C., and Hu, F.B. 2004. Sugar-sweetened beverages, weight gain, and incidence of type 2 diabetes in young and middle-aged women. *JAMA*, 292(8), 927–934.
Soderberg, S., Zimmet, P., Tuomilehto, J., de Courten, M., Dowse, G.K., Chitson, P., Gareeboo, H., Alberti, K., and Shaw, J.E. 2005. Increasing prevalence of type 2 diabetes mellitus in all ethnic groups in Mauritius. *Diabetic Med.*, 22(1), 61–68.
Soenen, S. and Westerterp-Plantenga, M.S. 2007. No differences in satiety or energy intake after high-fructose corn syrup, sucrose, or milk preloads. *Am. J. Clin. Nutr.*, 86(6), 1586–1594.
Southgate, D.A., Paul, A.A., Dean, A.C., and Christie, A.A. 1978. Free sugars in foods. *J. Hum. Nutr.*, 32(5), 335–347.
Stanhope, K.L., Medici, V., Bremer, A.A., Lee, V., Lam, H.D., Nunez, M.V., Chen, G.X., Keim, N.L., and Havel, P.J. 2015. A dose-response study of consuming high-fructose corn syrup-sweetened beverages on lipid/lipoprotein risk factors for cardiovascular disease in young adults. *Am. J. Clin. Nutr.*, 101(6), 1144–1154.
Stephen, A. M. 2006, *Impact of Carbohydrate Methodology on Dietary Intake.* Copenhagen.
Te, M.L., Mallard, S., and Mann, J. 2013. Dietary sugars and body weight: Systematic review and meta-analyses of randomised controlled trials and cohort studies. *BMJ*, 346, e7492.
Thompson, D.G., Wingate, D.L., Thomas, M., and Harrison, D. 1982. Gastric emptying as a determinant of the oral glucose tolerance test. *Gastroenterology*, 82(1), 51–55.
Trowell, H. 2006. Ischaemic heart disease and dietary fibre. *Am. J. Clin. Nutr.*, 25, 926–932.
Tuohy, K.M., Hinton, D.J., Davies, S.J., Crabbe, M.J., Gibson, G.R., and Ames, J.M. 2006. Metabolism of Maillard reaction products by the human gut microbiota—Implications for health. *Mol. Nutr. Food. Res.*, 50(9), 847–857.

U.S. Department of Agriculture and U.S. Department of Health and Human Services 2010. *Dietary Guidelines for Americans, 2010*, 7th ed. Washington, DC: U.S. Government Printing Office.

United States Department of Agriculture 2015. USDA National Nutrient Database for Standard Reference. http://www.ars.usda.gov/nutrientdata. (Accessed April 7, 2016.)

U.S. FDA 2006. FDA guidance for industry and FDA staff: Guidance on whole grain label statement. http://www.fda.gov/ohrms/dockets/98fr/06d-0066-gdl0001.pdf. (Accessed April 7, 2016.)

Vaaler, S., Hanssen, K.F., and Aagenaes, O. 1984. The effect of cooking upon the blood glucose response to ingested carrots and potatoes. *Diabetes Care*, 7(3), 221–223.

White, J.S., Foreyt, J.P., Melanson, K.J., and Angelopoulos, T.J. 2010. High-fructose corn syrup: Controversies and common sense. *Am. J. Lifestyle Med.*, 4, 515–520.

WHO/FAO 2003. *Diet, Nutrition and the Prevention of Chronic Disease. Report of a Joint WHO/FAO Expert Consultation.* Geneva, Switzerland: World Health Organisation.

Wiesenthal, S.R., Sandhu, H., McCall, R.H., Tchipashvili, V., Yoshii, H., Polonsky, K., Shi, Z.Q., Lewis, G.F., Mari, A., and Giacca, A. 1999. Free fatty acids impair hepatic insulin extraction in vivo. *Diabetes*, 48(4), 766–774.

Wolever, T.M. 2003. Carbohydrate and the regulation of blood glucose and metabolism. *Nutr. Rev.*, 61(5 Pt 2), S40–S48.

Wolever, T.M. 2006. Physiological mechanisms and observed health impacts related to the glycaemic index: Some observations. *Int. J. Obes.(Lond)*, 30(Suppl 3), S72–S78.

Wolever, T.M.S., Jenkins, D.J.A., Collier, G.R., Lee, R., Wong, G.S., and Josse, R.G. 1988. Metabolic response to test meals containing different carbohydrate foods.1. relationship between rate of digestion and plasma-insulin response. *Nutr. Res.*, 8(6), 573–581.

World Health Organization 2015, *Guideline: Sugars Intake for Adults and Children.* Geneva, Switzerland: World Health Organization.

Yang, Q., Zhang, Z., Gregg, E.W., Flanders, W.D., Merritt, R., and Hu, F.B. 2014. Added sugar intake and cardiovascular diseases mortality among US adults. *JAMA Intern. Med.*, 174(4), 516–524.

2 Common Criticisms of the Glycemic Index

Effie Viguiliouk, Viranda H. Jayalath, Vanessa Ha, and Thomas M.S. Wolever

CONTENTS

2.1 INTRODUCTION

The glycemic index (GI) has been subject to a number of criticisms, including but not limited to the following: (1) the GI methodology is not valid (Franz 1999; Pi-Sunyer 2002; DeVries 2007; Anderson 2008; Aziz 2009; Jones 2012); (2) GI is a poor predictor of healthy foods (Jones 2012) and carbohydrate quality (Slavin 2010); and (3) GI does not apply to mixed meals (Franz 1999; Pi-Sunyer 2002; Anderson 2008; Aziz 2009; Jones 2012; Wolever 2013). The following sections will address these criticisms and provide counterarguments.

2.2 THE GLYCEMIC INDEX METHODOLOGY IS NOT VALID

Concerns have been raised that the method to measure GI is nonstandardized (Aziz 2009), inaccurate, and imprecise (Franz 1999; Pi-Sunyer 2002; DeVries 2007; Anderson 2008; Aziz 2009; Jones 2012; Wolever 2013). With regard to the first concern, it should be noted that between 1998 and 2008, several documents published by various organizations and groups provided similar descriptions of the GI methodology (FAO 1998; Brouns et al. 2005; Wolever et al. 2003, 2008; Australian Standards Organization 2007; Aziz 2009), and since then, an official International Organization for Standardization (ISO) method to determine the GI of foods has been validated and published by the Food and Agriculture Organization of the United Nations (ISO 2010; Wolever 2013) (see Chapter 3). Therefore, an official standardized method to measure GI does exist; however, this does not mean that this method is always used correctly. Common errors of use include feeding food portions containing 50 g "total" carbohydrate instead of "available" carbohydrate; testing the reference food only "once" in each subject, instead of testing it at least twice; having less than ten subjects; using an imprecise method to measure glucose; and having a mean coefficient of variation of within-individual variation of area under the curve greater than 30% (Wolever 2013). Suggestions to help mitigate such errors include appropriate regulations consisting of education and enforced use of the correct methodology for measuring GI.

Other concerns regarding the inaccuracy and imprecision of GI have been raised because there is evidence that suggests: (1) high variation of the GI values in the international GI tables (Pi-Sunyer 2002); (2) various factors in food that affect GI (Pi-Sunyer 2002; Anderson 2008; Jones 2012); and (3) high day-to-day variation of glycemic responses between and within subjects (Franz 1999; Anderson 2008; Jones 2012; Wolever 2013). Although it is true that a high variation of the GI values exists within the international GI tables, some of this variation can be attributed to methodological errors, whereas most of the error results from real differences between foods within the same category that are not due to their chemical compositions. Some of the factors that can affect the GI value of food outside of its chemical composition include differences in variety, processing, and growing conditions; these factors are also relevant for other food properties such as micronutrient content. Although this presents some issues, it provides opportunities to reduce the GI of the diet without making major changes to the nature of the diet, by choosing a food with a lower or higher GI in the food group. For example, one could choose to cook dried legumes instead of using canned legumes, because the canning process has been shown to increase the GI of legumes (Wolever et al. 1987). In order to address these issues, it is important to identify a way that can provide reliable data on the GI of foods for consumers and health professionals, such as food labeling (see Chapter 12). Concerns regarding high day-to-day variation of glycemic responses between subjects stem from the quantity of food ingested at any one time, the frequency of eating, and the time period of eating. However, all these factors pertain to glycemic responses and not to GI. When properly measuring GI, these factors are controlled for, thus minimally influencing the resultant values. However, it is true that within-individual variation influences the accuracy and precision of measured GI values. Indeed, the GI methodology has been designed to minimize these effects, for example, by using the mean of two fasting blood samples when calculating the area under the curve (Wolever et al. 2006, Wolever 2013) and ensuring that the mean coefficient of variation of the reference food is less than 30% (Wolever et al. 2008).

2.3 THE GLYCEMIC INDEX IS A POOR PREDICTOR OF HEALTHY FOODS AND CARBOHYDRATE QUALITY

The GI was first clinically applied to the management of glycemic control and diabetes. However, a large body of evidence now exists that shows that GI has much broader implications in health and disease, including exercise performance (O'Reilly et al. 2010); cognitive function (Benton et al. 2003; Micha et al. 2010); pregnancy outcomes (Clapp 2002; Moses et al. 2006; Clapp and Lopez 2007; Chavarro et al. 2009; Marsh et al. 2010; Rhodes et al. 2010); weight maintenance (Chiu et al. 2011); risk for cardiovascular disease (Barclay et al. 2008; Mirrahimi et al. 2014); breast (Dong and Qin 2011); prostate (Shikany et al. 2011), colorectal, pancreatic, and other cancers (Barclay et al. 2008); depression (Mwamburi et al. 2011); and Parkinson's disease (Murakami et al. 2010). Despite this wealth of evidence supporting the health benefits of GI, its concept is still considered limited as a meaningful measure of carbohydrate quality. The primary factor suggested as limiting the use of GI to predict carbohydrate quality relates to the proposition that many healthy foods such as whole grains and starchy vegetables have high GI, whereas unhealthy foods such as sugary beverages and fructose have low GI. However, little evidence supports these notions. According to the data from published GI tables (Foster-Powell et al. 2002), the mean and distribution of GI between whole grain breads and all other breads do not differ, with the majority of breads considered to have medium to high GI. Similarly, starchy potatoes and sugary beverages cover a wide range of GI, with 80% and 90% of these products falling within medium- to high-GI categories. Furthermore, the misconceptions behind the delirious health consequences of fructose (derived from both sucrose and/or high-fructose corn syrup) are only supported by low-quality evidence from ecological studies (Bray et al. 2004) and animal models (Lee et al. 1994; Brunengraber et al. 2003; Dolan et al. 2010) and not by high-quality systematic reviews and meta-analyses of controlled trials in humans. The latter type of evidence suggests that moderate fructose consumption has no adverse effects on body weight (Sievenpiper et al. 2012), blood pressure (Ha et al. 2012), blood glucose (Cozma et al. 2012), or blood lipids (Sievenpiper et al. 2009). In fact, moderate fructose intakes may even benefit glycemic control and blood pressure (Cozma et al. 2012; Ha et al. 2012; Jayalath et al. 2014), supporting the health benefits predicted by its low GI. Overall, the results of these studies indicate that the issue is not with fructose but with consumption of excess energy.

Moreover, both whole grains and dietary fiber have been considered superior markers of carbohydrate quality than GI. However, a review of clinical trials of whole grains and GI suggests similar and complimentary cardiometabolic benefits for both dietary components (Wolever 2013), with low-GI diets showing greater benefits in diabetes (Jenkins et al. 2008; 2012). On the other hand, the health benefits of fiber depend on its type, where viscous fibers, which have a lower GI, tend to improve glycemia and cholesterol and nonviscous fibers, which have a higher GI, bulk stool (Wolever and Jenkins 1992). Thus, instead of considering fiber as a marker of carbohydrate quality, the GI of the fiber, which predicts its ability to reduce glycemic responses and elicit health benefits, should be considered. Overall, this evidence does not support the notion that fibers or whole grains are better predictors of carbohydrate quality than of GI.

2.4 THE GLYCEMIC INDEX DOES NOT APPLY TO MIXED MEALS

It is a common misconception that the GI of foods changes in mixed meals. For instance, it has previously been suggested that the GI of a mixed meal can drop by almost half with the addition of nuts (Jones 2012). It must be clarified that although the glycemic response may change, the GI of the carbohydrate food does not change. In fact, the addition or removal of other nutrients maintains the relative glycemic response predicted by GI; adding fat to a meal with potato (high-GI food) or with lentil (low-GI food) was shown to reduce the glycemic response by 40%–50% relative to each food without fat (Collier et al. 1984; Bornet et al. 1987; Henry et al. 2006). Moreover, the glycemic response elicited by mixed meals with equivalent macronutrient profiles containing carbohydrates with differing GIs is directly related to the meal's GI calculated using the individual food components (Collier et al. 1986; Wolever 1997). This supports the notion that GI remains an important predictor of glycemic response, independent of other macronutrients in mixed-meal scenarios.

Overall, these criticisms stem from misunderstanding or misinterpretation of GI. A number of issues need to be addressed before translating GI into practice; however, as discussed, these issues are not insurmountable.

REFERENCES

Anderson, G. H. 2008. The glycemic index: Clinical and public health significance, *Carbohydrate News (publication of the Canadian Sugar Institute*, http://www.sugar.ca/SUGAR/media/Sugar-Main/PDFs/CarboNews2008.pdf. (Accessed May 19, 2016.)

Australian Standards Organization. 2007. Glycemic Index of Foods AS4694 - 2007, http://infostore.saiglobal.com/store/Details.aspx?DocN=AS0733779662AT. (Accessed June 16, 2016.)

Aziz, A. 2009. The glycemic index: Methodological aspects related to the interpretation of health effects and to regulatory labeling, *J AOAC Int*, 92:879–87.

Barclay, A. W., Petocz, P., McMillan-Price, J., Flood, V. M., Prvan, T., Mitchell, P., Brand-Miller, J. C. 2008. Glycemic index, glycemic load, and chronic disease risk—A meta-analysis of observational studies, *Am J Clin Nutr*, 87:627–37.

Benton, D., Ruffin, M.-P., Lassel, T., Nabb, S., Messaoudi, M., Vinoy, S. et al. 2003. The delivery rate of dietary carbohydrates affects cognitive performance in both rats and humans, *Psychopharmacology (Berl)*, 166:86–90.

Bornet, F. R., Costagliola, D., Rizkalla, S. W., Blayo, A., Fontvieille, A. M., Haardt, M. J., Letanoux, M. et al. 1987. Insulinemic and glycemic indexes of six starch-rich foods taken alone and in a mixed meal by type 2 diabetics, *Am J Clin Nutr*, 45:588–95.

Bray, G. A., Nielsen, S. J., Popkin, B. M. 2004. Consumption of high-fructose corn syrup in beverages may play a role in the epidemic of obesity, *Am J Clin Nutr*, 79:537–43.

Brouns, F., Bjorck, I., Frayn, K. N., Gibbs, A. L., Lang, V., Slama, G., Wolever, T. M. 2005. Glycaemic index methodology, *Nutr Res Rev*, 18:145–71.

Brunengraber, D. Z., McCabe, B. J., Kasumov, T., Alexander, J. C., Chandramouli, V., Previs, S. F. 2003. Influence of diet on the modeling of adipose tissue triglycerides during growth, *Am J Physiol Endocrinol Metab*, 285:E917–E925.

Chavarro, J. E., Rich-Edwards, J. W., Rosner, B. A., Willett, W. C. 2009. A prospective study of dietary carbohydrate quantity and quality in relation to risk of ovulatory infertility, *Eur J Clin Nutr*, 63:78–86.

Chiu, C. J., Liu, S., Willett, W. C., Wolever, T. M., Brand-Miller, J. C., Barclay, A. W. et al. 2011. Informing food choices and health outcomes by use of the dietary glycemic index, *Nutr Rev*, 69:231–42.

Clapp, J. F. 2002. Maternal carbohydrate intake and pregnancy outcome, *Proc Nutr Soc*, 3rd., 61:45–50.

Clapp, J. F., Lopez, B. 2007. Low- versus high-glycemic index diets in women: Effects on caloric requirements, substrate utilization, and insulin sensitivity, *Metabol Synd Rel Disord*, 5:231–42.

Collier, G., McLean, A., O'Dea, K. 1984. Effect of co-ingestion of fat on the metabolic responses to slowly and rapidly absorbed carbohydrates, *Diabetologia*, 26:50–54.

Collier, G. R., Wolever, T. M., Wong, G. S., Josse, R. G. 1986. Prediction of glycemic response to mixed meals in noninsulin-dependent diabetic subjects, *Am J Clin Nutr*, 44:349–352.

Cozma, A. I., Sievenpiper, J. L., de Souza, R. J., Chiavaroli, L., Ha, V., Wang, D. D., Mirrahimi, A. et al. 2012. Effect of fructose on glycemic control in diabetes: A systematic review and meta-analysis of controlled feeding trials, *Diabetes Care*, 35:1611–1620.

DeVries, J. W. 2007. Glycemic index: The analytical perspective, *Cereal Foods World*, 52:45–49.

Dolan, L. C., Potter, S. M., Burdock, G. A. 2010. Evidence-based review on the effect of normal dietary consumption of fructose on blood lipids and body weight of overweight and obese individuals, *Crit Rev Food Sci Nutr*, 50:889–918.

Dong, J. Y., Qin, L. Q. 2011. Dietary glycemic index, glycemic load, and risk of breast cancer: Meta-analysis of prospective cohort studies, *Breast Cancer Res Treat*, 126:287–294.

FAO. 1998. *FAO Food and Nutrition Paper 66: Carbohydrates in Human Nutrition*. Rome, FAO.

Foster-Powell, K., Holt, S. H., Brand-Miller, J. C. 2002. International table of glycemic index and glycemic load values: 2002, *Am J Clin Nutr*, 76:5–56.

Franz, M. J. 1999. In defense of the American Diabetes Association's recommendations on the glycemic index, *Nutr Today*, 34:78–81.

Ha, V., Sievenpiper, J. L., de Souza, R. J., Chiavaroli, L., Wang, D. D., Cozma, A. I., Mirrahimi, A. et al. 2012. Effect of fructose on blood pressure: A systematic review and meta-analysis of controlled feeding trials, *Hypertension*, 59:787–795.

Henry, C. J., Lightowler, H. J., Kendall, F. L., Storey, M. 2006. The impact of the addition of toppings/fillings on the glycaemic response to commonly consumed carbohydrate foods, *Eur J Clin Nutr*, 60:763–769.

ISO. 2010. Food products - Determination of the glycaemic index (GI) and recommendation for food classification. *ISO 26642:2010*, Accessed May 19, 2016. http://www.iso.org/iso/catalogue_detail.htm?csnumber=43633.

Jayalath, V. H., Sievenpiper, J. L., de Souza, R. J., Ha, V., Mirrahimi, A., Santaren, I. D., Blanco Mejia, S., Di Buono, M. et al. 2014. Total fructose intake and risk of hypertension: A systematic review and meta-analysis of prospective cohorts, *J Am Coll Nutr*, 33:328–339.

Jenkins, D. J., Kendall, C. W., McKeown-Eyssen, G., Josse, R. G., Silverberg, J., Booth, G. L., Vidgen, E. et al. 2008. Effect of a low-glycemic index or a high-cereal fiber diet on type 2 diabetes: A randomized trial, *JAMA*, 300:2742–2753.

Jenkins, D. J., Kendall, C. W., Augustin, L. S., Mitchell, S., Sahye-Pudaruth, S., Blanco Mejia, S., Chiavaroli, L. et al. 2012. Effect of legumes as part of a low glycemic index diet on glycemic control and cardiovascular risk factors in type 2 diabetes mellitus: A randomized controlled trial, *Arch Intern Med*, 172:1653–1660.

Jones, J. M. 2012. Glycemic index: the state of the science, part 1: The measure and its variability, *Nutr Today*, 47:207–13.

Lee, W. N., Bassilian, S., Ajie, H. O., Schoeller, D. A., Edmond, J., Bergner, E. A. et al. 1994. In vivo measurement of fatty acids and cholesterol synthesis using D2O and mass isotopomer analysis, *Am J Physiol*, 266:E699–E708.

Marsh, K. A., Steinbeck, K. S., Atkinson, F. S., Petocz, P., Brand-Miller, J. C. 2010. Effect of a low glycemic index compared with a conventional healthy diet on polycystic ovary syndrome, *Am J Clin Nutr*, 92:83–92.

Micha, R., Rogers, P. J., Nelson, M. 2010. The glycaemic potency of breakfast and cognitive function in school children, *Eur J Clin Nutr*, 64:948–957.

Mirrahimi, A., Chiavaroli, L., Srichaikul, K., Augustin, L. S., Sievenpiper, J. L., Kendall, C. W., Jenkins, D. J. 2014. The role of glycemic index and glycemic load in cardiovascular disease and its risk factors: a review of the recent literature, *Curr Atheroscler Rep*, 16:381.

Moses, R. G., Luebcke, M., Davis, W. S., Coleman, K. J., Tapsell, L. C., Petocz, P., Brand-Miller, J. C. 2006. Effect of a low-glycemic-index diet during pregnancy on obstetric outcomes, *Am J Clin Nutr*, 84:807–812.

Murakami, K., Myake, Y., Sasaki, S., Tanaka, K., Fukushima, W., Kiyohara, C. et al. 2010. Dietary glycemic index is inversely associated with the risk of Parkinson's disease: A case-control study in Japan, *Nutrition*, 26:515–521.

Mwamburi, D. M., Liebson, E., Folstein, M., Bungay, K., Tucker, K. L., Qiu, W. Q. 2011. Depression and glycemic intake in the homebound elderly, *J Affect Disord*, 132:94–98.

O'Reilly, J., Wong, S. H., Chen, Y. 2010. Glycaemic index, glycaemic load and exercise performance, *Sports Med*, 40:27–39.

Pi-Sunyer, F. X. 2002. Glycemic index and disease, *Am J Clin Nutr*, 76:290S–298S.

Rhodes, E. T., Pawlak, D. B., Takoudes, T. C., Ebbeling, C. B., Feldman, H. A., Lovesky, M. M., Cooke, E. A. et al. 2010. Effects of a low-glycemic load diet in overweight and obese pregnant women: A pilot randomized controlled trial, *Am J Clin Nutr*, 92:1306–1315.

Shikany, J. M., Flood, A. P., Kitahara, C. M., Hsing, A. W., Mayer, T. E., Willcox, B. J. et al. 2011. Dietary carbohydrate, glycemic index, glycemic load, and risk of prostate cancer in the Prosate, Lung, Colorectal, and Ovarian Cancer Screening Trial (PLCO) cohort, *Cancer Causes Cont*, 22:995–1002.

Sievenpiper, J. L., Carleton, A. J., Chatha, S., Jiang, H. Y., de Souza, R. J., Beyene, J., Kendall, C. W., Jenkins, D. J. 2009. Heterogeneous effects of fructose on blood lipids in individuals with type 2 diabetes: Systematic review and meta-analysis of experimental trials in humans, *Diabetes Care*, 32:1930–1937.

Sievenpiper, J. L., de Souza, R. J., Mirrahimi, A., Yu, M. E., Carleton, A. J., Beyene, J., Chiavaroli, L. et al. 2012. Effect of fructose on body weight in controlled feeding trials: A systematic review and meta-analysis, *Ann Intern Med*, 156:291–304.

Slavin, J. 2010. Basic qualities of carbohydrates and GI/GL concept. In *Experimental Biology 2010*. Anaheim, CA.

Wolever, T. M. 1997. The glycemic index: Flogging a dead horse?, *Diabetes Care*, 20:452–456.

Wolever, T. M. 2013. Is glycaemic index (GI) a valid measure of carbohydrate quality?, *Eur J Clin Nutr*, 67:522–531.

Wolever, T. M., Brand-Miller, J. C., Abernethy, J., Astrup, A., Atkinson, F., Axelsen, M., Bjorck, I. et al. 2008. Measuring the glycemic index of foods: Interlaboratory study, *Am J Clin Nutr*, 87:247S-257S.

Wolever, T. M., Ip, B., Moghaddam, E. 2006. Measuring glycaemic responses: Duplicate fasting samples or duplicate measures of one fasting sample?, *Br J Nutr*, 96:799–802.

Wolever, T. M., Jenkins, D. J., Thompson, L. U., Wong, G. S. Josse, R. G. 1987. Effect of canning on the blood glucose response to beans in patients with type 2 diabetes, *Hum Nutr Clin Nutr*, 41:135–140.

Wolever, T. M., Vorster, H. H., Bjorck, I., Brand-Miller, J., Brighenti, F., Mann, J. I., Ramdath, D. D. et al. 2003. Determination of the glycaemic index of foods: interlaboratory study, *Eur J Clin Nutr*, 57:475–482.

Wolever, T. M. S., Jenkins, D. J. A. 1992. Effect of dietary fiber and foods on carbohydrate metabolism. In Spiller GA (ed.), *CRC Handbook of Dietary Fiber in Human Nutrition, 2nd edn.* CRC Press: Boca Raton, FL.

3 Measuring the Glycemic Index of Foods

Fiona S. Atkinson, Kai Lin Ek, and Jennie C. Brand-Miller

CONTENTS

3.1 INTRODUCTION

Historically, carbohydrates were classified only on the basis of their chemical structure into two categories: complex carbohydrates and simple sugars. Complex carbohydrates, such as those in bread and potatoes, were believed to be digested and absorbed slowly in the body, resulting in a gradual rise in postprandial blood glucose concentration. Conversely, simple sugars, such as table sugar and those in fruit, were thought to cause a rapid rise in glycemic response.

In the early 1980s, a new classification system for carbohydrates based on their physiological effects in the body was proposed first by Otto and Niklas (1980) and then by Jenkins et al. (1981). Jenkins and colleagues were responsible for the first comprehensive ranking of different carbohydrate-containing foods according to their glycemic responses, measured by the glycemic index (GI) (Jenkins et al. 1981). Their GI classification was designed to compare the relative effect of foods and beverages containing physiologically relevant amounts of carbohydrate on postprandial glycemia. The aim was to assist in the prevention and treatment of diabetes and other chronic diseases. Low-GI foods are classified as those that either are more slowly digested and absorbed or contain sugars (e.g., fructose and lactose) that inherently have a smaller impact on glycemia, resulting in a lower glycemic response. In contrast, high-GI foods produce a more rapid rise in glycemia and larger overall blood glucose response. Figure 3.1 depicts sample blood glucose response curves for a low- and a high-GI food.

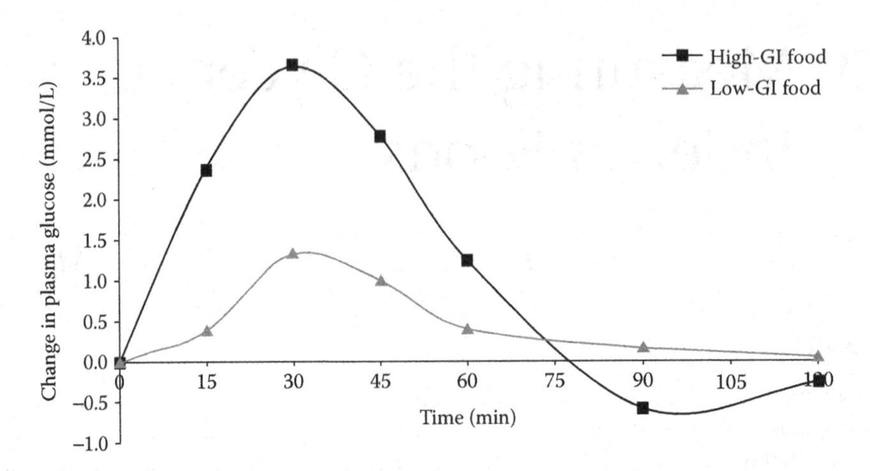

FIGURE 3.1 Sample blood glucose response curves for a low- and high-glycemic-index food.

The accuracy and reliability of GI values determined around the world are clearly important factors for the use of GI as a nutritional tool to guide food choices and their integration into dietary guidelines. The reproducibility of the methodology used for determining GI has been the subject of debate (Pi-Sunyer 2002, Monro 2003), and a need to standardize the measurement of GI values has been acknowledged. Some of the key concerns relate to the determination of "available" carbohydrate and the variability and reproducibility of results. Researchers have endeavored to address these concerns through studies to investigate the sources of variability in GI measurements between testing groups around the world (Wolever et al. 2003, 2008). In 2010, the International Organization for Standardization (ISO) published a GI testing methodology designed to provide a recognized and standardized procedure for measuring the GI values of food and beverages. This chapter explains and discusses the ISO methodology to determine the GI of foods and beverages, as well as factors that influence the GI.

3.2 CLASSIFICATION OF GLYCEMIC INDEX

In practice, carbohydrate-containing foods and beverages may be classified into low-, medium- and high-GI categories. Low-GI foods are those that have a GI value of 55 or less, medium-GI foods have a GI value between 56 and 69, and high-GI foods have a GI value of 70 or more (Atkinson et al. 2008). These GI categories apply only to individual foods or beverages and not to mixed meals or diets, in which case the range is smaller. Based on population data, Barclay et al. (2008) proposed that a low-GI meal or diet should have a GI value of 45 or less, whereas a high-GI meal or diet should have a GI value of 58 or more.

To avoid confusion, the GI value of a food should be reported on the glucose scale, whereby a glucose solution is the reference food (i.e., the GI value of glucose solution = 100). However, it is acceptable to use alternative foods as the reference, such as white bread or white rice, provided the GI value of that reference food is known, relative to glucose. A summary of the GI values of some common carbohydrate foods is listed in Table 3.1. Only foods that contain appreciable amounts of available carbohydrate (causing a rise in blood glucose) have a GI value. Therefore, protein- or fat-based foods, which contain no or little carbohydrate, such as meat, eggs, and oils, cannot be tested for GI. Similarly, many vegetables such as onion, broccoli, zucchini, and spinach contain low amounts of available carbohydrate and as such do not have GI values. In research studies, these types of foods are often coded as having a GI value of 0.

TABLE 3.1
Glycemic Index Values of Common Carbohydrate Foods

High-Carbohydrate Foods	GI	Breakfast Cereals	GI	Fruit and Fruit Products	GI
White wheat bread	75	Cornflakes	81	Apple	36
Wholemeal bread	74	Wheat flake biscuits	69	Orange	43
Specialty grain bread	53	Porridge, rolled oats	55	Banana	51
Unleavened wheat bread	70	Instant oat porridge	79	Pineapple	59
Wheat roti	62	Rice porridge	78	Watermelon	76
Chapatti	52	Muesli	57	Dates	42
Corn tortilla	46			Peaches, canned	43
White rice, boiled	73	**Vegetables**		Strawberry jam and/or jelly	49
Brown rice, boiled	68	Potato, boiled	78	Apple juice	41
Barley	28	Potato, instant mash	87	Orange juice	50
Sweet corn	52	Potato, french fries	63		
Spaghetti, white	49	Carrots, boiled	39	**Sugars**	
Spaghetti, wholemeal	48	Sweet potato, boiled	63	Fructose	15
Rice noodles	53	Pumpkin, boiled	64	Sucrose	65
Couscous	65			Glucose	103
		Legumes		Honey	61
Dairy Products and Alternatives		Chickpeas	28		
Milk, full fat	39	Kidney beans	24	**Snack Products**	
Ice cream	51	Lentils	32	Chocolate	40
Yoghurt, fruit	41	Soybeans	16	Potato chips/crisps	56
Soy milk	34			Soft drink/soda	59
Rice milk	86			Rice crackers/crisps	87

Source: Adapted from Atkinson et al. 2008, *Diabetes Care,* 31(12):2281–2283.
Note: Data are average results from the available values listed in the International Tables of GI and GL.

3.3 TESTING METHODOLOGY

The GI classifies carbohydrates on the basis of their physiological effects in the body. It compares the blood glucose responses elicited by a fixed amount of available carbohydrate from a test food with an equivalent available carbohydrate portion of a reference food. By definition, the GI value of a food or beverage must be measured in human volunteers and not by an *in vitro* assay; however, the rate of carbohydrate digestion or hydrolysis index can be assessed using *in vitro* methods (Englyst et al. 1996, 2003). Significant correlations are observed between *in vitro* starch hydrolysis assays and *in vivo* GI testing (Englyst et al. 1996). However, the results of *in vitro* studies should not be described as GI values (ISO 2010).

It is possible to mathematically estimate the GI value of a food on the basis of the component ingredients and nutritional information. However, the calculation does not adjust for potential *in vivo* interactions between ingredients or adequately correct for food factors that are known to lower glycemic responses (e.g., fat, protein, and soluble fiber). Theoretical calculations may be beneficial during product development but are not permitted by the ISO standard (ISO 2010) or government food-labeling authorities (e.g., Food Standards Australia New Zealand) for making GI claims. Important aspects of the GI testing methodology are summarized in the following sections. Readers are also directed to a thorough review of the scientific rationale for the GI methodology by Brouns and colleagues (Brouns et al. 2005).

3.3.1 Available Carbohydrate

Glycemic index testing is conducted by comparing the relative glucose responses of equal available carbohydrate portions of test foods with a reference food. Therefore, it is important to consider the determination of "available" carbohydrate. The ISO standard recommends the determination of available carbohydrate via direct measurement (ISO 2010). However, in practice, it can be difficult to accurately measure "available" carbohydrate. Carbohydrate by difference (100 – the percentage sum of moisture, protein, fat, fiber, and ash) is acceptable for the calculation of available carbohydrate, as this is the value often reported on food labels in many countries (ISO 2010). In some instances, total carbohydrate and fiber are shown on the food label, and fiber can be subtracted from the total to yield a measure of "available" carbohydrate. This method may not truly reflect the carbohydrate that is available for digestion and absorption *in vivo,* as some indigestible carbohydrates are not detected as fiber by using Association of Analytical Communities methods, and resistant starch assays can be problematic. However, most common foods contain minimal levels of resistant starch (<5%) or indigestible carbohydrates.

3.3.2 Reference Foods

Repeat testing of the reference food is an important part of determining a GI value, as it controls for variations in glucose tolerance from person to person, as well as from day to day. Glycemic responses to the same food can vary by more than 60% among healthy subjects; however, the GI value (the glycemic response of the test food relative to the reference food) is much less variable (Wolever et al. 1990). The day-to-day glycemic response to the same food in the same subject also varies, but a coefficient of variation (CV) of less than 25% is achievable for repeated food responses in the same individual. The CV is calculated by comparing the variability in glycemic response (determined by standard deviation) divided by the average glycemic response for a given individual (expressed as a percentage). The ISO standard stipulates that the "average" intraindividual CV (the day-to-day CV) for the group of subjects used in a given study should be 30% or less (ISO 2010).

A variety of reference foods have been utilized for GI testing studies (e.g., glucose, white bread, white rice, and other types of starchy foods, including traditional breads and potatoes) (Granfeldt et al. 1995a, Sugiyama et al. 2003, Ramdath et al. 2004, Atkinson et al. 2008). The most commonly used reference foods are a glucose solution and white bread, which are also generally recommended as the most appropriate (Brouns et al. 2005, ISO 2010), as they are relatively consistent products (in terms of both composition and GI) around the world (Atkinson et al. 2008). Some laboratories prefer white bread as the reference food over glucose solution, as white bread is more representative of a typical carbohydrate source.

It is acceptable to use alternative reference foods for GI studies, provided that the GI value for the alternative reference food is known and consistent, relative to glucose. The use of a starchy reference food, such as white bread, may be preferable when determining the GI values of starch-based foods to reduce between-subject variation (Venn et al. 2014). This is because the rate of starch digestion (but not glucose absorption) varies as a function of genetic variation in the salivary amylase gene (*AMY1*) copy number (Atkinson et al. 2014). Copy number variation results in individuals having a different number of copies of a gene present in their genome (in the case of the *AMY1* gene, humans have a range of between 2 and 16 copies [Perry et al. 2007]). Individuals with higher copy number of the *AMY1* gene digest starch more quickly than those with a lower copy number. Similarly, some studies have used sucrose as a reference food when determining the GI values of sweeteners that are used as sucrose substitutes in food manufacturing (Pelletier et al. 1994). Regardless of the reference food used, the final GI value should be reported relative to the glucose scale (glucose = 100). If results have been adjusted relative to the glucose scale, the conversion factor used for the alternative reference food should be stated (Brouns et al. 2005). For example, in our group of testers, white bread has a GI value of 70 when glucose is the reference food. If white bread has been used as the reference food, then the average GI value should be multiplied by 70/100 (or 0.7) for reporting purposes.

The reference food is used to account for the natural variation in glucose tolerance and metabolism between individuals. The reference food should be tested ideally three times in each subject on separate occasions within a 3-month period. Reference food tests for a given subject can be used in a subsequent study, provided the subject has not significantly altered his or her lifestyle habits (e.g., diet, exercise, and medication usage) and the subsequent GI study is conducted within 3 months (Brouns et al. 2005). The repeated testing of the reference food improves the precision of GI measurement (Wolever et al. 1991a, 2003) and provides a good estimation of the day-to-day variability in glucose tolerance in a subject. Within a study of several foods, it is best to conduct the three reference food sessions as the first, middle, and last tests, with the test foods randomized in between. Wolever and colleagues observed a statistically significant reduction in variability of mean GI with the use of at least two repeated reference food measurements, compared with the reference food that was measured on only one occasion (Wolever et al. 2003). The CV (the standard deviation divided by the mean, expressed as a percentage) for the repeated reference food sessions should be 30% or less for the subject group (ISO 2010).

3.3.3 Test Foods

Only foods that contain appreciable amounts of digestible carbohydrate are suitable for GI testing. The ISO method specifies that foods or beverages should contain a minimum of 10 g of available carbohydrate per serve (ISO 2010). As mentioned previously, available carbohydrate is defined as the carbohydrate that is accessible to be digested and absorbed by the body. Therefore, low-digestible carbohydrates, such as resistant starch, dietary fiber, and some sugar alcohols, should not be included in the determination of available carbohydrate. Certain sugar alcohols are partially absorbed (e.g., maltitol). In that instance, a percentage corresponding to the absorbable fraction of the sugar alcohol (e.g., 40% of maltitol is absorbed) (Livesey 2003) can be included in the determination of available carbohydrate. For example, if a product contains 7 g of maltitol/100 g, then 2.8 g of maltitol/100 g can be included as available carbohydrate for the calculation of the test portion.

Typically, foods are tested at a portion containing 50 g of digestible carbohydrate. This carbohydrate amount represents a large metabolic challenge. Increasing the amount of available carbohydrate produces a relatively linear dose–response increase in glucose response up to 50 g of available carbohydrate (Wolever and Bolognesi 1996b, Lee and Wolever 1998). The dose–response relationship begins to plateau at carbohydrate doses greater than 50 g, which means that additional carbohydrate does not produce a substantial increase in glucose incremental area under the curve (iAUC) (Jenkins et al. 1981).

Some carbohydrate foods, such as fruit, roots, and tubers, have a high water content, and therefore high volume relative to the amount of carbohydrate. It is acceptable to test such foods in portions containing 25 g of digestible carbohydrate. Reducing the carbohydrate dosage to 25 g helps minimize unrealistically large test portions for lower carbohydrate foods. It is not recommended to test products at amounts that contain less than 25 g of available carbohydrate because of the smaller fluctuations in glucose response elicited by lower carbohydrate doses.

The amount of available carbohydrate in the test food portion should be equivalent to the amount of available carbohydrate in the reference food. The test food or reference food portion should be completely consumed within 12 min. Typically, a standardized glass of 250 mL of water is served with all test foods and with the reference food (regardless of which reference food is used). The ISO method permits 250–500 mL of water, tea, or coffee to be consumed with the test food or reference food (ISO 2010). Nonnutritive sweetener and a small volume of milk (30 mL) may be added to the tea or coffee. Caffeine can acutely decrease insulin sensitivity (Graham et al. 2001), so it is preferable to use only plain water. The amount and type of fluid consumed with the reference or test foods should be standardized for all tests performed by a given subject.

Foods and beverages should be prepared for GI testing in the physical state in which they are normally consumed. For example, a rice or pasta product should be cooked according to the instructions on the food packet. In these instances, the 50 g carbohydrate portion should be weighed in the dry state and then that test portion should be cooked. Breakfast cereals should be consumed dry or with water instead of milk, because milk reduces glycemia. Similarly, powdered beverages should be prepared with water instead of milk, as the addition of milk proteins lowers the glycemic response (Petersen et al. 2009, Gunnerud et al. 2013). Added flavorings or other ingredients, such as salt, vinegar, butter, and herbs and spices, should be avoided, as these additional ingredients may influence the rate of gastric emptying and carbohydrate digestion.

Glucemic index testing should be conducted on individual foods rather than mixed meals. This is because mixed meals contain varying amounts of protein (Nuttall et al. 1984), fat (Collier and O'Dea 1983), soluble fiber (Wolever et al. 1991b), and other nutrients, which slow down carbohydrate digestion and absorption to varying degrees. As a result, mixed meals typically produce lower GI values than individual carbohydrate foods when tested against glucose or white bread (Atkinson et al. 2008). The relative glycemic-lowering effect of these nutrients can be different in individuals with differing glucose tolerance. However, it will never be possible to test every version of every mixed meal. For this reason, the GI values of mixed meals should be calculated mathematically by using the weighted average GI values for each of the component single ingredients. The weighting of each food is proportional to its contribution to the total available carbohydrate content. An example of GI calculation of a mixed meal is shown in Table 3.2. The GI value of whole diets can be estimated in the same way. Although this approach does not adjust for the potential influence of fat or protein on slowing the digestion of the carbohydrates, the calculated GI values of meals are consistent with the ranking of observed glycemic responses in experimental studies (Chew et al. 1988, Wolever and Bolognesi 1996a, Wolever et al. 2006).

3.3.4 Testing Subjects

Glycemic index is a property of carbohydrates in a given food and not of the subjects in which it is measured. Glycemic index values have been measured and reported in a range of subjects with differing levels of glucose tolerance (normal, type 1 diabetes, type 2 diabetes, gestational diabetes, etc.) (Atkinson et al. 2008). Within-subject variation (day-to-day variability) differs depending on the type of subjects included in a study. Individuals with type 2 diabetes or impaired glucose tolerance typically have lower within-subject variation than those with normal glucose tolerance (Wolever et al. 1998a, 1998b).

Numerous studies have shown that characteristics of the subject do not significantly influence the ranking of GI values among a group of foods: healthy versus diabetic individuals (Alkaabi et al. 2011), type 1 versus type 2 diabetes (Jenkins et al. 1986, Wolever et al. 1987), subjects with different ethnicities

TABLE 3.2
Sample Calculation of the Glycemic Index of a Mixed Meal

Meal	Serve (g)	Carbohydrate (g)	Carbohydrate Contribution (%)	GI	Meal GI[a]
Cornflakes	35	28	70	81	57
Milk	125	6	15	39	6
Strawberries	80	6	15	40	6
Meal total	210	40	100	–	69

Note: GI = glycemic index.
[a] Calculated as percentage carbohydrate contribution × GI (i.e., 0.7 × 81 = 57).

(Wolever et al. 2008), children versus adults (Wolever et al. 1988a), males versus females (Wolever et al. 2003), or subjects with differing body mass indexes (Wolever et al. 2008). Some variation in GI values measured in different groups has been observed, but the overall GI category is usually similar between subject groups. Some studies have reported important differences in the GI values of foods measured in different ethnic groups (Venn et al. 2010, Kataoka et al. 2013). However, this difference disappears if a starchy food such as white bread or rice is used as the reference food. Whatever the reference food, the final GI value should be expressed on the glucose scale to avoid confusion.

The ISO methodology stipulates the use of a minimum of ten healthy subjects with normal glucose tolerance (ISO 2010). In addition, subjects should not have any known food allergies and should not take any medications known to influence glucose tolerance or metabolism. There is no evidence that age affects GI testing, but typically healthy adults aged 18–65 years are recruited as testing subjects. Pregnancy increases insulin resistance and may precipitate gestational diabetes in predisposed individuals. Therefore, pregnant and lactating women are usually excluded from participating in GI testing. The precision and power to detect differences in GI values between foods are increased as the number of subjects used to determine the GI value is increased. Greater variability in GI is inherent for foods that have higher mean GI values, regardless of the number of subjects included in the study. Foods with GI values less than 55 usually show surprisingly low standard errors around the mean.

3.4 EXPERIMENTAL PROCEDURE

All GI testing studies must be approved by an appropriate human research ethics committee or institutional review board and abide by standards for the ethical conduct of research in humans.

3.4.1 Subject Preparation

Intuitively, strict control of subjects' eating and exercise habits on the day before a test session would be expected to minimize GI variability between subjects. However, studies do not support the strict standardization of these factors to reduce variability and improve reproducibility of results (Campbell et al. 2003, Wolever et al. 2003). In contrast, strict control of the evening meal, physical activity, and length of fast actually increased within-subject CV of glucose iAUC responses (Campbell et al. 2003).

All GI test sessions are conducted in the morning, after a 10–14 h overnight fast. Larger relative differences between postprandial responses to foods are observed in the morning compared with other times of day. In addition, morning testing helps minimize any intraindividual differences in food consumption or exercise habits before a test session (Brouns et al. 2005).

Providing a standardized evening meal does not appear to reduce intra- or interindividual variation (Campbell et al. 2003). Therefore, subjects are recommended to consume a high-carbohydrate evening meal before a test session, but the composition is not strictly specified. Moderate alcohol consumption the night before a test session is permitted. However, legumes (e.g., lentils, beans, and chickpeas) should not be consumed in the evening meal. Legumes are known to produce "second-meal" effects, such that they lower the postprandial glucose response at the next meal (Jenkins et al. 1982, Wolever et al. 1988b).

Acute physical activity is known to increase glucose tolerance by improving muscle glucose uptake, as well as increase insulin sensitivity for up to 2 days (Mikines et al. 1988). In the context of GI measurement, there is some evidence to show a trend of reductions in blood glucose concentrations during the 2 h test session after vigorous exercise (Campbell et al. 2003). Therefore, subjects are recommended to avoid any unusual, vigorous physical activity on the day before and to avoid exercise on the morning of a test session.

Randomization is used in clinical trials to remove treatment bias effects. Randomization of food presentation is not necessary for GI testing but can help reduce any potential order effects or seasonal variation in glucose tolerance. In most cases, the foods consumed as part of a GI study are commercial products that are unlikely to produce any carry-over effect on subsequent tests. A washout period of 1 day is likely to be sufficient between subsequent sessions to avoid any carry-over or "second-meal" effects (although experimental studies to support this have not been conducted). Researchers should consider that subjects who are not familiar with the testing procedures may feel anxious or stressed, until they are comfortable with the methodology (Brouns et al. 2005). Anxiety may influence postprandial glycemia via sympathetic and parasympathetic activations of hormones known to influence gastric emptying (e.g., cholecystokinin) and carbohydrate digestion (e.g., salivary α-amylase). Therefore, it would be advisable to repeat the reference food session at least twice (to assess a subject's usual day-to-day variability) before commencing the testing of foods. In practice, a subject's glucose iAUC is often unusual on his or her first test session, in which case the average of the second and third tests may have a lower CV than the average of the three tests. To minimize the potential effects of seasonal variation on glycemic responses, the number of foods included in a study should be limited, such that the study duration is under 3 months. Menstrual status has little, if any, effect on glucose tolerance and can be ignored (Bonora et al. 1987). Subjects who are unwell on the day of testing (e.g., respiratory infection) should be excluded.

3.4.2 Blood Collection and Analysis

Capillary blood is the "gold standard" for GI testing, as it is more sensitive to the acute, rapid changes in blood glucose after the consumption of a food than venous blood (Brouns et al. 2005). In addition, GI values determined using capillary blood collected from the fingertip show lower variability between subjects than the blood obtained by venous sampling (Wolever et al. 2003). Capillary blood typically shows greater fluctuations in postprandial glycemia, resulting in larger relative differences in glucose responses between foods (Granfeldt et al. 1995b). This is because the glucose is delivered to the tissues in the arterial and capillary system and reaches the venous system only after the tissues have absorbed the glucose they require.

Although capillary blood is preferable for GI testing, venous blood is also accepted in the ISO method (ISO 2010). There are differences in absolute glucose concentration measured in capillary versus venous blood (Granfeldt et al. 1995b). However, the GI value of the food is not affected if the blood sample type is consistent across all test sessions. This is because the relative difference in iAUC values between the two sampling forms is consistent for the reference food and test foods.

Blood samples are collected at regular intervals over 2 h for GI testing conducted in individuals with normal glucose tolerance. Two fasting samples are collected within 5 min and averaged to calculate the baseline glucose concentration. It is important to accurately determine the fasting, baseline glucose concentration for the iAUC calculations used to determine the GI value of a food. Additional blood samples are collected at 15, 30, 45, 60, 90, and 120 min after eating has commenced. Measurement over 3 h is preferable if testing is conducted in subjects with impaired glucose tolerance or diabetes, as the blood glucose response usually takes longer to return to baseline levels in these subject groups.

Glucose concentration can be measured in either whole blood or plasma. The choice of blood form should remain consistent across all tests. Testing laboratories often assay glucose concentration in duplicate in each blood sample, but it is not strictly required under the ISO method (ISO 2010). Data from the second interlaboratory study suggested that the measurement of two fasting blood samples and duplicate measurement at other time points tended to produce lower within-subject variability and lower group standard deviations for GI values (Wolever et al. 2008). Spectrophotometric or enzymatic assays are used to determine glucose concentration. Assay type was not found to have a significant effect on either the mean GI or the variability of GI in the first interlaboratory study (Wolever et al. 2003). The interassay CV for the assay method must be less than 3.6% (ISO 2010). Small glucometers are not suitable for GI testing because of their wider analytical measurement variation (Velangi et al. 2005).

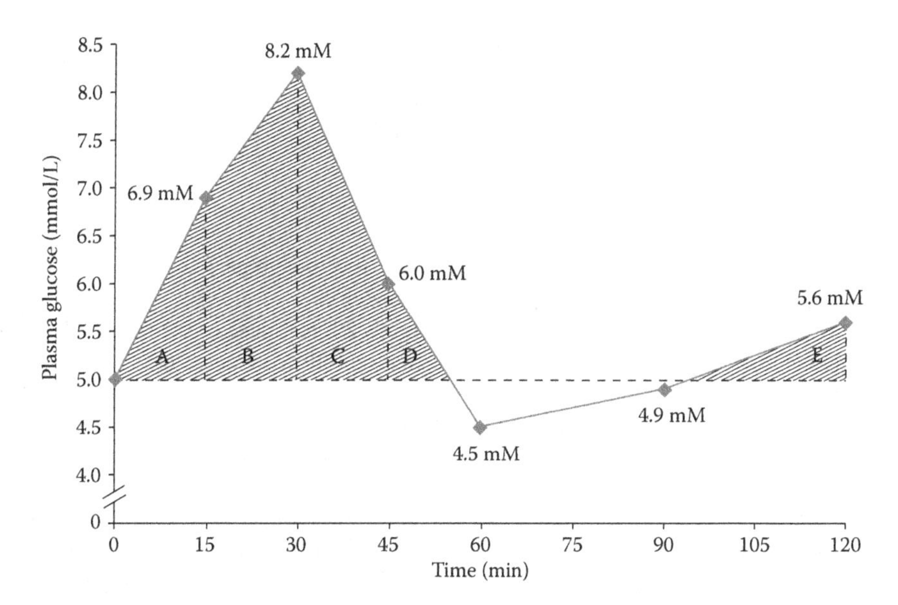

FIGURE 3.2 Representation of incremental area under the curve (iAUC). Only shaded areas above the baseline concentration (shown as a dotted line at SmM) are included in the iAUC calculation.

The iAUC is mathematically calculated from the blood glucose concentrations at each time point by using the trapezoid rule, and any negative area below the baseline (i.e. fasting) concentration is ignored (Food and Agriculture Organization of the United Nations 1998, ISO 2010). The iAUC describes the total increase in blood glucose during the 2 h test session in a subject, as a result of ingesting that particular test food (Figure 3.2).

As shown in Figure 3.2, the iAUC refers only to the shaded areas above the baseline. The iAUC for the plasma glucose response curve is calculated as follows. The iAUC for the 2 h glucose response is the sum of the areas labeled A, B, C, D, and E in Figure 3.2; these areas are made up of triangles and trapezoids.

Area A (triangle): (15 min concentration (conc) – fasting conc [time 0]) × time (min)/2
= (6.9 – 5) × 15/2
= 14.3 mmol/L.min

Area B (trapezoid): (15 min conc – 0 conc + 30 min conc – 0 conc) × time (min)/2
= (6.9 – 5 + 8.2 – 5) × 15/2
= 38.3 mmol/L.min

Area C (trapezoid): (30 min conc – 0 conc + 45 min conc – 0 conc) × time (min)/2
= (8.2 – 5 + 6 – 5) × 15/2
= 31.5 mmol/L.min

Area D (triangle): This triangle does not span between the two known time points (45 and 60 min); therefore, the usual time value of 15 min needs to be adjusted.
First, calculate the amount of time above baseline:
At 45 min, the concentration is 1 mmol/L above baseline
At 60 min, the concentration is 0.5 mmol/L below baseline
Therefore, the time can be expressed as t = 15 min × 1/(1 + 0.5) = 10
= (45 min conc – 0 conc) × 10/2
= (6 – 5) × 10/2
= 5.0 mmol/L.min

Area E (triangle): Similar to Area D, the time needs to be adjusted.

At 90 min, the concentration is 0.1 mmol/L below baseline

At 120 min, the concentration is 0.6 mmol/L above baseline

Therefore, the time can be expressed as $t = 30 \text{ min} \times 0.6/(0.1 + 0.6) = 25.7$

$= (120 \text{ min conc} - 0 \text{ conc}) \times 25.7/2$

$= (5.6 - 5) \times 25.7/2$

$= 7.7$ mmol/L.min

Therefore, the total iAUC for the blood glucose response over the 2 h period is the sum of the areas above baseline: 14.3 + 38.3 + 31.5 + 5.0 + 7.7 = 96.8 mM.min.

The GI value for a food is calculated for each subject's 2 h response to the test food divided by his or her average response for the reference food, using the following equation:

$$\text{GI} = \frac{\text{Plasma glucose iAUC value for test food}}{\text{Average iAUC value for the equal-carbohydrate portion of the reference food}} \times 100$$

The final GI value for a food or beverage is expressed as the average of the 10 subjects' individual GI values for that product. An individual GI value that falls two standard deviation (SD) outside the group mean GI is defined as an outlier and is removed from the final calculation. Glycemic index values are expressed to the nearest whole integer, with the standard error of the mean (SEM) reported (e.g. GI: 48 ± 5). Ideally, the SEM (a measure of precision) should be less than 10% of the mean GI value.

A sample dataset including the blood glucose responses for three reference foods and two test foods, in 10 healthy individuals, is shown in Table 3.3. In Table 3.3, subject 1 has a standard deviation of 32 for the three reference foods' iAUC results and an average glucose iAUC response of 232. That subject's CV for the repeated reference food sessions is 14% (= 32/232 × 100).

3.5 APPLICATION AND USE OF THE GLYCEMIC INDEX VALUE

The classification of foods and beverages on the basis of their physiological impact on blood glucose levels can assist in the prevention and management of a range of diseases (reviewed in this book) and assist consumers in making healthier food choices within a food category.

The GI has been used as a measure of carbohydrate "quality," comparing foods on a gram-for-gram basis of carbohydrate. The GI of a food does not change depending on the amount consumed. To account for difference in the quantity of carbohydrate in typical serving sizes, the glycemic load (GL) was proposed by Salmeron et al. (1997). The GL is defined as the mathematical product of GI and carbohydrate content ($\text{GL} = [\text{GI} \times g]/100$, where g is the weight of available carbohydrate consumed). Glycemic load therefore quantifies both carbohydrate quality and quantity, and its unit of measurement is gram. For example, if the GI value for a green apple is 40 and a standard serve of apple (one apple = 120 g) contains 16 g of available carbohydrate, then the GL of one apple is 6 g (GL = 40 × 16/100 = 6). The GL of a diet can be reduced by reducing either the GI of the component foods or the amount of carbohydrate consumed (although these two methods may produce different effects on health in the long term). The GL has been shown to predict the glycemic responses of individual foods and mixed meals (Bao et al. 2011).

The clinical utility of GI has been questioned, as foods are tested individually rather than in the context of mixed meals (Franz 1999, Pi-Sunyer 2002). The co-ingestion of fat, protein, fiber, and other nutrients or food factors (e.g., acidity) is known to influence the GI of a food. However, there is a good correlation between the calculated GI values for mixed meals and the observed postprandial responses (Bornet et al. 1987, Wolever et al. 2006). A mixed meal containing a higher-GI starchy carbohydrate will have a greater glycemic response than a similar meal containing a

TABLE 3.3
Sample Dataset for Three Reference Foods and Two Test Foods

Reference Food 1

Time (min)	1	2	3	4	5	6	7	8	9	10	Mean	SEM
0	5.3	5.0	5.3	5.2	5.3	5.1	5.2	5.3	5.2	5.3	5.2	0.0
15	7.0	7.5	6.9	7.8	8.2	7.9	6.5	6.5	6.8	9.0	7.4	0.3
30	10.2	9.4	8.3	10.8	7.8	9.1	9.7	8.8	8.5	8.8	9.1	0.3
45	10.7	8.4	8.1	10.3	6.1	7.9	7.1	8.5	7.5	8.2	8.3	0.4
60	9.0	6.5	7.5	8.1	5.8	7.2	6.2	7.3	6.1	7.5	7.1	0.3
90	5.1	5.9	6.5	5.5	5.2	6.6	6.1	5.0	4.4	5.6	5.6	0.2
120	4.1	4.8	5.4	4.3	5.4	6.0	5.6	5.2	3.9	4.1	4.9	0.2
iAUC	**260**	**213**	**198**	**270**	**104**	**250**	**171**	**160**	**122**	**206**	**195**	**18**

Reference Food 2

Time (min)	1	2	3	4	5	6	7	8	9	10	Mean	SEM
0	5.3	5.1	5.5	5.2	5.3	5.3	4.9	5.4	5.0	5.4	5.2	0.1
15	7.2	7.5	7.5	6.8	8.0	6.4	8.3	7.8	6.8	9.0	7.5	0.2
30	10.0	8.7	9.3	9.9	9.4	9.9	9.8	8.9	8.8	10.4	9.5	0.2
45	9.8	6.8	9.1	9.3	7.3	10.4	8.4	7.8	7.9	9.8	8.7	0.4
60	8.6	6.4	7.5	7.1	5.8	9.4	7.1	6.9	6.2	8.6	7.4	0.4
90	5.1	4.9	6.8	5.4	4.2	7.3	5.7	4.9	4.5	5.2	5.4	0.3
120	4.0	4.5	5.9	5.3	5.3	5.9	5.3	5.0	4.4	4.6	5.0	0.2
iAUC	**238**	**142**	**231**	**206**	**138**	**323**	**257**	**153**	**149**	**264**	**210**	**20**

Reference Food 3

Time (min)	1	2	3	4	5	6	7	8	9	10	Mean	SEM
0	5.2	5.0	5.2	5.4	5.1	5.2	5.1	4.9	4.9	5.5	5.2	0.1
15	6.9	8.4	6.4	8.2	8.1	8.5	8.6	8.4	6.4	8.9	7.9	0.3
30	9.7	8.6	8.6	10.4	9.2	9.7	8.7	7.3	8.6	10.2	9.1	0.3
45	9.3	6.7	7.8	9.1	6.3	8.8	7.3	7.2	7.5	9.4	7.9	0.4
60	7.4	6.6	7.0	7.9	5.5	7.4	6.7	6.3	6.0	8.0	6.9	0.3
90	4.6	5.5	5.9	4.3	5.6	6.8	5.4	6.1	4.5	4.1	5.3	0.3
120	3.7	4.2	5.5	4.1	5.9	5.8	4.4	5.0	4.4	4.0	4.7	0.3
iAUC	**197**	**177**	**174**	**217**	**161**	**278**	**181**	**192**	**137**	**223**	**194**	**12**

Summary of the Three Reference Food Sessions and Within-Subject Coefficient of Variation

	1	2	3	4	5	6	7	8	9	10
iAUCRef1	260	213	198	270	104	250	171	160	122	206
iAUCRef2	238	142	231	206	138	323	257	153	149	264
iAUCRef3	197	177	174	217	161	278	181	192	137	223
SD	32	36	29	34	29	37	47	21	14	30
Average iAUC	232	177	201	231	134	284	203	168	136	231
CV (%)	14	20	14	15	21	13	23	13	10	13

(Continued)

TABLE 3.3 (*Continued*)
Sample Dataset for Three Reference Foods and Two Test Foods

					Test Food 1							
Time (min)	1	2	3	4	5	6	7	8	9	10	Mean	SEM
0	5.2	5.0	5.3	5.2	5.2	5.3	5.0	5.2	5.0	5.3	**5.2**	**0.0**
15	5.5	5.5	6.1	7.0	6.0	5.6	7.5	6.2	5.2	5.6	**6.0**	**0.2**
30	7.6	7.6	6.9	8.1	7.6	6.6	7.9	6.3	6.8	7.3	**7.3**	**0.2**
45	8.5	7.1	6.0	7.1	5.0	6.3	6.6	5.9	7.5	8.6	**6.9**	**0.4**
60	7.4	6.2	5.9	6.2	5.2	6.0	5.9	6.0	6.2	7.4	**6.2**	**0.2**
90	5.5	5.3	5.0	4.7	5.4	6.2	5.1	5.0	4.4	5.4	**5.2**	**0.2**
120	4.3	5.0	5.5	4.4	5.8	6.0	4.8	5.0	4.5	5.1	**5.0**	**0.2**
iAUC	145	114	58	117	62	92	127	58	89	133	**99**	**10**
GI	**63**	**64**	**29**	**50**	**46**	**33**	**63**	**34**	**65**	**58**	**50**	**4**

					Test Food 2							
Time (min)	1	2	3	4	5	6	7	8	9	10	Mean	SEM
0	5.2	5.2	5.3	5.2	5.5	5.1	5.4	5.2	4.8	5.2	**5.2**	**0.1**
15	5.5	5.8	7.2	7.6	6.1	5.8	7.7	5.4	5.4	5.7	**6.2**	**0.3**
30	7.4	8.8	9.9	9.5	8.3	7.4	9.3	6.8	7.7	7.4	**8.3**	**0.3**
45	9.1	7.8	8.5	8.3	5.9	7.7	7.4	7.4	7.4	8.8	**7.8**	**0.3**
60	7.7	6.7	6.1	7.5	5.8	6.6	6.1	6.0	6.6	8.0	**6.7**	**0.2**
90	6.6	6.1	4.7	6.5	5.5	5.8	5.4	5.1	4.9	5.9	**5.7**	**0.2**
120	5.8	5.2	4.4	5.8	5.8	6.5	4.9	4.7	5.2	4.3	**5.3**	**0.2**
iAUC	203	163	158	247	68	160	139	77	141	173	**153**	**17**
GI	**88**	**92**	**79**	**107**	**51**	**56**	**68**	**46**	**104**	**75**	**76**	**7**

Note: GI, glycemic index; iAUC, incremental area under the curve; SEM, standard error of the mean.
The within-subject variation (coefficient of variation) for the repeated reference food sessions is calculated for each subject.

lower-GI carbohydrate, so the relative hierarchy of individual foods is maintained in the context of a meal. In addition, the glycemic response of a mixed meal can be reliably predicted from the GI values of the component foods (Chew et al. 1988, Wolever et al. 2006).

3.6 FOOD FACTORS THAT INFLUENCE GLYCEMIC INDEX

Physical and chemical properties, along with processing methods, influence the rate of gastric motility and carbohydrate digestion and absorption. Factors that are known to influence the GI include the nature of the starch present (Hoebler et al. 1999), particle size (Granfeldt et al. 1994), presence of other macronutrients (fat, protein, or soluble fiber) (Collier and O'Dea 1983, Nuttall et al. 1984, Wolever et al. 1991b), food form and texture (Haber et al. 1977), acidity (Ostman et al. 2005), and cooking and processing methods (Liljeberg et al. 1992a) (Table 3.4). Therefore, modifications to the ingredients and product formulation or the processing methods used to manufacture the food may warrant retesting of the food. In practice, flavoring components do not significantly alter GI values (e.g., different varieties of fruit yoghurt), but differences in fat, protein, carbohydrate, and fiber content of greater than 1% (1 g/100 g) suggest the need for separate or additional testing. The ISO standard permits "pair-testing" of close flavor variants, which means that five individuals test one flavor and five individuals test the other flavor, and the results are combined to give one GI value in 10 subjects for both flavors (ISO 2010).

TABLE 3.4
Food Factors That Influence the Glycemic Index of Foods

Factor	Effect on Glycemic Index
Degree of starch gelatinization[a]	Lower extent of gelatinization, slower starch digestion (Ross et al. 1987).
Amylose-to-amylopectin ratio[b]	Higher amylose content produces slower starch digestion (Hoebler et al. 1999).
Physical barrier	Presence of bran layer and/or intact grains results in slower starch digestion (Liljeberg et al. 1992b).
Particle size	Larger particle size or smaller surface-area-to-volume ratio results in slower starch digestion (Granfeldt et al. 1994).
Macronutrient–starch interaction in food matrix	The addition of fat or protein to a carbohydrate food slows gastric emptying and reduces enzymatic starch digestion (Collier and O'Dea 1983; Nuttall et al. 1984).
Fiber and viscosity	Viscous, soluble fiber reduces starch digestion by increasing viscosity of luminal contents. This slows enzymic action and access to absorptive surface (Wolever et al. 1991b).
Acidity/pH	Lower pH of food bolus leads to slower gastric emptying and slower starch digestion (Ostman et al. 2005).
Antinutrients/enzyme inhibitors	The presence of phytate or tannins can slow the rate of starch digestion (Yoon et al. 1983; Barrett et al. 2013).
Osmolarity and meal dilution	More concentrated carbohydrate solutions tend to show lower postprandial responses (Sievenpiper et al. 1998).

[a] Gelatinization refers to the swelling of starch granules in the presence of heat and water. This occurs to different extents, depending on the food in question. For example, the degree of starch gelatinization is lower in steel-cut porridge oats than in instant oats.

[b] Starch consists of two polymers of D-glucose joined together by glycosidic bonds: amylose is an essentially linear polysaccharide and amylopectin is a highly branched polysaccharide (see Chapter 1, Figures 1.1 and 1.2 for the structures of amylose and amylopectin). In general, starches with high amylose content are considered to be more resistant to enzymatic digestion and gelatinization during cooking, whereas high-amylopectin starches are more susceptible to digestion and heat. The proportions (ratio) of amylose and amylopectin vary from food to food.

3.7 CONCLUSION AND PERSPECTIVES

Standardization of the GI methodology is important to ensure the reliability and accuracy of published GI values and the consistency and reproducibility between laboratories around the world. Standardization is also central to ensuring the utility of GI as a tool for distinguishing the relative effects of different carbohydrates on human health. The GI of foods and beverages is only one aspect of a healthy diet, and eating plans should not be solely based on the GI. Other food characteristics, such as energy and micronutrient density or saturated fat and sodium content, should also be considered when making food choices.

REFERENCES

Alkaabi, J. M., B. Al-Dabbagh, S. Ahmad, H. F. Saadi, S. Gariballa, and M. A. Ghazali. 2011. Glycemic indices of five varieties of dates in healthy and diabetic subjects. *Nutrition Journal,* 10:59–59.

Atkinson, F. S., K. Foster-Powell, and J. C. Brand-Miller. 2008. International tables of glycemic index and glycemic load values: 2008. *Diabetes Care,* 31(12):2281–2283.

Atkinson, F. S., D. Hancock, P. Petocz, and J. C. Brand-Miller. 2014. Physiological significance of higher AMY1 gene copy number on postprandial responses to starchy foods in Caucasian adults. *Journal of Nutrition & Intermediary Metabolism,* 1:15.

Bao, J., F. Atkinson, P. Petocz, W. C. Willett, and J. C. Brand-Miller. 2011. Prediction of postprandial glycemia and insulinemia in lean, young, healthy adults: Glycemic load compared with carbohydrate content alone. *American Journal of Clinical Nutrition,* 93(5):984–996.

Barclay, A. W., P. Petocz, J. McMillan-Price, V. M. Flood, T. Prvan, P. Mitchell, and J. C. Brand-Miller. 2008. Glycemic index, glycemic load, and chronic disease risk—a metaanalysis of observational studies. *American Journal of Clinical Nutrition,* 87(3):627–637.

Barrett, A., T. Ndou, C. A. Hughey, C. Straut, A. Howell, Z. Dai, and G. Kaletunc. 2013. Inhibition of alpha-amylase and glucoamylase by tannins extracted from cocoa, pomegranates, cranberries, and grapes. *Journal of Agricultural & Food Chemistry,* 61(7):1477–1486.

Bonora, E., I. Zavaroni, O. Alpi, A. Pezzarossa, E. Dall'Aglio, C. Coscelli, and U. Butturini. 1987. Influence of the menstrual cycle on glucose tolerance and insulin secretion. *American Journal of Obstetrics and Gynecology,* 157(1):140–141.

Bornet, F. R., D. Costagliola, S. W. Rizkalla, A. Blayo, A. M. Fontvieille, M. J. Haardt, M. Letanoux, G. Tchobroutsky, and G. Slama. 1987. Insulinemic and glycemic indexes of six starch-rich foods taken alone and in a mixed meal by type 2 diabetics. *American Journal of Clinical Nutrition,* 45(3):588–595.

Brouns, F., I. Bjorck, K. N. Frayn, A. L. Gibbs, V. Lang, G. Slama, and T. M. S. Wolever. 2005. Glycaemic index methodology. *Nutrition Research Reviews,* 18(1):145–171.

Campbell, J. E., T. Glowczewski, and T. M. S. Wolever. 2003. Controlling subjects' prior diet and activities does not reduce within-subject variation of postprandial glycemic responses to foods. *Nutrition Research,* 23(5):621–629.

Chew, I., J. C. Brand, A. W. Thorburn, and A. S. Truswell. 1988. Application of glycemic index to mixed meals. *American Journal of Clinical Nutrition,* 47(1):53–56.

Collier, G. and K. O'Dea. 1983. The effect of coingestion of fat on the glucose, insulin, and gastric inhibitory polypeptide responses to carbohydrate and protein. *American Journal of Clinical Nutrition,* 37(6):941–944.

Englyst, H. N., J. Veenstra, and G. J. Hudson. 1996. Measurement of rapidly available glucose (RAG) in plant foods: a potential in vitro predictor of the glycaemic response. *British Journal of Nutrition,* 75(3):327–337.

Englyst, K. N., S. Vinoy, H. N. Englyst, and V. Lang. 2003. Glycaemic index of cereal products explained by their content of rapidly and slowly available glucose. *British Journal of Nutrition,* 89(3):329–339.

Food and Agriculture Organization of the United Nations. 1998. *FAO Food and Nutrition Paper 66: Carbohydrates in Human Nutrition.* Rome, Italy: Food and Agriculture Organization of the United Nations.

Franz, M. J. 1999. In defense of the American Diabetes Association's recommendations on the glycemic index. *Nutrition Today,* 34:78–81.

Graham, T. E., P. Sathasivam, M. Rowland, N. Marko, F. Greer, and D. Battram. 2001. Caffeine ingestion elevates plasma insulin response in humans during an oral glucose tolerance test. *Canadian Journal of Physiology & Pharmacology,* 79(7):559–565.

Granfeldt, Y., A. Drews, and I. Bjorck. 1995a. Arepas made from high amylose corn flour produce favorably low glucose and insulin responses in healthy humans. *Journal of Nutrition,* 125(3):459–465.

Granfeldt, Y., B. Hagander, and I. Bjorck. 1995b. Metabolic responses to starch in oat and wheat products. On the importance of food structure, incomplete gelatinization or presence of viscous dietary fibre. *European Journal of Clinical Nutrition,* 49(3):189–199.

Granfeldt, Y., H. Liljeberg, A. Drews, R. Newman, and I. Bjorck. 1994. Glucose and insulin responses to barley products: influence of food structure and amylose-amylopectin ratio. *American Journal of Clinical Nutrition,* 59(5):1075–1082.

Gunnerud, U. J., E. M. Ostman, and I. M. Bjorck. 2013. Effects of whey proteins on glycaemia and insulinaemia to an oral glucose load in healthy: A dose-response study. *European Journal of Clinical Nutrition,* 67(7):749–753.

Haber, G. B., K. W. Heaton, D. Murphy, and L. F. Burroughs. 1977. Depletion and disruption of dietary fibre: Effects on satiety, plasma-glucose, and serum-insulin. *The Lancet,* 2(8040):679–682.

Hoebler, C., A. Karinthi, H. Chiron, M. Champ, and J. L. Barry. 1999. Bioavailability of starch in bread rich in amylose: Metabolic responses in healthy subjects and starch structure. *European Journal of Clinical Nutrition,* 53(5):360–366.

International Organization for Standardization. 2010. ISO/FDIS 26642:2010. Food Products - Determination of the glycemic index (GI) and recommendation for food classification.

Jenkins, D. J., T. M. Wolever, A. L. Jenkins, C. Giordano, S. Giudici, L. U. Thompson, J. Kalmusky, R. G. Josse, and G. S. Wong. 1986. Low glycemic response to traditionally processed wheat and rye products: Bulgur and pumpernickel bread. *American Journal of Clinical Nutrition,* 43(4):516–520.

Jenkins, D. J., T. M. Wolever, R. H. Taylor, H. Barker, H. Fielden, J. M. Baldwin, A. C. Bowling, H. C. Newman, A. L. Jenkins, and D. V. Goff. 1981. Glycemic index of foods: A physiological basis for carbohydrate exchange. *American Journal of Clinical Nutrition,* 34(3):362–366.

Jenkins, D. J., T. M. Wolever, R. H. Taylor, C. Griffiths, K. Krzeminska, J. A. Lawrie, C. M. Bennett, D. V. Goff, D. L. Sarson, and S. R. Bloom. 1982. Slow release dietary carbohydrate improves second meal tolerance. *American Journal of Clinical Nutrition,* 35(6):1339–1346.

Kataoka, M., B. J. Venn, S. M. Williams, L. A. Te Morenga, I. M. Heemels, and J. I. Mann. 2013. Glycaemic responses to glucose and rice in people of Chinese and European ethnicity. *Diabetic Medicine,* 30(3):e101–e107.

Lee, B. M. and T. M. Wolever. 1998. Effect of glucose, sucrose and fructose on plasma glucose and insulin responses in normal humans: Comparison with white bread. *European Journal of Clinical Nutrition,* 52(12):924–928.

Liljeberg, H., Y. Granfeldt, and I. Bjorck. 1992a. Metabolic responses to starch in bread containing intact kernels versus milled flour. *European Journal of Clinical Nutrition,* 46(8):561–575.

Liljeberg, H., Y. Granfeldt, and I. Bjorck. 1992b. Metabolic responses to starch in bread containing intact kernels versus milled flour. *European Journal of Clinical Nutrition,* 46(8):561–575.

Livesey, G. 2003. Health potential of polyols as sugar replacers, with emphasis on low glycaemic properties. *Nutrition Research Reviews,* 16(2):163–191.

Mikines, K. J., B. Sonne, P. A. Farrell, B. Tronier, and H. Galbo. 1988. Effect of physical exercise on sensitivity and responsiveness to insulin in humans. *American Journal of Physiology,* 254(3 Pt 1):E248–E259.

Monro, J. 2003. Redefining the glycemic index for dietary management of postprandial glycemia. *Journal of Nutrition,* 133(12):4256–4258.

Nuttall, F. Q., A. D. Mooradian, M. C. Gannon, C. Billington, and P. Krezowski. 1984. Effect of protein ingestion on the glucose and insulin response to a standardized oral glucose load. *Diabetes Care,* 7(5):465–470.

Ostman, E., Y. Granfeldt, L. Persson, and I. Bjorck. 2005. Vinegar supplementation lowers glucose and insulin responses and increases satiety after a bread meal in healthy subjects. *European Journal of Clinical Nutrition,* 59(9):983–988.

Otto, H. and L. Niklas. 1980. Different glycemic responses to carbohydrate-containing foods: Implications for the dietary treatment of diabetes mellitus. *Hygiene (Geneve),* 38:3424–3429 (in French).

Pelletier, X., B. Hanesse, F. Bornet, and G. Debry. 1994. Glycaemic and insulinaemic responses in healthy volunteers upon ingestion of maltitol and hydrogenated glucose syrups. *Diabete et Metabolisme,* 20(3):291–296.

Perry, G. H., N. J. Dominy, K. G. Claw, A. S. Lee, H. Fiegler, R. Redon, J. Werner. 2007. Diet and the evolution of human amylase gene copy number variation. *Nature Genetics,* 39(10):1256–1260.

Petersen, B. L., L. S. Ward, E. D. Bastian, A. L. Jenkins, J. Campbell, and V. Vuksan. 2009. A whey protein supplement decreases post-prandial glycemia. *Nutrition Journal,* 8:47.

Pi-Sunyer, F. X. 2002. Glycemic index and disease. *American Journal of Clinical Nutrition,* 76(1):290S–298S.

Ramdath, D. D., R. L. Isaacs, S. Teelucksingh, and T. M. Wolever. 2004. Glycaemic index of selected staples commonly eaten in the Caribbean and the effects of boiling v. crushing. *British Journal of Nutrition,* 91(6):971–977.

Ross, S. W., J. C. Brand, A. W. Thorburn, and A. S. Truswell. 1987. Glycemic index of processed wheat products. *American Journal of Clinical Nutrition,* 46(4):631–635.

Salmeron, J., J. E. Manson, M. J. Stampfer, G. A. Colditz, A. L. Wing, and W. C. Willett. 1997. Dietary fiber, glycemic load, and risk of non-insulin-dependent diabetes mellitus in women. *JAMA-Journal of the American Medical Association,* 277(6):472–477.

Sievenpiper, J. L., V. Vuksan, E. Y. Wong, R. A. Mendelson, and C. Bruce-Thompson. 1998. Effect of meal dilution on the postprandial glycemic response: Implications for glycemic testing. *Diabetes Care,* 21(5):711–716.

Sugiyama, M., A. C. Tang, Y. Wakaki, and W. Koyama. 2003. Glycemic index of single and mixed meal foods among common Japanese foods with white rice as a reference food. *European Journal of Clinical Nutrition,* 57(6):743–752.

Velangi, A., G. Fernandes, and T. M. Wolever. 2005. Evaluation of a glucose meter for determining the glycemic responses of foods. *Clinica Chimica Acta,* 356(1–2):191–198.

Venn, B. J., M. Kataoka, and J. Mann. 2014. The use of different reference foods in determining the glycemic index of starchy and non-starchy test foods. *Nutrition Journal,* 13(50):1–6.

Venn, B. J., S. M. Williams, and J. I. Mann. 2010. Comparison of postprandial glycaemia in Asians and Caucasians. *Diabetic Medicine,* 27(10):1205–1208.

Wolever, T. M. and C. Bolognesi. 1996a. Prediction of glucose and insulin responses of normal subjects after consuming mixed meals varying in energy, protein, fat, carbohydrate and glycemic index. *Journal of Nutrition,* 126(11):2807–2812.

Wolever, T. M. and C. Bolognesi. 1996b. Source and amount of carbohydrate affect postprandial glucose and insulin in normal subjects. *Journal of Nutrition,* 126(11):2798–2806.

Wolever, T. M., J. C. Brand-Miller, J. Abernethy, A. Astrup, F. Atkinson, M. Axelsen, I. Bjorck et al. 2008. Measuring the glycemic index of foods: Interlaboratory study. *American Journal of Clinical Nutrition,* 87(1):247S–257S.

Wolever, T. M., J. L. Chiasson, A. Csima, J. A. Hunt, C. Palmason, S. A. Ross, and E. A. Ryan. 1998a. Variation of postprandial plasma glucose, palatability, and symptoms associated with a standardized mixed test meal versus 75 g oral glucose. *Diabetes Care,* 21(3):336–340.

Wolever, T. M., D. J. Jenkins, G. R. Collier, R. M. Ehrlich, R. G. Josse, G. S. Wong, and R. Lee. 1988a. The glycaemic index: Effect of age in insulin dependent diabetes mellitus. *Diabetes Research,* 7(2):71–74.

Wolever, T. M., D. J. Jenkins, A. L. Jenkins, and R. G. Josse. 1991a. The glycemic index: Methodology and clinical implications. *American Journal of Clinical Nutrition,* 54(5):846–854.

Wolever, T. M., D. J. Jenkins, R. G. Josse, G. S. Wong, and R. Lee. 1987. The glycemic index: Similarity of values derived in insulin-dependent and non-insulin-dependent diabetic patients. *Journal of the American College of Nutrition,* 6(4):295–305.

Wolever, T. M., D. J. Jenkins, A. M. Ocana, V. A. Rao, and G. R. Collier. 1988b. Second-meal effect: Low-glycemic-index foods eaten at dinner improve subsequent breakfast glycemic response. *American Journal of Clinical Nutrition,* 48(4):1041–1047.

Wolever, T. M., D. J. Jenkins, V. Vuksan, R. G. Josse, G. S. Wong, and A. L. Jenkins. 1990. Glycemic index of foods in individual subjects. *Diabetes Care,* 13(2):126–132.

Wolever, T. M., H. H. Vorster, I. Bjorck, J. Brand-Miller, F. Brighenti, J. I. Mann, D. D. Ramdath et al. 2003. Determination of the glycaemic index of foods: Interlaboratory study. *European Journal of Clinical Nutrition,* 57(3):475–482.

Wolever, T. M., V. Vuksan, H. Eshuis, P. Spadafora, R. D. Peterson, E. S. Chao, M. L. Storey, and D. J. Jenkins. 1991b. Effect of method of administration of psyllium on glycemic response and carbohydrate digestibility. *Journal of the American College of Nutrition,* 10(4):364–371.

Wolever, T. M., M. Yang, X. Y. Zeng, F. Atkinson, and J. C. Brand-Miller. 2006. Food glycemic index, as given in glycemic index tables, is a significant determinant of glycemic responses elicited by composite breakfast meals. *American Journal of Clinical Nutrition,* 83(6):1306–1312.

Wolever, T. M. S., J.-L. Chiasson, J. A. Hunt, C. Palmason, S. A. Ross, and E. A. Ryan. 1998b. Similarity of relative glycaemic but not relative insulinaemic responses in normal, IGT and diabetic subjects. *Nutrition Research,* 18(10):1667–1676.

Yoon, J. H., L. U. Thompson, and D. J. Jenkins. 1983. The effect of phytic acid on in vitro rate of starch digestibility and blood glucose response. *American Journal of Clinical Nutrition,* 38(6):835–842.

4 Glycemic Index and Diabetes Mellitus

Evidence on Prevention and Management and Implications on Insulin Resistance

Laura Chiavaroli, Livia S.A. Augustin, Cyril W.C. Kendall, and David J.A. Jenkins

CONTENTS

4.1 INTRODUCTION: BACKGROUND ON DIABETES AND THE CURRENT STATE

4.1.1 Diabetes

Diabetes is currently the fastest growing chronic disease worldwide, and it is widely acknowledged that both genes and the environment are important determinants in its development. Nevertheless, since changes in the gene pool and earlier detection cannot account for the recent rapid increase over the last 20 years in the incidence of diabetes, environmental changes are key to understanding this increase. The past few decades have seen dramatic changes in food production and processing, resulting in a marked rise in the availability of highly processed, energy dense but nutrient-poor foods. These nutritional changes have contributed to the obesity pandemic and accompanying rise in diabetes. With the recent doubling of diabetes globally, its projected increase in prevalence to 1 in 10 adults by 2040 and its heavy burden on healthcare costs (International Diabetes Federation 2013), there is a great need for targeting both the prevention and management of diabetes.

Although it is not the scope of this book to explain the pathophysiology of diabetes in detail, a brief explanation of type 1 and type 2 diabetes follows. Type 1 diabetes mellitus is characterized by the autoimmune destruction of pancreatic beta cells, which progressively decreases insulin secretory capacity, resulting in hyperglycemia and chronic inflammation, and in most cases, in the ultimate dependency on exogenous insulin (American Diabetes Association 2010). It is thought to be triggered by an infection; however, the causative environmental factors continue to be debated (Canadian Diabetes Association Clinical Practice Guidelines Expert Committee et al. 2013c). Type 2 diabetes mellitus results from the development of insulin resistance and subsequent decompensation of the pancreatic beta cells, leading to a relative lack of insulin, and thus causing hyperglycemia (Ohtsubo et al. 2011). Insulin resistance is a state where the body's cells fail to respond to insulin; thus, ineffective use of insulin results in elevated blood glucose concentration (Sesti 2006). Insulin resistance can result from a variety of factors, including obesity and excess caloric intake. These conditions lead to repeated exposure to excess glucose concentration, stimulating insulin secretion and elevations in triglycerides and free fatty acids, which in turn impair the insulin-mediated uptake of glucose (Roden et al. 1996, Koyama et al. 1997, Schinner et al. 2005). Other factors that have been associated with the development and progression of insulin resistance include a sedentary lifestyle and lack of physical activity (Balkau et al. 2008, Solomon and Thyfault 2013); chronic inflammation, which correlates with increases in circulating free fatty acids (Shi et al. 2006); and gut microbiota, which influences the inflammatory state of the body (Burcelin et al. 2012), as well as genetic factors (Harder et al. 2013, Ramirez et al. 2014). In uncontrolled diabetes, the resulting elevated blood glucose concentrations affect the vasculature throughout the entire body both at the microvascular level, increasing the risk of eye diseases (retinopathy) and kidney diseases (nephropathy), and at the macrovascular level, resulting in a near doubling of the risk of cardiovascular disease (CVD) and reduction in the lifespan of up to 10 years compared to people without diabetes (Manuel and Schultz 2004). Insulin resistance has also been a recognized feature in people with type 1 diabetes (DeFronzo et al. 1982) and has been associated with increased risk of microvascular and macrovascular complications (Kilpatrick et al. 2007). To reduce the risk of the associated complications in both type 1 and type 2 diabetes, there is a continued focus on the development of means to control elevated blood glucose concentration through both lifestyle and pharmaceutical means. Prospective cohort studies have demonstrated that good glycemic control in both type 1 and type 2 diabetes is associated with improved risk of microvascular complications, including retinopathy and nephropathy (Control Group et al. 2009, Boussageon et al. 2011, Hemmingsen et al. 2013, Fullerton et al. 2014), as is discussed in diabetes guidelines globally (The Diabetes Control and Complications Trial Research Group 1995, Stratton et al. 2000, Colagiuri S et al. 2009, Clinical Guidelines Task Force 2012, International Diabetes Federation 2012, Canadian Diabetes Association Clinical Practice Guidelines Expert Committee et al. 2013b, American Diabetes Association 2015). However, the results of three large randomized trials published in 2008 (ACCORD, ADVANCE, and VADT) (Action to Control Cardiovascular Risk in Diabetes Study Group et al. 2008, Advance Collaborative Group et al. 2008, Duckworth et al. 2009) failed to show significant CVD benefit for improved glycemic control over a period of 3–5 years. At about the same time, largely prompted by concern about cardiovascular safety of rosiglitazone and other anti-diabetic medications, the U.S. Food and Drug Administration (FDA) required demonstration of the cardiovascular safety of all new anti-diabetic agents (U.S. Food and Drug Administration 2008). Since then, longer term follow up of some of these trials (VADT and UKPDS) (Holman et al. 2008, Hayward et al. 2015), as well as the recently published EMPA REG OUTCOME™ study (Zinman et al. 2015) with the SGLT2 inhibitor empagliflozin, have demonstrated CVD benefit. Additionally, some anti-diabetic medications for intensive glycemic control have been demonstrated to confer a greater risk of hypoglycemia (Boussageon et al. 2011, Hemmingsen et al. 2013, Sardar et al. 2015), which has recently been suggested to contribute to the risk of diabetes complications (Gross et al. 2011). The use of diet and lifestyle factors for glycemic control, which usually has a more subtle effect, are of importance, and they may also be particularly beneficial in the prevention of diabetes in those at high risk (Knowler et al. 2002, Diabetes Prevention Program Research Group et al. 2009).

4.1.2 Carbohydrate Quality and Glycemia

Since both diabetes and prediabetes (insulin-resistant) are characterized by postprandial hyperglycemia, the metabolic effects of different carbohydrate foods and their absorption profiles (carbohydrate quality) are of great potential relevance. One way to classify the quality of carbohydrates is by the glycemic index (GI). The GI is a physiological classification of the available carbohydrate content in foods based on their postprandial blood glucose responses (Jenkins and Wolever 1981). The GI is defined as the glycemic response elicited by a portion of a carbohydrate-rich food compared to the response elicited by the same amount of carbohydrate from a standard or reference food. Therefore, foods that release their carbohydrates slowly, eliciting small rises in blood glucose are referred to as "low GI foods" (Augustin et al. 2015). High-GI foods, on the other hand, elicit higher glycemic and insulinemic responses and are considered fast release carbohydrates. The rise in blood glucose is influenced both by the type of carbohydrate (whether it is low or high GI) and by the amount of carbohydrate present in a serving. The glycemic load (GL) allows both the quality and quantity of carbohydrate to be accounted for. The GL is the product of GI and the total available carbohydrate content of a given amount of food (Augustin et al. 2015). Hence, if the amount of carbohydrate consumed is increased, the glycemic response and hence the GL will also increase, and the same would occur if a higher GI food were consumed. Therefore, since both GI (quality) and GL (quality and quantity) affect glycemia, their health effects are of great interest in the area of diabetes prevention and management.

4.2 GI AND DIABETES PREVENTION

4.2.1 Overview

Type 2 diabetes is thought to result from the toxic effects of chronically elevated levels of blood glucose and fatty acids on the pancreatic beta cells that release insulin. Initially, the beta cells can respond to greater fluxes in glucose by compensating with a greater secretion of insulin, which results in hyperinsulinemia (Festa et al. 2006). However, over time, beta-cell compensation to the chronic surplus in blood glucose is less successful. This is due to continuous increased release of free fatty acids that impair glucose-stimulated insulin secretion, thus leading to beta-cell dysfunction and damage, which results in further hyperglycemia, also called impaired glycemia and impaired glucose tolerance (IGT) for those at this stage (Ohtsubo et al. 2011). In the long term, these elevated glucose levels in IGT are toxic to the beta cells, leading to increased beta-cell failure and blood glucose concentrations further elevated to those considered to be characteristic of diabetes. Even at the upper end of normal glucose tolerance, impaired beta-cell function has been demonstrated to occur in those who are both lean and obese (Ferrannini et al. 2005). Thus, it is important to target prevention of any extreme rises in blood glucose concentration to reduce the risk of beta-cell failure and hence prevent the development of diabetes. Additionally, a high-GI diet has been shown to induce damage to pancreatic islet cells in animals (Pawlak et al. 2004). Therefore, low GI foods, which by definition elicit a lower blood glucose response, may represent a potential strategy to reduce the risk of developing diabetes.

4.2.2 Observational Evidence

Since 2000, multiple prospective cohort studies have explored the association between GI/GL and the risk of developing type 2 diabetes, and multiple systematic reviews and meta-analyses have collated these studies and assessed the overall effect. Of these, the most recent included three large cohort studies that included data from an additional 205,157 participants: the Nurses' Health Study, the Nurses' Health Study II, and the Health Professionals Follow-Up Study (Bhupathiraju et al. 2014). The meta-analysis for GI, which included 10 datasets from collated studies demonstrated that the risk of developing type 2 diabetes was 19% higher with higher GI compared to lower GI diets (Figure 4.1) (Bhupathiraju et al. 2014).

Similarly, the meta-analysis of the 14 datasets from collated studies with GL demonstrated a 13% increased risk of type 2 diabetes for higher GL diets when compared to lower GL diets (Figure 4.2) (Bhupathiraju et al. 2014).

Study	ES (95% CI)	% Weight
Krishnan et al. 2007	1.23 (1.05, 1.44)	6.44
Meyer et al. 2000	0.89 (0.72, 1.10)	3.58
Mosdol et al. 2007	0.94 (0.71, 1.23)	2.13
Rossi et al. 2013	1.14 (1.01, 1.30)	10.08
Sahyoun et al. 2008	1.00 (0.50, 2.00)	0.33
Sakurai et al. 2012	1.96 (1.04, 3.67)	0.40
Simila et al. 2011	0.87 (0.71, 1.07)	3.82
Sluijs et al. 2013, Denmark	1.03 (0.80, 1.32)	2.56
Sluijs et al. 2013, France	1.03 (0.73, 2.33)	0.48
Sluijs et al. 2013, Germany	0.94 (0.66, 1.34)	1.28
Sluijs et al. 2013, Italy	1.29 (0.96, 1.73)	1.85
Sluijs et al. 2013, Netherlands	0.80 (0.55, 1.16)	1.15
Sluijs et al. 2013, Spain	1.01 (0.85, 1.20)	5.40
Sluijs et al. 2013, Sweden	1.07 (0.85, 1.35)	3.00
Sluijs et al. 2013, United Kingdom	1.33 (0.88, 2.02)	0.93
van Woudenbergh et al. 2011	0.95 (0.75, 1.21)	2.81
Villegas et al. 2007	1.21 (1.03, 1.43)	5.97
Nurses' Heath Study	1.44 (1.33, 1.57)	23.34
Health Professionals Follow-Up Study	1.30 (1.15, 1.47)	10.66
Nurses' Health Study II	1.20 (1.08, 1.34)	13.80
Overall (I^2 = 68.5%, p < .0001)	**1.19 (1.14, 1.24)**	**100.00**

ES (95% CI)

0.272 1.00 3.67

Decreased risk Increased risk

FIGURE 4.1 Meta-analysis of prospective cohort studies investigating the association between GI and risk of type 2 diabetes. The pooled effect estimate is represented as a diamond. The p value is for an inverse-variance fixed-effects model. All data are presented as relative risks with 95% confidence intervals. ES, effect size; GI, glycemic index. (Adapted from Bhupathiraju, S.N. et al., *Am. J. Clin. Nutr.*, 100, 218–232, 2014. With permission.)

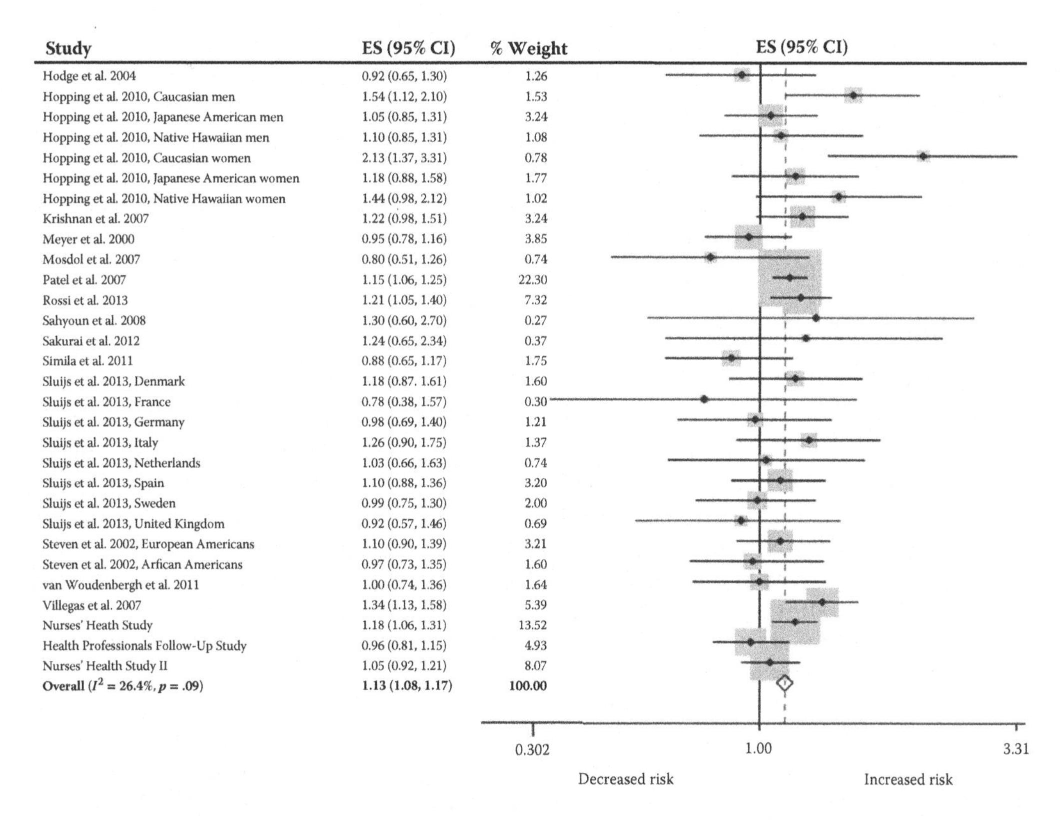

FIGURE 4.2 Meta-analysis of prospective cohort studies investigating the association between GL and risk of type 2 diabetes. The pooled effect estimate is represented as a diamond. The p-value is for an inverse-variance fixed-effects model. All data are presented as relative risks with 95% confidence intervals. ES, effect size; GL, glycemic load. (Adapted from Bhupathiraju, S.N. et al., *Am. J. Clin. Nutr.*, 100, 218–232, 2014. With permission.)

These results were independent of cereal fiber intake, which is noteworthy because intake of cereal fiber has been associated with a modest reduced risk of type 2 diabetes according to another recent systematic review and meta-analysis (Cho et al. 2013). Three previous systematic reviews and meta-analyses conducted on GI and diabetes risk also found similar effects (Barclay et al. 2008, Dong et al. 2011, Livesey et al. 2013). An additional meta-analysis by Sluijs et al. (2013), which was a nested case-cohort study performed in European countries, conversely, did not show any associations. However, the latter did not review studies in a systematic manner and thus did not include data from other studies performed in Europe, including four large European cohort studies (Mosdol et al. 2007, Simila et al. 2011, van Woudenbergh et al. 2011, Rossi et al. 2013). Additionally, not all cohort studies have found an association of GI/GL on risk of type 2 diabetes, including the Iowa Women's Health Study (Meyer et al. 2000), the Whitehall II Study (Mosdol et al. 2007), and the Atherosclerosis Risk in Communities (ARIC) study (Stevens et al. 2002), which may be related to their design. In these studies, the population included was older, and because they entered the study as healthy subjects, they might have also been healthier compared to their similar-aged peers. Furthermore, the tools used to assess GI were not specifically designed for this purpose and may not have been able to capture GI or GL accurately. For example, it is not clear from where the GI values were obtained from in the analysis of dietary intake in the Iowa Women's Health Study (Meyer et al. 2000), leaving doubts as to whether the correct dietary GI values were assigned to individual foods and if the proper GI calculations were performed. Furthermore, in the aforementioned cohorts, there may have been greater exposure to measurement error because only one baseline food frequency questionnaire (FFQ) was used. This is in contrast to the Nurses' Health Study I and II and the Health Professionals Follow-Up Study where FFQs were obtained every 4 years over the 24-, 18-, and 22-year follow-up periods, respectively, and used in the analyses (Bhupathiraju et al. 2014). Nevertheless, when data from all cohort studies are pooled together, including those that found no association, it is evident that overall, a significant association has been demonstrated for GI and GL and diabetes; thus, those consuming lower GI/GL diets may have a lower risk of developing type 2 diabetes (Bhupathiraju et al. 2014).

4.2.3 Clinical Trial Evidence

4.2.3.1 Overview

Although there have not yet been any specifically designed clinical trials on the effect of GI or GL on risk of diabetes, clinical trials have been conducted on the effects of the drug acarbose on diabetes development. Acarbose is an oral α-glucosidase inhibitor that reduces the rate of glucose absorption, effectively converting the diet to a low GI diet. The Study to Prevent Non-Insulin Dependent Diabetes Mellitus (STOP-NIDDM) showed that acarbose reduced progression to type 2 diabetes by 25% compared to a placebo in those with IGT (relative hazard ratio 0.75, 95% confidence interval (CI) 0.63–0.90, $p = .0015$) and significantly increased the reversion of IGT to normal glucose tolerance ($p < .001$) over 3 years (Chiasson et al. 2002). This study provides a proof-of-concept for low GI diets regarding diabetes prevention (Chiasson et al. 2002).

In addition to impaired fasting glucose and IGT, traits of the metabolic syndrome, including hypertension, dyslipidemia, abdominal obesity, and a proinflammatory state (Grundy et al. 2004), are independent predictors of the risk of developing type 2 diabetes (Hanefeld et al. 2009). Trials demonstrating an association between GI and GL and traits of the metabolic syndrome will be discussed separately in the following text. Clinical trials have demonstrated that those with the metabolic syndrome have a greater risk of developing type 2 diabetes. For example, in a secondary analysis of the STOP-NIDDM trial of 1368 participants with IGT (Hanefeld et al. 2009), participants were divided into those with and without the metabolic syndrome in each of the placebo and acarbose-treated groups. In both treatment groups, those who had the metabolic syndrome had a

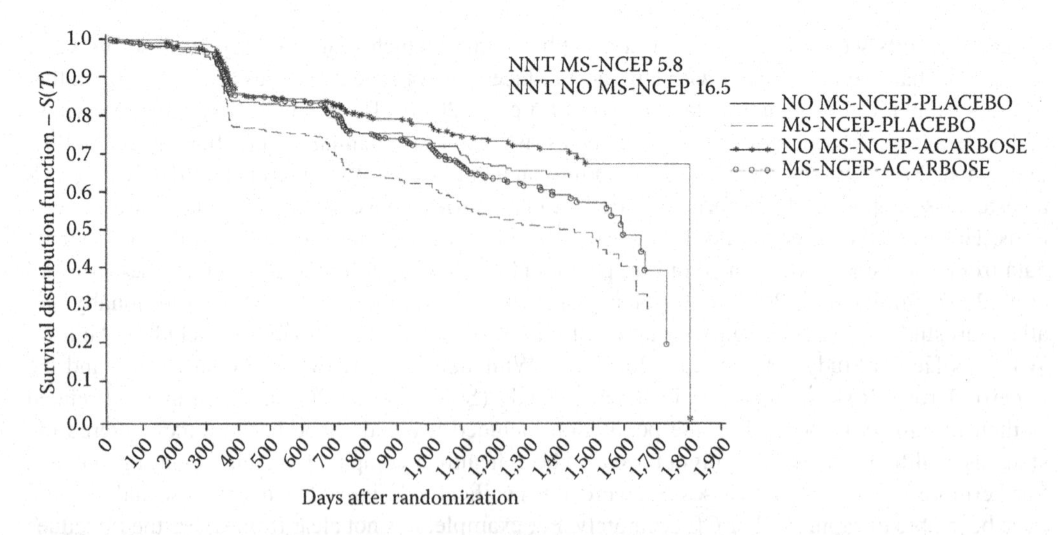

FIGURE 4.3 The effect of acarbose on incidence of diabetes in those with impaired glucose tolerance by metabolic syndrome status. MS, metabolic syndrome; NCEP, National Cholesterol Education Program; NNT, number needed to treat. (Reproduced from Hanefeld, M. et al., *Diab. Vasc. Dis. Res.*, 6, 32–37, 2009. With permission.)

higher incidence of diabetes than those without the metabolic syndrome (Hanefeld et al. 2009) (Figure 4.3). Of the four groups, those with the metabolic syndrome receiving the placebo treatment had the highest incidence of diabetes and those without the metabolic syndrome receiving the acarbose treatment had the lowest risk (Hanefeld et al. 2009). Interestingly, those with the metabolic syndrome who received the acarbose treatment appeared to have the same risk of developing diabetes as those without the metabolic syndrome who received the placebo treatment (Hanefeld et al. 2009) (Figure 4.3). This suggests that reducing postprandial glycemia, by either using acarbose or possibly using low GI diets, may reduce the risk of developing diabetes, especially in those with the metabolic syndrome.

4.2.3.2 Low-Density Lipoprotein-Cholesterol

It is of great interest to target LDL-C in people with diabetes because CVD is the leading cause of death in this population, and LDL-C is the primary target for CVD risk reduction. Low GI diets have been demonstrated to improve dyslipidemia, particularly LDL-C (Anderson et al. 2013, Stone et al. 2014). A systematic review and meta-analysis by Goff et al. (2013) of 28 randomized controlled trials with at least 4 weeks follow up demonstrated that low GI diets significantly reduced both total cholesterol (27 included trials; mean difference [MD] = −0.13 mmol/L, 95% CI −0.22 to −0.04, p = .004) and LDL-C (23 included trials; MD = −0.16 mmol/L, 95% CI −0.24 to −0.08, p < .0001) compared to high-GI diets (Figure 4.4).

Study	Mean Difference IV, Random (95% CI)	% Weight
Bouche et al. 2002	−0.39 (−1.14, 0.36)	1.0
Brand et al. 1991	−0.26 (−0.84, 0.32)	1.7
de Rougemont et al. 2007	−0.19 (−0.75, 0.37)	1.9
Frost et al. 1994	0.40 (−0.15, 0.95)	1.9
Frost et al. 1996	0.40 (−0.86, 0.86)	0.8
Frost et al. 2004	−0.21 (−0.61, 0.19)	3.7
Heilbronn et al. 2002	0.00 (−0.44, 0.44)	3.0
Jenkins et al. 2008	−0.15 (−0.40, 0.10)	9.2
Jimenez-Cruz et al. 2003	−0.20 (−0.70, 0.30)	2.4
Marsh et al. 2010	−0.02 (−0.44, 0.40)	3.4
Philippou et al. 2008	−0.18 (−0.67, 0.31)	2.4
Philippou et al. 2009	0.17 (−1.06, 0.26)	1.1
Rizkalla et al. 2004	−0.40 (−1.06, 0.26)	1.4
Shikany et al. 2009	0.14 (−0.33, 0.61)	2.6
Sichieri et al. 2007	−0.15 (−0.51, 0.21)	4.4
Sloth et al. 2004	−0.43 (−0.84, −0.02)	3.4
Tsihilas et al. 2000	−0.27 (−0.80, −0.26)	2.1
Venn et al. 2010	0.00 (−0.34, 0.34)	5.2
Wolever et al. 1992	−0.37 (−2.53, 1.79)	0.1
Wolever et al. 2003	0.00 (−0.61, 0.77)	1.3
Wolever et al. 2008	−0.08 (−0.29, 0.13)	12.8
Yusof et al. 2009	−0.26 (−0.61, 0.09)	4.8
Zhang et al. 2010	−0.26 (−0.40, 0.12)	29.2
Total (95% CI)	**−0.16 (−0.24, −0.08)**	**100.00**

Heterogeneity: Tau^2 = 0.00; Chi^2 = 14.35, df = 22 (p = .89): I^2 = 0%
Test for overall effect Z = 4.11 (p < .0001)

FIGURE 4.4 Meta-analysis of randomized controlled trials on the effect of low versus high-GI dietary interventions on LDL-C (mmol/L). The pooled effect estimate is represented as a diamond. The p value is for a generic inverse-variance random-effects model. All data are presented as effect estimates with 95% confidence intervals. CI, confidence interval; IV, inverse variance; GI, glycemic index; LDL-C, low density lipoprotein cholesterol; Mean Difference, mean difference in post intervention LDL-C between low GI and high-GI groups; SD, standard deviation. (Adapted from Goff, L.M. et al., *Nutr. Metab. Cardiovasc. Dis.*, 23, 1e10, 2013. With permission.)

Importantly, this reduction in LDL-C was observed independently of weight loss, which has been proven to improve cholesterol (Dattilo and Kris-Etherton 1992). In subgroup analyses by diabetes status, the reduction in LDL-C remained statistically significant in both those with and without diabetes (Goff et al. 2013). The reduction in LDL-C concentration seen following consumption of low GI diets may be due to the increased intake of dietary fiber, because subgroup analyses demonstrated significant reductions in LDL-C in those studies where low GI diets also contained significantly more fiber than high-GI diets ($p < .05$). Importantly, different subgroups are likely to contain other variables that differ beyond what they are divided on, which may act as confounders and influence the difference in observed effect(s) (Higgins 2011). Thus, the studies in the subgroup of low GI diets with significantly greater fiber intakes may also have, for example, greater differences in GIs, potentially driving the subgroup effect (Goff et al. 2013). Still, the effect of low GI diets on LDL-C may be in part driven by fiber, particularly viscous fiber. Indeed, low GI foods are characterized by a higher viscous fiber content, which is known for its cholesterol-lowering effects (Jenkins et al. 1993, U.S. Food and Drug Administration 1998, Wolever et al. 2010).

4.2.3.3 High-Density Lipoprotein-Cholesterol

Part of the contribution to the increased risk of CVD in those with diabetes is their low concentration of HDL-C (Goldbourt et al. 1997). In diabetes, low HDL-C is of particular concern because it is an independent predictor of coronary heart disease (CHD) morbidity and mortality (Gordon et al. 1989, Niskanen et al. 1998, Turner et al. 1998, Boden 2000, Gotto 2002, Drexel et al. 2005, Tenenbaum et al. 2006). Therefore, potential avenues to increase HDL-C are of interest. Although the systematic review and meta-analysis by Goff et al. (2013) found no effect of dietary GI on HDL-C, another systematic review and meta-analysis that included only longer term randomized controlled trials with at least 6 months follow up (n = 3 trials) demonstrated significant improvements in HDL-C (5% improvement; weighted mean difference [WMD] = 0.05 mmol/L, 95% CI 0.02 to 0.07, $p < .001$) with low GI diets (Ajala et al. 2013). Similar results have also been observed with acarbose (Oyama et al. 2008). In this respect, it may be important for studies to be of sufficient duration to capture changes in more slowly changing risk factors, such as HDL-C. The reader is referred to Chapter 5 for an extensive discussion on GI and CVD.

4.2.3.4 Weight Loss

Obesity is the single most frequent risk factor for the development of type 2 diabetes (Mokdad et al. 2003), and indeed, a substantial proportion of people with type 2 diabetes are overweight or obese. Additionally, in people with diabetes, a higher body mass index (BMI) is associated with increased mortality (Canadian Diabetes Association Clinical Practice Guidelines Expert Committee et al. 2013d). Weight loss is thus a primary target in guidelines to reduce diabetes risk (Canadian Diabetes Association Clinical Practice Guidelines Expert Committee et al. 2013c) and substantial benefits result from weight management. In light of these facts, the effect of low GI diets on weight loss has been assessed in people with and without diabetes. In a systematic review and meta-analysis that included only randomized controlled trials with the objective of weight loss in people without diabetes with a follow-up of at least 4 weeks, low GI diets were found to be significantly more effective for weight loss when compared to conventional energy-restricted diets (n = 4 trials), especially when the GL was lowered (Thomas et al. 2007). A more recent systematic review and meta-analysis by Schwingshackl and Hoffmann (2013), which included long-term randomized controlled trials with a minimum follow up of 6 months in obese individuals and of which approximately 30% of included trials were conducted in those with diabetes, found a similar reduction in body weight resulting from consumption of low GI/GL diets compared to high-GI/GL diets (n = 14 trials), although the effect did not reach statistical significance (p = .06). This outcome, however, is perhaps less remarkable because the majority of included trials were not intended for weight loss. Additionally, in a 22-week randomized trial of participants with type 2 diabetes instructed to follow either a vegan diet or the 2003 American Diabetes Association recommendations, the dietary GI was demonstrated to significantly predict changes in body weight after adjustments for various factors, including dietary fiber, energy, carbohydrate, and fat intake (Turner-McGrievy et al. 2011). Interestingly, in an exploratory analysis of three prospective cohorts from the United States (Nurses' Health Study, Nurses' Health Study II, and the Health Professionals Follow Up Study) of over 120,000 healthy men and women, increases in GL were independently associated with greater weight gain over an average 4-year follow up (Smith et al. 2015). This evidence suggests that a low GI/GL diet may be a useful dietary strategy for weight loss.

A number of physiological adaptations during weight loss can mitigate post weight loss success, including perturbations in appetite-regulating hormones and energy homeostasis (Greenway 2015). This has prompted the investigation of the effect of energy-restricted low GI/GL diets on factors that can impede success post weight loss. In a randomized parallel-design study of energy-restricted low GL or low fat diets in 39 overweight or obese young adults post 10% weight loss, resting energy expenditure decreased less, and less hunger was reported on the low GL compared to the low fat diet (Pereira et al. 2004). Of great interest is the result of the Diogenes trial, which was a randomized trial of 773 overweight adults from eight European countries given one of five ad libitum diets varying in protein content and GI over 26 weeks to assess the effect on weight regain after at least 8% body weight loss on a low calorie diet (Larsen et al. 2010). The study demonstrated that a low GI diet moderately high in protein prevented weight regain 6 months after the weight loss program where the effect of GI was independent of the effect of protein (Larsen et al. 2010). Although in a 12-month follow up on a subset of 256 study participants from 2 of the 8 participating countries, there was no observed difference between the diets varying in protein and GI, the authors note they were unable to objectively verify the small reported difference of five GI units between the high and low GI diet groups as obtained from the 3-day food records (Aller et al. 2014). Furthermore, in the additional 6-month follow up, participants were no longer provided with 80% of relevant foods free of charge as they had been in the first 6 months (Aller et al. 2014); thus, continued adherence to the diet may have been an issue in the follow up.

The potential for prevention of weight regain is particularly noteworthy because this is one of the greatest challenges with weight loss programs (Dansinger et al. 2007), and recently it has been debated as to whether programs specifically targeting weight loss are at all useful if not harmful in treating obesity because of the excess weight fluctuations that they may cause (Montani et al. 2006). Weight cycling has also been associated with increased incidence of diabetes (Delahanty et al. 2014); therefore, finding successful lifestyle changes, which may also result in weight loss without regain, which may include low GI/GL diets, may be particularly beneficial to reducing the risk of diabetes. The reader is referred to Chapter 6 for a detailed discussion of the effect of GI on obesity and weight management.

4.2.3.5 Inflammation

Markers of systemic inflammation, such as C-reactive protein (CRP), have been cross-sectionally associated with reduced insulin sensitivity and pancreatic beta-cell function and are thus targets of interest in those both at risk of and living with diabetes (Haffner et al. 2005, Barbarroja et al. 2012). There has been some evidence that low GI diets may reduce inflammation, which is particularly important in diabetes prevention and management because inflammation is also regarded to play a large role in the pathophysiology of obesity (Devaraj et al. 2009), and is an independent risk factor for CVD (Ridker and Morrow 2003). A recent systematic review of clinical trials found a more consistent anti-inflammatory benefit for low GI diets compared to high fiber and whole grain diets (Buyken et al. 2014). More specifically, low GI diets have been demonstrated to reduce CRP in a recent systematic review and meta-analysis of randomized controlled trials with ≤ 6 months follow up ($n = 7$ trials) (Schwingshackl and Hoffmann 2013). Of these trials, the randomized controlled trial with the longest follow up of 52 weeks by Wolever et al. (2008) was conducted in people with well-controlled type 2 diabetes and demonstrated that those on the low GI diet had a mean CRP 30% less than those on the high-GI diet. Furthermore, considering that a CRP level < 2 mg/L is a risk factor for CHD (Ridker et al. 2005) and the baseline CRP in the study by Wolever et al. (2008) was 2.64 mg/L, the 30% reduction drove CRP concentrations below the risk level, similar to the effect observed with the use of statins (Sommeijer et al. 2004, Yamada et al. 2006). Additionally, in 902 women with diabetes from the Nurses' Health Study, it was demonstrated that GI may reduce systemic inflammation through associations with reduced CRP (Qi et al. 2006), as well as increased adiponectin (Qi et al. 2005), which is known to have anti-inflammatory effects (Berg and Scherer 2005, Mantzoros et al. 2005). Although there are some observational trials that did not demonstrate significant correlations between inflammatory markers and GI/GL (Griffith et al. 2008, Vrolix and Mensink 2010), some have found borderline significance (Du et al. 2008), while other notably large trials, including the Women's Health Initiative (Levitan et al. 2008), found significant correlations between GI and CRP.

Since inflammation is associated with increased adipocytokine production from adipose tissue, which is recognized as a central mechanism underlying energy balance, obesity, and comorbidities, including cardiometabolic risk, it is also important to consider the effects of GI on these molecules. Adiponectin, which is inversely correlated with insulin resistance, glucose intolerance, dyslipidemia, and atherosclerosis (Ouchi et al. 2001, Esteve et al. 2009), is the most abundant adipocytokine found in the human body. Some studies on GI and GL have demonstrated beneficial effects, such as a 4-week randomized crossover trial by Neuhouser et al. (2012), which demonstrated that a low GL diet modestly increased adiponectin in addition to significantly reducing CRP concentrations compared to a high GL diet in 80 overweight individuals. Additionally, a longitudinal analysis of the PREDIMED cohort, where approximately 55% of the 511 high risk individuals had diabetes, demonstrated that after 1 year of follow up, those with greater increases in GI and GL showed greater reductions in adiponectin and leptin (Bullo et al. 2013), also implicated in energy balance and cardiometabolic risk (Bullo Bonet 2002). Furthermore, a 7-month randomized trial on acarbose in 188 individuals with diabetes demonstrated significant increases in plasma adiponectin, in addition to reductions in lipemia as well as body weight, which were significantly different from the control group with the exception of body weight (Derosa et al. 2011). Thus, GI may be effective in targeting inflammation as seen through effects on CRP and adipocytokines.

Overall, the potential multilevel effects of low GI/GL diets may work in combination to reduce the risk of developing diabetes.

4.2.4 GI and Insulin

Type 2 diabetes mellitus stems from the development of insulin resistance and a reduction in insulin secretion; thus, assessment of the effect of GI and GL on this significant hormone is imperative. C-peptide is a marker of insulin secretion and is secreted in equivalent units when the proinsulin molecule is cleaved to release insulin. Insulin demand, pancreatic stress, and high C-peptide concentration have been associated with insulin resistance and the development of diabetes and CVD (Haban et al. 2002). An assessment of healthy women from the Nurses' Health Study I and II demonstrated a positive association where higher GL was associated with higher C-peptide concentration (Wu et al. 2004). Additionally, the earliest clinical trials on low GI diets done in people with type 2 diabetes demonstrated reductions in urinary C-peptide, as well as reductions in fasting blood glucose and HbA1c when compared to high-GI diets (Burke et al. 1982, Jenkins et al. 1988). Furthermore, a recent systematic review and meta-analysis of trials in overweight and obese individuals with follow up greater than 6 months demonstrated significantly greater reductions in fasting insulin in those following low GI/GL diets compared to control diets (Schwingshackl and Hoffmann 2013).

More recently, clinical trials in individuals in the prediabetic phase have examined the effect of GI on insulin sensitivity and beta-cell function. A controlled clinical trial in 22 obese participants with prediabetes randomized to either a low or high-GI diet combined with an exercise program for 12 weeks demonstrated similar weight loss on both diets; however, postprandial hyperinsulinemia was reduced only on the low GI diet, whereas the high-GI diet demonstrated impaired beta-cell function despite significant weight loss (Solomon et al. 2010). Additional studies have demonstrated improvements in insulin sensitivity assessed by the HOmeostatic Model Assessment Index (HOMA-IR) on a low GI compared to a high-GI diet (Iannuzzi et al. 2009) and to a low fat diet (Juanola-Falgarona et al. 2014). Similar results, again using HOMA-IR, were found in the Framingham Offspring Study where increases in GI and GL were associated with increases in insulin resistance (McKeown et al. 2004). Furthermore, a 4-week randomized crossover clinical trial conducted in individuals with type 2 diabetes, where whole body peripheral insulin sensitivity was measured using the gold-standard euglycaemic hyperinsulinaemic clamp, reported insulin sensitivity to be significantly higher after the consumption of a low GI diet compared to after a high-GI diet (Rizkalla et al. 2004). Low GI and GL diets have been demonstrated in clinical trials to improve insulin sensitivity in both those with diabetes and in most, but not all, studies of healthy participants (Livesey et al. 2008), which is similar to what has been observed with acarbose (Derosa et al. 2011). A notable exception is a study by Sacks et al. (2014), where in a large, short-term (5 weeks) study of 163 overweight participants in their early 50s (mean age 53 years) with a relatively low incidence of metabolic syndrome (20%), no effect of GI was seen on HOMA-IR, insulin sensitivity, serum lipids, or blood pressure in DASH-type diets with either high or low level of carbohydrate. However, these discrepancies may be the result of short duration and the generally low risk of the participants. Overall, the weight of evidence suggests that where there is a sufficient level of risk, low GI/GL diets may reduce risk and improve the condition of type 2 diabetes by improving insulin sensitivity and reducing insulin resistance.

4.3 GI AND DIABETES TREATMENT

4.3.1 Overview

Diabetes is characterized by chronic hyperglycemia; thus, its treatment and management focuses specifically on how to best control these glycemic elevations. In addition to recommendations for pharmaceutical treatments, diabetes guidelines, including the Canadian, American, and European, among others, support the consumption of low GI carbohydrates for glycemic control (Mann et al. 2004, Diabetes U.K. Nutrition working group 2011, Italian Society of Human Nutrition [SINU] 2012, Canadian Diabetes Association Clinical Practice Guidelines Expert Committee et al. 2013a, Diabetes Australia 2014, Evert et al. 2014, International Diabetes Federation Guideline Development Group 2014) (Table 4.1). Without proper glycemic control, chronic hyperglycemia affects the vasculature at both the microvascular and macrovascular level resulting in whole-body complications. At the microvascular level, diabetic retinopathy (DR) has been found to be present in 21%–39% of patients at time of diagnosis of type 2 diabetes, and it is the leading cause of vision loss in Western nations (CNIB 2009, Canadian Diabetes Association Clinical Practice Guideline Expert Committee et al. 2013, Centers for Disease Control and Prevention [CDC] 2015). Diabetes is also the leading cause of kidney failure (The Kidney Foundation of Canada 2012, World Health Organization 2014). At the macrovascular level, CVD is the leading cause of death (Morrish et al. 2001, Public Health Agency of Canada 2011) and the leading driver of healthcare costs for people with diabetes (Simpson et al. 2003). Therefore, management strategies affecting glycemic control and preventing microvascular and macrovascular complications are of particular importance both

TABLE 4.1
Glycemic Index and Glycemic Load in Various Diabetes Guidelines

Organization	GI/GL-Related Content
Canadian Diabetes Association (CDA) 2013 (Canadian Diabetes Association Clinical Practice Guidelines Expert Committee et al. 2013a)	Choose food sources of a low glycemic index (GI).
American Diabetes Association (ADA) 2014 (Evert et al. 2014)	Substituting low GI foods for higher GI foods may be beneficial.
Diabetes and Nutrition Study Group (DNSG) of the European Association for the study of Diabetes (EASD) 2004 (Mann et al. 2004)	Low GI foods are suitable as carbohydrate-rich choices.
Italian Society of Human Nutrition (SINU) 2012 (Italian Society of Human Nutrition [SINU] 2012)	Preference for starchy food sources with low GI, particularly when the intake of carbohydrates is approaching the upper limit of intake, that is, 60% energy.
International Diabetes Federation (IDF) 2014 (International Diabetes Federation Guideline Development Group 2014)	Diets with a low glycaemic load are beneficial in improving glycaemic control. The use of GI can provide an additional benefit for diabetes control beyond that of carbohydrate counting.
Diabetes United Kingdom (U.K.) 2011 (Diabetes U.K. Nutrition working group 2011)	Diets of low glycaemic index/load and higher in dietary fiber and whole grains are protective.
Diabetes Australia 2014–2015 (Diabetes Australia 2014)	Some people with diabetes may require more intensive meal planning to ensure glycaemic control. They should have one high-fibre, low GI carbohydrate food at each meal.

for an improved quality of life for those living with diabetes and for the alleviation of the burden on healthcare systems.

4.3.2 Observational Evidence

4.3.2.1 CVD in Individuals with Type 2 Diabetes Mellitus

Prospective cohort studies exploring associations of GI and GL and management of diabetes complications, both at the microvascular and macrovascular levels, have been sparse and inconsistent. A recent assessment of the EPIC cohort of over 6000 individuals with confirmed type 2 diabetes from six European countries found no significant associations between baseline GI or GL and all-cause or CVD mortality after a median follow-up of 9.2 years (Burger et al. 2012). There was, however, a positive association between GL and mortality in the subgroup of normal weight individuals. It should be noted that there were important limitations of this prospective study because it relied on baseline dietary intake for the assessment of GI, which could lead to misclassifications due to dietary changes during the long follow-up period. Furthermore, the FFQs used were not specifically designed to measure GI or GL. In fact, in the overall assessment of EPIC GI methodology, it was concluded that ranking of participants based on GL values was acceptable; however, ranking according to GI was considered less reliable (van Bakel et al. 2009). This limitation also applies to the prospective ARIC study of 12, 251 healthy adults, aged 45–64 years at baseline with a follow up of 9 years, which found a positive association between GI and GL and CHD in the entire cohort but not in the diabetes subgroup. The association in the diabetes subgroup was positive but did not reach statistical significance; this, however, was limited by the small sample size of 1378 people with diabetes (Hardy et al. 2010). Another limitation with the use of a FFQ to assess GI and GL, which is probably an issue in other studies using FFQs, is misreporting, and specifically underreporting of snack-type and carbohydrate-rich foods, which is particularly common in those who are overweight. This could explain the lack of effect seen in the diabetes or obese subgroups (Heitmann and Lissner 1995). Interestingly, in another analysis of the EPIC cohort, examination of the association with intakes of legumes, which are a particularly low GI food, found significant reductions in all-cause and CVD mortality (Nothlings et al. 2008). Overall, prospective studies of CVD in individuals with diabetes are few and limited in their assessment of the association between GI and GL and all-cause or CVD mortality risk, and thus there remains a need for further exploration of any associations.

4.3.2.2 Retinopathy and Macular Degeneration

At the microvascular level, diabetes increases the risk of eye diseases, especially DR (The Diabetes Control and Complications Trial Research Group 1997, U.K. Prospective Diabetes Study [UKPDS] Group 1998). Age-related macular degeneration (AMD) is a leading cause of vision loss in the elderly. Studies suggest that older people with diabetes are more susceptible to AMD than those people without diabetes (Tumosa 2008). The risk of both DR and AMD may be greatly impacted by hyperglycemia (Chiu and Taylor 2011). To the best of our knowledge, there has been one observational study that assessed GI on retinal parameters and found that it was associated with both DR and AMD (Kaushik et al. 2008). The Blue Mountain Eye Study was a population-based cohort followed for 10 years, with retinal photographs taken at baseline and at 10-year follow up. A cross-sectional analysis of the 1952 participants who were re-examined at 10-year follow up found that a higher mean dietary GI was associated with a 77% increased 10-year risk of early AMD when comparing the highest and lowest quartiles of GI (relative risk = 1.77; 95% CI 1.13 to 2.78; p trend = .03). Early AMD is a recognized precursor of sight-threatening late AMD (Kaushik et al. 2008). In the same cohort, a doubling in the risk of stroke was demonstrated between the highest and lowest GI tertile, as well as a fivefold increased risk of stroke when the highest GI and the lowest cereal fiber tertile were combined and compared to the lowest GI and highest cereal fiber intake tertile (Kaushik et al. 2009). In addition, increasing GI and decreasing cereal fiber were associated with significant retinal (venular) vessel widening (p trend < .01), which is associated with markers of inflammation and endothelial dysfunction (Ikram et al. 2004, Klein et al. 2006, de Jong et al. 2007) and is known to predict stroke (Kaushik et al. 2009). Furthermore, the increased risk of stroke mortality associated with a higher GI diet was attenuated by 50% after accounting for variations in retinal venular caliber, and thus it is thought that the deleterious cerebrovascular effects from high-GI diets could operate partly by anatomic effects on the cerebral microvasculature (Kaushik et al. 2009). Concerning another area of the eye, GI was found to significantly predict the incident of cortical cataract in the 10-year follow up of the cohort from the Blue Mountains Eye Study (Tan et al. 2007). Thus, there is some evidence that GI may be associated with eye diseases; however, limited assessment has been done to date, calling for a well-designed study to assess any association. The reader is referred to Chapter 11 for a detailed discussion of GI and eye disease.

4.3.2.3 Kidneys

Although very limited, there is also some evidence from observational studies that GI may affect microvascular disease at the level of the kidneys. In a longitudinal analysis of the Blue Mountains Eye Study, participants in the highest GI quartile had a 55% increased likelihood of having moderate chronic kidney disease as defined by an estimated glomerular filtration rate (eGFR) of > 60 mL/min/1.73 m^2, compared with those in the first quartile (multivariable adjusted odds ratio = 1.55; 95% CI 1.07 to 2.26; p trend = .01) (Gopinath et al. 2011). This suggests that a low GI diet may confer some benefit at the level of the kidney.

Overall, from the prospective studies done to date, low GI/GL diets may provide some benefit to the microvascular and macrovascular complications associated with diabetes; however, there is a need for more well-designed observational studies and randomized controlled trials to specifically explore any associations.

4.3.3 Clinical Trial Evidence

4.3.3.1 Glycemic Control

The primary focus for management of diabetes is glycemic control. A recent systematic review and meta-analysis of randomized controlled clinical trials of < 6 months in those with type 2 diabetes demonstrated a significant improvement in HbA1c (MD = −0.14%, 95% CI −0.24 to −0.03%, $p < .008$) (Ajala et al. 2013). Although the reduction was small (0.14 HbA1c units), only three trials were included in this meta-analysis due to the restriction on length of follow up (Ajala et al. 2013). Of these three trials, two did not demonstrate a significant effect of GI. However, one of these trials, by Wolever et al. (2008), included 156 participants who commenced the study with already optimized HbA1c levels at baseline (mean of 6.1%) who did not yet require oral hypoglycemic medication, and the other study by Ma et al. (2008) of 40 participants with diabetes did not achieve a significant GI (or GL) difference between the two groups since the actual difference at 12 months was only four GI units. Their study did however demonstrate that significantly less anti-diabetic medication was required in those given the low GI dietary advice compared to those given the American Diabetes Association-recommended dietary advice. The one study of these three, the study by Jenkins et al. (2008), which did show a significant reduction of 0.5% HbA1c on the low GI diet, this being significantly lower than on the control high cereal fiber diet, had 210 participants with type 2 diabetes commence with a mean HbA1c level of 7.1% and achieved an 11 unit GI difference between the two groups. Thus, in participants with less well-controlled diabetes (baseline HbA1c between 6.6% and 8.5%) and with an achievement of a significant GI difference between treatment groups, the 0.5% reduction observed on the low GI diet versus the 0.2% on the control high cereal fiber diet demonstrates the effectiveness of the GI. This is so because a relative reduction of 0.3% is considered clinically significant by the FDA in assessing new drug therapies (U.S. Food and Drug Administration 2008), and 0.5% is comparable to the absolute decrease achieved through some anti-diabetic medications for type 2 diabetes (United Kingdom Prospective Diabetes Study [UKPDS] 1995, Holman et al. 1999). Another recent systematic review and meta-analysis that included 19 trials, which were either randomized controlled trials or case-control studies, in those with diabetes, where the shortest follow up was 2 weeks, also demonstrated significant benefits in both HbA1c (standardized mean difference [SMD] = −0.42, 95%CI −0.69 to −0.16, $p < .01$) and fructosamine (SMD= −0.44, 95% CI −0.82 to −0.06, $p = .02$) on low GI versus high-GI diets (Wang et al. 2014).

It has been criticized that it is difficult to isolate the beneficial effects of GI and GL from the benefits of dietary fiber because they are often studied in combination (Evert et al. 2014). However, some trials, such as that of Jenkins et al. (2008), controlled for dietary fiber in the low GI and control high cereal fiber diets, and the beneficial effects of low GI prevailed. Furthermore, another study that compared a low GI diet to a measured carbohydrate exchange diet in children with type 1 diabetes demonstrated that twice as many participants on the low GI diet reached acceptable HbA1c levels at 12 months compared to those on the carbohydrate exchange diet (Gilbertson et al. 2001). Overall, there is evidence that low GI diets reduce HbA1c in those with diabetes; however, more trials with stricter inclusion criteria for participants, a greater difference in GI between the treatment arms, and longer follow up are warranted to confirm this beneficial long-term effect of GI/GL on glycemic control.

In addition to the three aforementioned long-term studies, there are many shorter randomized controlled clinical trials that have been performed to assess the effect of GI and GL on glycemia. The systematic review and meta-analysis by Thomas and Elliott (2010) included 12 randomized controlled trials lasting < 4 weeks in individuals with diabetes whose glycemic control was not optimized at baseline and where glycemic control was the primary outcome. Seven of the twelve trials contained data (from 457 participants with diabetes) on HbA1c and demonstrated that low GI diets reduced HbA1c significantly more than the control diets by 0.43% (MD = −0.43%; 95% CI −0.69 to −0.17, $p = .001$) (Thomas and Elliott 2010) (Figure 4.5). Therefore, the overall effect observed in the meta-analysis is once more found to be close to what is considered clinically meaningful (U.S. Food and Drug Administration 2008).

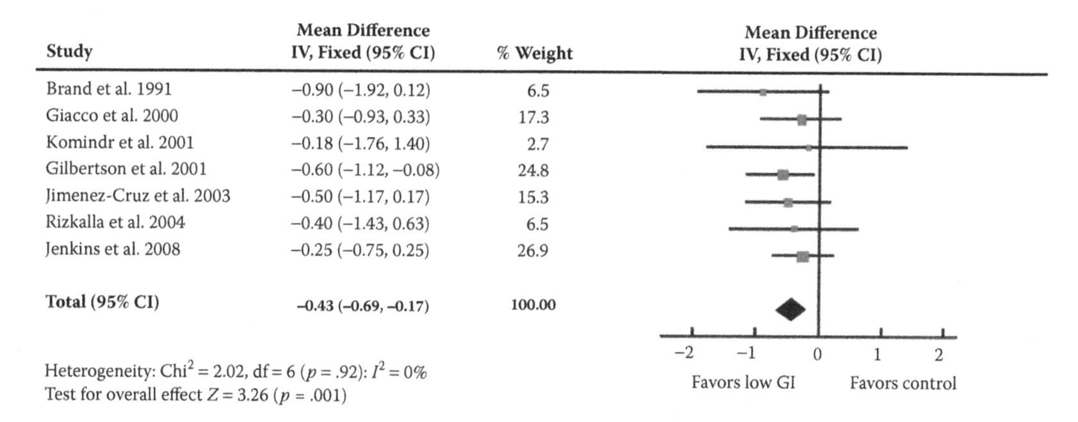

FIGURE 4.5 Meta-analysis of randomized controlled trials on the effect of a low GI diet compared to control diet (high GI or other) on HbA1c (%) in those with diabetes. The pooled effect estimate is represented as a diamond. The p-value is for a generic inverse-variance fixed-effects model. All data are presented as effect estimates with 95% confidence intervals. CI, confidence interval; IV, inverse variance; GI, glycemic index; HbA1c, hemoglobin A1c; SD, standard deviation. (Adapted from Thomas, D.E. and Elliott, E.J., *Br. J. Nutr.*, 104, 2010797–802. With permission.)

Furthermore, pooled analyses of four of the twelve trials that reported fructosamine (from 141 participants with diabetes) demonstrated a reduction in its concentration on a low versus a high-GI diet ($p = .05$), while one of the twelve identified trials in this systematic review and meta-analysis that measured glycosylated albumin demonstrated a significant reduction with a low GI ($p < .05$) but not a high-GI diet (Thomas and Elliott 2010). Taken together, these findings indicate that a low GI diet results in better medium to long-term glycemic control compared to a high-GI diet, supporting previous systematic reviews and meta-analyses, which have also concluded that low GI diets improve glycemic control (Brand-Miller et al. 2003, Livesey et al. 2008), including in those with type 1 diabetes (Collier et al. 1988, Giacco et al. 2000, Gilbertson et al. 2001).

In addition to these findings, pulses (dried leguminous seeds, including chickpeas, beans, peas, and lentils), which are particularly low in GI, have also been assessed within the context of a low GI diet. In a systematic review and meta-analysis conducted by Sievenpiper et al. (2009), pulses were demonstrated to significantly reduce markers of long-term glycemic control, including glycated proteins, measured by HbA1c or fructosamine, compared to a high-GI diet, in both individuals with and without diabetes (Figure 4.6).

Furthermore, low GL diets have been demonstrated to significantly reduce HbA1c compared to low-fat diets in a randomized trial of 79 obese participants with type 2 diabetes (low GL $-0.8\% \pm 1.3\%$ vs. low fat $-0.1\% \pm 0.2\%$; $p = .01$) in the context of long-term (40 weeks) hypocaloric diets resulting in similar weight loss (Fabricatore et al. 2011b).

The additional noteworthy benefit of a low GI diet over some anti-diabetic medications is that it reduces glycemia without the relevant adverse effects that are often associated with some anti-diabetic medications, specifically hypoglycemia, which has recently been suggested to contribute to the risk of diabetes complications (Gross et al. 2011). Two studies in the systematic review by Thomas and Elliott (2010) report on low GI diets and hypoglycemia in individuals with type 1 diabetes mellitus. One of these studies conducted in adults found significantly fewer episodes of hypoglycemia on the low GI, high-fiber diet compared to the high-GI, low-fiber diet (Giacco et al. 2000). The second (in children) found that although there were no significant differences in hypoglycemia, there were significantly fewer episodes of hyperglycemia reported on the low GI diet (Gilbertson et al. 2001). The latter study also reported that quality of life was significantly higher on the low GI diet compared to the standard of care, carbohydrate exchange diet, as assessed by difficulty in selecting

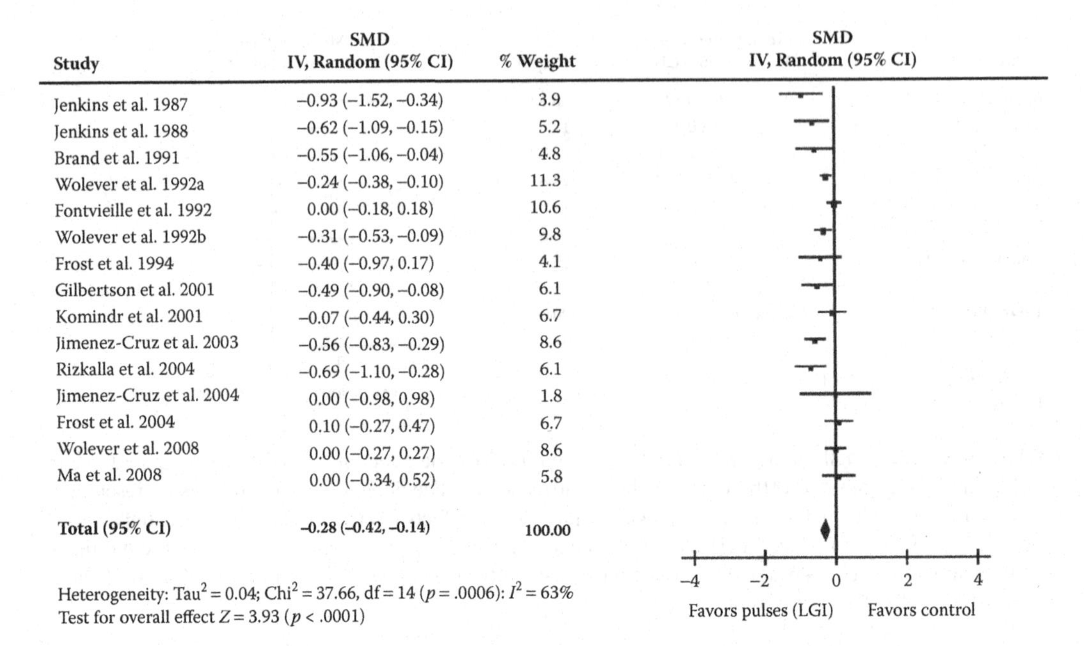

Study	SMD IV, Random (95% CI)	% Weight
Jenkins et al. 1987	−0.93 (−1.52, −0.34)	3.9
Jenkins et al. 1988	−0.62 (−1.09, −0.15)	5.2
Brand et al. 1991	−0.55 (−1.06, −0.04)	4.8
Wolever et al. 1992a	−0.24 (−0.38, −0.10)	11.3
Fontvieille et al. 1992	0.00 (−0.18, 0.18)	10.6
Wolever et al. 1992b	−0.31 (−0.53, −0.09)	9.8
Frost et al. 1994	−0.40 (−0.97, 0.17)	4.1
Gilbertson et al. 2001	−0.49 (−0.90, −0.08)	6.1
Komindr et al. 2001	−0.07 (−0.44, 0.30)	6.7
Jimenez-Cruz et al. 2003	−0.56 (−0.83, −0.29)	8.6
Rizkalla et al. 2004	−0.69 (−1.10, −0.28)	6.1
Jimenez-Cruz et al. 2004	0.00 (−0.98, 0.98)	1.8
Frost et al. 2004	0.10 (−0.27, 0.47)	6.7
Wolever et al. 2008	0.00 (−0.27, 0.27)	8.6
Ma et al. 2008	0.00 (−0.34, 0.52)	5.8
Total (95% CI)	**−0.28 (−0.42, −0.14)**	**100.00**

Heterogeneity: $Tau^2 = 0.04$; $Chi^2 = 37.66$, $df = 14$ ($p = .0006$): $I^2 = 63\%$
Test for overall effect $Z = 3.93$ ($p < .0001$)

FIGURE 4.6 Meta-analysis of randomized controlled trials on the effect of pulses as part of a low glycemic index diet compared to a high glycemic index diet on HbA1c (%) in those with and without diabetes. The pooled effect estimate is represented as a diamond. The p value is for a generic inverse-variance random-effects model. All data are presented as effect estimates with 95% confidence intervals. CI, confidence interval; HbA1c, hemoglobin A1c; IV, inverse variance; LGI, low glycemic index; SMD, standardized mean difference. (Adapted from Sievenpiper, J.L. et al., *Diabetologia,* 52, 1479–1495, 2009. With permission.) (References to included studies: Jenkins et al. 1988, Jenkins et al. 1987, Brand et al. 1991, Wolever et al. 1992a, b, 2008, Fontvieille et al. 1992, Frost et al. 1994, 2004, Gilbertson et al. 2001, Komindr et al. 2001, Jimenez-Cruz et al. 2003, Jimenez-Cruz et al. 2004, Rizkalla et al. 2004, Ma et al. 2008.)

meals (Gilbertson et al. 2001). Thus, a low GI diet may be useful in managing glycemic control in both type 1 and type 2 diabetes mellitus without the pharmacological risk of hypoglycemia.

4.3.3.2 Microvascular Disease

Tight glycemic control has been demonstrated to improve microvascular complications of diabetes (Boussageon et al. 2011). The Diabetes Control and Complications Trial (DCCT) in individuals with type 1 diabetes, randomized to receive either intensive or conventional treatment for glycemic control, found a significant relationship between HbA1c level and risk of microvascular complications, including retinopathy and nephropathy. Thus, better glycemic control was found to significantly reduce microvascular risk (Lachin et al. 2008). Furthermore, in those intensively treated participants who had provided dietary data, diets higher in fat and saturated fat and lower in carbohydrate were found to be associated with worse glycemic control, independently of exercise and BMI (Delahanty et al. 2009). This confirms that carbohydrate consumption per se may be of importance in diabetes management, as suggested by dietary guidelines (Mann et al. 2004, Diabetes U.K. Nutrition working group 2011, Italian Society of Human Nutrition [SINU] 2012, Canadian Diabetes Association Clinical Practice Guidelines Expert Committee et al. 2013a, Diabetes Australia 2014, Evert et al. 2014, International Diabetes Federation Guideline Development Group 2014). However, specific clinical trials on low GI diets directly assessing the effects on DR or nephropathy are lacking and necessary.

4.3.3.3 Macrovascular Disease

At the macrovascular level, although there is a lack of controlled clinical trials assessing the effects of GI and GL on cardiovascular risk in diabetes, a few trials, including some conducted with acarbose, suggest a potential benefit. A surrogate measure of CVD is endothelial function, which can be measured by flow-mediated dilation (FMD), a measure that has been demonstrated to be a predictor of CVD events (Yeboah et al. 2007, Rossi et al. 2008). In a 3-month randomized controlled clinical trial of high versus low GI weight loss diets matched for macronutrients and dietary fiber in 40 overweight and obese participants, FMD was significantly improved on the low GI diet compared to the high-GI diet ($p < .005$) (Buscemi et al. 2013).

Furthermore, a pilot study conducted in 38 men with at least 1 CHD risk factor randomized to a low or high-GI diet for 6 months along with healthy eating and weight loss advice, demonstrated that 24-h blood pressure was significantly improved in those on the low GI versus high-GI diet (Philippou et al. 2009). Additionally, the study demonstrated that carotid-femoral pulse wave velocity, which is a surrogate measure of arterial compliance (an index of the elasticity of large arteries and an important cardiovascular risk factor), was only significantly improved on the low GI diet (Philippou et al. 2009). FMD, 24-hour blood pressure and carotid-femoral pulse wave velocity are all measures of endothelial dysfunction resulting from insulin resistance, which reduces nitric oxide production and may be associated with increased production of reactive oxygen species, collectively leading to atherosclerosis (Giugliano et al. 1996, Brillante et al. 2009). Interestingly, a low GI diet has previously also been shown in 292 healthy adults to be associated with a reduction in oxidative stress compared to a high-GI diet (Hu et al. 2006, Ceriello and Ihnat 2010).

Another surrogate measure of CVD is carotid intima media thickness (CIMT), validated as a predictor of CVD risk, and is a preferred measure over FMD in clinical trials since measures are more consistent. Although its use in trial assessment has been debated, CIMT can be used reliably for diagnosis (Costanzo et al. 2012). In a 12-month clinical trial in those with type 2 diabetes randomized to receive a sulfonylurea with or without acarbose, a significant reduction in CIMT was demonstrated only in the group given acarbose (Oyama et al. 2008), thus indicating a potential reduction in arteriosclerotic risk. Furthermore, in a meta-analysis of randomized controlled trials on the effect of alpha-glucosidase inhibitors on CIMT, where 5 trials of 411 participants were identified, alpha-glucosidase therapy was associated with a significant reduction in the progression of CIMT and subgroup analyses demonstrated a significant effect both in those with type 2 diabetes ($n = 4$ trials) and those with IGT ($n = 1$ trial) (Geng et al. 2011). These data are in line with an international multicenter, double-blind, placebo-controlled trial of 1429 participants with IGT randomly assigned to receive either 100 mg of acarbose three times a day or placebo (Chiasson et al. 2003). Although this was a secondary analysis and in a small sample, acarbose was demonstrated to result in a 49% relative risk reduction in the development of CVD events (hazard ratio [HR] = 0.51, 95% CI 0.28 to 0.93, $p = .03$) and a 34% reduction in new cases of hypertension (HR = 0.66, 95% CI 0.49 to 0.89, $p = .006$) over 3 years, even after adjustment for major risk factors (Chiasson et al. 2003). A larger CVD event trial with acarbose in those with diabetes is currently underway. Additionally, a meta-analysis of seven randomized double-blind placebo-controlled acarbose studies with a minimum treatment duration of 52 weeks in individuals with type 2 diabetes demonstrated that acarbose showed favorable trends toward risk reduction in all categories of CVD, with a significant reduction for any CVD event (HR = 0.65, 95% CI 0.48 to 0.88, $p < .01$) (Hanefeld et al. 2004). Therefore, interventions that improve postprandial hyperglycemia, such as acarbose and thus potentially low GI diets, may improve cardiovascular risk.

Recently, the Spanish PREDIMED study of 7447 participants, which was a randomized trial of a low GI Mediterranean diet supplemented with extra virgin olive oil or nuts, compared to a low-fat diet for primary cardiovascular prevention, demonstrated that both supplemented Mediterranean diets significantly reduced incidence of major cardiovascular events over a median follow up of

4.8 years (Estruch et al. 2013). In a longitudinal analysis of 2866 participants without diabetes and at high risk of CVD, the Mediterranean diet interventions were associated with reductions in dietary GI and GL and were inversely associated with the GI and GL of the control diet group (Rodriguez-Rejon et al. 2014). Furthermore, when the data was assessed for associations with all-cause mortality, a high GI/GL was positively associated with all-cause mortality when comparing those in the highest to lowest quartile of GI and GL, over a median follow up of 4.7 years (Castro-Quezada et al. 2014). Therefore, a long-term trial assessing the effect of a low GI diet on CIMT by cardiovascular ultrasound or plaque volume by magnetic resonance imaging (MRI) in those with diabetes would be of great interest, in addition to a longer follow-up trial with CVD events being the primary outcome in high CVD risk individuals.

4.4 GI MECHANISMS OF ACTION

The main issue following consumption of a high GI or GL food or meal is that it results in a rapid rise in blood glucose which stimulates the production of insulin. This is exacerbated in overweight and/or insulin resistant individuals whose circulating free fatty acids are also elevated, resulting in postprandial hyperglycemia, hyperinsulinemia, and hyperlipidemia (Samuel and Shulman 2012). Over time, this increased demand on pancreatic beta cells may result in beta-cell dysfunction utimately lead to beta cell death (Jenkins and Wolever 1981, Willett et al. 2002, Pawlak et al. 2004), thus reducing the ability to secrete insulin in response to elevations in blood glucose. Conversely, low GI foods reduce the rate of carbohydrate absorption and would be expected to cause a lower rise in blood glucose compared to higher GI foods (Jenkins et al. 2002) (Figure 4.7).

This has been demonstrated in a study of free-living people with type 2 diabetes and obesity, where using a continuous glucose monitoring device and a simultaneous 3-day food record

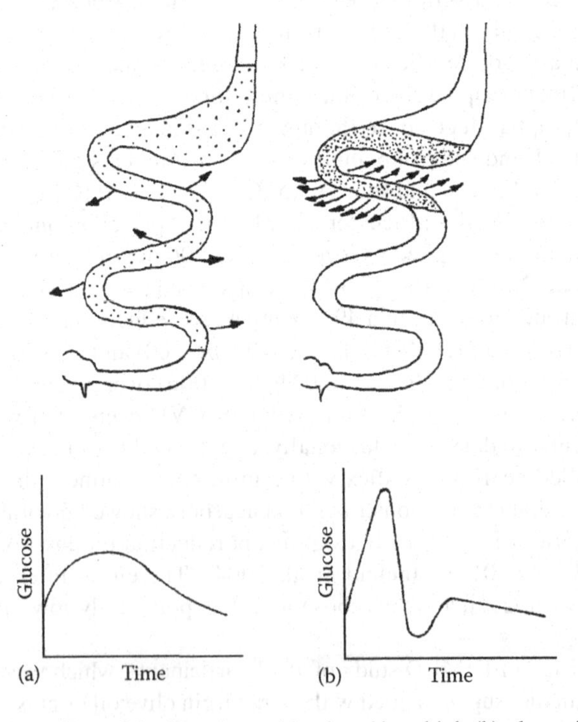

FIGURE 4.7 Hypothetical effect of feeding diets with a low (a) or high (b) glycemic index on gastrointestinal glucose absorption. (Adapted from Jenkins, D.J. et al., *Am. J. Clin. Nutr.*, 76, 266S–273S, 2002. With permission.)

(Fabricatore et al. 2011a), increasing dietary GI was shown to be positively associated with blood glucose area under the curve, mean glucose and hyperglycemic ranges, and negatively associated with euglycemic ranges (Fabricatore et al. 2011a). Dietary GI was also shown to be the strongest and the most consistent independent predictor of glycemic fluctuations (Fabricatore et al. 2011a). Thus, as a result of the consumption of a low GI diet, the reduction in glycemic fluctuations would lower the demand for insulin and thus reduce circulating insulin along with related gastrointestinal hormones, including the incretins, gastric inhibitory polypeptide (GIP), and glucagon-like peptide-1 (GLP-1) (Drucker 2015). Prolongation of glucose absorption and the longer but lower insulin concentration would maintain a longer suppression of free fatty acids, thereby improving cellular glucose metabolism while maintaining blood glucose concentration closer to baseline, despite continued absorption from the small intestine. This scenario has been demonstrated in healthy participants who sipped glucose over 4 h as opposed to drinking it in a bolus (Jenkins et al. 1990). Slowed absorption of glucose is relevant for both prevention and management of diabetes, as it helps prevent beta-cell exhaustion by reducing the insulin demand as well as minimizing oxidative stress and inflammation resulting from hyperglycemia. Furthermore, reduced insulin demand and improvement in insulin resistance are associated with prevention in the development of type 2 diabetes, better management of both type 1 and type 2 diabetes, and a reduction in the risk of microvascular and macrovascular complications (Kilpatrick et al. 2007).

The delayed absorption of carbohydrate in low GI foods through the above-described mechanisms can have multiple beneficial effects. First, it may affect body weight possibly due to increased satiety as shown in some studies (Ludwig 2000). Further to the possible mechanistic effect on body weight control, a low GI diet may reduce hunger by preventing hyperglycemia, since hyperinsulinemia that follows a high-GI/GL diet causes rapid reductions in blood glucose, depleting the metabolic fuels in the body, which in turn may stimulate hunger (Ludwig 2002). The reader is referred to Chapter 6 on GI and obesity prevention and management for further discussion of this issue. Second, there is evidence of a "second meal" effect where after consumption of a low GI meal, uptake of glucose after the subsequent meal is improved, possibly related to the prolonged suppression of free fatty acid concentrations (Jenkins et al. 1982, 1990). Third, it is hypothesized that at both the micro- and macrovascular levels, repeated occurrences of hyperglycemia and hypoglycemia (increased glycemic variability) may overwhelm the pathways by which glucose is metabolized, resulting in adverse reactions, including downregulation of genes involved in free radical detoxification, which result in formation of advanced glycation end products (AGEs) (Ceriello and Ihnat 2010). Glycemic variability has been demonstrated to activate oxidative stress (Brownlee and Hirsch 2006, Monnier et al. 2006, Ceriello and Ihnat 2010) whereas, by creating a more blunted and sustained glycemic response with a low GI diet, oxidative stress, as well as the production of AGEs, would be reduced. Furthermore, without the control of glycemic variability, AGEs, along with other molecules associated with oxidative damage and inflammation, may accumulate in the vasculature, altering cellular metabolism, causing dysfunction (glycating enzymes) and even cellular death, which contributes to the vascular complications of diabetes (Chiu and Taylor 2011). Overall, low GI diets may reduce the metabolic stress induced by rapid absorption of carbohydrates and may thus delay the progression of type 2 diabetes and the development of the associated vascular complications.

4.5 CONCLUSIONS AND PERSPECTIVES

Owing to the rapid rise in diabetes prevalence over the past few decades and the projected further increase over the next 20 years, as well as the many complications that develop as a result of diabetes, the quality and duration of life is severely diminished and the economic burden on our healthcare systems and individual patients is substantial. Thus, there is a need to find effective and sustainable prevention and treatment strategies for diabetes. Pharmacological strategies are being actively sought and many new drugs are being brought to market. Nevertheless, sustainable lifestyle changes, such as low GI diets, may be suitable to assist in both prevention and management of diabetes, possibly also allowing pharmacological therapy to be effective at lower doses with the subsequent lower risk of side effects. At this point in time, there is a lack of evidence on the effect of low GI diets on hard endpoints, particularly for CVD, which is the primary cause of death in diabetes. However, there is evidence that low GI diets may reduce the risk of diabetes and associated risk factors, including improving body weight and insulin resistance, and in clinical trials of participants with diabetes, improve glycemic control, CVD risk factors, and some diabetes-related complications. For these reasons, many international diabetes associations are now recommending low GI over high-GI carbohydrate choices (Table 4.1).

4.5.1 Recommendations for Future Research

As a result of the high global prevalence of diabetes, obesity, and the metabolic syndrome, there is a great need to identify strategies, specifically lifestyle changes, which may be effective in combating this challenge, for which there is growing evidence that low GI diets may be useful. Although there is evidence that low GI diets have been demonstrated to reduce the risk of diabetes and its associated conditions, including body weight and cholesterol, and specifically improve the control of blood glucose concentration, there is a great need for well-designed trials with harder endpoints. Observational studies exploring GI and GL on the management of diabetes complications are sparse and limited. The literature would benefit from a properly designed assessment of the association between GI/GL and diabetes complications including: (1) proper assessment of GI using validated FFQs in a cohort with diabetes, (2) FFQs to be collected at repeated time points over the duration of follow up for accurate representation, (3) proper assessment of the outcomes of interest, for example, DR using retinal photographs that are graded using specialized computer technology (Klein et al. 2006), and (4) longer follow up for better assessment of these outcomes.

Additionally, although there have been randomized controlled trials that have demonstrated benefit of low GI diets on glycemic control in diabetes, further trials, specifically assessing the hard endpoints of diabetes complications are warranted. These trials need to be specifically designed to assess both microvascular (DR and nephropathy) and macrovascular (cardiovascular development, CIMT and CVD events, and mortality) outcomes. A particularly useful trial would be one designed to assess plaque volume by MRI, including intraplaque hemorrhage and risk factors for plaque rupture, with longer follow up and CVD events being the primary outcome in high risk individuals (those with diabetes and the metabolic syndrome). For clinical trials, maintaining a significant difference in GI between the treatment groups, while holding all other variables constant, including dietary fiber, will also be an important consideration. Along these lines, it is necessary to provide consumers and health professionals with accurate and reliable information about the GI. This points to the need to develop GI education tools and make them widely available, as well as to have information on GI in food composition tables and food labels that should be updated at regular intervals (Augustin et al. 2015).

4.5.2 Recommendations for Dietary Choices for Those with Diabetes

Randomized controlled trials have fairly consistently shown a benefit of low GI diets on glycemic control in those with diabetes. Therefore, adopting a lower GI diet within the context of a healthy diet is advantageous, and the use of a low GI diet or low GI foods is recommended by diabetes guidelines internationally (Table 4.1). Examples of low GI dietary substitutions that could be implemented in a healthy diet are presented in Table 4.2. These modifications have been used in research (Jenkins et al. 2008, 2012, 2014) to reduce the GI of the diet by about 9–14 GI units and have demonstrated significant improvements in blood glucose control in diabetes.

TABLE 4.2
Example of Low GI Dietary Substitutions for a 2000 kcal Diet

		Portion Size	Choose	GI[a]	Instead of	GI[a]
7 servings	Cereal	⅓ cup dry	Steel cut oats	57	Instant oatmeal	83
			Oat bran	56	Cream of wheat	70
			All bran buds with psyllium	53	Pancakes	76
					Rice crisp cereal	82
	Pulses	½ cup cooked	Red, navy beans	39		
		or canned	Baked beans	56		
		low salt	Lentils	30		
			Chick peas	35		
	Other starchy	⅓ cup cooked	Pasta (al dente)	45	Rice noodles	62
	food	½ cup cooked	(White/whole wheat)	48	Rice	72
		½ cup cooked	Parboiled rice	53	Bread (white/whole	71
		½ cup cooked	Bulgur	28	wheat)	
		½ cup cooked	Barley	54		
			Quinoa[b]			
		⅓ cup cooked	Sweet potato/yam	54	Boiled potato	86
	Fruits	1 small	Apple	36	Banana	60
3 servings		1 cup	Orange	37	Melon	68
		1½ cups	Blueberries[b]	48	Watermelon	76
			Raspberries[b]	34	Pineapple	66
			Strawberries	40		
5+ servings	Vegetables	½ cup	All, especially eggplant and okra			
2 servings	Meat and dairy	60–90 g	Soy burgers/dogs	N/A	Fatty meats, sausage	N/A
	alternates	60–90 g	Tofu, seitan		Cream, ice cream, full	
		10	Tempeh, miso		fat yoghurt/milk	
		1–2	Nuts (almonds, walnuts,		Cheese > 15% fat	
		1 cup	pistachios, and hazel nuts)			
		1½ oz (45 g)	Eggs			
			Yoghurt (low fat, low sugar)			
			Skim or 1% milk			
			Soy beverage, fortified			
			Reduced fat cheese (<15% fat)			
	Snacks and	As listed above	Fruits, vegetables, andunsalted	above	Chips	63
	desserts		nuts	N/A	Popcorn	65
			Yoghurt (plain, low sugar)	19	Cakes	38–67
					Cookies (e.g., digestive)	59
	Spreads	1 tsp.	Peanut/almond butter	N/A	Butter	N/A
		1 tbsp.	Soft margarine Guacamole	N/A	Jam with sugar	50
		1 tsp	Hummus	N/A		
			Jam (no sugar reduced sugar)	6		
				26		
				51		
	Drinks		Water, tea, coffee, and	N/A	Fruit juice (e.g., orange	50
			sugar-free drinks	N/A	and cranberry)	59
			Low salt vegetable juice	31	Regular pop	63
			(e.g., tomato)			

Note: GI, glycemic index; GL, glycemic load; MF, milk fat. N/A, not applicable since the food is not a significant source of carbohydrates.

[a] GI values are presented on the glucose scale (to convert to the bread scale, multiply by 1.41). Classification: GI ≤ 55 = low GI; 56–69 = medium GI; ≥ 70 = high GI. GI values are approximate values obtained from an average of those tested and presented in the International Tables of GI and GL values (Atkinson, F. S. et al. 2008. *Diabetes Care*. 31:2281–2283).

[b] For these foods, GI testing was performed through the University of Toronto at Glycemic Index Laboratories, Canada.

It is advisable that those who are consuming a high-GI diet could make gradual dietary changes starting with replacing one high-GI food item with a low GI one at each meal, including the substitution of a high-GI fruit with a low GI fruit. The latter change has been shown to be associated with improvements in glycemic control (Jenkins et al. 2011). In order for the public to make low GI choices, they will require validated tools and education. This point further highlights the need for better validated GI education tools for both health professionals and the public.

REFERENCES

Action to Control Cardiovascular Risk in Diabetes Study Group, H. C. Gerstein, M. E. Miller, R. P. Byington, D. C. Goff, Jr., J. T. Bigger, J. B. Buseet al. 2008. Effects of intensive glucose lowering in type 2 diabetes. *N Engl J Med*, 358(24):2545–2559. doi: 10.1056/NEJMoa0802743.

Advance Collaborative Group, A. Patel, S. MacMahon, J. Chalmers, B. Neal, L. Billot, M. Woodward et al. 2008. Intensive blood glucose control and vascular outcomes in patients with type 2 diabetes. *N Engl J Med*, 358 (24):2560–2572. doi: 10.1056/NEJMoa0802987.

Ajala, O., P. English, and J. Pinkney. 2013. Systematic review and meta-analysis of different dietary approaches to the management of type 2 diabetes. *Am J Clin Nutr*, 97(3):505–516. doi: 10.3945/ajcn.112.042457.

Aller, E. E., T. M. Larsen, H. Claus, A. K. Lindroos, A. Kafatos, A. Pfeiffer, J. A. Martinez et al. 2014. Weight loss maintenance in overweight subjects on ad libitum diets with high or low protein content and glycemic index: The DIOGENES trial 12-month results. *Int J Obes (Lond)*, 38(12):1511–1517. doi: 10.1038/ijo.2014.52.

American Diabetes Association. 2010. Diagnosis and classification of diabetes mellitus. *Diabetes Care*, 33(Suppl 1):S62–S69. doi: 10.2337/dc10-S062.

American Diabetes Association. 2015. (6) Glycemic targets. *Diabetes Care*, 38(Suppl 1):S33–S40. doi: 10.2337/dc15-S009.

Anderson, T. J., J. Gregoire, R. A. Hegele, P. Couture, G. B. Mancini, R. McPherson, G. A. Francis et al. 2013. 2012 update of the Canadian Cardiovascular Society guidelines for the diagnosis and treatment of dyslipidemia for the prevention of cardiovascular disease in the adult. *Can J Cardiol*, 29(2):151–167. doi: 10.1016/j.cjca.2012.11.032.

Atkinson, F. S., K. Foster-Powell, and J. C. Brand-Miller. 2008. International tables of glycemic index and glycemic load values: 2008. *Diabetes Care*, 31(12):2281–2283.

Augustin, L. S., C. W. Kendall, D. J. Jenkins, W. C. Willett, A. Astrup, A. W. Barclay, I. Bjorck, J. C. et al. 2015. Glycemic index, glycemic load and glycemic response: An international scientific consensus summit from the international carbohydrate quality consortium (ICQC). *Nutr Metab Cardiovasc Dis*, 25(9):795–815. doi: 10.1016/j.numecd.2015.05.005.

Balkau, B., L. Mhamdi, J. M. Oppert, J. Nolan, A. Golay, F. Porcellati, M. Laakso, E. Ferrannini, and Egir-Risc Study Group. 2008. Physical activity and insulin sensitivity: The RISC study. *Diabetes*, 57(10):2613–2618. doi: 10.2337/db07-1605.

Barbarroja, N., C. Lopez-Pedrera, L. Garrido-Sanchez, M. D. Mayas, W. Oliva-Olivera, M. R. Bernal-Lopez, R. El Bekay, and F. J. Tinahones. 2012. Progression from high insulin resistance to type 2 diabetes does not entail additional visceral adipose tissue inflammation. *PLoS One*, 7(10):e48155. doi: 10.1371/journal.pone.0048155.

Barclay, A. W., P. Petocz, J. McMillan-Price, V. M. Flood, T. Prvan, P. Mitchell, and J. C. Brand-Miller. 2008. Glycemic index, glycemic load, and chronic disease risk—A meta-analysis of observational studies. *Am J Clin Nutr*, 87(3):627–637.

Berg, A. H. and P. E. Scherer. 2005. Adipose tissue, inflammation, and cardiovascular disease. *Circ Res*, 96(9):939–949. doi: 10.1161/01.RES.0000163635.62927.34.

Bhupathiraju, S. N., D. K. Tobias, V. S. Malik, A. Pan, A. Hruby, J. E. Manson, W. C. Willett, and F. B. Hu. 2014. Glycemic index, glycemic load, and risk of type 2 diabetes: Results from 3 large US cohorts and an updated meta-analysis. *Am J Clin Nutr*, 100(1):218–232. doi: 10.3945/ajcn.113.079533.

Boden, W. E. 2000. High-density lipoprotein cholesterol as an independent risk factor in cardiovascular disease: Assessing the data from Framingham to the Veterans Affairs High—Density Lipoprotein Intervention Trial. *Am J Cardiol*, 86(12A):19L–22L.

Bouche, C., S. W. Rizkalla, J. Luo, H. Vidal, A. Veronese, N. Pacher, C. Fouquet, V. Lang, and G. Slama. 2002. Five-week, low-glycemic index diet decreases total fat mass and improves plasma lipid profile in moderately overweight nondiabetic men. *Diabetes Care*, 25(5):822–828.

Boussageon, R., T. Bejan-Angoulvant, M. Saadatian-Elahi, S. Lafont, C. Bergeonneau, B. Kassai, S. Erpeldinger, J. M. Wright, F. Gueyffier, and C. Cornu. 2011. Effect of intensive glucose lowering treatment on all cause mortality, cardiovascular death, and microvascular events in type 2 diabetes: Meta-analysis of randomised controlled trials. *BMJ*, 343:d4169. doi: 10.1136/bmj.d4169.

Brand-Miller, J., S. Hayne, P. Petocz, and S. Colagiuri. 2003. Low-glycemic index diets in the management of diabetes: A meta-analysis of randomized controlled trials. *Diabetes Care*, 26(8):2261–2267.

Brand, J. C., S. Colagiuri, S. Crossman, A. Allen, D. C. Roberts, and A. S. Truswell. 1991. Low-glycemic index foods improve long-term glycemic control in NIDDM. *Diabetes Care*, 14(2):95–101.

Brillante, D. G., A. J. O'Sullivan, and L. G. Howes. 2009. Arterial stiffness in insulin resistance: The role of nitric oxide and angiotensin II receptors. *Vasc Health Risk Manag*, 5(1):73–78.

Brownlee, M. and I. B. Hirsch. 2006. Glycemic variability: A hemoglobin A1c-independent risk factor for diabetic complications. *JAMA*, 295(14):1707–1708. doi: 10.1001/jama.295.14.1707.

Bullo Bonet, M. 2002. Leptin in the regulation of energy balance. *Nutr Hosp*, 17(Suppl 1):42–48.

Bullo, M., R. Casas, M. P. Portillo, J. Basora, R. Estruch, A. Garcia-Arellano, A. Lasa, M. Juanola-Falgarona, F. Aros, and J. Salas-Salvado. 2013. Dietary glycemic index/load and peripheral adipokines and inflammatory markers in elderly subjects at high cardiovascular risk. *Nutr Metab Cardiovasc Dis*, 23(5):443–450. doi: 10.1016/j.numecd.2011.09.009.

Burcelin, R., L. Garidou, and C. Pomie. 2012. Immuno-microbiota cross and talk: The new paradigm of metabolic diseases. *Semin Immunol*, 24(1):67–74. doi: 10.1016/j.smim.2011.11.011.

Burger, K. N., J. W. Beulens, Y. T. van der Schouw, I. Sluijs, A. M. Spijkerman, D. Sluik, H. Boeing et al. 2012. Dietary fiber, carbohydrate quality and quantity, and mortality risk of individuals with diabetes mellitus. *PLoS One*, 7(8):e43127. doi: 10.1371/journal.pone.0043127.

Burke, B. J., M. Hartog, K. W. Heaton, and S. Hooper. 1982. Assessment of the metabolic effects of dietary carbohydrate and fibre by measuring urinary excretion of C-peptide. *Hum Nutr Clin Nutr*, 36(5):373–380.

Buscemi, S., L. Cosentino, G. Rosafio, M. Morgana, A. Mattina, D. Sprini, S. Verga, and G. B. Rini. 2013. Effects of hypocaloric diets with different glycemic indexes on endothelial function and glycemic variability in overweight and in obese adult patients at increased cardiovascular risk. *Clin Nutr*, 32(3):346–352. doi: 10.1016/j.clnu.2012.10.006.

Buyken, A. E., J. Goletzke, G. Joslowski, A. Felbick, G. Cheng, C. Herder, and J. C. Brand-Miller. 2014. Association between carbohydrate quality and inflammatory markers: Systematic review of observational and interventional studies. *Am J Clin Nutr*, 99(4):813–833. doi: 10.3945/ajcn.113.074252.

Canadian Diabetes Association Clinical Practice Guideline Expert Committee, S. R. Boyd, A. Advani, F. Altomare, and F. Stockl. 2013a. Retinopathy. *Can J Diabetes*, 37(Suppl 1):S137– S141. doi: 10.1016/j.jcjd.2013.01.038.

Canadian Diabetes Association Clinical Practice Guidelines Expert Committee, P. D. Dworatzek, K. Arcudi, R. Gougeon, N. Husein, J. L. Sievenpiper, and S. L. Williams. 2013a. Nutrition therapy. *Can J Diabetes*, 37(Suppl 1):S45–S55. doi: 10.1016/j.jcjd.2013.01.019.

Canadian Diabetes Association Clinical Practice Guidelines Expert Committee, S. A. Imran, R. Rabasa-Lhoret, and S. Ross. 2013b. Targets for glycemic control. *Can J Diabetes*, 37(Suppl 1):S31–S34. doi: 10.1016/j.jcjd.2013.01.016.

Canadian Diabetes Association Clinical Practice Guidelines Expert Committee, T. Ransom, R. Goldenberg, A. Mikalachki, A. P. Prebtani, and Z. Punthakee. 2013c. Reducing the risk of developing diabetes. *Can J Diabetes*, 37(Suppl 1):S16–S19. doi: 10.1016/j.jcjd.2013.01.013.

Canadian Diabetes Association Clinical Practice Guidelines Expert Committee, S. Wharton, A. M. Sharma, and D. C. Lau. 2013d. Weight management in diabetes. *Can J Diabetes*, 37(Suppl 1):S82– S86. doi: 10.1016/j.jcjd.2013.01.025.

Castro-Quezada, I., A. Sanchez-Villegas, R. Estruch, J. Salas-Salvado, D. Corella, H. Schroder, J. Alvarez-Perez et al. 2014. A high dietary glycemic index increases total mortality in a Mediterranean population at high cardiovascular risk. *PLoS One*, 9(9):e107968. doi: 10.1371/journal.pone.0107968.

Centers for Disease Control and Prevention (CDC). 2015. Vision Health Initiative. National Center for Health Statistics, Division of Health Interview Statistics, data from the National Health Interview Survey. http://www.cdc.gov/visionhealth/basic_information/eye_disorders.htm. (Accessed July 10, 2015.)

Ceriello, A. and M. A. Ihnat. 2010. Glycaemic variability: A new therapeutic challenge in diabetes and the critical care setting. *Diabet Med*, 27(8):862–867. doi: 10.1111/j.1464-5491.2010.02967.x.

Chiasson, J. L., R. G. Josse, R. Gomis, M. Hanefeld, A. Karasik, and M. Laakso. 2003. Acarbose treatment and the risk of cardiovascular disease and hypertension in patients with impaired glucose tolerance: The STOP-NIDDM trial. *JAMA*, 290(4):486–494.

Chiasson, J. L., R. G. Josse, R. Gomis, M. Hanefeld, A. Karasik, M. Laakso, and STOP-NIDDM Trail Research Group. 2002. Acarbose for prevention of type 2 diabetes mellitus: The STOP-NIDDM randomised trial. *Lancet*, 359(9323):2072–2077.

Chiu, C. J. and A. Taylor. 2011. Dietary hyperglycemia, glycemic index and metabolic retinal diseases. *Prog Retin Eye Res*, 30(1):18–53. doi: 10.1016/j.preteyeres.2010.09.001.

Cho, S. S., L. Qi, G. C. Fahey, Jr., and D. M. Klurfeld. 2013. Consumption of cereal fiber, mixtures of whole grains and bran, and whole grains and risk reduction in type 2 diabetes, obesity, and cardiovascular disease. *Am J Clin Nutr*, 98(2):594–619. doi: 10.3945/ajcn.113.067629.

CNIB. 2009. The cost of vision loss in Canada. CNIB and the Canadian Ophthalmological Society. Access Economics; 2009. http://www.cnib.ca/eng/cnib%20document%20library/research/covl_full_report.pdf. (Accessed July 10, 2015.)

Colagiuri S, Dickinson S, Girgis S, and Colagiuri R. 2009. *National Evidence Based Guideline for Blood Glucose Control in Type 2 Diabetes*. Diabetes Australia and the NHMRC. Canberra, Australia.

Collier, A., M. Jackson, R. M. Dawkes, D. Bell, and B. F. Clarke. 1988. Reduced free radical activity detected by decreased diene conjugates in insulin-dependent diabetic patients. *Diabet Med*, 5(8):747–749.

Control Group, F. M. Turnbull, C. Abraira, R. J. Anderson, R. P. Byington, J. P. Chalmers, W. C. Duckworth et al. 2009. Intensive glucose control and macrovascular outcomes in type 2 diabetes. *Diabetologia*, 52 (11):2288–2298. doi: 10.1007/s00125-009-1470-0.

Costanzo, P., J. G. Cleland, S. L. Atkin, E. Vassallo, and P. Perrone-Filardi. 2012. Use of carotid intima-media thickness regression to guide therapy and management of cardiac risks. *Curr Treat Options Cardiovasc Med*, 14(1):50–56. doi: 10.1007/s11936-011-0158-1.

Dansinger, M. L., A. Tatsioni, J. B. Wong, M. Chung, and E. M. Balk. 2007. Meta-analysis: The effect of dietary counseling for weight loss. *Ann Intern Med*, 147(1):41–50.

Dattilo, A. M. and P. M. Kris-Etherton. 1992. Effects of weight reduction on blood lipids and lipoproteins: A meta-analysis. *Am J Clin Nutr*, 56(2):320–328.

de Jong, F. J., M. K. Ikram, J. C. Witteman, A. Hofman, P. T. de Jong, and M. M. Breteler. 2007. Retinal vessel diameters and the role of inflammation in cerebrovascular disease. *Ann Neurol*, 61(5):491–495. doi: 10.1002/ana.21129.

de Rougemont, A., S. Normand, J. A. Nazare, M. R. Skilton, M. Sothier, S. Vinoy, and M. Laville. 2007. Beneficial effects of a 5-week low-glycaemic index regimen on weight control and cardiovascular risk factors in overweight non-diabetic subjects. *Br J Nutr*, 98(6):1288–1298. doi: 10.1017/S0007114507778674.

DeFronzo, R. A., R. Hendler, and D. Simonson. 1982. Insulin resistance is a prominent feature of insulin-dependent diabetes. *Diabetes*, 31(9):795–801.

Delahanty, L. M., D. M. Nathan, J. M. Lachin, F. B. Hu, P. A. Cleary, G. K. Ziegler, J. Wylie-Rosett, D. J. Wexler, and Diabetes Control Complications Trial/Epidemiology of Diabetes. 2009. Association of diet with glycated hemoglobin during intensive treatment of type 1 diabetes in the Diabetes Control and Complications Trial. *Am J Clin Nutr*, 89(2):518–524. doi: 10.3945/ajcn.2008.26498.

Delahanty, L. M., Q. Pan, K. A. Jablonski, V. R. Aroda, K. E. Watson, G. A. Bray, S. E. Kahn, J. C. Florez, L. Perreault, P. W. Franks, and Group Diabetes Prevention Program Research. 2014. Effects of weight loss, weight cycling, and weight loss maintenance on diabetes incidence and change in cardiometabolic traits in the Diabetes Prevention Program. *Diabetes Care*, 37(10):2738–2745. doi: 10.2337/dc14-0018.

Derosa, G., P. Maffioli, A. D'Angelo, E. Fogari, L. Bianchi, and A. F. Cicero. 2011. Acarbose on insulin resistance after an oral fat load: A double-blind, placebo controlled study. *J Diabetes Complications*, 25 (4):258–266. doi: 10.1016/j.jdiacomp.2011.01.003.

Devaraj, S., U. Singh, and I. Jialal. 2009. Human C-reactive protein and the metabolic syndrome. *Curr Opin Lipidol*, 20(3):182–189. doi: 10.1097/MOL.0b013e32832ac03e.

Diabetes Australia. 2014. General practice management of type 2 diabetes – 2014–15. Melbourne: The Royal Australian College of General Practitioners and Diabetes Australia. https://www.diabetesaustralia.com.au/best-practice-guidelines. (Accessed July 10, 2015.)

The Diabetes Control and Complications Trial Research Group. 1995. The relationship of glycemic exposure (HbA1c) to the risk of development and progression of retinopathy in the diabetes control and complications trial. *Diabetes*, 44(8):968–983.

The Diabetes Control and Complications Trial Research Group. 1997. Hypoglycemia in the Diabetes Control and Complications Trial. *Diabetes*, 46(2):271–286.

Diabetes Prevention Program Research Group, W. C. Knowler, S. E. Fowler, R. F. Hamman, C. A. Christophi, H. J. Hoffman, A. T. Brenneman et al. 2009. 10-year follow-up of diabetes incidence and weight loss in the Diabetes Prevention Program Outcomes Study. *Lancet*, 374(9702):1677–1686. doi: 10.1016/S0140-6736(09)61457-4.

Diabetes UK Nutrition working group. 2011. Evidence-based nutrition guidelines for the prevention and management of diabetes. https://www.diabetes.org.uk/nutrition-guidelines. (Accessed July 10, 2015.)
Dong, J. Y., L. Zhang, Y. H. Zhang, and L. Q. Qin. 2011. Dietary glycaemic index and glycaemic load in relation to the risk of type 2 diabetes: A meta-analysis of prospective cohort studies. *Br J Nutr*, 106(11):1649–1654. doi: 10.1017/S000711451100540X.
Drexel, H., S. Aczel, T. Marte, W. Benzer, P. Langer, W. Moll, and C. H. Saely. 2005. Is atherosclerosis in diabetes and impaired fasting glucose driven by elevated LDL cholesterol or by decreased HDL cholesterol? *Diabetes Care*, 28(1):101–107.
Drucker, D. J. 2015. Deciphering metabolic messages from the gut drives therapeutic innovation: The 2014 Banting Lecture. *Diabetes*, 64 (2):317–326. doi: 10.2337/db14-1514.
Du, H., A. Dl van der, M. M. van Bakel, C. J. van der Kallen, E. E. Blaak, M. M. van Greevenbroek, E. H. Jansen et al. 2008. Glycemic index and glycemic load in relation to food and nutrient intake and metabolic risk factors in a Dutch population. *Am J Clin Nutr*, 87(3):655–661.
Duckworth, W., C. Abraira, T. Moritz, D. Reda, N. Emanuele, P. D. Reaven, F. J. Zieve et al. 2009. Glucose control and vascular complications in veterans with type 2 diabetes. *N Engl J Med*, 360(2):129–139.
Esteve, E., W. Ricart, and J. M. Fernandez-Real. 2009. Adipocytokines and insulin resistance: The possible role of lipocalin-2, retinol binding protein-4, and adiponectin. *Diabetes Care*, 32(Suppl 2):S362–S367. doi: 10.2337/dc09-S340.
Estruch, R., E. Ros, J. Salas-Salvado, M. I. Covas, D. Corella, F. Aros, E. Gomez-Gracia et al. 2013. Primary prevention of cardiovascular disease with a Mediterranean diet. *N Engl J Med*, 368(14):1279–1290. doi: 10.1056/NEJMoa1200303.
Evert, A. B., J. L. Boucher, M. Cypress, S. A. Dunbar, M. J. Franz, E. J. Mayer-Davis, J. J. Neumiller et al. 2014. Nutrition therapy recommendations for the management of adults with diabetes. *Diabetes Care*, 37(Suppl 1):S120–S143. doi: 10.2337/dc14-S120.
Fabricatore, A. N., C. B. Ebbeling, T. A. Wadden, and D. S. Ludwig. 2011a. Continuous glucose monitoring to assess the ecologic validity of dietary glycemic index and glycemic load. *Am J Clin Nutr*, 94(6):1519–1524. doi: 10.3945/ajcn.111.020354.
Fabricatore, A. N., T. A. Wadden, C. B. Ebbeling, J. G. Thomas, V. A. Stallings, S. Schwartz, and D. S. Ludwig. 2011b. Targeting dietary fat or glycemic load in the treatment of obesity and type 2 diabetes: A randomized controlled trial. *Diabetes Res Clin Pract*, 92(1):37–45. doi: 10.1016/j.diabres.2010.12.016.
Ferrannini, E., A. Gastaldelli, Y. Miyazaki, M. Matsuda, A. Mari, and R. A. DeFronzo. 2005. beta-cell function in subjects spanning the range from normal glucose tolerance to overt diabetes: A new analysis. *J Clin Endocrinol Metab*, 90(1):493–500. doi: 10.1210/jc.2004-1133.
Festa, A., K. Williams, R. D'Agostino, Jr., L. E. Wagenknecht, and S. M. Haffner. 2006. The natural course of beta-cell function in nondiabetic and diabetic individuals: The Insulin Resistance Atherosclerosis Study. *Diabetes*, 55(4):1114–1120.
Fontvieille, A. M., S. W. Rizkalla, A. Penfornis, M. Acosta, F. R. Bornet, and G. Slama. 1992. The use of low glycaemic index foods improves metabolic control of diabetic patients over five weeks. *Diabet Med*, 9(5):444–450.
Frost, G., B. Keogh, D. Smith, K. Akinsanya, and A. Leeds. 1996. The effect of low-glycemic carbohydrate on insulin and glucose response in vivo and in vitro in patients with coronary heart disease. *Metabolism*, 45(6):669–72.
Frost, G. S., A. E. Brynes, C. Bovill-Taylor, and A. Dornhorst. 2004. A prospective randomised trial to determine the efficacy of a low glycaemic index diet given in addition to healthy eating and weight loss advice in patients with coronary heart disease. *Eur J Clin Nutr*, 58(1):121–127. doi: 10.1038/sj.ejcn.1601758.
Frost, G., J. Wilding, and J. Beecham. 1994. Dietary advice based on the glycaemic index improves dietary profile and metabolic control in type 2 diabetic patients. *Diabet Med*, 11(4):397–401.
Fullerton, B., K. Jeitler, M. Seitz, K. Horvath, A. Berghold, and A. Siebenhofer. 2014. Intensive glucose control versus conventional glucose control for type 1 diabetes mellitus. *Cochrane Database Syst Rev*, 2:CD009122. doi: 10.1002/14651858.CD009122.pub2.
Geng, D. F., D. M. Jin, W. Wu, C. Fang, and J. F. Wang. 2011. Effect of alpha-glucosidase inhibitors on the progression of carotid intima-media thickness: A meta-analysis of randomized controlled trials. *Atherosclerosis*, 218(1):214–219. doi: 10.1016/j.atherosclerosis.2011.05.004.
Giacco, R., M. Parillo, A. A. Rivellese, G. Lasorella, A. Giacco, L. D'Episcopo, and G. Riccardi. 2000. Long-term dietary treatment with increased amounts of fiber-rich low-glycemic index natural foods improves blood glucose control and reduces the number of hypoglycemic events in type 1 diabetic patients. *Diabetes Care*, 23(10):1461–1466.

Gilbertson, H. R., J. C. Brand-Miller, A. W. Thorburn, S. Evans, P. Chondros, and G. A. Werther. 2001. The effect of flexible low glycemic index dietary advice versus measured carbohydrate exchange diets on glycemic control in children with type 1 diabetes. *Diabetes Care*, 24(7):1137–1143.

Giugliano, D., A. Ceriello, and G. Paolisso. 1996. Oxidative stress and diabetic vascular complications. *Diabetes Care*, 19(3):257–267.

Goff, L. M., D. E. Cowland, L. Hooper, and G. S. Frost. 2013. Low glycaemic index diets and blood lipids: A systematic review and meta-analysis of randomised controlled trials. *Nutr Metab Cardiovasc Dis*, 23(1):1–10. doi: 10.1016/j.numecd.2012.06.002.

Goldbourt, U., S. Yaari, and J. H. Medalie. 1997. Isolated low HDL cholesterol as a risk factor for coronary heart disease mortality. A 21-year follow-up of 8000 men. *Arterioscler Thromb Vasc Biol*, 17(1):107–113.

Gopinath, B., D. C. Harris, V. M. Flood, G. Burlutsky, J. Brand-Miller, and P. Mitchell. 2011. Carbohydrate nutrition is associated with the 5-year incidence of chronic kidney disease. *J Nutr*, 141(3):433–439. doi: 10.3945/jn.110.134304.

Gordon, D. J., J. L. Probstfield, R. J. Garrison, J. D. Neaton, W. P. Castelli, J. D. Knoke, D. R. Jacobs, Jr., S. Bangdiwala, and H. A. Tyroler. 1989. High-density lipoprotein cholesterol and cardiovascular disease. Four prospective American studies. *Circulation*, 79(1):8–15.

Gotto, A. M., Jr. 2002. High-density lipoprotein cholesterol and triglycerides as therapeutic targets for preventing and treating coronary artery disease. *Am Heart J*, 144(6 Suppl):S33–S42. doi: 10.1067/mhj.2002.130301.

Greenway, F. L. 2015. Physiological adaptations to weight loss and factors favouring weight regain. *Int J Obes (Lond)*, 39(8):1188–1196. doi: 10.1038/ijo.2015.59.

Griffith, J. A., Y. Ma, L. Chasan-Taber, B. C. Olendzki, D. E. Chiriboga, E. J. Stanek, 3rd, P. A. Merriam, and I. S. Ockene. 2008. Association between dietary glycemic index, glycemic load, and high-sensitivity C-reactive protein. *Nutrition*, 24(5):401–406. doi: 10.1016/j.nut.2007.12.017.

Gross, J. L., C. K. Kramer, C. B. Leitao, N. Hawkins, L. V. Viana, B. D. Schaan, L. C. Pinto, T. C. Rodrigues, M. J. Azevedo, Diabetes, and Group Endocrinology Meta-analysis. 2011. Effect of antihyperglycemic agents added to metformin and a sulfonylurea on glycemic control and weight gain in type 2 diabetes: A network meta-analysis. *Ann Intern Med*, 154(10):672–679. doi: 10.7326/0003-4819-154-10-201105170-00007.

Grundy, S. M., H. B. Brewer, Jr., J. I. Cleeman, S. C. Smith, Jr., and C. Lenfant. 2004. Definition of metabolic syndrome: Report of the National Heart, Lung, and Blood Institute/American Heart Association conference on scientific issues related to definition. *Circulation*, 109(3):433–438.

Haban, P., R. Simoncic, E. Zidekova, and L. Ozdin. 2002. Role of fasting serum C-peptide as a predictor of cardiovascular risk associated with the metabolic X-syndrome. *Med Sci Monit*, 8(3):CR175–CR179.

Haffner, S., M. Temprosa, J. Crandall, S. Fowler, R. Goldberg, E. Horton, S. Marcovina et al. 2005. Intensive lifestyle intervention or metformin on inflammation and coagulation in participants with impaired glucose tolerance. *Diabetes*, 54(5):1566–1572.

Hanefeld, M., M. Cagatay, T. Petrowitsch, D. Neuser, D. Petzinna, and M. Rupp. 2004. Acarbose reduces the risk for myocardial infarction in type 2 diabetic patients: Meta-analysis of seven long-term studies. *Eur Heart J*, 25(1):10–16. doi: S0195668x03004688 [pii].

Hanefeld, M., A. Karasik, C. Koehler, T. Westermeier, and J. L. Chiasson. 2009. Metabolic syndrome and its single traits as risk factors for diabetes in people with impaired glucose tolerance: The STOP-NIDDM trial. *Diab Vasc Dis Res*, 6(1):32–37. doi: 10.3132/dvdr.2009.006.

Harder, M. N., R. Ribel-Madsen, J. M. Justesen, T. Sparso, E. A. Andersson, N. Grarup, T. Jorgensen, A. Linneberg, T. Hansen, and O. Pedersen. 2013. Type 2 diabetes risk alleles near BCAR1 and in ANK1 associate with decreased beta-cell function whereas risk alleles near ANKRD55 and GRB14 associate with decreased insulin sensitivity in the Danish Inter99 cohort. *J Clin Endocrinol Metab*, 98(4):E801–E806. doi: 10.1210/jc.2012-4169.

Hardy, D. S., D. M. Hoelscher, C. Aragaki, J. Stevens, L. M. Steffen, J. S. Pankow, and E. Boerwinkle. 2010. Association of glycemic index and glycemic load with risk of incident coronary heart disease among Whites and African Americans with and without type 2 diabetes: The Atherosclerosis Risk in Communities study. *Ann Epidemiol*, 20(8):610–616. doi: 10.1016/j.annepidem.2010.05.008.

Hayward, R. A., P. D. Reaven, W. L. Wiitala, G. D. Bahn, D. J. Reda, L. Ge, M. McCarren, W. C. Duckworth, N. V. Emanuele, and Vadt Investigators. 2015. Follow-up of glycemic control and cardiovascular outcomes in type 2 diabetes. *N Engl J Med*, 372(23):2197–2206. doi: 10.1056/NEJMoa1414266.

Heilbronn, L. K., M. Noakes, and P. M. Clifton. 2002. The effect of high- and low-glycemic index energy restricted diets on plasma lipid and glucose profiles in type 2 diabetic subjects with varying glycemic control. *J Am Coll Nutr*, 21(2):120–127.

Heitmann, B. L. and L. Lissner. 1995. Dietary underreporting by obese individuals—Is it specific or non-specific? *BMJ*, 311(7011):986–989.

Hemmingsen, B., S. S. Lund, C. Gluud, A. Vaag, T. P. Almdal, C. Hemmingsen, and J. Wetterslev. 2013. Targeting intensive glycaemic control versus targeting conventional glycaemic control for type 2 diabetes mellitus. *Cochrane Database Syst Rev*, 11:CD008143. doi: 10.1002/14651858.CD008143.pub3.

Higgins, J. P. 2011. Cochrane Handbook for Systematic Reviews of Interventions Version 5.1.0. The Cochrane Collaboration; 2011. In: The Cochrane Collaboration. (Accessed July 10, 2015.)

Hodge, A. M., D. R. English, K. O'Dea, and G. G. Giles. 2004. Glycemic index and dietary fiber and the risk of type 2 diabetes. *Diabetes Care*, 27(11):2701–2706.

Holman, R. R., C. A. Cull, and R. C. Turner. 1999. A randomized double-blind trial of acarbose in type 2 diabetes shows improved glycemic control over 3 years (U.K. Prospective Diabetes Study 44). *Diabetes Care*, 22(6):960–964.

Holman, R. R., S. K. Paul, M. A. Bethel, D. R. Matthews, and H. A. Neil. 2008. 10-year follow-up of intensive glucose control in type 2 diabetes. *N Engl J Med*, 359(15):1577–1589. doi: 10.1056/NEJMoa0806470.

Hopping, B. N., E. Erber, A. Grandinetti, M. Verheus, L. N. Kolonel, and G. Maskarinec. 2010. Dietary fiber, magnesium, and glycemic load alter risk of type 2 diabetes in a multiethnic cohort in Hawaii. *J Nutr*, 140(1):68–74. doi: 10.3945/jn.109.112441.

Hu, Y., G. Block, E. P. Norkus, J. D. Morrow, M. Dietrich, and M. Hudes. 2006. Relations of glycemic index and glycemic load with plasma oxidative stress markers. *Am J Clin Nutr*, 84(1):70–76; quiz 266–267.

Iannuzzi, A., M. R. Licenziati, M. Vacca, D. De Marco, G. Cinquegrana, M. Laccetti, A. Bresciani et al. 2009. Comparison of two diets of varying glycemic index on carotid subclinical atherosclerosis in obese children. *Heart Vessels*, 24(6):419–424. doi: 10.1007/s00380-008-1138-6.

Ikram, M. K., F. J. de Jong, J. R. Vingerling, J. C. Witteman, A. Hofman, M. M. Breteler, and P. T. de Jong. 2004. Are retinal arteriolar or venular diameters associated with markers for cardiovascular disorders? The Rotterdam Study. *Invest Ophthalmol Vis Sci*, 45(7):2129–2134.

International Diabetes Federation 2012 Clinical Guidelines Task Force. 2012. Global Guidelines for Type 2 Diabetes. http://www.idf.org. (Accessed July 10, 2015.)

International Diabetes Federation. 2013. International Diabetes Federation (IDF) Diabetes Atlas 6th Ed. http://www.idf.org/diabetesatlas. (Accessed July 10, 2015.)

International Diabetes Federation Guideline Development Group. 2014. Guideline for management of postmeal glucose in diabetes. *Diabetes Res Clin Pract*, 103(2):256–268. doi: 10.1016/j.diabres.2012.08.002.

Italian Society of Human Nutrition (SINU). 2012. Livelli di Assunzione di Riferimento di Nutrienti ed energia per la popolazione italiana. (Reference levels of intake of nutrients and energy for the Italian population). http://www.sinu.it/documenti/20121016_LARN_bologna_sintesi_prefinale.pdf. (Accessed July 10, 2015.)

Jenkins, D. J., C. W. Kendall, L. S. Augustin, S. Franceschi, M. Hamidi, A. Marchie, A. L. Jenkins, and M. Axelsen. 2002. Glycemic index: Overview of implications in health and disease. *Am J Clin Nutr*, 76(1):266S–273S.

Jenkins, D. J., C. W. Kendall, L. S. Augustin, S. Mitchell, S. Sahye-Pudaruth, S. Blanco Mejia, L. Chiavaroli et al. 2012. Effect of legumes as part of a low glycemic index diet on glycemic control and cardiovascular risk factors in type 2 diabetes mellitus: A randomized controlled trial. *Arch Intern Med*, 172(21):1653–1660. doi: 10.1001/2013.jamainternmed.70.

Jenkins, D. J., C. W. Kendall, G. McKeown-Eyssen, R. G. Josse, J. Silverberg, G. L. Booth, E. Vidgen et al. 2008. Effect of a low-glycemic index or a high-cereal fiber diet on type 2 diabetes: A randomized trial. *JAMA*, 300(23):2742–2753.

Jenkins, D. J., C. W. Kendall, V. Vuksan, D. Faulkner, L. S. Augustin, S. Mitchell, C. Ireland et al. 2014. Effect of lowering the glycemic load with canola oil on glycemic control and cardiovascular risk factors: A randomized controlled trial. *Diabetes Care*, 37(7):1806–1814. doi: 10.2337/dc13-2990.

Jenkins, D. J., K. Srichaikul, C. W. Kendall, J. L. Sievenpiper, S. Abdulnour, A. Mirrahimi, C. Meneses et al. 2011. The relation of low glycaemic index fruit consumption to glycaemic control and risk factors for coronary heart disease in type 2 diabetes. *Diabetologia*, 54(2):271–279. doi: 10.1007/s00125-010-1927-1.

Jenkins, D. J. and T. M. Wolever. 1981. Slow release carbohydrate and the treatment of diabetes. *Proc Nutr Soc*, 40(2):227–235.

Jenkins, D. J., T. M. Wolever, G. Buckley, K. Y. Lam, S. Giudici, J. Kalmusky, A. L. Jenkins, R. L. Patten, J. Bird, G. S. Wong, and et al. 1988. Low-glycemic-index starchy foods in the diabetic diet. *Am J Clin Nutr*, 48(2):248–254.

Jenkins, D. J., T. M. Wolever, G. R. Collier, A. Ocana, A. V. Rao, G. Buckley, Y. Lam, A. Mayer, and L. U. Thompson. 1987. Metabolic effects of a low-glycemic-index diet. *Am J Clin Nutr*, 46(6):968–975.

Jenkins, D. J., T. M. Wolever, A. M. Ocana, V. Vuksan, S. C. Cunnane, M. Jenkins, G. S. Wong, W. Singer, S. R. Bloom, L. M. Blendis, and et al. 1990. Metabolic effects of reducing rate of glucose ingestion by single bolus versus continuous sipping. *Diabetes*, 39(7):775–781.

Jenkins, D. J., T. M. Wolever, A. V. Rao, R. A. Hegele, S. J. Mitchell, T. P. Ransom, D. L. Boctor, P. J. Spadafora, A. L. Jenkins, C. Mehling, and et al. 1993. Effect on blood lipids of very high intakes of fiber in diets low in saturated fat and cholesterol. *N Engl J Med*, 329(1):21–26. doi: 10.1056/NEJM199307013290104.

Jenkins, D. J., T. M. Wolever, R. H. Taylor, C. Griffiths, K. Krzeminska, J. A. Lawrie, C. M. Bennett, D. V. Goff, D. L. Sarson, and S. R. Bloom. 1982. Slow release dietary carbohydrate improves second meal tolerance. *Am J Clin Nutr*, 35(6):1339–1346.

Jimenez-Cruz, A., M. Bacardi-Gascon, W. H. Turnbull, P. Rosales-Garay, and I. Severino-Lugo. 2003. A flexible, low-glycemic index mexican-style diet in overweight and obese subjects with type 2 diabetes improves metabolic parameters during a 6-week treatment period. *Diabetes Care*, 26(7):1967–1970.

Jimenez-Cruz, A., W. H. Turnbull, M. Bacardi-Gascon, and P. Rosales-Garay. 2004. A high-fiber, moderate-glycemic-index, Mexican style diet improves dyslipidemia in individuals with type 2 diabetes. *Nutr Res*, 24:19–27.

Juanola-Falgarona, M., J. Salas-Salvado, N. Ibarrola-Jurado, A. Rabassa-Soler, A. Diaz-Lopez, M. Guasch-Ferre, P. Hernandez-Alonso, R. Balanza, and M. Bullo. 2014. Effect of the glycemic index of the diet on weight loss, modulation of satiety, inflammation, and other metabolic risk factors: A randomized controlled trial. *Am J Clin Nutr*, 100(1):27–35. doi: 10.3945/ajcn.113.081216.

Kaushik, S., J. J. Wang, V. Flood, J. S. Tan, A. W. Barclay, T. Y. Wong, J. Brand-Miller, and P. Mitchell. 2008. Dietary glycemic index and the risk of age-related macular degeneration. *Am J Clin Nutr*, 88(4):1104–1110.

Kaushik, S., J. J. Wang, T. Y. Wong, V. Flood, A. Barclay, J. Brand-Miller, and P. Mitchell. 2009. Glycemic index, retinal vascular caliber, and stroke mortality. *Stroke*, 40(1):206–212. doi: 10.1161/STROKEAHA.108.513812.

The Kidney Foundation of Canada. 2012. Facing the Facts. The Kidney Foundation of Canada. National Office - Public Policy. http://www.kidney.ca. (Accessed July 10, 2015.)

Kilpatrick, E. S., A. S. Rigby, and S. L. Atkin. 2007. Insulin resistance, the metabolic syndrome, and complication risk in type 1 diabetes: "double diabetes" in the Diabetes Control and Complications Trial. *Diabetes Care*, 30(3):707–712. doi: 10.2337/dc06 - 1982.

Klein, R., B. E. Klein, M. D. Knudtson, T. Y. Wong, and M. Y. Tsai. 2006. Are inflammatory factors related to retinal vessel caliber? The Beaver Dam Eye Study. *Arch Ophthalmol*, 124 (1):87–94. doi: 10.1001/archopht.124.1.87.

Klein, R., B. E. Klein, S. E. Moss, T. Y. Wong, and A. R. Sharrett. 2006. Retinal vascular caliber in persons with type 2 diabetes: The Wisconsin Epidemiological Study of Diabetic Retinopathy: XX. *Ophthalmology*, 113(9):1488–1498. doi: 10.1016/j.ophtha.2006.03.028.

Knowler, W. C., E. Barrett-Connor, S. E. Fowler, R. F. Hamman, J. M. Lachin, E. A. Walker, D. M. Nathan, and Group Diabetes Prevention Program Research. 2002. Reduction in the incidence of type 2 diabetes with lifestyle intervention or metformin. *N Engl J Med*, 346(6):393–403. doi: 10.1056/NEJMoa012512.

Komindr, S., S. Ingsriswang, N. Lerdvuthisopon, and A. Boontawee. 2001. Effect of long-term intake of Asian food with different glycemic indices on diabetic control and protein conservation in type 2 diabetic patients. *J Med Assoc Thai*, 84(1):85–97.

Koyama, K., G. Chen, Y. Lee, and R. H. Unger. 1997. Tissue triglycerides, insulin resistance, and insulin production: Implications for hyperinsulinemia of obesity. *Am J Physiol*, 273(4 Pt 1):E708–E713.

Krishnan, S., L. Rosenberg, M. Singer, F. B. Hu, L. Djousse, L. A. Cupples, and J. R. Palmer. 2007. Glycemic index, glycemic load, and cereal fiber intake and risk of type 2 diabetes in US black women. *Arch Intern Med*, 167(21):2304–2309. doi: 10.1001/archinte.167.21.2304.

Lachin, J. M., S. Genuth, D. M. Nathan, B. Zinman, B. N. Rutledge, and Dcct Edic Research Group. 2008. Effect of glycemic exposure on the risk of microvascular complications in the diabetes control and complications trial—Revisited. *Diabetes*, 57(4):995–1001. doi: 10.2337/db07-1618.

Larsen, T. M., S. M. Dalskov, M. van Baak, S. A. Jebb, A. Papadaki, A. F. Pfeiffer, J. A. Martinez et al. 2010. Diets with high or low protein content and glycemic index for weight-loss maintenance. *N Engl J Med*, 363(22):2102–2113. doi: 10.1056/NEJMoa1007137.

Levitan, E. B., N. R. Cook, M. J. Stampfer, P. M. Ridker, K. M. Rexrode, J. E. Buring, J. E. Manson, and S. Liu. 2008. Dietary glycemic index, dietary glycemic load, blood lipids, and C-reactive protein. *Metabolism*, 57(3):437–443. doi: 10.1016/j.metabol.2007.11.002.

Livesey, G., R. Taylor, T. Hulshof, and J. Howlett. 2008. Glycemic response and health—a systematic review and meta-analysis: Relations between dietary glycemic properties and health outcomes. *Am J Clin Nutr*, 87(1):258S–268S.

Livesey, G., R. Taylor, H. Livesey, and S. Liu. 2013. Is there a dose-response relation of dietary glycemic load to risk of type 2 diabetes? Meta-analysis of prospective cohort studies. *Am J Clin Nutr*, 97(3):584–96. doi: 10.3945/ajcn.112.041467.

Ludwig, D. S. 2000. Dietary glycemic index and obesity. *J Nutr*, 130(2S Suppl):280S–283S.

Ludwig, D. S. 2002. The glycemic index: Physiological mechanisms relating to obesity, diabetes, and cardiovascular disease. *JAMA*, 287(18):2414–2423. doi: jsc10297 [pii].

Ma, Y., B. C. Olendzki, P. A. Merriam, D. E. Chiriboga, A. L. Culver, W. Li, J. R. Hebert, I. S. Ockene, J. A. Griffith, and S. L. Pagoto. 2008. A randomized clinical trial comparing low-glycemic index versus ADA dietary education among individuals with type 2 diabetes. *Nutrition*, 24(1):45–56. doi: 10.1016/j.nut.2007.10.008.

Mann, J. I., I. De Leeuw, K. Hermansen, B. Karamanos, B. Karlstrom, N. Katsilambros, G. Riccardi et al. 2004. Evidence-based nutritional approaches to the treatment and prevention of diabetes mellitus. *Nutr Metab Cardiovasc Dis*, 14(6):373–94.

Mantzoros, C. S., T. Li, J. E. Manson, J. B. Meigs, and F. B. Hu. 2005. Circulating adiponectin levels are associated with better glycemic control, more favorable lipid profile, and reduced inflammation in women with type 2 diabetes. *J Clin Endocrinol Metab*, 90(8):4542–4548. doi: 10.1210/jc.2005-0372.

Manuel, D. G. and S. E. Schultz. 2004. Health-related quality of life and health-adjusted life expectancy of people with diabetes in Ontario, Canada, 1996–1997. *Diabetes Care*, 27(2):407–414.

Marsh, K. A., K. S. Steinbeck, F. S. Atkinson, P. Petocz, and J. C. Brand-Miller. 2010. Effect of a low glycemic index compared with a conventional healthy diet on polycystic ovary syndrome. *Am J Clin Nutr*, 92(1):83–92. doi: 10.3945/ajcn.2010.29261.

McKeown, N. M., J. B. Meigs, S. Liu, E. Saltzman, P. W. Wilson, and P. F. Jacques. 2004. Carbohydrate nutrition, insulin resistance, and the prevalence of the metabolic syndrome in the Framingham Offspring Cohort. *Diabetes Care*, 27(2):538–546.

Meyer, K. A., L. H. Kushi, D. R. Jacobs, Jr., J. Slavin, T. A. Sellers, and A. R. Folsom. 2000. Carbohydrates, dietary fiber, and incident type 2 diabetes in older women. *Am J Clin Nutr*, 71(4):921–930.

Mokdad, A. H., E. S. Ford, B. A. Bowman, W. H. Dietz, F. Vinicor, V. S. Bales, and J. S. Marks. 2003. Prevalence of obesity, diabetes, and obesity-related health risk factors, 2001. *JAMA*, 289(1):76–79.

Monnier, L., E. Mas, C. Ginet, F. Michel, L. Villon, J. P. Cristol, and C. Colette. 2006. Activation of oxidative stress by acute glucose fluctuations compared with sustained chronic hyperglycemia in patients with type 2 diabetes. *JAMA*, 295(14):1681–1687. doi: 10.1001/jama.295.14.1681.

Montani, J. P., A. K. Viecelli, A. Prevot, and A. G. Dulloo. 2006. Weight cycling during growth and beyond as a risk factor for later cardiovascular diseases: The "repeated overshoot" theory. *Int J Obes (Lond)*, 30(Suppl 4):S58–S66. doi: 10.1038/sj.ijo.0803520.

Morrish, N. J., S. L. Wang, L. K. Stevens, J. H. Fuller, and H. Keen. 2001. Mortality and causes of death in the WHO Multinational Study of Vascular Disease in Diabetes. *Diabetologia*, 44(Suppl 2):S14–S21.

Mosdol, A., D. R. Witte, G. Frost, M. G. Marmot, and E. J. Brunner. 2007. Dietary glycemic index and glycemic load are associated with high-density-lipoprotein cholesterol at baseline but not with increased risk of diabetes in the Whitehall II study. *Am J Clin Nutr*, 86(4):988–994.

Neuhouser, M. L., Y. Schwarz, C. Wang, K. Breymeyer, G. Coronado, C. Y. Wang, K. Noar, X. Song, and J. W. Lampe. 2012. A low-glycemic load diet reduces serum C-reactive protein and modestly increases adiponectin in overweight and obese adults. *J Nutr*, 142(2):369–374. doi: 10.3945/jn.111.149807.

Niskanen, L., A. Turpeinen, I. Penttila, and M. I. Uusitupa. 1998. Hyperglycemia and compositional lipoprotein abnormalities as predictors of cardiovascular mortality in type 2 diabetes: A 15-year follow-up from the time of diagnosis. *Diabetes Care*, 21(11):1861–1869.

Nothlings, U., M. B. Schulze, C. Weikert, H. Boeing, Y. T. van der Schouw, C. Bamia, V. Benetou et al. 2008. Intake of vegetables, legumes, and fruit, and risk for all-cause, cardiovascular, and cancer mortality in a European diabetic population. *J Nutr*, 138(4):775–781.

Ohtsubo, K., M. Z. Chen, J. M. Olefsky, and J. D. Marth. 2011. Pathway to diabetes through attenuation of pancreatic beta cell glycosylation and glucose transport. *Nat Med*, 17(9):1067–1075. doi: 10.1038/nm.2414.

Ouchi, N., S. Kihara, Y. Arita, M. Nishida, A. Matsuyama, Y. Okamoto, M. Ishigami et al. 2001. Adipocyte-derived plasma protein, adiponectin, suppresses lipid accumulation and class A scavenger receptor expression in human monocyte-derived macrophages. *Circulation*, 103(8):1057–1063.

Oyama, T., A. Saiki, K. Endoh, N. Ban, D. Nagayama, M. Ohhira, N. Koide, Y. Miyashita, and K. Shirai. 2008. Effect of acarbose, an alpha-glucosidase inhibitor, on serum lipoprotein lipase mass levels and common carotid artery intima-media thickness in type 2 diabetes mellitus treated by sulfonylurea. *J Atheroscler Thromb*, 15(3):154–159. doi: JST.JSTAGE/jat/E549 [pii].

Patel, A. V., M. L. McCullough, A. L. Pavluck, E. J. Jacobs, M. J. Thun, and E. E. Calle. 2007. Glycemic load, glycemic index, and carbohydrate intake in relation to pancreatic cancer risk in a large US cohort. *Cancer Causes Control*, 18(3):287–294. doi: 10.1007/s10552-006-0081-z.

Pawlak, D. B., J. A. Kushner, and D. S. Ludwig. 2004. Effects of dietary glycaemic index on adiposity, glucose homoeostasis, and plasma lipids in animals. *Lancet*, 364(9436):778–785. doi: 10.1016/S0140-6736(04)16937-7.

Pereira, M. A., J. Swain, A. B. Goldfine, N. Rifai, and D. S. Ludwig. 2004. Effects of a low-glycemic load diet on resting energy expenditure and heart disease risk factors during weight loss. *JAMA*, 292(20):2482–2490. doi: 10.1001/jama.292.20.2482.

Peters, S. A., H. M. den Ruijter, D. E. Grobbee, and M. L. Bots. 2013. Results from a carotid intima-media thickness trial as a decision tool for launching a large-scale morbidity and mortality trial. *Circ Cardiovasc Imaging*, 6(1):20–25. doi: 10.1161/CIRCIMAGING.112.978114.

Philippou, E., C. Bovill-Taylor, C. Rajkumar, M. L. Vampa, E. Ntatsaki, A. E. Brynes, M. Hickson, and G. S. Frost. 2009. Preliminary report: The effect of a 6-month dietary glycemic index manipulation in addition to healthy eating advice and weight loss on arterial compliance and 24-hour ambulatory blood pressure in men: A pilot study. *Metabolism*, 58(12):1703–1708. doi: 10.1016/j.metabol.2009.05.026.

Philippou, E., B. M. McGowan, A. E. Brynes, A. Dornhorst, A. R. Leeds, and G. S. Frost. 2008. The effect of a 12-week low glycaemic index diet on heart disease risk factors and 24 h glycaemic response in healthy middle-aged volunteers at risk of heart disease: A pilot study. *Eur J Clin Nutr*, 62(1):145–149. doi: 10.1038/sj.ejcn.1602688.

Public Health Agency of Canada. 2011. Unpublished analysis using 2008/09 data from the Canadian Chronic Disease Surveillance System (Public Health Agency of Canada). http://www.phac-aspc.gc.ca/cd-mc/cvd-mcv/index-eng.php. (Accessed July 10, 2015.)

Qi, L., E. Rimm, S. Liu, N. Rifai, and F. B. Hu. 2005. Dietary glycemic index, glycemic load, cereal fiber, and plasma adiponectin concentration in diabetic men. *Diabetes Care*, 28(5):1022–1028.

Qi, L., R. M. van Dam, S. Liu, M. Franz, C. Mantzoros, and F. B. Hu. 2006. Whole-grain, bran, and cereal fiber intakes and markers of systemic inflammation in diabetic women. *Diabetes Care*, 29(2):207–211.

Ramirez, C. E., M. M. Shuey, G. L. Milne, K. Gilbert, N. Hui, C. Yu, J. M. Luther, and N. J. Brown. 2014. Arg287Gln variant of EPHX2 and epoxyeicosatrienoic acids are associated with insulin sensitivity in humans. *Prostaglandins Other Lipid Mediat*, 113–115:38–44. doi: 10.1016/j.prostaglandins.2014.08.001.

Ridker, P. M., C. P. Cannon, D. Morrow, N. Rifai, L. M. Rose, C. H. McCabe, M. A. Pfeffer, E. Braunwald, and Pravastatin or Atorvastatin Evaluation and Infection Therapy-Thrombolysis in Myocardial Infarction 22 (PROVE IT-TIMI 22) Investigators. 2005. C-reactive protein levels and outcomes after statin therapy. *N Engl J Med*, 352(1):20–28. doi: 10.1056/NEJMoa042378.

Ridker, P. M. and D. A. Morrow. 2003. C-reactive protein, inflammation, and coronary risk. *Cardiol Clin*, 21(3):315–325.

Rizkalla, S. W., L. Taghrid, M. Laromiguiere, D. Huet, J. Boillot, A. Rigoir, F. Elgrably, and G. Slama. 2004. Improved plasma glucose control, whole-body glucose utilization, and lipid profile on a low-glycemic index diet in type 2 diabetic men: A randomized controlled trial. *Diabetes Care*, 27(8):1866–1872.

Roden, M., T. B. Price, G. Perseghin, K. F. Petersen, D. L. Rothman, G. W. Cline, and G. I. Shulman. 1996. Mechanism of free fatty acid-induced insulin resistance in humans. *J Clin Invest*, 97(12):2859–2865. doi: 10.1172/JCI118742.

Rodriguez-Rejon, A. I., I. Castro-Quezada, C. Ruano-Rodriguez, M. D. Ruiz-Lopez, A. Sanchez-Villegas, E. Toledo, R. Artacho et al. 2014. Effect of a Mediterranean Diet Intervention on Dietary Glycemic Load and Dietary Glycemic Index: The PREDIMED Study. *J Nutr Metab*, 2014:985373. doi: 10.1155/2014/985373.

Rossi, M., F. Turati, P. Lagiou, D. Trichopoulos, L. S. Augustin, C. La Vecchia, and A. Trichopoulou. 2013. Mediterranean diet and glycaemic load in relation to incidence of type 2 diabetes: Results from the Greek cohort of the population-based European Prospective Investigation into Cancer and Nutrition (EPIC). *Diabetologia*, 56(11):2405–2413. doi: 10.1007/s00125-013-3013-y.

Rossi, R., A. Nuzzo, G. Origliani, and M. G. Modena. 2008. Prognostic role of flow-mediated dilation and cardiac risk factors in post-menopausal women. *J Am Coll Cardiol*, 51(10):997–1002. doi: 10.1016/j.jacc.2007.11.044.

Sacks, F. M., V. J. Carey, C. A. Anderson, E. R. 3. r. d. Miller, T. Copeland, J. Charleston, B. J. Harshfield et al. 2014. Effects of high vs low glycemic index of dietary carbohydrate on cardiovascular disease risk factors and insulin sensitivity: The OmniCarb randomized clinical trial. *JAMA*, 312(23):2531–2541. doi: 10.1001/jama.2014.16658.

Sahyoun, N. R., A. L. Anderson, F. A. Tylavsky, J. S. Lee, D. E. Sellmeyer, T. B. Harris, and Health Aging and Body Composition Study. 2008. Dietary glycemic index and glycemic load and the risk of type 2 diabetes in older adults. *Am J Clin Nutr*, 87(1):126–131.

Sakurai, M., K. Nakamura, K. Miura, T. Takamura, K. Yoshita, Y. Morikawa, M. Ishizaki et al. 2012. Dietary glycemic index and risk of type 2 diabetes mellitus in middle-aged Japanese men. *Metabolism* 61(1):47–55. doi: 10.1016/j.metabol.2011.05.015.

Samuel, V. T. and G. I. Shulman. 2012. Mechanisms for insulin resistance: Common threads and missing links. *Cell*, 148(5):852–871. doi: 10.1016/j.cell.2012.02.017.

Sardar, P., J. A. Udell, S. Chatterjee, S. Bansilal, D. Mukherjee, and M. E. Farkouh. 2015. Effect of Intensive Versus Standard Blood Glucose Control in Patients With Type 2 Diabetes Mellitus in Different Regions of the World: Systematic Review and Meta-analysis of Randomized Controlled Trials. *J Am Heart Assoc*, 4(5). doi: 10.1161/JAHA.114.001577.

Schinner, S., W. A. Scherbaum, S. R. Bornstein, and A. Barthel. 2005. Molecular mechanisms of insulin resistance. *Diabet Med*, 22(6):674–682. doi: 10.1111/j.1464-5491.2005.01566.x.

Schwingshackl, L. and G. Hoffmann. 2013. Long-term effects of low glycemic index/load vs. high glycemic index/load diets on parameters of obesity and obesity-associated risks: A systematic review and meta-analysis. *Nutr Metab Cardiovasc Dis*, 23(8):699–706. doi: 10.1016/j.numecd.2013.04.008.

Sesti, G. 2006. Pathophysiology of insulin resistance. *Best Pract Res Clin Endocrinol Metab*, 20(4):665–679. doi: 10.1016/j.beem.2006.09.007.

Shi, H., M. V. Kokoeva, K. Inouye, I. Tzameli, H. Yin, and J. S. Flier. 2006. TLR4 links innate immunity and fatty acid-induced insulin resistance. *J Clin Invest*, 116(11):3015–3025. doi: 10.1172/JCI28898.

Shikany, J. M., R. P. Phadke, D. T. Redden, and B. A. Gower. 2009. Effects of low- and high-glycemic index/glycemic load diets on coronary heart disease risk factors in overweight/obese men. *Metabolism*, 58(12):1793–1801. doi: 10.1016/j.metabol.2009.06.006.

Sichieri, R., A. S. Moura, V. Genelhu, F. Hu, and W. C. Willett. 2007. An 18-mo randomized trial of a low-glycemic-index diet and weight change in Brazilian women. *Am J Clin Nutr*, 86(3):707–713.

Sievenpiper, J. L., C. W. Kendall, A. Esfahani, J. M. Wong, A. J. Carleton, H. Y. Jiang, R. P. Bazinet, E. Vidgen, and D. J. Jenkins. 2009. Effect of non-oil-seed pulses on glycaemic control: A systematic review and meta-analysis of randomised controlled experimental trials in people with and without diabetes. *Diabetologia*, 52(8):1479–1495. doi: 10.1007/s00125-009-1395-7.

Simila, M. E., L. M. Valsta, J. P. Kontto, D. Albanes, and J. Virtamo. 2011. Low-, medium- and high-glycaemic index carbohydrates and risk of type 2 diabetes in men. *Br J Nutr*, 105(8):1258–1264. doi: 10.1017/S000711451000485X.

Simpson, S. H., P. Corabian, P. Jacobs, and J. A. Johnson. 2003. The cost of major comorbidity in people with diabetes mellitus. *CMAJ*, 168(13):1661–1667.

Sloth, B., I. Krog-Mikkelsen, A. Flint, I. Tetens, I. Bjorck, S. Vinoy, H. Elmstahl, A. Astrup, V. Lang, and A. Raben. 2004. No difference in body weight decrease between a low-glycemic-index and a high-glycemic-index diet but reduced LDL cholesterol after 10-wk ad libitum intake of the low-glycemic-index diet. *Am J Clin Nutr*, 80(2):337–347.

Sluijs, I., J. W. Beulens, Y. T. van der Schouw, A. DI van der, G. Buckland, A. Kuijsten, M. B. Schulze et al. 2013. Dietary glycemic index, glycemic load, and digestible carbohydrate intake are not associated with risk of type 2 diabetes in eight European countries. *J Nutr*, 143(1):93–99. doi: 10.3945/jn.112.165605.

Smith, J. D., T. Hou, D. S. Ludwig, E. B. Rimm, W. Willett, F. B. Hu, and D. Mozaffarian. 2015. Changes in intake of protein foods, carbohydrate amount and quality, and long-term weight change: Results from 3 prospective cohorts. *Am J Clin Nutr*, 101(6):1216–1224. doi: 10.3945/ajcn.114.100867.

Solomon, T. P., J. M. Haus, K. R. Kelly, M. D. Cook, J. Filion, M. Rocco, S. R. Kashyap, R. M. Watanabe, H. Barkoukis, and J. P. Kirwan. 2010. A low-glycemic index diet combined with exercise reduces insulin resistance, postprandial hyperinsulinemia, and glucose-dependent insulinotropic polypeptide responses in obese, prediabetic humans. *Am J Clin Nutr*, 92(6):1359–1368. doi: 10.3945/ajcn.2010.29771.

Solomon, T. P. and J. P. Thyfault. 2013. Type 2 diabetes sits in a chair. *Diabetes Obes Metab*, 15(11):987–992. doi: 10.1111/dom.12105.

Sommeijer, D. W., M. R. MacGillavry, J. C. Meijers, A. P. Van Zanten, P. H. Reitsma, and H. Ten Cate. 2004. Anti-inflammatory and anticoagulant effects of pravastatin in patients with type 2 diabetes. *Diabetes Care*, 27(2):468–473.

Stevens, J., K. Ahn, Juhaeri, D. Houston, L. Steffan, and D. Couper. 2002. Dietary fiber intake and glycemic index and incidence of diabetes in African-American and white adults: The ARIC study. *Diabetes Care*, 25(10):1715–1721.

Stone, N. J., J. G. Robinson, A. H. Lichtenstein, C. N. Bairey Merz, C. B. Blum, R. H. Eckel, A. C. Goldberg et al. 2014. 2013 ACC/AHA guideline on the treatment of blood cholesterol to reduce atherosclerotic cardiovascular risk in adults: A report of the American College of Cardiology/American Heart Association Task Force on Practice Guidelines. *Circulation*, 129(25 Suppl 2):S1–45. doi: 10.1161/01.cir.0000437738.63853.7a.

Stratton, I. M., A. I. Adler, H. A. Neil, D. R. Matthews, S. E. Manley, C. A. Cull, D. Hadden, R. C. Turner, and R. R. Holman. 2000. Association of glycaemia with macrovascular and microvascular complications of type 2 diabetes (UKPDS 35): Prospective observational study. *BMJ*, 321(7258):405–412.

Tan, J., J. J. Wang, V. Flood, S. Kaushik, A. Barclay, J. Brand-Miller, and P. Mitchell. 2007. Carbohydrate nutrition, glycemic index, and the 10-y incidence of cataract. *Am J Clin Nutr*, 86(5):1502–1508.

Tenenbaum, A., E. Z. Fisman, M. Motro, and Y. Adler. 2006. Atherogenic dyslipidemia in metabolic syndrome and type 2 diabetes: Therapeutic options beyond statins. *Cardiovasc Diabetol*, 5:20. doi: 10.1186/1475-2840-5-20.

Thomas, D. E. and E. J. Elliott. 2010. The use of low-glycaemic index diets in diabetes control. *Br J Nutr*, 104(6):797–802. doi: 10.1017/S0007114510001534.

Thomas, D. E., E. J. Elliott, and L. Baur. 2007. Low glycaemic index or low glycaemic load diets for overweight and obesity. *Cochrane Database Syst Rev*, (3):CD005105. doi: 10.1002/14651858.CD005105.pub2.

Tsihlias, E. B., A. L. Gibbs, M. I. McBurney, and T. M. Wolever. 2000. Comparison of high- and low-glycemic-index breakfast cereals with monounsaturated fat in the long-term dietary management of type 2 diabetes. *Am J Clin Nutr*, 72(2):439–449.

Tumosa, N. 2008. Eye disease and the older diabetic. *Clin Geriatr Med*, 24(3):515–527, vii. doi: 10.1016/j.cger.2008.03.002.

Turner-McGrievy, G. M., D. J. Jenkins, N. D. Barnard, J. Cohen, L. Gloede, and A. A. Green. 2011. Decreases in dietary glycemic index are related to weight loss among individuals following therapeutic diets for type 2 diabetes. *J Nutr*, 141(8):1469–1474. doi: 10.3945/jn.111.140921.

Turner, R. C., H. Millns, H. A. Neil, I. M. Stratton, S. E. Manley, D. R. Matthews, and R. R. Holman. 1998. Risk factors for coronary artery disease in non-insulin dependent diabetes mellitus: United Kingdom Prospective Diabetes Study (UKPDS: 23). *BMJ*, 316(7134):823–828.

UK Prospective Diabetes Study (UKPDS) Group. 1998. Effect of intensive blood-glucose control with metformin on complications in overweight patients with type 2 diabetes (UKPDS 34). *Lancet*, 352(9131):854–865.

United Kingdom Prospective Diabetes Study (UKPDS). 1995. 13: Relative efficacy of randomly allocated diet, sulphonylurea, insulin, or metformin in patients with newly diagnosed non-insulin dependent diabetes followed for three years. *BMJ*, 310(6972):83–88.

US Food and Drug Administration. 1998. *Food Labeling: Health Claims; Soluble Fiber from Certain Foods and Coronary Heart Disease*. Rockville, MD. Docket No. 96P-0338.

US Food and Drug Administration. 2008. Guidance for industry: Diabetes mellitus: Developing drugs and therapeutic biologics for treatment and prevention. http://www.fda.gov/cder/guidance/7630dft.pdf. (Accessed July 10, 2015.)

van Bakel, M. M., N. Slimani, E. J. Feskens, H. Du, J. W. Beulens, Y. T. van der Schouw, F. Brighenti et al. 2009. Methodological challenges in the application of the glycemic index in epidemiological studies using data from the European Prospective Investigation into Cancer and Nutrition. *J Nutr*, 139 (3):568–575. doi: 10.3945/jn.108.097121.

van Woudenbergh, G. J., A. Kuijsten, E. J. Sijbrands, A. Hofman, J. C. Witteman, and E. J. Feskens. 2011. Glycemic index and glycemic load and their association with C-reactive protein and incident type 2 diabetes. *J Nutr Metab*, 2011:623076. doi: 10.1155/2011/623076.

Venn, B. J., T. Perry, T. J. Green, C. M. Skeaff, W. Aitken, N. J. Moore, J. I. Mann et al. 2010. The effect of increasing consumption of pulses and whole grains in obese people: A randomized controlled trial. *J Am Coll Nutr*, 29(4):365–372.

Villegas, R., S. Liu, Y. T. Gao, G. Yang, H. Li, W. Zheng, and X. O. Shu. 2007. Prospective study of dietary carbohydrates, glycemic index, glycemic load, and incidence of type 2 diabetes mellitus in middle-aged Chinese women. *Arch Intern Med*, 167(21):2310–2316. doi: 10.1001/archinte.167.21.2310.

Vrolix, R. and R. P. Mensink. 2010. Effects of glycemic load on metabolic risk markers in subjects at increased risk of developing metabolic syndrome. *Am J Clin Nutr*, 92(2):366–374. doi: 10.3945/ajcn.2009.28339.

Wang, Q., W. Xia, Z. Zhao, and H. Zhang. 2014. Effects comparison between low glycemic index diets and high glycemic index diets on HbA1c and fructosamine for patients with diabetes: A systematic review and meta-analysis. *Prim Care Diabetes*, doi: 10.1016/j.pcd.2014.10.008.

Willett, W., J. Manson, and S. Liu. 2002. Glycemic index, glycemic load, and risk of type 2 diabetes. *Am J Clin Nutr*, 76(1):274S–280S.

Wolever, T. M., A. L. Gibbs, C. Mehling, J. L. Chiasson, P. W. Connelly, R. G. Josse, L. A. Leiter, P. Maheux, R. Rabasa-Lhoret, N. W. Rodger et al. 2008. The Canadian trial of carbohydrates in diabetes (CCD), a 1-y controlled trial of low-glycemic-index dietary carbohydrate in type 2 diabetes: No effect on glycated hemoglobin but reduction in C-reactive protein. *Am J Clin Nutr*, 87(1):114–125. doi: 87/1/114 [pii].

Wolever, T. M., D. J. Jenkins, V. Vuksan, A. L. Jenkins, G. C. Buckley, G. S. Wong, and R. G. Josse. 1992a. Beneficial effect of a low glycaemic index diet in type 2 diabetes. *Diabet Med*, 9(5):451–458.

Wolever, T. M., D. J. Jenkins, V. Vuksan, A. L. Jenkins, G. S. Wong, and R. G. Josse. 1992b. Beneficial effect of low-glycemic index diet in overweight NIDDM subjects. *Diabetes Care*, 15(4):562–564.

Wolever, T. M. and C. Mehling. 2003. Long-term effect of varying the source or amount of dietary carbohydrate on postprandial plasma glucose, insulin, triacylglycerol, and free fatty acid concentrations in subjects with impaired glucose tolerance. *Am J Clin Nutr*, 77(3):612–621.

Wolever, T. M., S. M. Tosh, A. L. Gibbs, J. Brand-Miller, A. M. Duncan, V. Hart, B. Lamarche, B. A. Thomson, R. Duss, and P. J. Wood. 2010. Physicochemical properties of oat beta-glucan influence its ability to reduce serum LDL cholesterol in humans: A randomized clinical trial. *Am J Clin Nutr*, 92(4):723–732. doi: 10.3945/ajcn.2010.29174.

World Health Organization. 2014. *WHO 2014 Global Status Report on Noncommunicable Diseases*. Geneva, Switzerland: WHO Press.

Wu, T., E. Giovannucci, T. Pischon, S. E. Hankinson, J. Ma, N. Rifai, and E. B. Rimm. 2004. Fructose, glycemic load, and quantity and quality of carbohydrate in relation to plasma C-peptide concentrations in US women. *Am J Clin Nutr*, 80(4):1043–1049.

Yamada, S., T. Yanagawa, K. Sasamoto, A. Araki, M. Miyao, and T. Yamanouchi. 2006. Atorvastatin lowers plasma low-density lipoprotein cholesterol and C-reactive protein in Japanese type 2 diabetic patients. *Metabolism*, 55(1):67–71. doi: 10.1016/j.metabol.2005.07.017.

Yeboah, J., J. R. Crouse, F. C. Hsu, G. L. Burke, and D. M. Herrington. 2007. Brachial flow-mediated dilation predicts incident cardiovascular events in older adults: The cardiovascular health study. *Circulation*, 115(18):2390–2397. doi: 10.1161/CIRCULATIONAHA.106.678276.

Yusof, B. N., R. A. Talib, N. A. Kamaruddin, N. A. Karim, K. Chinna, and H. Gilbertson. 2009. A low-GI diet is associated with a short-term improvement of glycaemic control in Asian patients with type 2 diabetes. *Diabetes Obes Metab*, 11(4):387–396. doi: 10.1111/j.1463-1326.2008.00984.x.

Zhang, Z., E. Lanza, P. M. Kris-Etherton, N. H. Colburn, D. Bagshaw, M. J. Rovine, J. S. Ulbrecht, G. Bobe, R. S. Chapkin, and T. J. Hartman. 2010. A high legume low glycemic index diet improves serum lipid profiles in men. *Lipids*, 45(9):765–775. doi: 10.1007/s11745-010-3463-7.

Zinman, B., C. Wanner, J. M. Lachin, D. Fitchett, E. Bluhmki, S. Hantel, M. Mattheus et al. 2015. Empagliflozin, cardiovascular outcomes, and mortality in type 2 diabetes. *N Engl J Med*, doi: 10.1056/NEJMoa1504720.

5 Glycemic Index and Cardiovascular Disease Risk Prevention and Management

Vanessa Ha, Effie Viguiliouk,* Arash Mirrahimi, John L. Sievenpiper, Russell J. de Souza, Cyril W.C. Kendall, David J.A. Jenkins, and Thomas M.S. Wolever*

CONTENTS

5.1 INTRODUCTION

Public health has shifted its focus from fat intake back to carbohydrate intake as an important marker of dietary quality to manage cardiovascular health. The glycemic index (GI) is a relative ranking of carbohydrates in foods according to how they affect fasting blood glucose (FBG) (Jenkins et al., 1981). It has been gaining attention for its clinical utility in managing chronic diseases, including cardiovascular disease (CVD) (Mitchell, 2008). Meta-analyses have consistently reported a reduced

* Shared first authorship.

cardiovascular risk when comparing the highest with the lowest quantile of GI intakes (Fan et al., 2012; Mirrahimi et al., 2012). There is also strong consistent evidence that GI benefits low-density lipoprotein cholesterol (LDL-C) (Fleming and Godwin, 2013; Goff et al., 2013), type 2 diabetes (T2DM), and diabetes risk factors (Ajala et al., 2013). However, the evidence for the effects of GI on other cardiometabolic outcomes has been less consistent. Systematic reviews and meta-analyses have suggested that GI may improve body weight only in overweight/obese people and the effects on blood pressure are mixed (Schwingshackl and Hoffmann, 2013). Despite inconsistencies in the data, sufficient positive findings have emerged to suggest that the dietary GI is of potential importance in the prevention and treatment of cardiovascular disease. These benefits have led to the inclusion of GI on food labels in Australia, the United Kingdom, and South Africa to guide consumers for food purchases (Mitchell, 2008) (see Chapter 12).

The importance of blood glucose in cardiovascular risk management has been recognized. Fluctuations in blood glucose after a meal have been linked to increased oxidative stress (Monnier et al., 2006), a process involved in the build-up of atheromatosis (Singh et al., 2005). Therefore, a reduced rate of glucose absorption after the consumption of low-GI foods will reduce the postprandial rise in blood glucose. Ideally, health guidelines have set plasma glucose levels at 2-h time point after a meal at or below 7.8 mmol/L (140 mg/dl), and values above this concentration are considered to indicate the presence of impaired glucose tolerance (American Diabetes Association, 2015; Goldenberg and Punthakee, 2013). Mitigating the risk of adverse outcomes associated with elevated postprandial glucose is an important target for population health.

GI has a long history of being used in research and clinical practice for managing elevated postprandial glucose. In this context, low-GI foods have also been shown to improve clinically established targets for cardiovascular health. Prospective cohort studies have consistently reported a protective association between intakes of low- and high-GI foods on coronary heart disease (CHD) (Fan et al., 2012; Mirrahimi et al., 2012), and some clinical trials have demonstrated improvements of cardiovascular risk factors in specific individuals (Ajala et al., 2013; Fleming and Godwin, 2013; Goff et al., 2013; Schwingshackl and Hoffmann, 2013). However, there are also a handful of clinical trials that did not show an effect of GI on cardiovascular risk. Part of this inconsistent finding is due to the study sample used (Brand-Miller et al., 2015), achieved GI difference between the low- and high-GI study groups, and the duration of follow-up (Brand-Miller et al., 2015). The utility of GI is best seen in participants who are at high risk for CVD (e.g., hypercholesterolemic, hypertensive, overweight/obese, and/or people living with diabetes), in which case a sufficient GI difference between diets is achieved and follow-up duration is greater than 24 weeks (or 6 months). This chapter will review the evidence from prospective cohort studies and clinical trials that assess the relationship between GI and cardiovascular health.

5.2 GLOBAL BURDEN OF CARDIOVASCULAR DISEASE

CVD is a major public health concern. The two most common types of CVD and most modifiable by dietary interventions are CHD and stroke (Boden-Albala and Sacco, 2000; Stampfer et al., 2000). The prevalence of CHD and stroke has decreased in high-income countries in the last 30 years; however, the global burden of both CHD and stroke still remains high (Yusuf et al., 2001). The burden is largely attributable to low- and middle-income countries (LMIC), as their socioeconomic status continues to change with increasing urbanization and industrialization (Yusuf et al., 2001). In 1990, almost 80% of all CVD deaths occurred in developing countries, with 8 million deaths attributable to CVD in LMIC, whereas in the same year, 5.3 million deaths due to CVD were recorded in high-income countries (Yusuf et al., 2001). By 2020, it is estimated that this discrepancy will become far larger, where CVD deaths in LMIC will increase to 19 million and CVD deaths in high-income countries will remain relatively stable at 6 million (Yusuf et al., 2001)—a 140% increase in cardiovascular deaths in LMIC in contrast to the 13% increase in high-income countries. The increasing burden of CVD in LMIC is likely because of changes in the lifestyle and a lack of accessibility to health resources that are needed for the prevention and management of CVD risk that are not always available in LMIC (Yusuf et al., 2001). Therefore, effective interventions for reducing the growing burden of CVD are important for public health.

5.2.1 Risk Factors for Cardiovascular Disease

Most CHD and stroke events are caused by the formation of atheromatosis, which is a plaque that develops along the lining of arterial walls. The process of plaque formation starts during childhood and is usually advanced by the time symptoms occur (Munro and Cotran, 1988). Atheromatosis starts with the uptake of LDL-C into the endothelial layer of the blood vessels. The LDL-C is more prone to oxidation once inside the arterial walls, where it becomes an inflammatory molecule (ox-LDL-C) when oxidized. In response, endothelial cells of the arterial walls attract monocytes, which become macrophages when activated. It has been proposed that ox-LDL-C is more likely to be taken up by macrophages via scavenger receptors and deposit as atheromatous plaques, as the macrophages die and become foam cells, leading to increased incidence of cardiovascular events (Singh et al., 2005).

Many risk factors for CHD and stroke have been identified to help modulate the formation of atheromatosis. Broadly, cardiovascular risk factors are classified into two categories: (1) nonmodifiable risk factors, which are fixed and cannot be altered, such as age, sex, and family history and (2) modifiable risk factors, which are dynamic and to some extent can be altered through changes in lifestyle and medication. The major modifiable risk factors of cardiovascular risk are considered to be dyslipidemia, hypertension, diabetes mellitus, and overweight/obesity (Stamler et al., 1999; Wilson et al., 1998; Yusuf et al., 2004). Along with cigarette smoking, these major risk factors have been reported to explain 92% of CHD deaths in the United States (Stamler et al., 1999). Similarly, the Framingham Heart Study (FHS) reported that 75%–77% of cardiovascular risk can be largely predicted by these same risk factors (Wilson et al., 1998). Screening and managing these conditions form the basis of many published guidelines of risk assessment and reduction strategies (American Diabetes Association, 2014; American Heart Association, 2009, 2011, 2013; Anderson et al., 2013; Canadian Diabetes Association, 2013; Canadian Hypertension Education Plan, 2015; Greenland et al., 2010; Joint British Societies-3, 2014; Joint National Committee-8, 2014; National Cholesterol Education Program, 2002; National Heart Foundation of Australia and the Cardiac Society of Australia and New Zealand, 2005).

5.2.1.1 Blood Lipids, Dyslipidemia, and Cardiovascular Disease

Dyslipidemia is a major cause of CHD and stroke because of the direct role that blood lipids play in the formation of atheromatosis. Generally, blood lipids can be classified into two groups: (1) atherogenic lipids, including LDL-C, intermediate-density lipoprotein cholesterol, very-low-density lipoprotein cholesterol, and chylomicrons and (2) nonatherogenic lipids, including high-density lipoprotein cholesterol (HDL-C) (National Cholesterol Education Program, 2002). It is proposed that the atherogenic lipids contribute to atheromatosis (Blaha et al., 2008). On the contrary, nonatherogenic HDL-C is protective of this process through its reverse cholesterol transport function (fats and cholesterol are transported out of the blood vessels and into the liver for metabolism) as well as through inhibition of monocyte migration, increased nitric oxide production (relaxes blood vessels), inhibition of the coagulation cascade, and antioxidative activity (Mearns, 2011). There is strong and consistent evidence from prospective cohort studies that apolipoprotein B (Apo-B) and apolipoprotein A (Apo-A), the proteins found on atherogenic and nonatherogenic lipid particles, respectively, are better predictors for cardiovascular risk (Barter and Rye, 2006; Barter et al., 2006). As there is only one Apo-B or Apo-A protein on each lipid particle, the measurement of these proteins are a better reflection of the actual number of circulating lipid particles in the blood (Barter and Rye, 2006; Barter et al., 2006). As a result, higher concentrations of Apo-B or Apo-A would correspond to higher circulating concentrations of the respective lipid particles.

The importance of dyslipidemia in cardiovascular risk has been well established. The FHS was the first study to identify that individuals who had elevated concentrations of cholesterol were at increased risk for heart disease (Joint British Socieities-3, 2014). These findings have been consistently confirmed in more expansive and rigorous epidemiological studies. The INTERHEART study, a case-control study of 52 countries with approximately 30,000 enrolled participants, identified that almost 50% of acute myocardial infarctions (MIs) can be prevented by modifying dyslipidemia (Yusuf et al., 2004), and similarly, the prospective cohort study, Multiple Risk Factor Intervention Trial, found that there was an inverse relationship between elevated cholesterol concentration and stroke risk in American men who were followed for 6 years (Iso et al., 1989). Recent genetic epidemiological studies have further demonstrated the importance of dyslipidemia in cardiovascular health. Findings from classic genetic studies suggest that early exposure to excessive LDL-C, which is often the result of mutations in the LDL-C receptor (occurring in genetic disorders such as familial hypercholesterolemia), results in early atherothrombosis (Ridker, 2014). On the basis of these consistent findings of the importance of lipids in cardiovascular health, dyslipidemia has been widely regarded as an important predictor of CVD.

Of all the lipids involved in cardiovascular health, LDL-C has been traditionally considered the most important. It is the only lipid that can be targeted by medication. Statins (also called 3-hydroxy-3-methylglutaryl-coenzyme A [HMG-CoA] reductase inhibitors), which work to suppress HMG-CoA reductase, a hepatic enzyme that plays a role in cholesterol synthesis, is a proof of this concept (Nissen and Wolski, 2007; Ray et al., 2010). On average, statins can lower LDL-C by 1.8 mmol/L (70 mg/dL), which translates into an estimated 60% decrease in the number of cardiac events (heart attack and sudden cardiac death) and a 17% reduced risk of stroke after long-term treatment (Law et al., 2003). Furthermore, a large meta-analysis that was undertaken by the Cholesterol Treatment Trialists' Collaboration reported that for every 1 mmol/L reduction in LDL-C, CHD risk is reduced by 20% (Mihaylova et al., 2012).

Heart health guidelines have established targets for lipids for the management of cardiovascular health. All major guidelines have set LDL-C as the primary target for managing dyslipidemia (American Heart Association, 2009, 2011, 2013; Anderson et al., 2013; Greenland et al., 2010; Joint British Societies-3, 2014; National Cholesterol Education Program, 2002; National Heart Foundation of Australia and the Cardiac Society of Australia and New Zealand, 2005). The Canadian guideline has also recently established non-HDL-C, which reflects all circulating atherogenic lipids and Apo-B as the alternate primary targets (Anderson et al., 2013).

5.2.1.2 Blood Pressure, Hypertension, and Cardiovascular Disease

Elevated blood pressure or hypertension is another major risk factor for CHD (Chobanian et al., 2003; Hackam et al., 2013) and stroke (National Heart, Lung and Blood Institute, 2014; Lawes et al., 2008). There are two measurements that are used clinically to assess blood pressure: (1) systolic blood pressure (SBP), which is the pressure reflected in the arteries when the heart is pumping blood and (2) diastolic blood pressure (DBP), which is the pressure reflected in the arteries when the heart is relaxed (Canadian Hypertension Education Plan, 2014; Chobanian et al., 2003; Hackam et al., 2013; Joint British Societies-3, 2014). Other indications of blood pressure are mean arterial pressure (the average of SBP and DBP) and pulse pressure (the difference between SBP and DBP), but these are not used clinically (Canadian Hypertension Education Plan, 2014; Chobanian et al., 2003; Hackam et al., 2013; Joint British Societies-3, 2014). Elevated blood pressure is a serious concern, because it reflects the level of resistance that the heart must overcome to pump blood into circulation, which, if not managed appropriately, can lead to major complications of the heart, kidneys, eyes, and brain over time (Mensah, 2002).

Similar to dyslipidemia, hypertension is a well-recognized risk factor of CHD and stroke. The FHS was the first to identify that elevated blood pressure is a significant predictor of cardiovascular events and mortality (Kannel et al., 1971). Since then, many studies have shown similar strong results in a range of patient populations and age groups (Mourad, 2008). The same previous INTERHEART study found that the population attributable risk for hypertension was 17.1% for MI (Yusuf et al., 2004), and other studies have found that the population attributable risk was greater than 55% for stroke (Lawes et al., 2008). Furthermore, meta-analyses of prospective cohort studies and randomized controlled trials (RCTs) have shown a consistent dose–response relationship between blood pressure and cardiovascular risk. In a recent meta-analysis of 61 prospective cohort studies involving 1 million adults, stroke mortality risk was reduced between 64% (ages 40–49 years) and 33% (ages 80–89 years) for every 20 mmHg SBP reduction and between 65% (ages 40–49 years) and 37% (ages 80–89 years) for every 10 mmHg DBP reduction. Similarly, ischemic heart disease mortality risk was reduced between 51% (ages 40–49 years) and 33% (ages 80–89 years) for every 20 mmHg SBP reduction and between 53% (ages 40–49 years) and 37% for every 10 mmHg DBP reduction (Lewington et al., 2002). Similar findings for the relationship between SBP and cardiovascular risk have also been found in meta-analyses of RCTs, but the effect estimates are smaller than those reported in prospective cohort studies, in which an average reduction of 12–13 mmHg in SBP over 4 years was associated with a 21% reduction in CHD, 37% reduction in stroke, and 25% reduction in total cardiovascular mortality (He and Whelton, 1999).

The predictive ability of SBP and DBP in cardiovascular risk has led to the development of recommendations to manage blood pressure. The blood pressure targets for individuals living without diabetes is 120/80 mmHg (SBP/DBP), whereas targets for individuals who are living with diabetes is set higher at 130/90 mmHg (Chobanian et al., 2003; Hackam et al., 2013; Joint British Socieities-3, 2014; National Heart Foundation of Australia and the Cardiac Society of Australia and New Zealand, 2005).

5.2.1.3 Body Weight, Overweight/Obesity, and Cardiovascular Disease

Overweight/obesity has become a global epidemic (Caballero, 2007) and in the past 10 years, dramatic increases in overweight/obesity have occurred in both children and adults (Poirier et al., 2006). Several methods of characterizing overweight/obesity have been developed, including body weight, percentage body fat, waist circumference, and waist-to-hip ratio, but the method that is most clinically used is body mass index (BMI), which is a function of an individual's body weight and height. Excessive weight gain is thought to be a function of the law of thermodynamics, where weight gain occurs as a result of positive energy balance (e.g., energy input is greater than output) (Caballero, 2007). Indeed, a lifestyle pattern of excessive food intake and sedentary habits is already prevalent in high-income countries and will become more prevalent as LMIC shifts toward greater economic prosperity (Yusuf et al., 2001). The effects of overweight/obesity are profound. Besides an altered metabolic profile, a variety of adaptations/alterations in cardiac structure and function occurs in the individual as adipose tissue accumulates in excess amounts, even in the absence of comorbidities (Caballero, 2007). Hence, overweight/obesity affects the heart through its influence on known risk factors such as dyslipidemia, hypertension, glucose intolerance, inflammatory markers, and the prothrombotic state (Caballero, 2007).

The importance of excessive body weight as a marker of overall health was recognized in the 1930s, but its relation to cardiovascular health was not established until the 1950s (Caballero, 2007). Using the body weight data collected by the Metropolitan Life Insurance Company, Breslow was the first to propose a direct link between the increasing prevalence of obesity and the increasing rates of CVD in the U.S. population (Breslow, 1952), a theme that was re-emphasized by the U.S. government in reports in the 1960s and 1970s (Caballero, 2007). More recent studies have also confirmed this relationship between overweight/obesity and cardiovascular risk. The INTERHEART study, which was conducted in 52 countries, found that the reduction of abdominal obesity could reduce greater than 30% of acute MIs, and similar results were also found for stroke risk (Yusuf et al., 2004). Furthermore, weight loss trials have reported that weight loss of even 5%–10% of body weight could produce a modest reduction in cardiovascular risk, regardless of individual's health status (Wing et al., 2011).

All cardiovascular health organizations support that a healthy body weight should be maintained for optimal heart health (American Diabetes Association, 2014; American Heart Association, 2009, 2011, 2013; Anderson et al., 2013; Canadian Diabetes Association, 2013; Canadian Hypertension Education

Plan, 2015; Greenland et al., 2010; Joint British Societies-3, 2014; Joint National Committee-8, 2014; National Cholesterol Education Program, 2002; National Heart Foundation of Australia and the Cardiac Society of Australia and New Zealand, 2005). Recommendations have been made that individuals should aim for a BMI between 18.5 kg/m^2 and 24.9 kg/m^2 for optimal health. Individuals with a BMI greater than 25 kg/m2 and greater than 30 kg/m2 are considered overweight and obese respectively, and individuals with these values of BMI are highly encouraged by health organizations to modify lifestyle patterns to reduce BMI and therefore the prevention of chronic diseases (American Diabetes Association, 2014; American Heart Association, 2009, 2011, 2013; Anderson et al., 2013; Canadian Diabetes Association, 2013; Canadian Hypertension Education Plan, 2015; Greenland et al., 2010; Joint British Societies-3, 2014; Joint National Committee-8, 2014; National Cholesterol Education Program, 2002; National Heart Foundation of Australia and the Cardiac Society of Australia and New Zealand, 2005).

5.2.1.4 Glycemic Control, Diabetes Mellitus, and Cardiovascular Disease

CVD is a major complication of diabetes mellitus (American Diabetes Association, 2015; Canadian Diabetes Association, 2013). Diabetes increases the risk of CVD between 4 times and 10 times, depending on the population being studied (Mazzone, 2010), and about 75% of deaths of individuals with diabetes are due to coronary artery disease (Luscher et al., 2003). There are several diabetes classifications, most of which fall under the following three categories: (1) type 1 diabetes, which usually develops during childhood or adolescence and is characterized by little or no insulin production; (2) T2DM, which usually develops during adulthood and is characterized by insulin resistance and a progressive decline in pancreatic β-cell function; and (3) gestational diabetes, which develops during pregnancy and is characterized by insulin resistance (American Diabetes Association, 2015; Australia Diabetes Society, 2012; National Institute for Care and Excellence, 2009; Goldenberg and Punthakee, 2013). Type 2 diabetes is the most common type of diabetes, with approximately 80% of the burden found in LMIC, where the prevalence is projected to continue to grow as LMIC becomes more urbanized and adopts more Western lifestyle patterns (Maruthur, 2013). The biochemical pathway linking CVD and diabetes remains unclear, but it is primarily thought to be via the higher inflammation and blood glycemia, leading to an increased oxidative environment and thus increasing the likelihood of the formation of atheromatosis (Dokken, 2008).

The relation of diabetes and CVD is well established. Similar to the previous risk factors, the FHS was the first study to identify that diabetes was a major risk factor for CVD (Kannel and McGee, 1979). Since then, multiple prospective cohort studies have been able to confirm the increased cardiovascular risk associated with diabetes. The INTERHEART study found that diabetes contributed to almost 10% of all acute MIs (Yusuf et al., 2004), and the Northern Manhattan Study, a prospective multiethnic cohort study of individuals living in Northern Manhattan, found that diabetes contributes to approximately 20% of stroke (Willey et al., 2014). In further support, a meta-analysis of RCTs (n = 5 trials and 33,040 participants) found that intensive glycemic control compared with standard of care resulted in significant improvements in cardiovascular risk. The pooled analysis demonstrated that intensive glycemic control compared with the control reduced nonfatal MI by 17% and CHD events by 15% (Ray et al., 2009). The relation of glycemia and vascular risk appears to be nonlinear. In another meta-analysis of prospective cohort studies, a modest J-shaped association between FBG and vascular risk was found. Compared with individuals with FBG concentrations ranging from 3.90 to 5.59 mmol/L (which was not associated with increased vascular risk), individuals with FBG concentrations less than 3.9, 5.60–6.09, and 6.10–6.99 mmol/L had 7%, 11%, and 17% increased risk, respectively (Sarwar et al., 2010).

Although diabetes organizations recognize the impact diabetes has on cardiovascular risk, each of the guidelines has its own approach with regard to minimizing cardiovascular risk for individuals living with diabetes (American Diabetes Association, 2015; Canadian Diabetes Association, 2013; Australian Diabetes Society, 2012; National Institute for Care and Excellence, 2009). The Canadian Diabetes Association recommends that glycemic control should aim for an HbA1c level of 7% or less in order to reduce the risk of microvascular complications (including retinopathy, nephropathy, and neuropathy) and possibly, also macrovascular complications (including CVD) (Canadian Diabetes

Association, 2013). In contrast, the Australian Diabetes Society (ADS) focuses on only managing glycemia to prevent macrovascular complications, where it recommends that FBG should be less than 10 mmol/L (Australian Diabetes Society, 2012). Both the American Diabetes Association (ADA) and the U.K.'s National Institute for Care and Excellence have taken a more comprehensive approach in their diabetes recommendations to manage cardiovascular health (American Diabetes Association, 2015; National Institute for Care and Excellence, 2009). Both guidelines outline specific blood pressure, blood lipids, and glycemia targets (American Diabetes Association, 2015; National Institute for Care and Excellence, 2009). Overall, all diabetes associations recognize the need for individuals living with diabetes to take extra steps to better manage their cardiometabolic health.

5.2.1.5 Other Emerging Cardiovascular Risk Factors

Although most cardiovascular risk can be explained by conventional risk factors, the search for additional risk factors continues in an attempt to address residual risk. Four important emerging risk factors have been identified are as follows: C-reactive protein (CRP), lipoprotein (a) [Lp(a)], fibrinogen, and homocysteine (Hackam and Anand, 2003). With the exception of homocysteine, all three of the previous emerging risk factors have been established to be involved with acute inflammatory response, thus linking them to the formation of arterial plaque build-up (atheromatosis), whereas the biological function of homocysteine is still unknown (Hackam and Anand, 2003). The independent associations of these emerging risk factors have been supported from epidemiological and basic sciences; however, with regard to CRP, there has been a lack of evidence to demonstrate the specificity of the risk factor to CVD, and RCTs have been lacking to show that targeting individuals with high levels of any of these risk factors improves the prevalence of CVD or that lowering the levels of these risk factors lowers cardiovascular risk (Hackam and Anand, 2003). Furthermore, studies showing that are limited the addition of any of these risk factors adds substantial information to the current global assessments for cardiovascular risk, such as the widely used Framingham Risk Score (Buckley et al., 2009; Clarke et al., 2010; Hackam and Anand, 2003; Nordestgaard et al., 2010). The lack of certainty on the impact of CRP, Lp(a), fibrinogen, and homocysteine has been reflected in current cardiovascular guidelines by the absence of recommendations for these risk factors (American Heart Association, 2011; Anderson et al., 2013; Joint British Societies-3, 2014; National Vascular Disease Prevention Alliance, 2009).

5.3 PREVENTION AND MANAGEMENT OF CARDIOVASCULAR DISEASE

Since the burden of CVD is high, effective interventions to prevent and manage CVD are important to public health. Medications and lifestyle choices (e.g., smoking, physical activity, and diet) are preferred methods for cardiovascular health management.

5.3.1 Medication

The availability of medications to manage the risk of CVD has grown in parallel with the increasing prevalence of CVD. Although most of these medications have been proven to be safe and effective, they are not all well tolerated by some individuals and recent studies have found they do not always deliver their anticipated benefits. For example, statins, the most commonly prescribed cholesterol-lowering medication, can elevate muscle or liver enzymes (Blaier et al., 2011), and a recent meta-analysis has not shown statin to reduce all-cause mortality in a high-risk prevention setting (Ray et al., 2010); diuretics, a common blood pressure-lowering medication increased the risk of hyper- and hypokalemia and has been shown to increase mortality risk in individuals with acute renal failure (Mehta et al., 2002); orlistat, the only U.S. Food and Drug Administration (FDA)-approved weight-loss medication, has not shown long-term benefits (Redberg and Katz, 2012); and metformin, the most commonly prescribed glycemia-lowering medication, can increase build-up of lactic acid, which can lead to muscle pain or weakness (Kritchevsky and Story, 1974). Furthermore, although medication has become more affordable over the last few decades, there is still a large gap in healthcare accessibility and affordability in LMIC (Yusuf et al., 2001) and even within high-income countries such as the United States (Morgan and Kennedy, 2010). Therefore, other approaches for the prevention and management of cardiovascular risk are still needed.

5.3.2 Smoking

Smoking is a major risk factor for cardiovascular events, and thus, smoking cessation is an important intervention in the prevention and management of cardiovascular health. Smoking cessation strategies include quitting without assistance; medication, including nicotine replacement therapy and varenicline; and behavioral counseling. A meta-analysis of 41 RCTs found that the combination of medication and behavioural counseling was the most effective approach for increasing smoking cessation rates (Stead and Lancaster, 2012). Many pathophysiological changes caused by smoking can be reversed or improved by smoking cessation. A meta-analysis of 20 prospective cohort studies found a 36% reduction in relative risk (RR) of mortality for patients with CHD who quit smoking compared with those who continued smoking (Critchley and Capewell, 2003). RCTs have also reported similar results, where the Multiple Risk Factor Intervention Trial found a 62% risk reduction in CHD mortality in those who successfully quit smoking compared with those who did not after a 3-year follow-up period (Ockene et al., 1990). Although smoking is the number one predictor for cardiovascular health, accounting for 35.7% of all acute MIs (Yusuf et al., 2004), the importance of smoking cessation to reduce cardiovascular risk needs to be better emphasized, as studies have shown that the number of smokers is increasing, with greater than 80% of them currently residing in LMIC (Erhardt, 2009). Nevertheless, over time, the consumption of fatty and refined carbohydrate foods combined with a more sedentary lifestyle becomes more prevalent, as the countries becomes more affluent (Jenkins et al., 2002). Thus, diet and exercise become even more important interventions for the management of cardiovascular risk.

5.3.3 Physical Activity and Diet

Further optimization of cardiovascular health involves consistent physical activity and healthy eating. As metabolism is a function of the input and output of energy, physical activity and diet are important factors to consider in cardiovascular health. The current Western lifestyle characterized by sedentary habits and a Western diet characterized by a higher intake of processed meat, red meat, butter, high-fat dairy products, eggs, and refined grains (Hu, 2002) represent a surge of excess energy. The picture emerges of an overweight population challenged by an excess of rapidly absorbed food and lack of physical activity, resulting in adiposity, which predisposes one to cardiometabolic diseases. The Western lifestyle of the twenty-first century may thus be viewed as the nexus for the major chronic diseases.

5.4 GLYCEMIC INDEX

GI has been gaining public health attention as a dietary strategy to reduce cardiometabolic risk. The concept was developed by Dr. David Jenkins and his team at the University of Toronto in 1981 (Jenkins et al., 1981) and is used as an indication of the food's effect on a person's blood glucose concentration after consumption. High-GI foods produce a sharp spike in blood glucose after consumption, which has been linked to increased cardiovascular risk factors and oxidative stress, whereas low-GI foods produce a smaller rise in blood glucose, which in turn has been associated with better cardiovascular health (Ludwig, 2002).

5.5 CURRENT DIETARY GUIDELINES ON GLYCEMIC INDEX

Healthy eating recommendations and disease prevention guidelines recognize the importance of carbohydrate food choices in the prevention and management of cardiometabolic risk (American

Diabetes Association, 2014; American Heart Association, 2009, 2011, 2013; Anderson et al., 2013; Canadian Diabetes Association, 2013; Canadian Hypertension Education Plan, 2015; Greenland et al., 2010; Joint British Societies-3, 2014; Joint National Committee-8, 2014; National Cholesterol Education Program, 2002; National Heart Foundation of Australia and the Cardiac Society of Australia and New Zealand, 2005). Although many guidelines have made a distinction on both the type and quantity of carbohydrates consumed, only a few guidelines have made specific recommendations to include the use of GI and glycemic load (GL) in making healthy choices regarding carbohydrate foods. These guidelines include the diabetes associations (European Association for the Study of Diabetes, ADS, Canadian Diabetes Association, and ADA), National Institute for Care and Excellence, and the World Health Organization/Food and Agriculture Organization (Table 5.1).

With the exception of the ADS, the GI and GL recommendations made by the diabetes associations are based on the glycemic improvements observed in feeding trials and observational studies. These health organizations have found a consistent reduction in HbA1c between 0.4% and 0.5% when comparing low-GI diets with high-GIs diets in feeding trials and an increased diabetes risk with higher GI intake in prospective cohort studies. Although the beneficial glycemic effect is smaller than other dietary interventions, the European Association for the Study of Diabetes found this effect to be important, as the effect is above and beyond most of what other dietary interventions can achieve (e.g., reduction in total carbohydrate intake and increase in dietary fiber intake) (Mann et al., 2004). Furthermore, this HbA1c reduction of 0.4%–0.5% exceeds the clinically meaningful threshold of 0.3% or more proposed by FDA for the development of new drugs for diabetes (Food and Drug Administration, 2002). Taken together, there is strong evidence to support a glycemic benefit with lower GI intakes.

5.6 EFFECTS OF THE GLYCEMIC INDEX ON RISK FACTORS OF CARDIOVASCULAR DISEASE

Although the benefits of following a low-GI diet have been well established for the management of blood sugars (Brand-Miller et al., 2003), there has been a great deal of interest in understanding the relation between GI and other CVD risk factors. As diabetes predisposes individuals to vascular disease (Haffner et al., 1998), following a low-GI diet may represent a possible dietary therapy that may be used in conjunction with other preventative measures and/or treatments to help individuals manage their CVD risk. Both prospective cohort studies and controlled dietary trials have examined the relationship between GI and CVD risk factors and incident CVD cases, which will be reviewed in the following sections.

5.6.1 Glycemic Index, Blood Lipids, and Dyslipidemia

In acute studies of low-GI diets compared with high-GI or other control diets, where follow-up duration was less than 24 weeks, consistent improvements in total cholesterol (TC) and LDL-C were reported. A systematic review and meta-analysis of four RCTs consisting of overweight and obese individuals ($n = 212$) found that low-GI diets significantly improved TC and LDL-C in comparison with high-GI diets over an average 9-week follow-up duration, without significantly affecting HDL-C or triglyceride (TG) concentrations (Fleming and Godwin, 2013) (Figure 5.1). These findings were consistent with those of an updated systematic review and meta-analysis of 28 RCTs consisting of individuals with various health conditions (including diabetes, CHD, and overweight or obese; $n = 1272$). This study also found that low-GI diets significantly improved TC and LDL-C in comparison with control diets (high-GI, "normal," or "healthy-eating" diet) over an average 18-week duration, which was seen independent of weight loss (Figure 5.1) (Goff et al., 2013). Of particularly importance, the greatest improvements in LDL-C were seen in trials, with a larger difference in GI between intervention and control although, these improvements may be restricted to trials of shorter duration (<24 weeks) (Goff et al., 2013).

TABLE 5.1
Recommendations on Glycemic Index and Glycemic Load in Dietary Guidelines

Guideline	Carbohyrate	Fiber	Glycemic Index and/or Load
		General Dietary Advice	
IOM 2002	45%–65% E	For adults $\leq$50 years of age, 26 g/d (women) 38 g/d (men) For adults >50 years of age, 21 g/d (women) 30 g/d (men)	–
WHO/FAO 2002 and 2007	55%–75% E	>25 g/d	Can be indicative of food quality but should not be the sole determinant
NHMRC 2013	45%–65% E	Increase consumption of cereal foods	Lack of information on GI
USDA 2015	45%–65% E	25 g/d (women) 38 g/d (men)	Not necessary to consider for weight management
		Cardiovascular Recommendations	
AHA 2009 (overweight and obesity)	–	–	Insufficient evidence to determine whehter GI or GL affects lipids or BP
AHA 2013 (lifestyle guideline)	–	–	High and low GL produce a comparable weight loss
		Dyslipidemia Recommendations	
NCEP- ATP III 2002	<60% E	5–10 g/d of viscous fiber	Not a widely accepted practicle means for CHO food choices
AHA 2011	–	Increase intake	The role of GI remains controversial
CCS 2012	–	>10 g/d	–
		Hypertension Recommendations	
JNC 8 2014	–	–	–
CHEP 2015	–		–
		Diabetes Recommendations	
EASD 2004	45%–65% E	>40 g/d	Low-GI foods are suitable as CHO food choice
NICE 2009	–	Increase intake	Increase low-GI foods
ADC 2012	–	Increase intake	Increase nutritious low-GI foods
CDA 2013	$\geq$45% E if regular diet ~60% E if CHO is low-GI or high-fiber	For adults $\leq$50 years of age, 26 g/d (women) 38 g/d (men) For adults >50 years of age, 21 g/d (women) 30 g/d (men)	Replacement of low-GL foods for higher-Gl may modestly improve glycemic control
ADA 2014	–	25 g/d (women) 38 g/d (men)	Replacement of low-GL foods for higher-GL may modestly improve glycemic control

Abbreviations: % E, percentage of total daily energy intake; g/d, grams per day; BP, blood pressure; GI, glycemic index; GL, glycemic load; ADA, American Diabetes Association; ADC, Australian Diabetes Council; AHA, American Heart Association; CDA, Canadian Diabetes Association; CHO, carbohydrate; CHEP, Canadian Hypertension Education Plan; CCS, Canadian Cardiovascular Society; EASD, European Association for the Study of Diabetes; IOM, Institute of Medicine; JNC 8, Eighth Joint National Committee; NCEP-ATP, National Cholesterol Educatipn Plan-Adult Treatment Plan; NHMRC, Austrialian National Health Medical Research Council; UK, United Kingdom; USDA, United States Department of Agriculture; WHO/FAO, World Health Organization/Food and Agriculture Organization.

Blood Lipid End Point	SRMA	No. RCTs	n	Participant Characteristics	Achieved GI, Control	Achieved GI, Intervention	Follow-up Duration, wks	Pooled Effect Estimates, MD (95% CI), mmol/L	I^2
TC	Fleming et al. 2013	4	212	Mixed lipid status	~74.5	~43.7	5–12	−0.27 (−0.44, −0.10)	0%
	Goff et al. 2013	27	1441	Mixed lipid status	~63.5	~47.0	4–52	−0.13 (−0.22, −0.04)	0%
	Schwingshackl et al. 2013	13	2271	Mixed lipid status	~64.2	~52.8	24–68	−0.03 (−0.15, 0.08)	44%
	Ajala et al. 2013	–	–	–	–	–	–	–	–
LDL-C	Fleming et al. 2013	4	212	Mixed lipid status	~74.5	~43.7	5–12	−0.23 (−0.39, −0.06)	0%
	Goff et al. 2013	23	1281	Mixed lipid status	~63.4	~47.3	4–52	−0.16 (−0.24, −0.08)	0%
	Schwingshackl et al. 2013	14	2344	Mixed lipid status	~64.3	~52.4	24–68	−0.01 (−0.12, 0.10)	54%
	Ajala et al. 2013	–	–	–	–	–	–	–	–
HDL-C	Fleming et al. 2013	4	212	Mixed lipid status	~74.5	~43.7	5–12	0.09 (−0.06, 0.23)	78%
	Goff et al. 2013	24	1331	Mixed lipid status	~63.4	~47.1	4–52	−0.03 (−0.06, 0.00)	0%
	Schwingshackl et al. 2013	14	2344	Mixed lipid status	~64.3	~52.4	24–68	0.02 (−0.01, 0.04)	0%
	Ajala et al. 2013	3	357	Mixed lipid status	~81.8	~72.8	12–48	0.05 (0.02, 0.07)	–
TG	Fleming et al. 2013	4	212	Mixed lipid status	~74.5	~43.7	5–12	−0.15 (−0.48, 0.18)	84%
	Goff et al. 2013	27	1412	Mixed lipid status	~63.5	~46.5	4–52	0.01 (−0.06, 0.08)	0%
	Schwingshackl et al. 2013	14	2344	Mixed lipid status	~64.3	~52.4	24–68	−0.01 (−0.07, 0.05)	0%
	Ajala et al. 2013	–	–	–	–	–	–	–	–

−1 −0.5 0 0.5 1
Favors low GI **Favors control**

FIGURE 5.1 Summary of most recent systematic reviews and meta-analyses of RCTs looking at the effect of GI on blood lipid endpoints. Achieved GI, average GI of intervention or control arm across all trials included in the meta-analysis; MD, mean difference; mixed lipid status, meta-analysis included participants with and without elevated blood lipids; n, number of participants; No., number; SRMA, systematic review and meta-analysis; TC, total cholesterol. *I^2 refers to the degree of interstudy heterogeneity, where 0%–40%: might not be important heterogeneity; 30%–60%: moderate heterogeneity; 50%–90%: may be substantial heterogeneity; and 75%–100%: considerable heterogeneity. (From Higgins, J. P. T. and S. Green (editors). 2011. *Cochrane Handbook for Systematic Reviews of Interventions Version 5.1.0* (updated March 2011). The Cochrane Collaboration, Oxford. Available from http://handbook.cochrane.org/. With Permission.)

In contrast to the findings from the acute studies of less than 24 weeks, longer-term RCTs with follow-up duration of 24 weeks or more have not found consistent blood lipid effects. A third systematic review and meta-analysis of three RCTs consisting of individuals with T2DM ($n = 357$) and a follow-up duration of 6 months or more found that low-GI diets did not significantly lower LDL-C and TG levels but significantly improved HDL-C in comparison with control diets (high-GI, high-fiber, or ADA diet) (Ajala et al., 2013) (Figure 5.1). This lack of effect on LDL-C and TG has also been reported in another systematic review and meta-analysis of 14 RCTs consisting of overweight and obese individuals with and without diabetes ($n = 2325$), which again restricted its analysis to studies with a minimum 6-month follow-up duration (Schwingshackl and Hoffmann, 2013).

This meta-analysis showed that the combined effects of low-GI and low-GL diets did not have any effects on TC, LDL-C, HDL-C, or TG concentrations in comparison with the combined effects of high-GI and high-GL diets (Schwingshackl and Hoffmann, 2013) (Figure 5.1). This lack of effect on blood lipids may be due to the small difference in GI achieved between intervention and control across the trials, which consisted of a GI difference of approximately 8 units in both meta-analyses (Ajala et al., 2013; Schwingshackl and Hoffmann, 2013). This small difference in GI achieved within studies with a longer follow-up duration may reflect the participants' greater difficulty to comply with dietary interventions over time, a threat to validity that has been reported in many other dietary studies and is supported by data from more recent longer-term RCTs (Aller et al., 2014; Juanola-Falgarona et al., 2014). For example, in the GLYNDIET study, a 6-month RCT conducted in overweight and obese participants ($n = 81$) with at least one risk factor of the metabolic syndrome, no significant differences in TC, LDL-C, and HDL-C were found between those on a low-GI diet and those on a high-GI diet. The intention of this study was to achieve a GI difference of 28 units between intervention and control; however, the actual GI difference achieved at the end of study was only seven units (Juanola-Falgarona et al., 2014). This was also seen in a 12-month RCT conducted in overweight and obese individuals ($n = 256$) at eight study centers of the Diet, obesity, and genes (Diogenes) study. It found no difference in effect on TC, LDL-C, HDL-C, or TG concentrations between those on a low-GI diet and those on a high-GI diet, and the achieved GI difference between the two diets was only 5.1 units (Aller et al., 2014). Taken together, the current evidence suggests that low-GI diets compared with control diets improve TC and LDL-C at the start of studies, but in longer-term RCTs of follow-up duration greater than 24 weeks, these improvements are lost likely as a result of lost compliance to dietary interventions.

There are, however, notable exceptions to the above remark, where a greater GI difference is needed to achieve improvements on blood lipids. The OmniCarb study, an RCT conducted in healthy overweight adults ($n = 163$), did not find TC and LDL-C improvements, even though it achieved a GI difference of approximately 25 units between diets. Although this GI difference is considered large, the follow-up duration was much shorter (5 weeks) (Sacks et al., 2014). On the contrary, studies with both longer follow-up durations of 3 and 6 months and larger GI differences between 12.6 units and 19 units have reported improvements in TC, LDL-C, and TC:HDL-C ratio (Jenkins et al., 2014; Philippou et al., 2009). Therefore, longer-term dietary trials with larger GI differences between intervention and control diets are needed to clarify these results.

Traditional foods with low-GI have resulted in short-term improvements on blood lipids. A systematic review and meta-analysis of eight RCTs in healthy individuals ($n = 253$) that compared the effect of barley consumption with control diets found significant improvements in TC (mean difference [MD] = −0.29 mmol/L; 95% CI: −0.39, −0.19 mmol/L; $p < .00001$) and LDL-C (MD = −0.26 mmol/L; 95% CI: −0.34, −0.19 mmol/L; $p < .00001$) (AbuMweis et al., 2010). Likewise, dietary pulses (beans, chickpeas, lentils, and peas), another traditional low-GI food, have also demonstrated TC and LDL-C lowering benefits. This was shown in a systematic review and meta-analysis of 26 RCTs ($n = 1037$) conducted in individuals with hyperlipidemia, normal lipid levels, or both, which found that dietary pulse intake significantly lowered LDL-C (MD = −0.17 mmol/L; 95% CI: −0.25, −0.09 mmol/L; $p < .0001$) over a median of approximately 6-week follow-up duration (Ha et al., 2014). Although the median follow-up duration of all these meta-analyses was greater than 3 weeks, a duration that satisfies the minimum follow-up requirement issued by FDA for the scientific evaluation of lipid-lowering health claims (Center for Drug Evaluation and Research, 2008), it is unclear whether these effects can be sustained over a longer time duration (e.g., 3 months). Therefore, longer trials are needed to better assess the effect of low-GI foods on blood lipids.

Several mechanisms have been proposed for the modification of blood lipids by low-GI diets. First, the typical high-fiber content of low-GI diets may bring about reductions in bile acid and cholesterol reabsorption from the ileum, which may inhibit hepatic cholesterol synthesis (Augustin et al., 2002; Jenkins et al., 1993; Kritchevsky and Story, 1974). Second, low-GI diets may lower the activity of insulin-stimulated HMG-CoA reductase, the rate-limiting enzyme in cholesterol synthesis, as a result of a reduced rate of carbohydrate absorption (Augustin et al., 2002; Rodwell et al., 1976). Third, resistant low-GI starches can give rise to by-products of colonic fermentation, such as the short-chain fatty acid propionate, which has been shown to inhibit cholesterol synthesis (Augustin et al., 2002; Illman et al., 1988; Wright et al., 1990).

Overall, the results of the most recent studies discussed in this section show that low-GI diets improve blood lipids over the short term, which appear to be greater in trials with greater differences in GI between intervention and control, whereas the lack of effect in longer-term trials may be due to compliance issues and small achieved differences in GI. Therefore, longer-term dietary trials with larger GI differences are needed to better understand the effect of low-GI diets on blood lipids.

5.6.2 Glycemic Index, Blood Pressure, and Hypertension

Only one systematic review and meta-analysis of RCTs has examined the effects of GI and GL on blood pressure. This pooled analysis of 11 RCTs consisting of overweight and obese individuals with and without diabetes (n = 1576) and a follow-up duration of 6 months or more found no significant differences between high-GI/GL diets and low-GI/GL diets on SBP and DBP (Figure 5.2) (Schwingshackl and Hoffmann, 2013). Consistent with these findings are those from several RCTs that have been conducted since the publication of this meta-analysis. The Diogenes trial, which was conducted in overweight and obese individuals (n = 256) over a 12-month follow-up duration, reported no differences in SBP and DBP between low-GI and high-GI diets (Aller et al., 2014). The study participants, however, had healthy blood pressure values (<120 mmHg SBP and <80 mmHg DBP), which makes it more difficult to achieve any significant improvements (Aller et al., 2014). Similar findings have also been reported by RCTs conducted in overweight and obese children and adolescents (Iannuzzi et al., 2009; Rouhani et al., 2013). One exception to this pattern was the OmniCarb trial, which found no blood pressure effect even though the participants' baseline values for blood pressure exceeded clinical targets of 120 mmHg for SBP and 80 mmHg for DBP (Sacks et al., 2014). This may be due to the short 5-week follow-up duration (Sacks et al., 2014), which may or may not be long enough to detect significant changes in blood pressure. Therefore, future trials should be of longer follow-up duration and focus on examining the effect of low-GI diets in individuals with less optimal blood pressure.

Despite these findings in otherwise-healthy individuals, low-GI diets appear to have a positive effect on blood pressure in overweight and obese adults with T2DM. One RCT (n = 121) that achieved a low-GI diet through increased dietary pulse consumption found greater reduction in SBP when compared with a high-fiber diet (MD = 4.5 mmHg; 95% CI: −7.0, −2.1 mmHg; $p < .001$) (Jenkins et al., 2012). Similarly, in another RCT (n = 141) that compared a low-GL diet containing higher monounsaturated fatty acid (MUFA) and α-linolenic acid (ALA) content with a whole-grain diet, SBP improvement was observed in those who had the greatest benefits in glycemic control (Jenkins et al., 2014). Overall, the results of these studies support the beneficial effect of low-GI diets on blood pressure in individuals with more than one CVD risk factor; however, more trials are needed to further verify these findings.

Blood Pressure End Point	SRMA	No. RCTs	*n*	Participant Characteristics	Achieved GI, Control	Achieved GI, Intervention	Follow-up Duration, wks	Pooled Effect Estimates, MD (95% CI), mmHg	I^2
SBP	Schwingshackl et al. 2013	11	2034	Mixed hypertensive status	~62.5	~51.7	24–68	0.08 (−1.12, 1.28)	0%
DBP	Schwingshackl et al. 2013	11	2034	Mixed hypertensive status	~62.5	~51.7	24–68	−0.75 (−1.71, 0.21)	13%

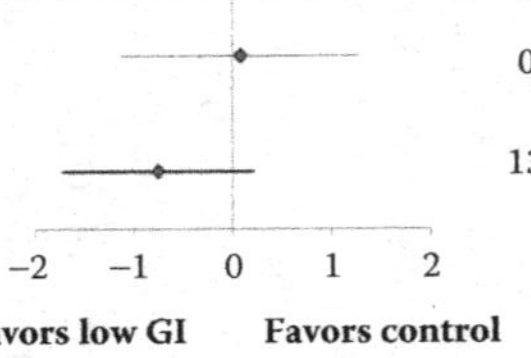

FIGURE 5.2 Summary of most recent systematic reviews and meta-analyses of RCTs looking at the effect of GI on blood pressure endpoints. Achieved GI, average GI of intervention or control arm across all trials included in the meta-analysis; DBP, diastolic blood pressure; MD, mean difference; mixed hypertensive status, meta-analysis included participants with and without elevated blood pressure; *n*, number of participants; No., number; SBP, systolic blood pressure; SRMA, systematic review and meta-analysis. *I^2 refers to the degree of interstudy heterogeneity, where 0%–40%: might not be important heterogeneity; 30%–60%: moderate heterogeneity; 50%–90%: may be substantial heterogeneity; and 75%–100%: considerable heterogeneity. (From Higgins, J. P. T. and S. Green (editors). 2011. *Cochrane Handbook for Systematic Reviews of Interventions Version 5.1.0* (updated March 2011). The Cochrane Collaboration, Oxford. Available from http://handbook.cochrane.org/. With Permission.)

Dietary pulses and temperate climate foods, which are traditional low-GI foods, have been found to improve blood pressure. One systematic review and meta-analysis of eight RCTs (n = 554) that looked at the effect of pulse consumption in individuals with various health conditions (overweight or obese, pre-metabolic syndrome, T2DM, etc.) found that incorporating approximately 162 d serving of dietary pulses per day over a median 10-week follow-up duration significantly reduced SBP (MD = −2.25 mmHg; 95% CI: −4.22, −0.28 mmHg; p = .03), without significantly affecting DBP (Jayalath et al., 2014). These findings appear to be consistent with those reported from large observational studies using data collected from National Health and Nutrition Examination Survey (Bazzano et al., 2001; Papanikolaou and Fulgoni, 2008), one of which found that consumption of legumes four times a week lowered the risk of CHD and CVD by 22% and 11%, respectively (Bazzano et al., 2001). Temperate climate fruits (apples, pears, citrus fruit, berries, and fruits from the *Prunus* family), which are low-GI foods, have also been shown to potentially lower blood pressure (Jenkins et al., 2011). In a secondary analysis of a 6-month RCT advising individuals with T2DM (n = 152) to follow a low-GI or high-fiber diet, which also included advice on fruit consumption, it was shown that higher intake of temperate climate fruits significantly predicted reductions in SBP (r = −0.183; p = .024) and CHD risk (r = −0.213; p = .008) (Jenkins et al., 2011). Therefore, higher intakes of specific low-GI foods, such as dietary pulses and temperate climate fruits, appear to have beneficial effects on blood pressure.

5.6.3 Glycemic Index, Body Weight, and Obesity

The most recent systematic reviews and meta-analyses of RCTs assessing the effect of low-GI diets in comparison with control diets on body weight outcomes do not appear to show any overall significant effects (Figure 5.3). A systematic review and meta-analysis of 14 long-term RCTs (≥24 weeks) consisting of overweight and obese individuals with and without diabetes (n = 2325) showed that low-GI/low-GL diets did not significantly alter body weight, fat mass, and waist circumference in comparison with high-GI/high-GL diets (Figure 5.3) (Schwingshackl and Hoffmann, 2013). A similar lack of effect on body weight has also been found for individuals with T2DM (n = 357) (Figure 5.3) (Ajala et al., 2013). These findings are also consistent with recent results from several RCTs identified outside of these meta-analyses. For example, a 3-month low-GL diet emphasizing ALA and MUFA did not significantly alter body weight or waist circumference in comparison with a whole-grain diet in a group of overweight and obese individuals with T2DM (n = 141) (Jenkins et al., 2014). However, both diets showed significant reductions in body weight and waist circumference at the end of the 3-month period, indicating that a low-GL diet may be beneficial for weight loss but not above and beyond the body weight effect seen with a whole-grain diet (Jenkins et al., 2014). The OmniCarb trial conducted in overweight adults (n = 163) residing in the United States that looked at the effect of low- and high-GI diets in the context of the healthy DASH diet found no body weight difference between the two GI diets; however, participants did lose 1 kg of body weight in each arm over the 5-week study duration (Sacks et al., 2014). Again, this demonstrates that following a low-GI diet may not produce any additional weight loss benefits when compared with other healthy diets, but in itself, it still produces meaningful weight reduction.

There is an indication that obese individuals may derive greater benefit from a low-GI diet. In a meta-analysis of RCTs, a low GI/GL diet compared with a high GI/GL diet showed significant weight loss in obese individuals with a BMI of 30 kg/m^2 or more (both MD = −1.26 kg; 95% CI: −2.17, −0.34 kg), but a similar significant weight loss effect was not seen for normal weight or overweight people (Schwingshackl and Hoffmann, 2013).

Prospective cohort studies that looked at the relationship between GI and obesity risk have shown mixed findings. The Seguimiento Universidad de Navarra cohort, which was conducted in a Spanish university student cohort over a 5-year follow-up duration (n = 9267), found no

Body Weight End Point	SRMA	No. RCTs	n	Participant Characteristics	Achieved GI, Control	Achieved GI, Intervention	Follow-up Duration, wks	Pooled Effect Estimates, MD (95% CI)	I^2
Body weight (kg)	Schwingshackl et al. 2013	14	2325	Overweight or obese	~64.2	~52.4	24–68	−0.62 (−1.28, 0.03)	0%
	Ajala et al. 2013	3	357	Overweight or obese	~81.8	~72.8	12–48	1.39 (−1.58, 4.36)	–
Waist circumference (cm)	Schwingshackl et al. 2013	8	1726	Overweight or obese	~61.8	~55.9	24–68	0.06 (−0.83, 0.96)	0%
	Ajala et al. 2013	–	–	–	–	–	–	–	–
Fat mass (kg)	Schwingshackl et al. 2013	5	868	Overweight or obese	~62.0	~52.2	26–68	−0.56 (−1.24, 0.12)	0%
	Ajala et al. 2013	–	–	–	–	–	–	–	–

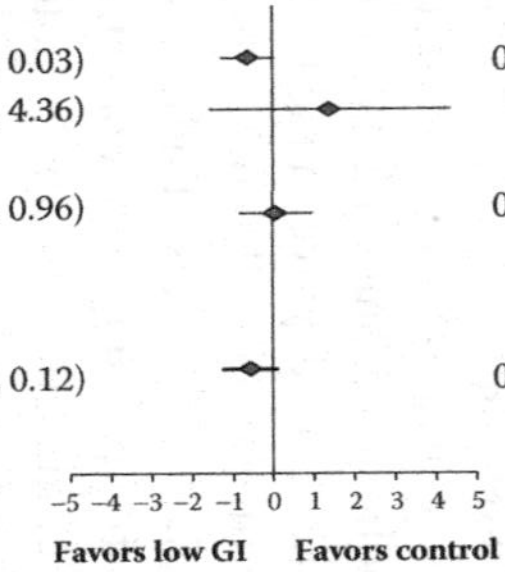

FIGURE 5.3 Summary of most recent systematic reviews and meta-analyses of RCTs looking at the effect of GI on body weight endpoints. Achieved GI, average GI of intervention or control arm across all trials included in the meta-analysis; MD, mean difference; *n*, number of participants; No., number; SRMA, systematic review and meta-analysis. *I^2 refers to the degree of inter-study heterogeneity, where 0%–40%: might not be important heterogeneity; 30%–60%: moderate heterogeneity; 50%–90%: may be substantial heterogeneity; and 75%–100%: considerable heterogeneity. (From Higgins, J. P. T. and S. Green (editors). 2011. *Cochrane Handbook for Systematic Reviews of Interventions Version 5.1.0* (updated March 2011). The Cochrane Collaboration, Oxford. Available from http://handbook.cochrane.org/. With Permission.)

significant association between higher GI/GL and risk of becoming overweight or obese (de la Fuente-Arrillaga et al., 2014). This was further confirmed by a study part of the Diogenes project conducted across five countries in Europe ($n = 89{,}432$) over a mean follow-up duration of 6.5 years, which found no overall significant association between GI and weight gain (MD = 0.084 kg per year; 95% CI: −0.005, 0.172 kg) and between GL and weight gain (MD = 0.01 kg per year; 95% CI: −0.064, 0.084 kg) (Du et al., 2009). In contrast to these findings, the American Seasonal Variation of Blood Cholesterol Study, a prospective study conducted in healthy adults in central Massachusetts ($n = 572$) over a 1-year period, found a significant positive association between GI and BMI, where BMI increased by 0.04 kg/m^2 per year (95% CI: 0.01, 0.07 kg/m^2) for every five-unit increase in GI (Ma et al., 2005). This was consistent with the findings of a 6-year prospective cohort study commissioned by the World Health Organization, which consisted of a subsample of men and women from the Danish Monitoring Trends and Determinants in Cardiovascular Disease study ($n = 376$), where the authors reported significant positive associations between GI and changes in body weight, body fat percentage, and waist circumference in women but not in men (Hare-Bruun et al., 2006).

Overall, the results from RCTs and prospective cohort studies indicate that low-GI diets may be beneficial for weight loss but may not produce any additional benefits when compared with other healthy diets. These studies also indicate that low-GI diets may be of greater benefit in specific subsets of the population (e.g., obese individuals and women). Therefore, future research should focus on assessing the effect of low-GI diets in the context of typically consumed background diets (e.g., Western diet) and within specific subsets of the population, in order to clarify the findings from current studies (see also Chapter 6).

5.6.4 Glycemic Index, Glycemic Control, and Diabetes

Low-GI diets have been shown to be beneficial for glycemic control in individuals with diabetes. Earlier meta-analyses of RCTs conducted in individuals with diabetes comparing low- with high-GI diets have shown significant improvements in fructosamine and HbA1c (Brand-Miller et al., 2003; Thomas and Elliott, 2010). These findings were consistent with an updated systematic review and meta-analysis of 19 RCTs conducted in individuals with type 1 diabetes and T2DM ($n = 840$), which reported similar reductions in fructosamine and HbA1c when comparing low- with high-GI diets over a median 9-week follow-up duration (Wang et al., 2015) (Figure 5.4). The reduction in HbA1c reported in this meta-analysis, as well as in previous meta-analyses, exceeds the clinically meaningful threshold of 0.3% or more, proposed by FDA for the development of new drugs for diabetes (FDA, 2009). Therefore, following a low-GI diet can have a clinically meaningful impact on the management of glycemia in individuals with diabetes.

These improvements in HbA1c have also been sustained in longer-term RCTs. This was shown in a systematic review and meta-analysis of three RCTs for 24 weeks or more, conducted in individuals with T2DM ($n = 357$), which compared low-GI diets with other types of diets (high-fiber diet, ADA diet, etc.) (Figure 5.4) (Ajala et al., 2013). As HbA1c reflects the average blood glucose concentration of the preceding 3 months (~90 days or 12 weeks) (Saudek et al., 2005), these results provide stronger support for the beneficial effects of low-GI diets on long-term glycemic control in individuals with diabetes. However, these findings were not consistent with a systematic review and meta-analysis of 14 long-term RCTs conducted in overweight and obese individuals ($n = 2325$), which showed that low-GI diets did not significantly alter HbA1c and FBG despite significantly lowering fasting insulin (Figure 5.4) (Schwingshackl and Hoffmann, 2013). However, this lack of an improvement in markers of glucose control may be due to the mixed inclusion of participants, where both individuals with diabetes and non-diabetes were grouped together, thus possibly diluting the findings toward the null, as the majority of included trials were conducted in individuals without diabetes (10 out of 14 RCTs) (Schwingshackl and Hoffmann, 2013).

Glycemic Control End Point	SRMA	No. RCTs	*n*	Participant Characteristics	Achieved GI, Control	Achieved GI, Intervention	Follow-up Duration, wks	Pooled Effect Estimates, MD (95% CI)	I^2
HbA1c (%)	Schwingshackl et al. 2013	4	486	Mixed diabetes status	~64.8	~72.9	24–52	−0.09 (−0.52, 0.33)	72%
	Ajala et al. 2013	3	357	Diabetes	~81.8	~72.8	12–48	−0.14 (−0.23, −0.03)	80%
	Wang et al. 2014	15	738	Diabetes	NA	NA	2–144	−0.42 (−0.69, −0.16)	64%
Fructosamine (mmol/L)	Schwingshackl et al. 2013	–	–	–	–	–	–	–	–
	Ajala et al. 2013	–	–	–	–	–	–		–
	Wang et al. 2014	9	148	Diabetes	NA	NA	2–12	−0.44 (−0.82, −0.06)	50%
Fasting glucose (mmol/L)	Schwingshackl et al. 2013	11	2059	Mixed diabetes status	~54.2	~63.4	26–68	0.03 (−0.07, 0.12)	52%
	Ajala et al. 2013	–	–	–	–	–	–	–	–
	Wang et al. 2014	–	–	–	–	–	–	–	–
Fasting insulin (pmol/L)	Schwingshackl et al. 2013	9	1741	Mixed diabetes status	~53.4	~62.7	24–68	−5.16 (−8.45, −1.88)	48%
	Ajala et al. 2013	–	–	–	–	–	–	–	–
	Wang et al. 2014	–	–	–	–	–	–	–	–

FIGURE 5.4 Summary of most recent systematic reviews and meta-analyses of RCTs looking at the effect of GI on glycemic control endpoints. Achieved GI, average GI of intervention or control arm across all trials included in the meta-analysis; MD, mean difference; mixed diabetes status, meta-analysis included participants with and without diabetes; n, number of participants; NA, data not available; No., number; SRMA, systematic review and meta-analysis. *I^2 refers to the degree of interstudy heterogeneity, where 0%–40%: might not be important heterogeneity; 30%–60%: moderate heterogeneity; 50%–90%: may be substantial heterogeneity; and 75%–100%: considerable heterogeneity. (From Higgins, J. P. T. and S. Green (editors). 2011. Cochrane Handbook for Systematic Reviews of Interventions Version 5.1.0 (updated March 2011). The Cochrane Collaboration, Oxford. Available from http://handbook.cochrane.org/. With Permission.)

More recent RCTs conducted in overweight and obese individuals showed an absence of improvement in glycemic control, which may be due to insufficient differences in GI between treatment and control. In the GLYNDIET study (n = 122), a 6-month RCT comparing a low with a high-GI diet, with a GI difference of 7, no significant differences were found between the two diets in glycemic control and insulin sensitivity parameters (Juanola-Falgarona et al., 2014). Likewise, the Diogenes study (n = 256), a 12-month RCT conducted at eight study centers across Europe, which compared the effect of low-GI to high-GI diets with an achieved GI difference of 7, reported no significant differences between the two diets with regard to FBG, fasting insulin, and fructosamine (Aller et al., 2014). In contrast to these findings, RCTs that have achieved a higher GI difference (>15) reported greater improvements in glycemic control. A 3-month RCT with an achieved GI difference of 17, which compared a low-GI diet emphasizing dietary pulse intake with a high-fiber diet in predominantly overweight and obese individuals with T2DM (n = 121), showed improvements in HbA1c (MD = −0.2%; 95% CI: −0.3%, −0.1%) and fasting glucose (Jenkins et al., 2012). Similarly, another 3-month RCT conducted in a similar group of individuals with a GI difference of 52, which compared a low-GL diet emphasizing MUFA and ALA with a wholegrain diet, also showed improvements in HbA1c (MD = −0.16; 95% CI: −0.25, −0.06) (Jenkins et al., 2014). Again, one exception to these glycemic improvements, despite a sufficient GI difference of greater than 15, is the OmniCarb study, which was a 5-week RCT conducted in overweight individuals (n = 163) comparing a low- with a high-GI diet in the context of healthy background diets based on the DASH diet (Sacks et al., 2014). However, its eligibility criteria included both individuals with and without diabetes, and similar to the previously mentioned meta-analysis (Schwingshackl and Hoffmann, 2013), a lack of an effect on glycemic control was possibly demonstrated because in individuals without diabetes glycemic control is already well managed.

The effect of diets containing specific low-GI foods has also been investigated in several RCTs, which overall have shown to have glycemic control benefits. In a systematic review and meta-analysis of 41 RCTs (n = 1674) that looked at the effect of dietary pulses in individuals from different health groups (e.g., type 1 diabetes and T2DM, normoglycemia, and/or hypercholesterolemia), significant reductions were found on glycemic parameters (such as FBG, fructosamine, HbA1c, and fasting insulin) when dietary pulses were incorporated into the diet alone, in the context of a low-GI diet and in the context of a high-fiber diet (Sievenpiper et al., 2009). Temperate climate fruits, which are low-GI foods, have also been shown to be associated with improvements in HbA1c (r = −0.206; p = .011) in a secondary analysis of a 6-month RCT conducted in individuals with T2DM (n = 152). This analysis also showed that the percentage change in HbA1c was reduced by 0.5% (95% CI: −0.2, −0.8%) when comparing the highest with the lowest quartile of low-GI fruit intake. Overall, these results indicate that incorporating specific low-GI foods into the diet or in the context of specific diets can be beneficial for glycemic control.

Evidence from systematic reviews and meta-analyses of prospective cohort studies suggests that higher GI and GL are associated with T2DM risk. Earlier meta-analyses of prospective cohort studies showed a significant association between GI, GL, and the risk of T2DM when comparing the highest with the lowest GI intakes (Barclay et al., 2008; Dong et al., 2011). These findings have been further confirmed in the most recent systematic review and meta-analysis of 10 prospective cohort studies that reported that higher GI and GL intakes are significantly associated with T2DM (RR: 1.19; 95% CI: 1.14, 1.24 and RR: 1.13; 95% CI: 1.08, 1.17, respectively) (Bhupathiraju et al., 2014). Two other recent systematic reviews and meta-analyses of prospective cohort studies, which looked at the dose–response relationship between GI, GL, and T2DM risk, reported that those consuming higher-GI, -GL diets were associated with significantly higher T2DM risk (Greenwood et al., 2013). Therefore, these findings indicate that consumption of lower-GI and -GL diets may be beneficial for the prevention of T2DM.

Several physiologic mechanisms have been proposed to explain the positive association between GI, GL, and T2DM. High-GI and -GL diets produce higher concentration of blood glucose, which stimulates an increased production of insulin. Consumption of such diets over the course of several years can put a greater demand on the pancreatic β-cells, which can eventually lead to β-cell exhaustion and failure (Jenkins et al., 1981; Pawlak et al., 2004; Willett et al., 2002). High-GI diets could also lead to increased release of postprandial nonesterified fatty acids, which can directly increase insulin resistance (Ludwig, 2002) and eventually lead to a higher risk for developing T2DM (Dong et al., 2011). Furthermore, acarbose, an oral α-glucosidase inhibitors, acts similarly to low-GI diets in that it slows the rate of carbohydrate absorption, providing a 'proof-of-concept' for low GI diets (Bhupathiraju et al., 2014). In the STOP-NIDDM trial, a multicenter double-blind, placebo-controlled RCT (n = 1368), acarbose was shown to reduce the risk of T2DM by 25% over a mean follow-up of 3 years (Chiasson et al., 2002). It was also shown to significantly reduce the risk for MI (HR = 0.36; 95% CI: 0.16, 0.80) and any cardiovascular event (Hanefeld et al., 2004). Given that low-GI diets and acarbose share the same property of slowing carbohydrate absorption, this provides stronger support for the ability of low-GI diets to reduce diabetes and cardiovascular risks (see also Chapter 4).

5.7 GLYCEMIC INDEX AND CARDIOVASCULAR DISEASE

A beneficial association between GI and heart disease risk has been demonstrated, especially in women. The most recent systematic reviews and meta-analyses of prospective cohort studies comparing the highest to lowest categories of GI and GL intakes reported that higher GI and GL increased the risk for heart disease by 19%–26% for higher GI and 35%–69% for higher GL in women, but not in men (Dong et al., 2012; Fan et al., 2012; Ma et al., 2012; Mirrahimi et al., 2012). Furthermore, these meta-analyses reported a sex and weight interaction, such that overweight and obese women consuming highest-GI diets have the greatest risk of heart disease (Fan et al., 2012). The reason for the observed sex differences is unclear. There is some evidence that the lipid profile in women is more sensitive to high-GI diets, where women tend to have higher HDL-C concentrations, which is heart disease protective (Gordon et al., 1989; Knopp et al., 2005). High-GI diets, however, tend to reduce HDL-C while increasing TG concentrations, thus increasing heart disease risk disproportionately in women (Matthews et al., 1989). Therefore, more research is needed to clarify these sex differences.

In terms of the association between GI, GL, and stroke risk, the results have been less consistent. In two systematic reviews and meta-analyses of prospective cohort studies, no significant associations were found between GI and overall stroke risk (Cai et al., 2015; Fan et al., 2012); however, when comparing the highest and the lowest categories of GL intake, higher GL was significantly associated with 19% higher stroke risk. Therefore, these results suggest that both the quality and the amount of carbohydrates consumed may significantly impact the development of stroke. Future research should focus on identifying the mechanism of GL and stroke, and more prospective cohort studies are needed to verify the results of these two meta-analyses.

5.8 FUTURE RESEARCH DIRECTIONS

Future research is needed to address the existing uncertainties and limitations in the current body of evidence on the effect of low-GI diets on cardiovascular risk factors and events. In particular, longer-term RCTs (≥24-week follow-up duration) conducted in individuals at risk for CVD, with prescribed diets consisting of larger GI differences (>15) between the intervention and control arms, are required to further clarify the reported findings. As compliance is a common issue in dietary trials, it is suggested that future RCTs are designed to be fully or partially metabolically controlled by providing all foods or key study foods to participants. This would allow investigators to achieve larger GI differences between intervention and control and to control for different methods of preparation (boiling, baking, roasting, frying, etc.), which can largely influence the

GI of foods (Bahado-Singh et al., 2006, 2011; Wolever et al., 1987). In order to achieve larger GI differences, it is recommended that foods with distinct differences in GI be provided to participants, such as steel-cut oats, dietary pulses, parboiled rice, and breads made from pumpernickel or stoneground flours to the low-GI/intervention arm and instant oats, cream of wheat, white rice, and white or brown bread to the high-GI/control arm. Similar approaches have been used by several long-term RCTs conducted in individuals with diabetes, which achieved large differences in GI and significant improvements in various cardiovascular risk factors (Jenkins et al., 2008, 2012, 2014). In addition, as many of the same foods that are available on the market can largely vary in their GI, industry collaborations are recommended for the development of study foods, in order to ensure distinct differences in GI.

In a real-world setting, following a low-GI diet may be one strategy that can be combined with standard therapy to reduce one's risk for CVD and to improve CVD management. Given that there is an overall high consumption of high-GI foods, such as refined grains (Halkjaer et al., 2009; Phillips et al., 2015), and low consumption of low-GI foods, such as pulses (Mitchell et al., 2009), in Western and European countries, there is ample room to incorporate low-GI foods into one's diet. Education about low-GI foods and cooking practices that helps maintain the GI of a food would be useful for encouraging patients and consumers to consume a low-GI diet. The inclusion of GI on food labels would also be useful in helping consumers identify low-GI food sources. Such practices have already been implemented in some countries, such as Australia and the United Kingdom (Mitchell, 2008), and efforts to enforce labeling in other countries, such as Canada, are currently ongoing (Wolever, 2013) (see Chapter 12).

5.9 CONCLUSIONS

Overall, low-GI diets appear to have beneficial effects on blood lipids in acute RCTs, body weight in certain groups of the population. Many trials, however, were of short follow-up duration (<24 weeks) and had a small GI difference between the intervention and control arms (<15 units). In prospective cohort studies, lower GI intakes were shown to lower diabetes risk. It appears also that low GI intakes may have differential associations to heart disease risk based on sex, where women appear to benefit more from lower GI intakes. Given the high prevalence and increasing burden of CVD, effective interventions that focus on modifiable risk factors, such as diet, remain important. Therefore, future research should focus on designing longer trials with larger GI differences in individuals with higher CVD risk in order to clarify the findings reported from the current body of evidence.

REFERENCES

AbuMweis, S. S., S. Jew, and N. P. Ames. 2010. Beta-glucan from barley and its lipid-lowering capacity: A meta-analysis of randomized, controlled trials. *Eur J Clin Nutr,* 64(12):1472–1480.

Ajala, O., P. English, and J. Pinkney. 2013. Systematic review and meta-analysis of different dietary approaches to the management of type 2 diabetes. *Am J Clin Nutr,* 97(3):505–516.

Aller, E. E., T. M. Larsen, H. Claus, A. K. Lindroos, A. Kafatos, A. Pfeiffer, J. A. Martinez et al. 2014. Weight loss maintenance in overweight subjects on ad libitum diets with high or low protein content and glycemic index: The DIOGENES trial 12-month results. *Int J Obes (Lond),* 38(12):1511–1517.

American Diabetes Association. 2015. Standards of medical care in diabetes—2015. *Diabetes Care,* 38 (Suppl 1):S1–S93.

American Heart Association. 2009. Harmonizing the metabolic syndrome: A joint interim statement of the international diabetes federation task force on epidemiology and prevention; national heart, lung, and blood institute; American Heart Association; World Heart Federation; International Atherosclerosis Society; and International Association for the study of obesity. *Circulation,* 120:1640–1645.

American Heart Association. 2011. Triglycerides and cardiovascular disease: A scientific statement from the American Heart Association. *Circulation,* 123:2292–2333.

American Heart Association. 2014. 2013 AHA/ACC/TOS guideline for the management of overweight and obesity in adults: A report of the American College of Cardiology/American Heart Association task force on practice guidelines and the obesity society. *Circulation,* 129(Suppl 2):S102–S138.

Anderson, T. J., J. Gregoire, R. A. Hegele, P. Couture, G. B. Mancini, R. McPherson, G. A. Francis et al. 2013. 2012 update of the Canadian Cardiovascular Society guidelines for the diagnosis and treatment of dyslipidemia for the prevention of cardiovascular disease in the adult. *Can J Cardiol,* 29(2):151–167.

Augustin, L. S., S. Franceschi, D. J. Jenkins, C. W. Kendall, and C. La Vecchia. 2002. Glycemic index in chronic disease: A review. *Eur J Clin Nutr,* 56(11):1049–1071.

Australian Diabetes Society. 2012. Australian Diabetes Council. Catering Guidelines.

Bahado-Singh, P. S., C. K. Riley, A. O. Wheatley, and H. I. Lowe. 2011. Relationship between processing method and the glycemic indices of ten sweet potato (*Ipomoea batatas*) cultivars commonly consumed in Jamaica. *J Nutr Metab,* 2011:584832.

Bahado-Singh, P. S., A. O. Wheatley, M. H. Ahmad, E. Y. Morrison, and H. N. Asemota. 2006. Food processing methods influence the glycaemic indices of some commonly eaten West Indian carbohydrate-rich foods. *Br J Nutr,* 96(3):476–481.

Barclay, A. W., P. Petocz, J. McMillan-Price, V. M. Flood, T. Prvan, P. Mitchell, and J. C. Brand-Miller. 2008. Glycemic index, glycemic load, and chronic disease risk–a meta-analysis of observational studies. *Am J Clin Nutr,* 87(3):627–637.

Barter, P. J., C. M. Ballantyne, R. Carmena, M. Castro Cabezas, M. J. Chapman, P. Couture, J. de Graaf et al. 2006. Apo B versus cholesterol in estimating cardiovascular risk and in guiding therapy: Report of the thirty-person/ten-country panel. *J Intern Med,* 259(3):247–258.

Barter, P. J. and K. A. Rye. 2006. The rationale for using apoA-I as a clinical marker of cardiovascular risk. *J Intern Med,* 259(5):447–454.

Bazzano, L. A., J. He, L. G. Ogden, C. Loria, S. Vupputuri, L. Myers, and P. K. Whelton. 2001. Legume consumption and risk of coronary heart disease in US men and women: NHANES I epidemiologic follow-up study. *Arch Intern Med,* 161(21):2573–2578.

Bhupathiraju, S. N., D. K. Tobias, V. S. Malik, A. Pan, A. Hruby, J. E. Manson, W. C. Willett, and F. B. Hu. 2014. Glycemic index, glycemic load, and risk of type 2 diabetes: Results from 3 large US cohorts and an updated meta-analysis. *Am J Clin Nutr,* 100(1):218–232.

Blaha, M. J., R. S. Blumenthal, E. A. Brinton, and T. A. Jacobson. 2008. The importance of non-HDL cholesterol reporting in lipid management. *J Clin Lipidol,* 2(4):267–273.

Blaier, O., M. Lishner, and A. Elis. 2011. Managing statin-induced muscle toxicity in a lipid clinic. *J Clin Pharm Ther,* 36(3):336–341.

Boden-Albala, B. and R. L. Sacco. 2000. Lifestyle factors and stroke risk: Exercise, alcohol, diet, obesity, smoking, drug use, and stress. *Curr Atheroscler Rep,* 2(2):160–166.

Brand-Miller, J., A. Astrup, and A. E. Buyken. 2015. Low vs high glycemic index diet. *JAMA,* 313(13):1371–1372.

Brand-Miller, J., S. Hayne, P. Petocz, and S. Colagiuri. 2003. Low-glycemic index diets in the management of diabetes: A meta-analysis of randomized controlled trials. *Diabetes Care,* 26 (8):2261–2267.

Breslow, L. 1952. Public health aspects of weight control. *Am J Public Health Nations Health,* 42 (9):1116–1120.

Buckley, D. I., R. Fu, M. Freeman, K. Rogers, and M. Helfand. 2009. C-reactive protein as a risk factor for coronary heart disease: A systematic review and meta-analyses for the U.S. Preventive Services Task Force. *Ann Intern Med,* 151(7):483–495.

Caballero, B. 2007. The global epidemic of obesity: An overview. *Epidemiol Rev,* 29:1–5.

Cai, X., C. Wang, S. Wang, G. Cao, C. Jin, J. Yu, X. Li et al. 2015. Carbohydrate intake, glycemic index, glycemic load, and stroke: A meta-analysis of prospective cohort studies. *Asia Pac J Public Health,* 27(5):486–496.

Canadian Diabetes Association. 2013. Canadian Diabetes Association 2013 Clinical Practice Guidelines for the Prevention and Management of Diabetes in Canada. *Can J Diabetes*, 37(suppl 1):S1–S212.

Center for Drug Evaluation and Research. 2008. Guidance for industry: Diabetes Mellitus: Developing Drugs and Therapeutic Biologics for Treatment and Prevention (DRAFT GUIDANCE). Rockville, MD, U.S. Department of Health and Human Services Food and Drug Administration, pp. 1–30.

Chiasson, J. L., R. G. Josse, R. Gomis, M. Hanefeld, A. Karasik, and M. Laakso. 2002. Acarbose for prevention of type 2 diabetes mellitus: The STOP-NIDDM randomised trial. *Lancet,* 359(9323):2072–2077.

Chobanian, A. V., G. L. Bakris, H. R. Black, W. C. Cushman, L. A. Green, J. L. Izzo, Jr., D. W. Jones et al. 2003. Seventh report of the Joint National Committee on Prevention, Detection, Evaluation, and Treatment of High Blood Pressure. *Hypertension,* 42(6):1206–1252.

Clarke, R., J. Halsey, S. Lewington, E. Lonn, J. Armitage, J. E. Manson et al. 2010. Effects of lowering homocysteine levels with B vitamins on cardiovascular disease, cancer, and cause-specific mortality: Meta-analysis of 8 randomized trials involving 37 485 individuals. *Arch Intern Med,* 170(18):1622–1631.

Critchley, J. A. and S. Capewell. 2003. Mortality risk reduction associated with smoking cessation in patients with coronary heart disease: A systematic review. *JAMA,* 290(1):86–97.

de la Fuente-Arrillaga, C., M. A. Martinez-Gonzalez, I. Zazpe, Z. Vazquez-Ruiz, S. Benito-Corchon, and M. Bes-Rastrollo. 2014. Glycemic load, glycemic index, bread and incidence of overweight/obesity in a Mediterranean cohort: The SUN project. *BMC Public Health,* 14:1091.

Dokken B. B., V. Saengsirisuwan, J. S. Kim, M. K. Teachy, and E. J. Henriksen. 2008. Oxidative stress-induced insulin resistance in rat skeletal muscle: Role of glycogen synthase kinase-3. *Am J Physiol Endocrinol Metab,* 294(3):E615–E621.

Dong, J. Y., L. Zhang, Y. H. Zhang, and L. Q. Qin. 2011. Dietary glycaemic index and glycaemic load in relation to the risk of type 2 diabetes: A meta-analysis of prospective cohort studies. *Br J Nutr,* 106(11):1649–1654.

Du, H., A. D. van der, M. M. van Bakel, N. Slimani, N. G. Forouhi, N. J. Wareham, J. Halkjaer et al. 2009. Dietary glycaemic index, glycaemic load and subsequent changes of weight and waist circumference in European men and women. *Int J Obes (Lond),* 33:1280–1288.

Erhardt, L. 2009. Cigarette smoking: An undertreated risk factor for cardiovascular disease. *Atherosclerosis,* 205(1):23–32.

Fan, J., Y. Song, Y. Wang, R. Hui, and W. Zhang. 2012. Dietary glycemic index, glycemic load, and risk of coronary heart disease, stroke, and stroke mortality: A systematic review with meta-analysis. *PLoS One,* 7(12):e52182.

Fleming, P. and M. Godwin. 2013. Low-glycaemic index diets in the management of blood lipids: A systematic review and meta-analysis. *Fam Pract,* 30(5):485–491.

Goff, L. M., D. E. Cowland, L. Hooper, and G. S. Frost. 2013. Low glycaemic index diets and blood lipids: A systematic review and meta-analysis of randomised controlled trials. *Nutr Metab Cardiovasc Dis,* 23(1):1–10.

Gordon, D. J., J. L. Probstfield, R. J. Garrison, J. D. Neaton, W. P. Castelli, J. D. Knoke, D. R. Jacobs Jr., S. Bangdiwala, and H. A. Tyroler. 1989. High-density lipoprotein cholesterol and cardiovascular disease: Four prospective American studies. *Circulation,* 79(1):8–15.

Greenland, P., J. S. Alpert, G. A. Beller, E. J. Benjamin, M. J. Budoff, Z. A. Fayad, E. Foster et al. 2010. 2010 ACCF/AHA Guideline for Assessment of Cardiovascular Risk in Asymptomatic Adults: Executive Summary. *Circulation,* 122:2748–2764.

Greenwood, D. C., D. E. Threapleton, C. E. Evans, C. L. Cleghorn, C. Nykjaer, C. Woodhead, and V. J. Burley. 2013. Glycemic index, glycemic load, carbohydrates, and type 2 diabetes: Systematic review and dose-response meta-analysis of prospective studies. *Diabetes Care,* 36(12):4166–4171.

Ha, V., J. L. Sievenpiper, R. J. de Souza, V. H. Jayalath, A. Mirrahimi, A. Agarwal, L. Chiavaroli et al. 2014. Effect of dietary pulse intake on established therapeutic lipid targets for cardiovascular risk reduction: A systematic review and meta-analysis of randomized controlled trials. *CMAJ,* 186(8):E252–E262.

Hackam, D. G. and S. S. Anand. 2003. Emerging risk factors for atherosclerotic vascular disease: A critical review of the evidence. *JAMA,* 290(7):932–940.

Hackam, D. G., R. R. Quinn, P. Ravani, D. M. Rabi, K. Dasgupta, S. S. Daskalopoulou, N. A. Khan et al. 2013. The 2013 Canadian Hypertension Education Program recommendations for blood pressure measurement, diagnosis, assessment of risk, prevention, and treatment of hypertension. *Can J Cardiol,* 29(5):528–542.

Haffner, S. M., S. Lehto, T. Ronnemaa, K. Pyorala, and M. Laakso. 1998. Mortality from coronary heart disease in subjects with type 2 diabetes and in nondiabetic subjects with and without prior myocardial infarction. *N Engl J Med,* 339(4):229–234.

Halkjaer, J., A. Olsen, L. J. Bjerregaard, G. Deharveng, A. Tjonneland, A. A. Welch, F. L. Crowe et al. 2009. Intake of total, animal and plant proteins, and their food sources in 10 countries in the European Prospective Investigation into Cancer and Nutrition. *Eur J Clin Nutr,* 63(Suppl 4):S16–S36.

Hanefeld, M., M. Cagatay, T. Petrowitsch, D. Neuser, D. Petzinna, and M. Rupp. 2004. Acarbose reduces the risk for myocardial infarction in type 2 diabetic patients: Meta-analysis of seven long-term studies. *Eur Heart J,* 25(1):10–16.

Hare-Bruun, H., A. Flint, and B. L. Heitmann. 2006. Glycemic index and glycemic load in relation to changes in body weight, body fat distribution, and body composition in adult Danes. *Am J Clin Nutr,* 84(4):871–879.

He, J. and P. K. Whelton. 1999. Elevated systolic blood pressure and risk of cardiovascular and renal disease: Overview of evidence from observational epidemiologic studies and randomized controlled trials. *Am Heart J,* 138(3 Pt 2):211–219.

Higgins, J. P. T. and S. Green (editors). 2011. *Cochrane Handbook for Systematic Reviews of Interventions Version 5.1.0* (updated March 2011). The Cochrane Collaboration, Oxford. Available from http://handbook.cochrane.org/. (Accessed June 16, 2016.)

Hu, F. B. 2002. Dietary pattern analysis: A new direction in nutritional epidemiology. *Curr Opin Lipidol,* 13(1):3–9.

Iannuzzi, A., M. R. Licenziati, M. Vacca, D. De Marco, G. Cinquegrana, M. Laccetti, A. Bresciani et al. 2009. Comparison of two diets of varying glycemic index on carotid subclinical atherosclerosis in obese children. *Heart Vessels,* 24(6):419–424.

Illman, R. J., D. L. Topping, G. H. McIntosh, R. P. Trimble, G. B. Storer, M. N. Taylor, and B. Q. Cheng. 1988. Hypocholesterolaemic effects of dietary propionate: Studies in whole animals and perfused rat liver. *Ann Nutr Metab,* 32(2):95–107.

Iso, H., D. R. Jacobs, Jr., D. Wentworth, J. D. Neaton, and J. D. Cohen. 1989. Serum cholesterol levels and six-year mortality from stroke in 350,977 men screened for the multiple risk factor intervention trial. *N Engl J Med,* 320(14):904–910.

Jayalath, V. H., R. J. de Souza, J. L. Sievenpiper, V. Ha, L. Chiavaroli, A. Mirrahimi, M. Di Buono et al. 2014. Effect of dietary pulses on blood pressure: A systematic review and meta-analysis of controlled feeding trials. *Am J Hypertens,* 27(1):56–64.

Jenkins, D. J., C. W. Kendall, L. S. Augustin, S. Franceschi, M. Hamidi, A. Marchie, A. L. Jenkins, and M. Axelsen. 2002. Glycemic index: Overview of implications in health and disease. *Am J Clin Nutr,* 76, 266S–273S.

Jenkins, D. J., C. W. Kendall, L. S. Augustin, S. Mitchell, S. Sahye-Pudaruth, S. Blanco Mejia, L. Chiavaroli et al. 2012. Effect of legumes as part of a low glycemic index diet on glycemic control and cardiovascular risk factors in type 2 diabetes mellitus: A randomized controlled trial. *Arch Intern Med,* 172(21):1653–1660.

Jenkins, D. J., C. W. Kendall, V. Vuksan, D. Faulkner, L. S. Augustin, S. Mitchell, C. Ireland et al. 2014. Effect of lowering the glycemic load with canola oil on glycemic control and cardiovascular risk factors: A randomized controlled trial. *Diabetes Care,* 37(7):1806–1814.

Jenkins, D. J., K. Srichaikul, C. W. Kendall, J. L. Sievenpiper, S. Abdulnour, A. Mirrahimi, C. Meneses et al. 2011. The relation of low glycaemic index fruit consumption to glycaemic control and risk factors for coronary heart disease in type 2 diabetes. *Diabetologia,* 54(2):271–279.

Jenkins, D. J., T. M. Wolever, A. V. Rao, R. A. Hegele, S. J. Mitchell, T. P. Ransom, D. L. Boctor, P. J. Spadafora, A. L. Jenkins, C. Mehling et al. 1993. Effect on blood lipids of very high intakes of fiber in diets low in saturated fat and cholesterol. *N Engl J Med,* 329(1):21–26.

Jenkins, D. J., T. M. Wolever, R. H. Taylor, H. Barker, H. Fielden, J. M. Baldwin, A. C. Bowling, H. C. Newman, A. L. Jenkins, and D. V. Goff. 1981. Glycemic index of foods: A physiological basis for carbohydrate exchange. *Am J Clin Nutr,* 34(3):362–366.

Joint British Societies-3. 2014. Joint British Societies' consensus recommendations for the prevention of cardiovascular disease (JBS3). *Heart,* 100:ii1–ii67.

Joint National Committee-8. 2014. 2014 Evidence-Based Guideline for the Management of High Blood Pressure in Adults Report From the Panel Members Appointed to the Eighth Joint National Committee (JNC 8). *JAMA,* 311(5):507–520.

Juanola-Falgarona, M., J. Salas-Salvado, N. Ibarrola-Jurado, A. Rabassa-Soler, A. Diaz-Lopez, M. Guasch-Ferre, P. Hernandez-Alonso, R. Balanza, and M. Bullo. 2014. Effect of the glycemic index of the diet on weight loss, modulation of satiety, inflammation, and other metabolic risk factors: A randomized controlled trial. *Am J Clin Nutr,* 100(1):27–35.

Kannel, W. B. and D. L. McGee. 1979. Diabetes and cardiovascular disease: The Framingham study. *JAMA,* 241(19):2035–2038.

Kannel, W. B., T. Gordon, and M. J. Schwartz. 1971. Systolic versus diastolic blood pressure and risk of coronary heart disease. The Framingham study. *Am J Cardiol,* 27(4):335–346.

Knopp, R. H., P. Paramsothy, B. M. Retzlaff, B. Fish, C. Walden, A. Dowdy, C. Tsunehara, K. Aikawa, M. C. Cheung. 2005. Gender differences in lipoprotein metabolism and dietary response: Basis in hormonal differences and implications for cardiovascular disease. *Curr Atheroscler Rep,* 7(6):472–479.

Kritchevsky, D. and J. A. Story. 1974. Binding of bile salts in vitro by nonnutritive fiber. *J Nutr,* 104(4):458–462.

Law, M. R., N. J. Wald, and A. R. Rudnicka. 2003. Quantifying effect of statins on low density lipoprotein cholesterol, ischaemic heart disease, and stroke: Systematic review and meta-analysis. *BMJ,* 326(7404):1423.

Lawes, C. M., S. Vander Hoorn, and A. Rodgers. 2008. Global burden of blood-pressure-related disease, 2001. *Lancet,* 371(9623):1513–1518.

Lewington, S., R. Clarke, N. Qizilbash, R. Peto, and R. Collins. 2002. Age-specific relevance of usual blood pressure to vascular mortality: A meta-analysis of individual data for one million adults in 61 prospective studies. *Lancet,* 360(9349):1903–1913.

Ludwig, D. S. 2002. The glycemic index: Physiological mechanisms relating to obesity, diabetes, and cardiovascular disease. *JAMA,* 287(18):2414–2423.

Luscher, T. F., M. A. Creager, J. A. Beckman, and F. Cosentino. 2003. Diabetes and vascular disease: Pathophysiology, clinical consequences, and medical therapy: Part II. *Circulation,* 108(13):1655–1661.

Ma, X. Y., J. P. Liu, and Z. Y. Song. 2012. Glycemic load, glycemic index and risk of cardiovascular diseases: Meta-analyses of prospective studies. *Atherosclerosis,* 223(2):491–496.

Ma Y., B. Olendzki, D. Chiriboga, J. R. Hebert, Y. Li, W. Li, M. Campbell, K. Gendreau, and I. S. Ockene. 2005. Association between dietary carbohydrates and body weight. *Am J Epidemiol,* 161(4):359–367.

Mann, J. I., I. De Leeuw, K. Hermansen, B. Karamanos, B. Karlstrom, N. Katsilambros, G. Riccardi et al. 2004. Evidence-based nutritional approaches to the treatment and prevention of diabetes mellitus. *Nutr Metab Cardiovasc Dis,* 14(6):373–394.

Maruthur, N. M. 2013. The growing prevalence of type 2 diabetes: Increased incidence or improved survival? *Curr Diab Rep,* 13(6):786–794.

Matthews, K. A., E. Meilahn, L. H. Kuller, S. F. Kelsey, A. W. Caggiula, and R. R. Wing. 1989. Menopause and risk factors for coronary heart disease. *N Engl J Med,* 321(10):641.

Mazzone, T. 2010. Intensive glucose lowering and cardiovascular disease prevention in diabetes: Reconciling the recent clinical trial data. *Circulation,* 122(21):2201–2211.

Mearns, B. M. 2011. Targeting levels and functions of blood lipids in the prevention of CVD. *Nat Rev Cardiol,* 8(4):179–180.

Mehta, R. L., M. T. Pascual, S. Soroko, and G. M. Chertow. 2002. Diuretics, mortality, and nonrecovery of renal function in acute renal failure. *JAMA,* 288(20):2547–2553.

Mensah, G. A. 2002. Clinical hypertension. *Cardiol Clin,* 20(2):xiii–xiv.

Mihaylova, B., J. Emberson, L. Blackwell, A. Keech, J. Simes, E. H. Barnes, M. Voysey, A. Gray, R. Collins, and C. Baigent. 2012. The effects of lowering LDL cholesterol with statin therapy in people at low risk of vascular disease: Meta-analysis of individual data from 27 randomised trials. *Lancet,* 380(9841):581–590.

Mirrahimi, A., R. J. de Souza, L. Chiavaroli, J. L. Sievenpiper, J. Beyene, A. J. Hanley, L. S. A. Augustin, C. W. C. Kendall, and D. J. A. Jenkins. 2012. Associations of Glycemic Index and Load With Coronary Heart Disease Events: A Systematic Review and Meta-Analysis of Prospective Cohorts. *JAHA,* 1:e000752.

Mitchell, H. L. 2008. The glycemic index concept in action. *Am J Clin Nutr,* 87(suppl):244S–246S.

Mitchell, D. C., F. R. Lawrence, T. J. Hartman, and J. M. Curran. 2009. Consumption of dry beans, peas, and lentils could improve diet quality in the US population. *J Am Diet Assoc,* 109(5):909–913.

Monnier, L., E. Mas, C. Cinet, F. Michel, L. Villon, J. Cristol, and C. Colette. 2006. Activation of oxidative stress by acute glucose fluctuations compared with sustained chronic hyperglycemia in patients with type 2 diabetes. *JAMA,* 295:1681–1687.

Morgan, S. and J. Kennedy. 2010. Prescription Drug Accessibility and Affordability in the United States and Abroad. *Commonwealth Fund pub,* 1408(89):1.

Mourad, J. J. 2008. The evolution of systolic blood pressure as a strong predictor of cardiovascular risk and the effectiveness of fixed-dose ARB/CCB combinations in lowering levels of this preferential target. *Vasc Health Risk Manag,* 4(6):1315–1325.

Munro, J. M. and R. S. Cotran. 1988. The pathogenesis of atherosclerosis: Atherogenesis and inflammation. *Lab Invest,* 58(3):249–261.

National Cholesterol Education Program. 2002. National Cholesterol Education Program Expert Panel on Detection, Evaluation, and Treatment of High Blood Cholesterol in Adults (Adult Treatment Panel III). *Circulation,* 106:3143.

National Heart Foundation of Australia and the Cardiac Society of Australia and New Zealand. 2005. Position statement on lipid management-2005. *Heart Lung Circ,* 14:275–291.

National Heart, Lung and Blood Institute. 2014. *Who is at Risk for a Stroke?* https://www.nhlbi.nih.gov/health/health-topics/topics/stroke/atrisk. (Accessed October 15, 2015.)

National Institute for Health and Care Excellence. 2009. Type 2 diabetes: The management of type 2 diabetes. Accessed via nice.org.uk/guidance/cg87

National Vascular Disease Prevention Alliance. 2009. *Guidelines for the Assessment of Absolute Cardiovascular Disease Risk.*

Nissen, S. E. and K. Wolski. 2007. Effect of rosiglitazone on the risk of myocardial infarction and death from cardiovascular causes. *N Engl J Med,* 356(24):2457–2471.

Nordestgaard, B. G., M. J. Chapman, K. Ray, J. Boren, F. Andreotti, G. F. Watts, H. Ginsberg et al. 2010. Lipoprotein(a) as a cardiovascular risk factor: Current status. *Eur Heart J,* 31(23):2844–2853.

Ockene, J. K., L. H. Kuller, K. H. Svendsen, and E. Meilahn. 1990. The relationship of smoking cessation to coronary heart disease and lung cancer in the Multiple Risk Factor Intervention Trial (MRFIT). *Am J Public Health,* 80(8):954–958.

Papanikolaou, Y. and V. L. Fulgoni, 3rd. 2008. Bean consumption is associated with greater nutrient intake, reduced systolic blood pressure, lower body weight, and a smaller waist circumference in adults: Results from the National Health and Nutrition Examination Survey 1999–2002. *J Am Coll Nutr,* 27(5):569–576.

Pawlak, D. B., J. A. Kushner, and D. S. Ludwig. 2004. Effects of dietary glycaemic index on adiposity, glucose homoeostasis, and plasma lipids in animals. *Lancet,* 364(9436):778–785.

Philippou, E., C. Bovill-Taylor, C. Rajkumar, M. L. Vampa, E. Ntatsaki, A. E. Brynes, M. Hickson, and G. S. Frost. 2009. Preliminary report: the effect of a 6-month dietary glycemic index manipulation in addition to healthy eating advice and weight loss on arterial compliance and 24-hour ambulatory blood pressure in men: A pilot study. *Metabolism,* 58(12):1703–1708.

Phillips, S. M., V. L. Fulgoni, 3rd, R. P. Heaney, T. A. Nicklas, J. L. Slavin, and C. M. Weaver. 2015. Commonly consumed protein foods contribute to nutrient intake, diet quality, and nutrient adequacy. *Am J Clin Nutr,* epub ahead of print.

Poirier, P., T. D. Giles, G. A. Bray, Y. Hong, J. S. Stern, F. X. Pi-Sunyer, and R. H. Eckel. 2006. Obesity and cardiovascular disease: Pathophysiology, evaluation, and effect of weight loss: An update of the 1997 American Heart Association Scientific Statement on Obesity and Heart Disease from the Obesity Committee of the Council on Nutrition, Physical Activity, and Metabolism. *Circulation,* 113(6):898–918.

Ray, K. K., S. R. Seshasai, S. Erqou, P. Sever, J. W. Jukema, I. Ford, and N. Sattar. 2010. Statins and all-cause mortality in high-risk primary prevention: A meta-analysis of 11 randomized controlled trials involving 65,229 participants. *Arch Intern Med,* 170(12):1024–1031.

Ray, K. K., S. R. Seshasai, S. Wijesuriya, R. Sivakumaran, S. Nethercott, D. Preiss, S. Erqou, and N. Sattar. 2009. Effect of intensive control of glucose on cardiovascular outcomes and death in patients with diabetes mellitus: A meta-analysis of randomised controlled trials. *Lancet,* 373(9677):1765–1772.

Redberg, R. F. and M. H. Katz. 2012. Reassessing benefits and risks of statins. *N Engl J Med,* 367(8):776.

Ridker, P. M. 2014. LDL cholesterol: Controversies and future therapeutic directions. *Lancet,* 384(9943):607–617.

Rodwell, V. W., J. L. Nordstrom, and J. J. Mitschelen. 1976. Regulation of HMG-CoA reductase. *Adv Lipid Res,* 14:1–74.

Rouhani, M. H., R. Kelishadi, M. Hashemipour, A. Esmaillzadeh, and L. Azadbakht. 2013. The effect of low glycemic index diet on body weight status and blood pressure in overweight adolescent girls: A randomized clinical trial. *Nutr Res Pract,* 7(5):385–392.

Sacks, F. M., V. J. Carey, C. A. Anderson, E. R. Miller, 3rd, T. Copeland, J. Charleston, B. J. Harshfield et al. 2014. Effects of high vs low glycemic index of dietary carbohydrate on cardiovascular disease risk factors and insulin sensitivity: The OmniCarb randomized clinical trial. *JAMA,* 312(23):2531–2541.

Sarwar, N., P. Gao, S. R. Seshasai, R. Gobin, S. Kaptoge, E. Di Angelantonio, E. Ingelsson et al. 2010. Diabetes mellitus, fasting blood glucose concentration, and risk of vascular disease: A collaborative meta-analysis of 102 prospective studies. *Lancet,* 375(9733):2215–2222.

Saudek, C. D., R. R. Kalyani, and R. L. Derr. 2005. Assessment of glycemia in diabetes mellitus: Hemoglobin A1c. *J Assoc Physicians India,* 53:299–305.

Schwingshackl, L. and G. Hoffmann. 2013. Long-term effects of low glycemic index/load vs. high glycemic index/load diets on parameters of obesity and obesity-associated risks: A systematic review and meta-analysis. *Nutr Metab Cardiovasc Dis,* 23(8):699–706.

Sievenpiper, J. L., C. W. Kendall, A. Esfahani, J. M. Wong, A. J. Carleton, H. Y. Jiang, R. P. Bazinet, E. Vidgen, and D. J. Jenkins. 2009. Effect of non-oil-seed pulses on glycaemic control: A systematic review and meta-analysis of randomised controlled experimental trials in people with and without diabetes. *Diabetologia,* 52(8):1479–1495.

Singh, U., S. Devaraj, and I. Jialal. 2005. Vitamin E, oxidative stress, and inflammation. *Annu Rev Nutr,* 25:151–174.

Stamler, J., R. Stamler, J. D. Neaton, D. Wentworth, M. L. Daviglus, D. Garside, A. R. Dyer, K. Liu, and P. Greenland. 1999. Low risk-factor profile and long-term cardiovascular and noncardiovascular mortality and life expectancy: findings for 5 large cohorts of young adult and middle-aged men and women. *JAMA,* 282(21):2012–2018.

Stampfer, M. J., F. B. Hu, J. E. Manson, E. B. Rimm, and W. C. Willett. 2000. Primary prevention of coronary heart disease in women through diet and lifestyle. *N Engl J Med,* 343(1):16–22.

Stead, L. F. and T. Lancaster. 2012. Combined pharmacotherapy and behavioural interventions for smoking cessation. *Cochrane Database Syst Rev,* 10:CD008286.

Thomas, D. E. and E. J. Elliott. 2010. The use of low-glycaemic index diets in diabetes control. *Br J Nutr,* 104(6):797–802.

U.S. Department of Health and Human Services and U.S. Department of Agriculture. 2015. Dietary Guidelines for Americans, 8th Edition. http://health.gov/dietaryguidelines/2015/guidelines/.

Wang Q., W. Xia. Z. Zhao, and H. Zhang. 2015. Effects comparison between low glycemic index diets and high glycemic index diets on HbA1c and fructosamine for patients with diabetes: A systematic review and meta-analysis. *Prim Care Diabetes,* 9(5):362–369.

Willett, W., J. Manson, and S. Liu. 2002. Glycemic index, glycemic load, and risk of type 2 diabetes. *Am J Clin Nutr,* 76(1):274S–280S.

Willey, J. Z., Y. P. Moon, E. Kahn, C. J. Rodriguez, T. Rundek, K. Cheung, R. L. Sacco, and M. S. Elkind. 2014. Population attributable risks of hypertension and diabetes for cardiovascular disease and stroke in the northern Manhattan study. *J Am Heart Assoc,* 3(5):e001106.

Wilson, P. W., R. B. D'Agostino, D. Levy, A. M. Belanger, H. Silbershatz, and W. B. Kannel. 1998. Prediction of coronary heart disease using risk factor categories. *Circulation,* 97(18):1837–1847.

Wing, R. R., W. Lang, T. A. Wadden, M. Safford, W. C. Knowler, A. G. Bertoni, J. O. Hill, F. L. Brancati, A. Peters, and L. Wagenknecht. 2011. Benefits of modest weight loss in improving cardiovascular risk factors in overweight and obese individuals with type 2 diabetes. *Diabetes Care,* 34(7):1481–1486.

Wolever, T. M. 2013. Glycemic index claims on food labels: Review of Health Canada's evaluation. *Eur J Clin Nutr,* 67(12):1229–1233.

Wolever, T. M., D. J. Jenkins, L. U. Thompson, G. S. Wong, and R. G. Josse. 1987. Effect of canning on the blood glucose response to beans in patients with type 2 diabetes. *Hum Nutr Clin Nutr,* 41(2):135–140.

Wright, R. S., J. W. Anderson, and S. R. Bridges. 1990. Propionate inhibits hepatocyte lipid synthesis. *Proc Soc Exp Biol Med,* 195(1):26–29.

Yusuf, S., S. Hawken, S. Ounpuu, T. Dans, A. Avezum, F. Lanas, M. McQueen, A. Budaj, P. Pais, J. Varigos, and L. Lisheng. 2004. Effect of potentially modifiable risk factors associated with myocardial infarction in 52 countries (the INTERHEART study): Case-control study. *Lancet,* 364(9438):937–952.

Yusuf, S., S. Reddy, S. Ounpuu, and S. Anand. 2001. Global burden of cardiovascular diseases: part I: General considerations, the epidemiologic transition, risk factors, and impact of urbanization. *Circulation,* 104(22):2746–2753.

6 Glycemic Index in Preventing and Managing Obesity

Implications for Appetite and Body Weight Regulation

Anne Raben, Signe Nyby, and Martí Juanola-Falgarona

CONTENTS

6.1 INTRODUCTION: BACKGROUND AND RATIONALE

In Europe, the prevalence of obesity (body mass index [BMI] > 30 kg/m^2) has tripled in many countries since the 1980s, and the number continues to rise. Presently, more than 50% of the population are overweight (BMI > 25 kg/m^2) and more than 20% are obese [1]. This amounts to more than 200 million overweight or obese Europeans.

In the United States, the prevalence of overweight and obesity is 69%, and the figure for obesity alone is as high as 35% (or 79 million adults) [2]. In addition, childhood obesity is increasing at an alarming pace. Obesity is the most important known risk factor for type 2 diabetes, but obesity also gives rise to other serious complications such as cardiovascular diseases, hypertension, certain cancers (particularly in breast and colon), as well as psychosocial problems (e.g., depression, anxiety, loneliness, discrimination, and mobbing). Further health consequences of obesity include dyslipidemia, insulin resistance, osteoarthritis, sleep apnea, asthma, lower back pain, gallbladder disease, reproductive hormone abnormalities, polycystic ovarian syndrome, impaired fertility, and childbirth complications. Taking action against the current obesity pandemic is therefore most important. A major approach is to initiate changes in food intake and eating behavior.

The main goals of obesity treatment include sustained weight loss, with a primary focus on abdominal obesity, improvement of obesity-related health risks and quality of life, and reduction of mortality. Intentional weight loss is normally associated with reduced mortality, improved blood pressure and lipid profile, better mental health, and enhanced quality of life [3]. Thus, a modest weight loss of 5%–10% significantly reduces obesity-related risks [3,4]. Lifestyle management, including diet and physical activity, is recommended as the first-line treatment for obesity and its metabolic consequences. The key element of obesity treatment is, therefore, to help patients develop healthy lifestyle habits through the improvement of dietary and physical activity, which will lead to a gradual weight loss.

Up to now, numerous nutritional strategies have been proposed to deal with obesity with the majority of the international societies studying obesity recommending low-energy diets as the most valid therapy for obesity treatment [5–11]. Although low-energy diets do not have a specific definition, the scientific community and health professionals have established low-energy diets as those with a reduction of of daily calorie needs between 500 kcal/d and 1000 kcal/d and with a total energy intake greater than 800 kcal/d. However, macronutrient composition of the low-calorie diet is still a matter of debate, although it seems of less importance when caloric intake is controlled. There is an intense debate about the different diets and macronutrient proportions that are most effective for treating overweight or obesity. Several trials assessing dietary composition have been conducted aiming to improve both weight loss and weight maintenance.

In the past several decades, high-carbohydrate, low-fat diets have been recommended as "healthy" and have been prescribed as the primary approach of dietary intervention in obesity treatment [6,9,10,11]. Supportive of this are a number of dietary intervention trials that have shown that a high-carbohydrate, high-fiber, low-fat diet eaten *ad libitum* can cause a spontaneous weight loss, especially in overweight subjects [12–15]. According to previous and newer meta-analyses, a reduction of 10% in the proportion of energy from fat is associated with a reduction in body weight of 2.0–2.8 kg over 6 months [16]. Such a weight loss may seem small, but when compared with the gradual increase in body weight that many people now experience over time, a weight loss of even a few kilograms over 6 months is important, especially when no energy restriction is involved in achieving this weight loss. A spontaneous reduction in energy intake due to a low energy density (great volume) and a high-fiber intake is probably a major reason why such a diet decreases and helps maintain body weight in the long term.

However, the effects may also differ depending on whether fat is substituted by carbohydrate or protein. Thus, protein has been found to be even more efficient than carbohydrate in producing spontaneous weight loss on an *ad libitum* fat-reduced diet [17,18].

The persistence of the obesity epidemic among Western developed countries and the rising cases of obesity in emergent countries have forced the scientific community to evaluate new dietary strategies to overcome this epidemic. Low-carbohydrate diets have been proposed as a valid alternative to low-fat diets. A great number of trials and several meta-analyses have compared the effects of low-fat and low-carbohydrate diets on weight loss [19–21], concluding that low-carbohydrate diets exert, at least, the same effect as traditional low-fat diets. A switch in regulatory hormones (e.g., insulin and glucagon) and substrate metabolism (e.g., fat oxidation and storage) can explain some of these effects.

Considering carbohydrates, it has been suggested that low-glycemic-index (GI) foods increase satiety and reduce body weight compared with high-GI foods [22,23]; however, controversies still exist [24–26]. In this chapter, the short- and long-term effects of changing GI in the diet for appetite regulation, energy balance, and body weight regulation will be addressed. Studies in both adults and children will be considered; however, most studies have been conducted in the adult population.

6.2 ACUTE EFFECTS OF DIETARY GI ON APPETITE REGULATION AND ENERGY BALANCE

For weight maintenance, an energy balance must persist, meaning that energy intake must equal energy expenditure (EE). Although diet-induced thermogenesis may vary slightly according to macronutrient composition, dietary composition probably influences energy intake more than EE [27]. Macronutrients compete with each other in an oxidative hierarchy with the order: alcohol > protein > carbohydrate > fat. A high oxidation rate may promote satiety; therefore, a satiety hierarchy of the same order has been proposed [27]. However, this has not been proven correct in all studies [28].

Another view is that energy density, rather than macronutrient-specific mechanisms, determines energy intake [29]; hence, overeating may be encouraged by energy-dense foods. The question is how GI and glycemic load (GL) affect food intake.

6.2.1 Effects of GI on Appetite Regulation

It has been suggested that low-GI foods, which produce longer and slower blood glucose responses, increase satiety compared with high-GI foods. Thus, high-GI foods would increase hunger and lower satiety because of a rapid, transient increase in blood glucose, followed by a hyperinsulinemic response and then a decline in blood glucose concentration [30]. On the other hand, high-GI foods may suppress energy intake through acute carbohydrate-induced satiating mechanisms, increased hepatic glycogen stores, oxidation in the peripheral tissues, or satiating hormones, such as gastric inhibitory polypeptide, glucagon-like peptide-1 (GLP-1), and insulin.

A systematic review written by Raben back in 2002 identified 31 short-term studies (<1 day) comparing the effects of high- and low-GI foods or meals on appetite, energy intake, and EE. In 15 studies, low-GI foods were associated with greater satiety or reduced hunger, whereas reduced satiety or no differences were seen in the remaining 16 studies. Furthermore, in seven studies, low-GI foods reduced *ad libitum* energy intake, but this could not be found in eight other studies [24].

In a more recent review from 2007, Bornet and coworkers identified 25 short-term human intervention studies that tested either single food items (six items with pure carbohydrate) or complete meals [31]. Interestingly, the overall finding was that both high- and low-GI food items suppressed appetite and food intake, but the time courses seemed to differ. Within the first hours, an early short-term satiating effect was observed with high-GI carbohydrates, resulting in decreased food intake 60–90 min after consumption. For low-GI carbohydrates, a later satiating effect was found, with a reduced food intake 2–6 h after the ingestion of the preload [32]. This observation of a time pattern for the satiating effect of high- and low-GI foods is very plausible and could be closer to the truth than most of the previous and current statements of a "black or white" perception on the role of GI in appetite regulation.

An important aspect is also the amount of carbohydrate actually eaten in a meal. GI is determined from 50 g available carbohydrate, but this may mean quite a large amount for some foods. For instance, 100 g boiled potato contains only about 10 g available carbohydrates. Therefore, although GI is high (78 for boiled potatoes), the GL of boiled potato is relatively small (GL: 15) compared with that for instance pasta (GL: 23), despite the fact that pasta has a lower GI value (GI: 49).

It is worth noting that potatoes, a high-quality carbohydrate source, including vitamins, minerals, antioxidants, and dietary fiber (if consumed with the peal), have achieved a poor reputation in the population and thus make an interesting case for research deserving more attention.

In 1995, Holt and colleagues generated a satiety index based on the rated appetite sensations after intake of 1000 kJ of potatoes, rice, pasta, and various other carbohydrate sources. Compared with white pasta (119 ± 35) and rice (138 ± 31), boiled potatoes (323 ± 51) produced more than twice as high a satiety index [33].

However, in four later studies, satiety ratings were not different after intake of potatoes compared with other carbohydrate sources [34–37]. A possible explanation is that in the latter studies, only carbohydrate-equivalent intakes (50 g) were compared. Although Erdmann et al. [35] found no difference in satiety after rice, pasta, or potato meals, total energy intake was significantly lower after the potato meal (2177 kJ) compared with other meals with the same amount of carbohydrate (pasta: 3174 kJ and rice: 2829 kJ). The postprandial satiety rating is affected by the energy densities of the carbohydrate sources, and as boiled potatoes were the least energy dense of these three meals, they provided more volume and satiation for less energy. This would suggest that intake of boiled potatoes may not be associated with long-term weight gain.

The importance of factors other than glucose response for feelings of satiety (e.g., insulin and gut hormones) has been investigated in several meal test studies. However, conflicting results have been shown. In a study by Flint et al. 3-h glucose, insulin, appetite, and subsequent energy intake were assessed in 28 healthy, normal-weight adult men consuming up to 14 typical European breakfasts varying in GI, energy, and macronutrients. Each meal contained 50 g carbohydrate. The glycemic response was unrelated to appetite sensations, whereas the insulinemic response was positively associated with postprandial fullness. The glycemic, but not the insulinemic, response was positively associated with energy intake at lunch [38]. This study does not support the contention that postprandial glycemic response has an important effect on short-term appetite sensations, but a low GI meal may reduce energy intake in a subsequent meal. In contrast, postprandial insulin seemed to affect short-term appetite sensations.

Likewise, in a later meta-analysis of seven different meal test studies ($n = 137$), it was found that insulin, but not glucose, was associated with short-term appetite regulation in healthy participants. Interestingly, this relationship seemed to be disrupted in overweight and obese subjects [39].

In another study, Reynolds et al. found that adults who consumed low-GI meals during the whole day (10 h) had lower glucose and insulin profiles than those who consumed high-GI meals, but there were no significant differences in subsequent food intake [40]. Similarly, Alfenas and Mattes and Aston et al. investigated the effects of high- and low-GI foods over multiple days and found no significant differences in energy intake measured either acutely or over the whole study period [41,42].

To support this, Makris and colleagues observed no differential effect of high- or low-GI meals on energy intake in a subsequent *ad libitum* meal or in self-reported hunger, satiety, and prospective energy intake. The authors concluded that there were no effects of GI on appetite or energy intake 4 h after breakfast. Together, their findings suggested that subsequent energy intake cannot be predicted solely by the glycemic effect of a previously consumed meal. It is more likely determined by a variety of internal factors mediating energy intake [43].

In addition, in support of the above was a study by Kristensen et al. [44]. They compared the effects of wholemeal bread and wholemeal pasta on glycemic response, appetite, and *ad libitum* food intake of 4 test meals in 20 normal-weight adults. They found that wholemeal bread, but not wholemeal pasta, increased satiety compared with refined breads, but the effect was unrelated to glycemic response and was not associated with reduced energy intake. Finally, Burton-Freeman et al. conducted a randomized crossover study with 22 overweight women (20–50 years of age). They found that a high-GI meal resulted in greater overall satiety and less hunger, desire to eat, and prospective food consumption compared with low-GI meals, but no difference in the sensation of fullness was found [45].

The above findings are in contrast to prevalent statements in scientific and lay literature claiming low-GI foods to be superior to high-GI foods in managing appetite and body weight. However, as mentioned above, the time course may be important for the observed effects. Furthermore, normal-weight subjects may respond differently than overweight subjects. These methodological issues need to be considered when evaluating the effects of GI on appetite regulation.

6.2.2 Effects of GI on Energy Balance

Another factor to consider is whether high-GI carbohydrates stimulate EE, an effect that could counteract a possible increase in energy intake. In addition, oxidation of the different macronutrients could be different, and therefore, this is also important to consider.

With regard to EE, diet-induced thermogenesis is different between the main macronutrients, normally in the following order: protein > carbohydrate > fat. Considering the different types of carbohydrates, it has been shown that in an acute situation, an increased intake of sucrose stimulates thermogenesis, as compared with glucose or starch [46–48]. However, the effect of GI *per se* has not been studied to a great extent.

One study evaluated the glycemic effect on fuel oxidation using isolated carbohydrates [49]. In total, 12 obese women were included in a randomized crossover design, with two test meals (breakfast + lunch). High- or low-GI meals of similar energy and macronutrient distribution were provided on separate days. Fuel oxidation was measured in a respiratory chamber for 10 h, and glucose, free fatty acids, insulin, and glucagon samples were taken for 5 h after breakfast. This study showed that glucose and insulin changed significantly in response to the different glycemic breakfasts, as expected. However, carbohydrate and fat oxidations were not different after the low- and high-GI breakfasts. Thus, this study showed that dietary glycemic characteristics were unable to modify the fuel partitioning in sedentary obese women.

In 2006, an overview was published by Diaz et al. [50]. They concluded that several studies comparing the effects of meals with different GI for hours, days, or weeks failed to demonstrate any differential effect on fuel partitioning, when either substrate oxidation or body composition measurements were performed. Thus, the GI-induced differences in blood parameters were not sufficient in magnitude and/or duration to modify fuel oxidation.

Krog-Mikkelsen et al. concluded on the basis of a human intervention study with 29 healthy, overweight women that a low-GI meal did not affect postprandial EE or substrate oxidation rates differently, compared with a high-GI meal (4-h meal test) [51]. The breakfast meals were given after 10 weeks' intervention [51] and differed in GI but were otherwise equal in total energy, macronutrient composition, fiber content, and energy density. The low-GI meal did result in significantly lower plasma glucose, serum insulin, GLP-1, and gastric inhibitory polypeptide concentrations than the high-GI meal, and ratings of fullness were slightly higher after the low-GI meal. However, no differences were seen in postprandial GLP-2, glucagon, leptin, ghrelin, or *ad libitum* energy intake at lunch. Thus, no effects were seen for the expending side of energy balance, although differences in blood parameters could have mediated such effects. It can be speculated that adaptation to the diets had taken place after 10 weeks or perhaps that the differences in blood parameters were not large enough to produce a difference in EE and substrate oxidation.

In line with the above studies, the long-term Carbohydrate Ratio Manipulation in European National Diets (CARMEN) trial observed no differences in 24-h EE, postprandial thermogenesis, or basal metabolic rate after 6-month *ad libitum* diets high in simple carbohydrates, complex carbohydrates, or fat [52]. Carbohydrate and fat oxidations, adjusted for energy balance, increased and decreased, respectively, on both carbohydrate-rich diets, but the changes were not different between these two diets. The shift in the oxidation pattern thus closely reflected the fat and carbohydrate intake in these overweight and obese subjects, but the type of carbohydrate did not matter.

Overall, the data from human intervention studies does not provide convincing evidence that low-GI meals have more positive effects on appetite regulation and energy balance than high-GI meals. However, the discrepancies between studies may be due to differences in design and methodology, including the timing of the postprandial measurements, amount of carbohydrate, energy, and volume of the test meal. Furthermore, study population characteristics, degree of standardization regarding study procedure and confounding factors, and inevitably, but perhaps, decisive day-to-day variation (e.g., appetite regulation) complicate the comparison of data obtained from different studies. An additional factor could be that GI is an indicator of the quality of glycemic carbohydrates but not of a whole meal, which can be affected by other factors such as fat and protein contents. Therefore, isolated carbohydrates are not comparable to mixed meals, in which other food components influence the glycemic response [53].

6.3 EFFECT OF DIETARY GI ON WEIGHT LOSS AND WEIGHT MAINTENANCE

6.3.1 GI and Weight Loss in Adults

6.3.1.1 Population Studies

Several prospective cohort studies have investigated the link between dietary GI and GL with anthropometrical measurements and with increased risk of obesity [54–66]. The most investigated anthropometrical measurement in this context is BMI; however, waist circumference has also been evaluated.

A number of studies have linked both GI and GL with BMI, but with inconsistent results [54,55,59,60,63,65,67]. Ma and colleagues were the first to assess the associations between the type of carbohydrates and BMI in 572 healthy American adults. Body mass index was found to be positively associated with GI but not with GL [54]. Similar results were found in a prospective cohort study, including 185 men and 191 women, from the Danish arm of the Monitoring Trends and Determinants in Cardiovascular Disease study (MONICA). The authors found significant positive associations between baseline GI and 6-year changes in body weight and percentage body fat among women but not among men [68].

These results were also found in a prospective cohort study, including 3931 Japanese young adults. Murakami et al. found a positive association not only between GI and BMI (lowest vs. highest quintiles: 20.8 and 21.2 kg/m^2, p for trend = .03) but also between GL and BMI (lowest vs. highest quintiles: 20.5 and 21.5 kg/m^2, p for trend = .0005) [65]. However, other investigators have found inverse [55,59,60] or no [57,63] associations between BMI and GI or GL. Two studies conducted in Mediterranean populations (Spain and Italy) found inverse associations between GI or GL and BMI. Mendez and coworkers were the first to report this inverse association in 8195 Spanish adults [55]. After adjusting for total energy intake, mean difference in BMI between the highest and lowest GL tertile was −0.71 kg/m^2 ($p < .05$) for women, which means a higher BMI in the lowest GL tertile. No significant association was found in men. In a similar analysis, Rossi et al. also found an inverse association between GL or GI and BMI. Compared with the lowest tertile, the coefficient for the highest tertile of GI was −0.46 (−0.74, −0.19) among men and −0.81 (−1.13, −0.49) among women. Regression coefficients for GL were −0.79 (−1.14, −0.45) among men and −1.33 (−1.73, −0.94) among women. The same authors also analyzed the correlation between GI or GL and waist-to-hip ratio but did not find any significant results [59].

Although the majority of these population studies have analyzed the associations between baseline GI or GL and BMI or weight change, a recent study has evaluated the associations between 4-year changes in GI or GL and 4-year weight change over a 16- to 24-year follow-up. This study included 120,784 healthy men and women from three different prospective U.S. cohorts (Nurses' Health Study, Nurses' Health Study II, and Health Professionals Follow-Up Study) [69]. The authors found a significant positive relationship between both total dietary GL and GI and weight gain during follow-up. After adjusting for multiple variables, each 50-unit increase in GL was associated with +0.42 kg (95% CI: 0.24 kg, 0.60 kg) greater weight gain every 4 years and each 5-unit increase in GI was associated with +0.35 kg (95% CI: 0.25 kg, 0.45 kg) greater weight gain.

The effect of different types of carbohydrate on waist circumference has also been evaluated in four studies, but with inconsistent results [56–58,63]. Two of the four studies found a positive association between GI and waist circumference [56,57] but the other two did not [58,63]. In a cohort of 89,432 participants, aged 20–78 years, from five European countries, Du and collaborators observed that with every 10-point increase in GI, waist circumference increased by 0.19 cm per year (95% CI: 0.11, 0.27) [57]. GI has also been associated with a large weight girth in a cohort with 10,912 participants from the Cooper Center Longitudinal Study [70]. In this study, men and women consuming the highest quintile of energy-adjusted GI had a 27% (95% CI: 1.07, 1.51) and 74% (95% CI: 1.04, 2.89) higher risk of large waist girth than those consuming the lowest, energy-adjusted GI quintile. Conversely, however, GL was inversely associated with a large waist girth (OR: 0.52; 95% CI: 0.43, 0.63) in men, but not in women.

Finally, GL was negatively associated with obesity prevalence in 1078 Korean men and women. Thus, participants in the highest tertile of GL had a 50% lower risk of being obese compared with those in the lowest GL tertile [60].

In summary, a relatively large number of epidemiological studies have evaluated the associations between GI or GL and obesity-related parameters, but with inconsistent results. More studies with longer follow-up periods and larger population are needed in order to understand the potential benefits of GI and GL for body weight regulation.

6.3.1.2 Intervention Trials

The usefulness of the GI and GL concepts to reduce body weight has been investigated in a large number of intervention trials varying in length, approaches, and populations. The few systematic reviews and meta-analyses published to date have found a modest beneficial effect of low-GI and -GL diets in comparison with high-GI and -GL diets or low-fat diets; however, there is a significant amount of inconsistency in the current findings [71–73]. In 2007, Thomas et al. published the first meta-analysis, including 202 participants from six different studies. Here, a significantly greater weight loss was reported in participants consuming the low-GI diets compared with those consuming the control diets. However, the magnitude was modest (1.1 kg difference) and the control diet was of mixed nature, including high-fat diets and other diets that did not only differ in GI [72].

In 2011, Esfahani identified 23 clinical trials that examined low-GI and -GL diets and weight loss as the primary outcome measure. In general, the studies showed much inconsistency in their findings [71]. A few studies found significantly greater weight loss on the low-GI and -GL diets, whereas most of the other studies showed only a nonsignificant trend, in favor of low-GI and -GL diets. This suggests that factors other than GI and GL played a role. The authors concluded that there is a need for more long-term randomized controlled trials (RCTs) that not only focus on weight loss but also on weight maintenance and body composition.

In general, the majority of clinical trials conducted to date to assess the effect of GI and GL on weight loss have used a parallel design and have compared low-GI and -GL diets with either a low-fat or a high-GI or -GL diet. Furthermore, they have included healthy overweight or obese participants with or without energy restriction. Table 6.1 presents an overview of these studies.

Of the 21 identified clinical trials, 13 studies were energy-restricted, five did not restrict energy intake, and three varied in dietary approach. Of these studies, five found a significant beneficial effect of GI or GL on weight loss [74–79]. One of them is the study conducted by Abete and collaborators, which randomized 32 participants (14 females and 18 males), to either a low-GI or a high-GI diet, both of which were energy-restricted, for 8 weeks. Results showed that participants allocated to the low-GI diet had a significantly greater reduction in body weight than the high-GI group; however, the differences were small (–7.5% vs. –5.3%, respectively) [74].

More recently, Juanola-Falgarona et al. conducted a 6-month randomized, parallel, controlled clinical trial, the "GLYNDIET" study, including 122 overweight and obese adults that were randomly assigned to one of the following three isocaloric energy-restricted diets: (1) a moderate-carbohydrate, high-GI diet (HGI), (2) a moderate-carbohydrate, low-GI diet (LGI), and (3) a low-fat, high-GI diet (LF). After 6 months, reductions in BMI were greater in the LGI group than in the LF group, whereas in the HGI group, reductions in BMI did not differ significantly from those in the other two groups (Figure 6.1) [80]. Fasting insulin, HOMA-IR, and HOMA-Beta cell function followed a similar pattern, but no other differences were observed in waist circumference, body composition, fasting or postprandial appetite sensations, blood lipids, or inflammatory markers after 6 months. Therefore, this study does not support a role of dietary GI *per se* in body weight regulation and risk factors for metabolic diseases. The GLYNDIET study was of a reasonably long duration and was performed in large groups of subjects. However, the energy restriction and isocaloric design might have eliminated the possible differences between diets of high and low GI, which could perhaps have been seen if an *ad libitum* design had been used.

The rest of the clinical trials conducted to date also did not see significant differences between intervention groups; however, the majority of them found a beneficial trend in the low-GI and -GL interventions [81–92]. Only the study of Bellisle et al. found greater body weight reductions in the control group, which followed the standard Weight Watcher plan [93].

Three more trials evaluated the effects of GI on weight loss with different approaches. All three were clinical trials with multiple interventions, combining GI with other weight loss strategies. However, none of them found significant differences between the interventions [94,96].

TABLE 6.1
Summary Table of Clinical Trials Evaluating the Effect of Dietary GI on Weight Loss in Adults

Authors	Subjects	Duration	Population	Design	Age (Year)	BMI (kg/m²)	Intervention	Weight Loss (kg)
				Energy-Restricted Studies				
Slabber et al. (1994)	30 f	12 weeks	Obese hyperinsulinemic participants	Parallel	35.2 ± 1.1	34.8 ± 0.8	Low GI vs. energy restricted diet	−7.41 ± 4.23 vs. −9.34 ± 2.49
Pereira et al. (2004)	39 (30 f; 9 m)	Varied	Overweight or obese participants	Parallel	30.5 ± 0.9	91.5 ± 2.3[a]	Low GL vs. low fat	−9.6 ± 0.3 in 65.2 ± 3.3 vs. −9.5 ± 0.3 in 69.4 ± 3.8
Raatz et al. (2005)	29 (24 f; 5 m)	12 weeks	Obese participants	Parallel	18–70	36.3 ± 1.0	Low GI vs. high GI vs. high fat	−9.95 ± 1.4 vs. −9.3 ± 1.3 vs. −8.4 ± 1.5
Thompson et al. (2005)	90 (77 f; 13 m) (72 completers)	48 weeks	Obese participants	Parallel	41.4 ± 0.9	43.8 ± 0.3	High calcium/ low GI vs. high calcium vs. moderate calcium/moderate Fiber (MCMF)	−8.8 ± 1.42 vs. −8.8 ± 1.37 vs. −9.1 ± 1.30
McMillan-Price et al. (2006)	129 (98 f; 31 m)	12 weeks	Overweight or obese participants	Parallel	31.8 ± 0.8	31.2 ± 0.4	High-carb/high GI vs. high-carb/low GI vs. high protein/high GI vs. high protein/low GI	−3.7 ± 0.5 vs. −4.8 ± 0.5 vs. −5.3 ± 0.5 vs. −4.4 ± 0.5
Pittas et al. (2006)	32 (25 f; 7 m)	6 months	Overweight participants	Parallel	34.7 ± 0.9	27.6 ± 0.3	Low GL (53) vs. high GL (86)	−7.7 vs. −7.2
Das et al. (2007)	34 (26 f; 8 m) (29 completers)	6 months	Overweight participants	Parallel	34.5 ± 0.9	27.6 ± 0.2	Low GI (52) vs. high GI (85)	−10.4 ± 1.1% vs. −9.1 ± 1.1%
Maki et al. (2007)	86 (58 f; 28 m) (84 completers)	12 weeks	Overweight or obese participants	Parallel	49.7 ± 1.18	31.9 ± 0.4	Low GL (46) vs. low fat (51)	−4.9 ± 0.5 vs. −2.5 ± 0.5
Sichieri et al. (2007)	203 f (123 completers)	18 months	Overweight participants	Parallel	37.3 ± 0.3	26.8 ± 0.1	Low GI (40) vs. high GI (79)	−0.41 ± 0.37 vs. −0.26 ± 0.46
Bellisle et al. (2007)	96 f (65 completers)	12 weeks	Overweight or obese participants	Parallel	45.7 ± 1.6	30.3 ± 0.5	Low GI weight watchers vs. standard weight watchers	−4.0 ± 3.1 vs. −4.5 ± 3.4

(Continued)

TABLE 6.1 (*Continued*)
Summary Table of Clinical Trials Evaluating the Effect of Dietary GI on Weight Loss in Adults

Authors	Subjects	Duration	Population	Design	Age (Year)	BMI (kg/m²)	Intervention	Weight Loss (kg)
Abete et al. (2008)	32 (14 f; 18 m)	8 weeks	Obese participants	Parallel	36 ± 1.2	32.5 ± 0.8	Low GI (40–45) vs. high GI (60–65)	−7.5 ± 0.73% vs. −5.3 ± 0.65%
Buscemi et al. (2013)	40 (21 f; 19 m)	3 months	Obese participants	Parallel	50 ± 11.3	93.5 ± 22.5[a]	Low GI (46) vs. high GI (57)	−2.8 ± 8.8 vs. −2.6 ± 7.0
Goss et al. (2013)	59 (32 f; 27 m)	8 weeks	Overweight participants	Parallel	21–50	31.7 ± 2.1	Low GL vs. high GL	−6.1 ± 3.9 vs. −4.3 ± 0.8
Juanola-Falgarona et al. (2014)	121 (97 f; 24 m)	6 months	Overweight or obese participants	Parallel	43.5 ± 1.1	31.0 ± 0.5	Low GI vs. high GI vs. low fat (high GL)	−2.45 ± 0.27 vs. −2.30 ± 0.27 vs. −1.43 ± 0.27
Isocaloric or *Ad Libitum* Studies								
Bouché et al. (2002)	11 m	5 weeks	Healthy participants	Crossover	46 ± 3	28 ± 1.0	Low GI vs. high GI	−0.3 ± 3.3 vs. 0.5 ± 3.3
Sloth et al. (2004)	45 f	10 weeks	Overweight participants	Parallel	29.8 ± 0.9	27.6 ± 0.2	Low GI vs. high GI	−1.9 ± 0.5 vs. −1.3 ± 0.3
Ebbeling et al. (2005)	34 (30 f; 4 m) (23 completers)	6 months	Obese participants	Parallel	28.4 ± 1.0	32.5 ± 1.2	Low GL vs. low fat	−8.4 ± 1.5% vs. −7.8 ± 1.5%
De Rougemont et al. (2007)	38 (18 f; 20 m)	5 weeks	Overweight participants	Parallel	38.4 ± 1.5	27.4 ± 0.2	Low GI (46.5) vs. high GI (66.3)	−1.1 ± 0.3 vs. −0.2 ± 0.2
Retterstol et al. (2009)	16 m	4 weeks	Overweight or obese participants	Crossover	36–66	30.4 (26.6–34.9) Median (range)	Low GI vs. low-fat vs. high GI	−2.4 (range: −3.9 to −1.4) vs. 0 vs. −1.4 kg (range: −3.6 to 0.2)
Combined Strategies Studies								
Melanson et al. (2012)	157 (138 f; 19 m)	12 weeks	Overweight or obese participants	Parallel	38.7 ± 6.7	31.8 ± 2.2	Low GI vs. low energy density vs. portion control	−3.39 ± 2.76 vs−4.14 ± 3.64 vs. −3.73 ± 2.84
Lagerpusch et al. (2013)	32 m	6 weeks	Healthy participants	Parallel	25.5 ± 3.9	23.5 ± 2.0	Low GL vs. high GL	−4.2 ± 0.9 (mean difference between interventions)
Shyam et al. (2013)	77 f	6 months	Overweight participants with previous GDM	Parallel	31.2 ± 2.1	26.4 ± 4.6	Low GI vs. health diet	−1.3 ± 3.4 vs. −0.1 ± 3.5

Note: GI, Glycemic index; GL, Glycemic load; F, Female; M, Male.
[a] Expressed in kilogram.

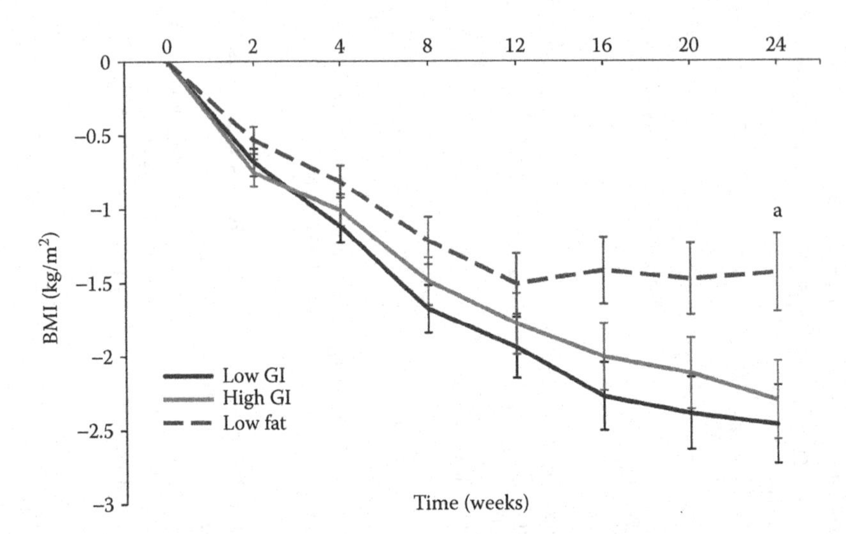

FIGURE 6.1 Changes in BMI during the 6-month follow-up for each intervention group. Total $n = 121$. ANOVA models were used to assess differences between intervention groups. The $p < .05$ between low-GI and low-fat groups. The p value of changes in BMI at the end of the intervention was .012; pairwise comparisons: low-GI group compared with high-GI group, $p = 1.000$; low-GI group compared with low-fat group, $p = .016$; high-GI group compared with low-fat group, $p = .061$. ANOVA, analysis of variance; BMI, body mass index; GI, glycemic index. (Data from Juanola-Falgarona M. et al. *Am J Clin Nutr*, 2014:100:27–35.)

Interestingly, Randolph et al. [97] showed that even with a high daily intake of potatoes, a weight loss could be induced. In a 12-week study, subjects were randomized to receive dietary advice for either a high or low GI intake, with energy restriction and instructions to consume 5–7 servings of potatoes per week. At the end of the intervention period, the diets had the same GI and there were no differences in weight loss between the groups. The study is interesting as there was no differential effect on body weight of a high daily potato intake, as previously indicated in epidemiological studies [98,99].

However, intervention studies with an isocaloric or hypocaloric design cannot reveal how GI might affect appetite and body weight in a real-life situation; therefore, it is relevant to consider studies using an *ad libitum* design.

The large-scale, long-term, randomized, controlled multicenter CARMEN trial involved a total of 316 overweight subjects in five different countries [100]. Here, it was found that 6 months' *ad libitum* intake of low-fat diets rich in either simple or complex carbohydrates reduced body weight and fat mass by 1.6–2.4 kg compared with a higher-fat, control diet, with no significant differences between the simple and complex carbohydrate diets.

Quite often, important aspects such as macronutrient composition, fiber content, energy content, and energy density of the LGI and HGI meals or diets are not well matched. Foods with an LGI tend to be rich in fiber and have a low energy density, so these factors should ideally be kept constant when testing the effect of GI *per se*. The few existing studies in which the diets compared are kept similar in macronutrient composition, dietary fiber, and energy density, did not show consistent results. Furthermore, diets are often energy fixed. If *ad libitum* energy intake and fluctuations in body weight and ensuing changes in health are allowed, a more real-life situation is achieved, making results easier to apply to the public. There have been very few long-term intervention studies, with diets matched for macronutrient composition, fiber content, energy content, and energy density, investigating the effect of GI in healthy participants [32,81,89], and the evidence of a beneficial effect of longer-term diets is therefore inconclusive.

In a previous *ad libitum* study, in which macronutrients, dietary fiber, and energy density were well matched and only GI was manipulated, there were no significant differences in 10 weeks' body weight or fat mass in the overweight study subjects [89]. Thus, energy intake, body weight, and fat mass decreased similarly on the high- and low-GI diets. In a subsample, there were also no differences in 24-h EE or substrate oxidation rates. However, after 10 weeks on the low-GI diet, fasting low-density lipoprotein cholesterol, postprandial plasma glucose, serum insulin, and GLP-1 were significantly reduced, compared with a high-GI diet [51].

Although some of the trials evaluating the effect of GI on weight loss have found a small beneficial effect, the effects are not consistent. Discrepancies in methodology and approach make it difficult to get a clear view of the role of GI as a potential nutritional tool to fight obesity.

6.3.2 Effects of Dietary GI on Weight Maintenance after Weight Loss

In the last century, the scientific and medical community focused mainly on how to achieve a significant weight loss through a wide variety of dietary interventions. However, in the past 10–15 years, more attention has been paid to secondary prevention of weight regain in overweight or obese individuals who had achieved a desired weight loss in order to reduce the adverse consequences of obesity. Regaining nearly half of the lost weight after 1 year is usual, and most of the individuals who had reduced their body weight acquire their initial weight within 3–5 years [101]. According to the data from the National Health and Nutrition Examination Survey (1999–2006), only one in six overweight and obese adults report to have ever maintained weight loss of at least 10% for 1 year. The scientific community considers it a great achievement when a person sustains even 5%–10% of his or her weight loss [102]. Actually, weight maintenance is defined as weight change up to 3% of the actual body weight after weight loss [103].

One possible explanation for poor long-term weight maintenance results could be attributed to a behavioral component and reduced motivation to achieve compliance to an energy-restricted dietary treatment over time. Therefore, using behavior modification tools seem most important for maintaining any change in lifestyle patterns [104]. An alternative explanation could be metabolic adaptation, specifically a reduction in EE (adaptive thermogenesis) and compensatory changes in a number of appetite regulatory peptides that promote weight regain [105,106].

To our knowledge, only four trials have evaluated the effect of dietary GI or GL on weight maintenance as the main objective [107–110]. Three of these conducted similar trials consisting of two phases. First, they included a weight loss phase in which participants were encouraged to lose between 5% and 12.5% of the initial weight. This was a prerequisite for being randomized to the second phase. In the second phase, participants were randomized to one of the interventions for weight maintenance. This second phase usually compared a low-GI diet with other control diets in a parallel design. Only the study of Ebbeling and coworkers designed a crossover intervention [108].

The first study investigating the possible beneficial effect of GI on weight maintenance was the study conducted by Sloth et al. They enrolled 154 participants in an initial 8-week low-energy diet part of the trial. After 8-week low-energy diet and a 2- to 3-week refeeding period, 131 subjects were randomized to three diets for 6 months: a moderate-fat diet (35–45 E% [E%] fat), high in monounsaturated fat, with low GI; a low-fat diet (20–30 fat); and a control (35 E% fat). After 6 months, there were no differences between the interventions [107].

Similarly, Ebbeling and coworkers designed a three-way crossover trial, including 21 overweight or obese participants. After achieving at least 10% weight loss, participants were allocated to a low-fat diet (60% of energy from carbohydrate, 20% from fat, 20% from protein; high GL), a low-GI diet (40% from carbohydrate, 40% from fat, and 20% from protein; moderate GL), and a very-low-carbohydrate diet (10% from carbohydrate, 60% from fat, and 30% from protein; low GL) for 4 weeks each. Similar to the results observed in the previous study, body weight did not differ significantly between the three interventions after the weight maintenance phase [108].

The third study investigating the potential beneficial effect of GI on weight maintenance after weight loss was conducted by Philippou and coworkers in 42 overweight or obese participants. After an initial weight-loss phase of at least 5%, participants were randomized to either a high-GI or a low-GI diet. After 4 months of weight maintenance, the groups did not differ in body weight (high-GI group: 0.3 kg; low-GI group: −0.7 kg, $p = .3$) [109].

To date, the longest trial regarding this matter is the Diogenes study. The Diogenes study is a pan-European, randomized, controlled multicenter trial that investigated how different combinations of GI and dietary protein could prevent weight regain after weight loss in free-living conditions [110]. A design that included both the *ad libitum* principle and weight maintenance after weight loss was used. Families with at least one overweight or obese parent (18–65 years) and at least one child (5–18 years) were enrolled from eight European countries. This trial was designed as a 6-month intervention trial, in which families were randomized to one of five arms: normal-protein/low-GI diet; normal-protein, high-GI; high-protein, low-GI diet; high-protein, high-GI diet; and control diet with medium protein content and no specific instructions on GI, after an initial 8-week low-calorie diet (adults only).

In Diogenes study, it was shown that after 6-month weight maintenance phase, a combination of an *ad libitum* low-GI, high-protein diet maintained body weight loss better and had a favorable effect on glycemic control and insulin sensitivity than other protein and GI combinations [110,111]. Looking at GI only, mean weight gain was about 1 kg less in the low-GI groups than in the high-GI groups ($p < .05$) at the end of the 6-month intervention (Figure 6.2). Additional analyses also

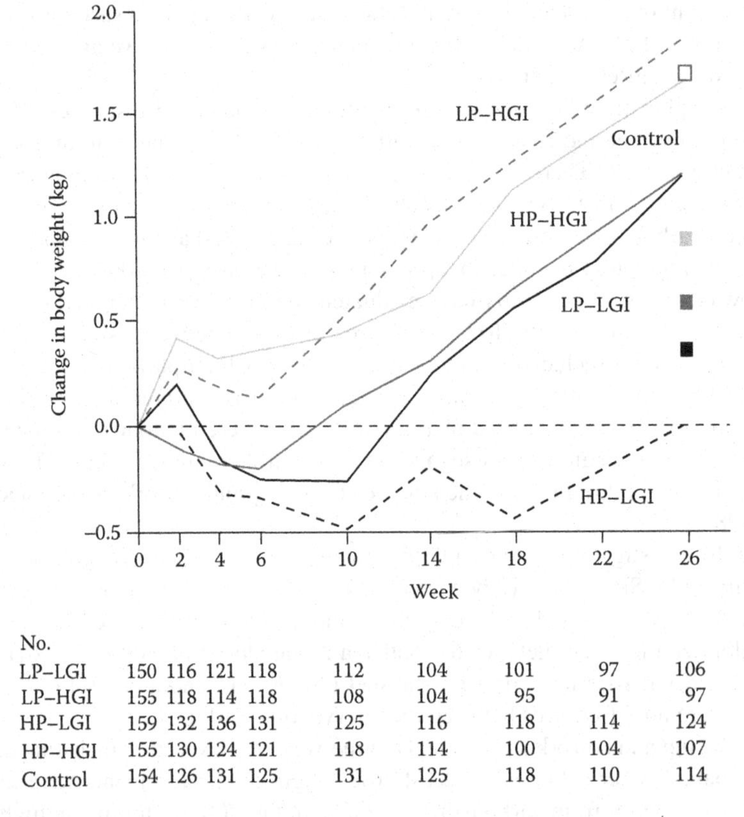

No.									
LP–LGI	150	116	121	118	112	104	101	97	106
LP–HGI	155	118	114	118	108	104	95	91	97
HP–LGI	159	132	136	131	125	116	118	114	124
HP–HGI	155	130	124	121	118	114	100	104	107
Control	154	126	131	125	131	125	118	110	114

FIGURE 6.2 Changes in body weight for each of the dietary groups during the weight-maintenance intervention, adjusted for body mass index at randomization, weight loss during the low-calorie-diet phase, sex, family type (single-parent family, two-parent family with one parent as participant, or two-parent family with both parents as participants), center, and age at screening, on the basis of an intention-to-treat mixed-model analysis. The changes in body weight from randomization to week 26 among participants who completed the intervention are also shown (boxes). All participants who underwent randomization and for whom data on weight at the time of randomization were available were included. HGI, high glycemic index; HP, high protein; LGI, low glycemic index; LP, low protein. (Data from Larsen T.M. et al. *N Engl J Med*, 2010:363:2102–2113.)

showed that low-GI groups were more likely to achieve a further weight loss of more than 5% compared with the high-GI groups (odd ratio: 2.54; $p = .003$). However, the 12-month follow-up data did not support these results and actually showed a reverse picture. Thus, the role of GI for body weight maintenance was not clear anymore [112].

The combined effects of GI, protein, and other lifestyle factors on 3-year weight maintenance after weight loss (8-week low-calorie diet) and the development of type 2 diabetes in prediabetic overweight subjects are currently being studied in the "PREVIEW" project (PREVention of diabetes through lifestyle Intervention and population studies in Europe and around the World). This EU-FP7 project involves both a 3-year RCT and analyses of data from large cohort studies (http://www.previewstudy.com) [113]. A total of about 2350 adults and 150 children or adolescents have been enrolled and will be followed for 3 and 2 years, respectively. The project will end in 2018 and is expected to provide much more knowledge on the role of both GI and protein in body weight maintenance, metabolic risk factors, and incidence of type 2 diabetes.

6.3.2.1 GI and Body Weight Regulation in Children and Adolescents

Childhood and adolescence are critical periods in which healthy eating habits should be taught in order to promote healthy eating habits. Overweight and obesity in youth are important public health concerns and are of particular interest because of possible long-term associations with adult weight status and morbidity [114].

Only a handful of trials have investigated the potential beneficial effects of low GI or GL on weight loss in children and adolescents [115–119]. From the five identified trials, the majority used a parallel design and compared either isocaloric low-GI or low-GL diets with low-fat diets. Armeno and coworkers used energy-restricted diets and a standard healthy diet as a control [118]. Although only two of the five reported studies showed significant reductions in body weight with low-GI and -GL diets [115,116], the majority of them found beneficial effects in other anthropometric variables such as percentage of body fat or waist circumference.

In the Diogenes trial, data from 465 children showed that the low-protein, high-GI group increased body fat percentage significantly more than the other groups. Furthermore, the percentage of overweight/obese children decreased in the high-protein, low-GI group [120]. However, the conclusion was that neither GI nor protein had an isolated effect on body composition.

6.4 METHODOLOGICAL AND ANALYTICAL PITFALLS

When reviewing the literature on cross-sectional surveys and longitudinal studies, a number of common methodological and analytical flaws can be identified. These must be taken into consideration in order to achieve a consistent picture of the relationship between dietary GI, GL, and body weight. A source of possible error, more important than nonrepresentative sampling, lies in the difficult task of self-observation and reporting of food intake, but also of body weight and height.

It is well established that a major pitfall is the systematic underreporting of energy by overweight and obese individuals, which has been clearly demonstrated by simultaneous measurement of free-living EE, by the doubly labeled water method, and of energy intake [121–123]. Further selective underreporting of foods is most likely also taking place, making interpretation of dietary records and recall very complicated [124].

Besides underreporting of energy intake, overweight and obese subjects have a larger propensity to underreport their weight and to overreport their height [125,126]. This has an influence on the BMI and has been shown to produce significant errors in estimating the prevalence of overweight and obese subjects; therefore, weight and height should preferably be measured by the investigators instead of the participants, and appropriate corrections should be made [127].

Furthermore, it is important to realize that population studies cannot reveal the exact causes of overweight. Thus, people with clinical conditions may change dietary habits, and thereby, spurious associations or reverse causality can arise. Instead, RCTs should be given more consideration when evaluating how a certain dietary pattern may affect body weight and human health.

On the other hand, when assessing the results of intervention studies, it is important to consider the study design and study subjects and identify if only the GI/GL or several other factors have been changed in order to manipulate the diet. Keeping all dietary factors fixed, but one, is a demanding challenge in food and nutrition research. If real foods are used as they are normally eaten, several factors beyond the one studied (e.g., GI) will normally differ. If one specific characteristic of a meal or diet (e.g., GI) is investigated and all other factors are kept identical, this will often mean the investigation of less natural or adapted foods, which would not normally be eaten in real life. Both types of studies have a purpose, depending on whether the focus is on mechanisms or on real-life situations. However, these differences in purpose and outcome must be considered and decided upon each time before a dietary intervention study is conducted—and also be considered carefully when results from such studies are evaluated.

6.5 CONCLUSION

Results from numerous short- and long-term studies have been published, but the overall picture for GI, appetite, and body weight regulation is not clear. In some cases, low-GI diets have been proven better than high-GI diets, but lack of well-matched control diets have often muddied the picture. Furthermore, methodological problems, in general, with the GI concept could explain the lack of consistent findings. It is also possible that the impact of different GI diets differs between more- and less vulnerable individuals (e.g., subjects +/− obesity, obesity-prone, +/− impaired glucose tolerance). Last but not least, it is possible that GI and GL are indicators of a different dietary pattern and/or a different lifestyle in the investigated population and that the results are therefore confounded by these differences.

REFERENCES

1. World Health Organization. Country profiles on nutrition, physical activity and obesity in the 53 WHO European Region Member States Methodology and summary. WHO Regional Office for Europe, Copenhagen, Denmark (2013).
2. Ogden C.L., Carroll M.D., Kit B.K., and Flegal K.M. Prevalence of Childhood and Adult Obesity in the United States, 2011–2012. *JAMA* (2014):311(8):806–814. doi:10.1001/jama.2014.732.
3. Van Gaal L.F., Wauters M.A., and De Leeuw I.H. The beneficial effects of modest weight loss on cardiovascular risk factors. *Int J Obes Relat Metab Disord* (1997):21(1):5–9.
4. Mertens I.L. and Van Gaal L.F. Overweight, obesity, and blood pressure: the effects of modest weight reduction. *Obes Res* (2000):8:270–278.
5. Lau D.C.W., Douketis J.D., Morrison K.M., Hramiak I.M., Sharma A.M., and Ur E. 2006 Canadian clinical practice guidelines on the management and prevention of obesity in adults and children [summary]. *CMAJ* (2007):176:1–13.
6. Salas-Salvadó J., Rubio M.A., Barbany M., and Moreno B. SEEDO 2007 Consensus for the evaluation of overweight and obesity and the establishment of therapeutic intervention criteria. *Med Clin (Barc)* (2007):128:184–196.
7. Arrizabalaga J.J., Masmiquel L., Vidal J. et al. Overweight and obesity in adults: Recommendations and treatment algorithms. *Med Clin (Barc)* (2004):122(3):104–110.
8. National Heart, Lung and Blood Institute. The practical guide. Identification, Evaluation, and Treatment of Overweight and Obesity in Adults. National Institutes of Health, Bethesda, MD (2000).
9. Seagle H.M., Strain G.W., Makris A., and Reeves R.S. Position of the American Dietetic Association: weight management. *J Am Diet Assoc* (2009):109:330–346.
10. Tsigos C., Hainer V., Basdevant A. et al. Management of obesity in adults: European clinical practice guidelines. *Obes Facts* (2008):1:106–116.
11. World Health Organization. The challenge of obesity in the WHO European Region and the strategies for response: WHO Library Cataloguing-in-Publication (2007).

12. Prewitt T.E., Schmeisser D., Bowen P.E. et al. Changes in body weight, body composition, and energy intake in women fed high- and low-fat diets, *Am J Clin Nutr* (1991):54:304–310.
13. Bray G.A. and Popkin B.M. Dietary fat intake does affect obesity! *Am J Clin Nutr* (1998): 68:1157–1173.
14. Yu-Poth S., Zhao G., Etherton T., Naglak M., Jonnalagadda S., and Kris-Etherton P.M., Effects of the National Cholesterol Education Program's Step I and Step II dietary intervention programs on cardiovascular disease risk factors: a meta-analysis, *Am J Clin Nutr* (1999):69:581–582.
15. Astrup A., Grunwald G.K., Melanseon E.L., Saris W.H., and Hill J.O. The role of low-fat diets in body weight control: a meta-analysis of *ad libitum* dietary intervention studies, *Int J Obes Relat Metab Disord* (2000):24:1545–1552.
16. Hooper L., Abdelhamid A., Moore H.J., Douthwaite W., Skeaff M., and Summerbell C.D. Effect of reducing total fat intake on body weight: systematic review and meta-analysis of randomized controlled trials and cohort studies. *BMJ* (2012):345:e7666. doi: 10.1136/bmj.e7666.
17. Skov A.R.,Toubro S., Rønn B., Holm L., and Astrup A. Randomized trial on protein vs carbohydrate in ad libitum fat reduced diet for the treatment of obesity. *Int J Obesity* (1999):23:528–536.
18. Leidy H.J., Clifton P.M., Astrup A. et al. The role of protein in weight loss and maintenance. *Am J Clin Nutr* (2015). doi: 10.3945/ajcn.114.084038.
19. Hession M., Rolland C., Kulkarni U., Wise A., and Broom J. Systematic review of randomized controlled trials of low-carbohydrate vs. low-fat/low-calorie diets in the management of obesity and its comorbidities. *Obes Rev* (2009):10:36–50.
20. Levine M.J., Jones J.M., and Lineback D.R. Low-carbohydrate diets: Assessing the science and knowledge gaps, summary of an ILSI North America Workshop. *J Am Diet Assoc* (2006):106:2086–2094.
21. Bravata D.M., Sanders L., and Huang J. Efficacy and safety of low-carbohydrate diets: A systematic review. *JAMA* (2003):289:1837–1850.
22. Roberts S.B. High-glycemic index foods, hunger, and obesity: Is there a connection? *Nutr Rev* (2000):58:163–169.
23. Ludwig D.S. Dietary glycemic index and obesity. *J Nutr* (2000):130: 280–283.
24. Raben A. Should obese patients be counselled to follow low-glycemic index diet. No. *Obes Rev* (2002):3:245–256.
25. Tagliabue A., Christensen N.J., Madsen J., Holst J.J., and Astrup A. Resistant starch: The effect on postprandial glycemia, hormonal response and satiety, *Am J Clin Nutr* (1994):60:544–551.
26. Raben A. Glycemic index and metabolic risks – how strong is the evidence? Editorial. *Am J Clin Nutr* (2014):100(1):1–3.
27. Stubbs J., Raben A., and Westerterp-Plantenga M.S. Macronutrient metabolism and appetite. In Westerterp-Plantenga M.S., Steffens A.B., and Tremblay A. (eds.) *Regulation of Food Intake and Energy Expenditure* (1999), Edra, Milano, pp. 59–85.
28. Raben A., Agerholm-Larsen L., Flint A., Holst J.J., and Astrup A. Meals with similar energy densities but rich in protein, fat, carbohydrate, or alcohol have different effects on energy expenditure and substrate metabolism but not on appetite and energy intake. *Am J Clin Nutr* (2003):77:91–100.
29. Prentice A.M. and Jebb S.A., Fast foods, energy density and obesity: A possible mechanistic link. *Obes Rev* (2003):4:187–194.
30. Niwano Y., Adachi T., and Kashimura J. Is glycemic index of food a feasible predictor of appetite, hunger, and satiety? *J Nutr Sci Vitamonil* (2009):55:201–207.
31. Bornet F.R.J., Jardy-Gennetier A.E., Jacquet N., and Stowell J. Glycaemic response to food: impact on satiety and long-term weight regulation. *Appetite* (2007):49(3):535–553.
32. Anderson G.H., Catherine N.L., and Woodend D.M. Inverse association between the effect of carbohydrates on blood glucose and subsequent short-term food intake in young men. *Am J Clin Nutr* (2002):76:1023–1030.
33. Holt S.H., Miller J.C., Petrcz P., and Farmakalidis E. A satiety index of common foods. *Eur J Clin Nutr* (1995):49(9):675–690.
34. Erdmann J., Hebeisen Y., Lippl F., Wagenpfeil S., and Schusdziarra V. Food intake and plasma ghrelin response during potato-, rice- and pasta-rich test meals. *Eur J Nutr* (2007):46(4):196–203.
35. Leeman M., Ostman E., and Bjorck I. Glycaemic and satiating properties of potato products. *Eur J Clin Nutr* (2008):62(1):87–95.
36. Geliebter A., I.-Ching Lee M., Abdillahi M. and Jones J. Satiety following intake of potatoes and other carbohydrate test meals. *Ann Nutr Metab* (2013):62:37–43.
37. Kaplan R.J. and Greenwood C.E. Influence of dietary carbohydrates and glycaemic response on subjective appetite and food intake in healthy elderly persons. *Int J Food Sci Nutr* (2002):53(4):305–316.

38. Flint A., Møller B.K., Raben A. et al. Glycemic and inculinemic responses as determinants of appetite in humans. *Am J Clin Nutr* (2006):84:1365–1373.
39. Flint A., Gregersen N.T., Gluud L.L. et al. Associations between postprandial insulin and blood glucose responses, appetite sensations and energy intake in normal weight and overweight individuals: A meta-analysis of meal-test studies. *Br J Nutr* (2007):98:17–25.
40. Reynolds R.C., Stockmann K.S., Atkinson F.S., Denyer G.S., and Brand-Miller J.C. Effect of the glycemic index of carbohydrates on day-log (10 h) profiles of plasma glucose, insulin, cholecystokinin and ghrelin. *Eur J Clin Nutr* (2009):63:872–878.
41. Alfenas R.C. and Mattes R.D. Influence of glycemic index/load on glycemic response, appetite, and food intake in healthy humans. *Diabetes Care* (2005):28:2123–2129.
42. Aston L.M., Stokes C.S., and Jebb S.A. No effect of a diet with a reduced glyceamic index on satiety, energy intake and body weight in overweight and obese women. *Int J Obes* (2008):32:160–165.
43. Makris A.P., Borradaile K.E., Oliver T.L. et al. The individual and combined effects of glycemic index and protein on glycemic response, hunger, and energy intake. *Obesity* (2011):19:2365–2373.
44. Kristensen, M., Jensen, M.G., Riboldi G. et al. Wholegrain vs. refined wheat bread and pasta. Effect on postprandial glycemia, appetite and subsequent ad libitum energy intake in young healthy adults. *Appetite* (2010):54:163–169.
45. Burton-Freeman, B.M. and Keim, N.L. Glycemic index, cholecystokinin, satiety and disinhibition: Is there an unappreciated paradox for overweight women? *Int J Obes* (2008):32:1647–1654.
46. Tappy L., Randin J., Felber J. et al. Comparison of thermogenic effect of fructose and glucose in normal humans. *Am. J. Physiol* (1986):13:717–724.
47. Blaak E.E. and Saris W.H.M. Health aspects of various digestible carbohydrates. *Nutr Res* (1995):15:1547–1573.
48. Raben A., Kiens B., and Richter E.A. Differences in glycaemia, hormonal response and energy expenditure after a meal rich in mono- and disaccharides compared to a meal rich in polysaccharides in physically fit and sedentary subjects. *Clin Phys* (1994):14:267–280.
49. Diaz E.O., Galgani J.E., Aguirre C.A., Atwater I.J., and Burrows R. Effect of glycemic index on whole-body substrate oxidation in obese women. *Int J Obes* (2005):29:108–114.
50. Díaz E.O., Galgani J.E., Aguirre C.A. Glycaemic index effects on fuel partitioning in humans Review. *Obes Rev* (2006):7:219–226.
51. Krog-Mikkelsen I., Sloth B., Dimitrov D. et al. A low glycemic index diet does not affect postprandial energy metabolism but decreases postprandial insulinemia and increases fullness rating in healthy women. *J Nutr* (2011):141:1679–1684.
52. Vasilaras T., Raben A., and Astrup A. Twenty-four hour energy expenditure and substrate oxidation before and after 6 months' *ad libitum* intake of a diet rich in simple or complex carbohydrates or a habitual diet. *Int J Obes* (2001):25:954–965.
53. Flint A., Møller B.K., Raben A., Pedersen D., Tetens I., Holst J.J., and Astrup A. The use of glycaemic index tables to predict glycaemic index of composite breakfast meals. *Br J Nutr* (2004):91:979–989.
54. Ma Y., Olendzki B., Chiriboga D. et al. Association between dietary carbohydrates and body weight. *Am J Epidemiol* (2005):161:359–67.
55. Mendez M.A., Covas M.I., Marrugat J., Vila J., and Schroder H. Glycemic load, glycemic index, and body mass index in Spanish adults. *Am J Clin Nutr* (2009):89:316–22.
56. Culberson A., Kafai M.R., and Ganji V. Glycemic load is associated with HDL cholesterol but not with the other components and prevalence of metabolic syndrome in the third National Health and Nutrition Examination Survey, 1988 - 1994. *Int Arch Med* (2009):2:3.
57. Du H., van der A.D.L., van Bakel M.M.E. et al. Dietary glycaemic index, glycaemic load and subsequent changes of weight and waist circumference in European men and women. *Int J Obes* (2009):33:1280–1288.
58. Finley C.E., Barlow C.E., Halton T.L., and Haskell W.L. Glycemic index, glycemic load, and prevalence of the metabolic syndrome in the Cooper center longitudinal study. *J Am Diet Assoc* (2010):110:1820–9.
59. Rossi M., Bosetti C., Talamini R. et al. Glycemic index and glycemic load in relation to body mass index and waist to hip ratio. *Eur J Nutr* (2010):49:459–464.
60. Youn S., Woo H.D., Cho Y.A., Shin A., Chang N., and Kim J. Association between dietary carbohydrate, glycemic index, glycemic load, and the prevalence of obesity in Korean men and women. *Nutr Res* (2012):32:153–159.
61. Murakami K., McCaffrey T.A., and Livingstone M.B.E. Associations of dietary glycaemic index and glycaemic load with food and nutrient intake and general and central obesity in British adults. *Br J Nutr* (2013):110:2047–57.

62. Song S., Lee J., Song W.O., Paik H.Y., and Song Y. Carbohydrate intake and refined-grain consumption are associated with metabolic syndrome in the Korean adult population. *J Acad Nutr Diet* (2013):114:1:54–62.
63. Goto M., Morita A., Goto A. et al. Dietary glycemic index and glycemic load in relation to HbA1c in Japanese obese adults: a cross-sectional analysis of the Saku Control Obesity Program. *Nutr Metab* (2012):9:79.
64. Hosseinpour-Niazi S., Sohrab G., Asghari G., Mirmiran P., Moslehi N., and Azizi F. Dietary glycemic index, glycemic load, and cardiovascular disease risk factors: Tehran Lipid and Glucose Study. *Arch Iran Med* (2013):16:401–407.
65. Murakami K., Sasaki S., Okubo H., Takahashi Y., Hosoi Y., and Itabashi M. Dietary fiber intake, dietary glycemic index and load, and body mass index: a cross-sectional study of 3931 Japanese women aged 18–20 years. *Eur J Clin Nutr* (2007):61:986–995.
66. Smith J.D., Hou T., Ludwig D.S. et al. Changes in intake of protein foods, carbohydrate amount and quality, and long-term weight change: Results from 3 prospective cohorts. *Am J Clin Nutr* (2015):101(6):1216–1224.
67. Murakami K., Miyake Y., Sasaki S., Tanaka K., and Arakawa M. Dietary glycemic index and glycemic load in relation to risk of overweight in Japanese children and adolescents: The Ryukyus Child Health Study. *Int J Obes* (2011):35:925–936.
68. Hare-Bruun H., Flint A., and Heitmann B.L. Glycemic index and glycemic load in relation to changes in body weight, body fat distribution, and body composition in adult Danes. *Am J Clin Nutr* (2006):84:871–879.
69. Smith J.D., Hou T., Ludwig D.S. et al. Changes in intake of protein foods, carbohydrate amount and quality, and long-term weight change: results from 3 prospective cohorts. *Am J Clin Nutr* (2015):101(6):1216–1224. doi: 10.3945/ajcn.114.100867.
70. Finley C.E., Barlow C.E., Halton T.L. and Haskell W.L. Glycemic index, glycemic load, and prevalence of the metabolic syndrome in the cooper center longitudinal study. *J Am Diet Assoc.* (2010):110:1820–9.
71. Esfahani A., Wong J.M., Mirrahimi A., Villa C.R., and Kendall C.W. The application of the glycemic index and glycemic load in weight loss: A review of the clinical evidence. *IUBMB Life* (2011):63:7–13.
72. Thomas D.E., Elliott E.J., and Baur L. Low glycaemic index or low glycaemic load diets for overweight and obesity. *Cochrane Database Syst Rev* (2007):3:CD005105.
73. Livesey G., Taylor R., Hulshof T., and Howlett J. Glycemic response and health—a systematic review and meta-analysis: relations between dietary glycemic properties and health outcomes. *Am J Clin Nutr* (2008):87(1):258–268.
74. Abete I., Parra D., and Martinez J.A. Energy-restricted diets based on a distinct food selection affecting the glycemic index induce different weight loss and oxidative response. *Clin Nutr* (2008):27:545–551.
75. De Rougemont A., Normand S., Nazare J.A. et al. Beneficial effects of a 5-week low-glycaemic index regimen on weight control and cardiovascular risk factors in overweight non-diabetic subjects. *Br J Nutr* (2007):98:1288–1298.
76. Maki K.C., Rains T.M., Kaden V.N., Raneri K.R., and Davidson M.H. Effects of a reduced-glycemicload diet on body weight, body composition, and cardiovascular disease risk markers in overweight and obese adults. *Am J Clin Nutr* (2007):85:724–734.
77. Slabber M., Barnard H.C., Kuyl J.M., Dannhauser A., and Schall R. Effects of a low-insulinresponse, energy-restricted diet on weight loss and plasma insulin concentrations in hyperinsulinemic obese females. *Am J Clin Nutr* (1994):60:48–53.
78. Salinardi T.C., Batra P., Roberts S.B. et al. Lifestyle intervention reduces body weight and improves cardiometabolic risk factors in worksites. *Am J Clin Nutr* (2013):97(4):667–676. doi: 10.3945/ajcn.112.046995.
79. Shyam S., Arshad F., Abdul Ghani R. et al. Low glycaemic index diets improve glucose tolerance and body weight in women with previous history of gestational diabetes: a six months randomized trial. *Nutr J* (2013):12:68. doi: 10.1186/1475-2891-12-68.
80. Juanola-Falgarona M., Salas-Salvadó J., Ibarrola-Jurado N. et al. Effect of the glycemic index of the diet on weight loss, modulation of satiety, inflammation, and other metabolic risk factors: A randomized controlled trial. *Am J Clin Nutr* (2014):100(1):27–35.
81. Sichieri R., Moura A.S., Genelhu V., Hu F., and Willett W.C. An 18-mo randomized trial of a low-glycemic-index diet and weight change in Brazilian women. *Am J Clin Nutr* (2007):86:707–713.
82. Retterstol K., Hennig C.B., and Iversen P.O. Improved plasma lipids and body weight in overweight/obese patients with type III hyperlipoproteinemia after 4 weeks on a low glycemic diet. *Clin Nutr* (2009):28:213–215.

83. Pereira M.A., Swain J., Goldfine A.B., Rifai N., and Ludwig D.S. Effects of a low-glycemic load diet on resting energy expenditure and heart disease risk factors during weight loss. *JAMA* (2004):292:2482–2490.
84. Bouche C., Rizkalla S.W., Luo J. et al. Five-week, low-glycemic index diet decreases total fat mass and improves plasma lipid profile in moderately overweight nondiabetic men. *Diabetes Care* (2002):25:822–828.
85. Das S.K., Gilhooly C.H., Golden J.K. et al. Long-term effects of 2 energy-restricted diets differing in glycemic load on dietary adherence, body composition, and metabolism in CALERIE: a 1-y randomized controlled trial. *Am J Clin Nutr* (2007):85:1023–1030.
86. Ebbeling C.B., Leidig M.M., Sinclair K.B., Seger-Shippee L.G., Feldman H.A. and Ludwig D.S. Effects of an ad libitum low-glycemic load diet on cardiovascular disease risk factors in obese young adults. *Am J Clin Nutr* (2005):81:976–982.
87. Pittas A.G., Roberts S.B., Das S.K. et al. The effects of the dietary glycemic load on type 2 diabetes risk factors during weight loss. *Obesity (Silver Spring)* (2006):14:2200–2209.
88. Raatz S.K., Torkelson C.J., Redmon J.B. et al. Reduced glycemic index and glycemic load diets do not increase the effects of energy restriction on weight loss and insulin sensitivity in obese men and women. *J Nutr* (2005):135:2387–2391.
89. Sloth B., Krog-Mikkelsen I., Flint A. et al. No difference in body weight decrease between a low-glycemic-index and a high-glycemic-index diet but reduced LDL cholesterol after 10-wk ad libitum intake of the low-glycemic-index diet. *Am J Clin Nutr* (2004):80:337–347.
90. Lagerpusch M., Enderle J., Eggeling B. et al. Carbohydrate quality and quantity affect glucose and lipid metabolism during weight regain in healthy men. *J Nutr* 2013:143:1593–1601.
91. Goss A.M., Goree L.L., Ellis A.C. et al. Effects of diet macronutrient composition on body composition and fat distribution during weight maintenance and weight loss. *Obesity (Silver Spring)* (2013):21:1139–1142.
92. Buscemi S., Cosentino L., Rosafio G. et al. Effects of hypocaloric diets with different glycemic indexes on endothelial function and glycemic variability in overweight and in obese adult patients at increased cardiovascular risk. *Clin Nutr* (2013):32:346–352.
93. Bellisle F., Dalix A.M., De Assis M.A. et al. Motivational effects of 12-week moderately restrictive diets with or without special attention to the Glycaemic Index of foods. *Br J Nutr* (2007):97(4):790–798.
94. McMillan-Price J., Petocz P., Atkinson F. et al. Comparison of 4 diets of varying glycemic load on weight loss and cardiovascular risk reduction in overweight and obese young adults: A randomized controlled trial. *Arch Intern Med* (2006):166:1466–1475.
95. Thompson W.G., Rostad Holdman N., Janzow D.J., Slezak J.M., Morris K.L. and Zemel M.B. Effect of energy-reduced diets high in dairy products and fiber on weight loss in obese adults. *Obes Res* (2005):13:1344–1353.
96. Melanson K.J., Summers A., Nguyen V. et al. Body composition, dietary composition, and components of metabolic syndrome in overweight and obese adults after a 12-week trial on dietary treatments focused on portion control, energy density, or glycemic index. *Nutr J* (2012):11:57.
97. Randolph J.M., Edirisinghe I., Masoni A.M., Kappagoda T., and Burton-Freeman B. Potatoes, glycemic index, and weight loss in free-living individuals: practical implications. *J Am Coll Nutr* (2014):33(5):375–384.
98. Liu S and Willett W.C. Dietary glycemic load and atherothrombotic risk. *Curr Atheroscler Rep* (2002):6:454–461.
99. Halton T.L, Willett W.C., Liu S., Manson J.E., Stampfer M.J., and Hu F.B. Potato and french fry consumption and risk of type 2 diabetes in women. *Am J Clin Nutr* (2006);83(2):284–290.
100. Saris W.H.M., Astrup A., Prentice A.M. et al. Randomized controlled trial of changes in dietary carbohydrate/fat ratio and simple vs. complex carbohydrates on body weight and blood lipids: The CARMEN study. *Int J Obes* (2000):24:1310–1318.
101. Legenbauer T.M., de Zwaan M., Mühlhans B., Petrak F., and Herpertz S. Do mental disorders and eating patterns affect long-term weight loss maintenance? *Gen Hosp Psychiatry* (2010):32(2):132–140.
102. LeCheminant J.D., Jacobsen D.J., Hall M.A., and Donnelly J.E, J. A comparison of meal replacements and medication in weight maintenance after weight loss. *Am Coll Nutr* (2005):24(5):347–353.
103. Kraschnewski J.L., Boan J., Esposito J. et al. Long-term weight loss maintenance in the United States. *Int J Obes* (2010):34(11):1644–1654.
104. Montesi L., El Ghoch M., Brodosi L., Calugi S., Marchesini G., and Dalle Grave R. Long-term weight loss maintenance for obesity: a multidisciplinary approach. *Diabetes Metab Syndr Obes* (2016):9:37–46.
105. Leibel R.L., Rosenbaum M., and Hirsch J. Changes in energy expenditure resulting from altered body weight. *N Engl J Med* (1995):332(10):621–628.

106. Sumithran P., Prendergast L.A., Delbridge E. et al. Long-term persistence of hormonal adaptations to weight loss. *N Engl J Med* (2011):365(17):1597–1604.
107. Sloth B., Due A., Larsen T.M., Holst J.J., Heding A., and Astrup A. The effect of a high-MUFA, low-glycaemic index diet and a low-fat diet on appetite and glucose metabolism during a 6-month weight maintenance period. *Br J Nutr* (2009):101(12):1846–1858.
108. Ebbeling C.B., Swain J.F., Feldman H.A. et al. Effects of dietary composition on energy expenditure during weight-loss maintenance. *JAMA* (2012):307(24):2627–2634.
109. Philippou E., Neary N.M., Chaudhri O. et al. The effect of dietary glycemic index on weight maintenance in overweight subjects: a pilot study. *Obesity (Silver Spring)* (2009):17(2):396–401.
110. Larsen T.M., Dalskov S.-M., van Baak M. et al. Diets with high or low protein content and glycemic index for weight-loss maintenance. *N Engl J Med* (2010):363(22):2102–2113.
111. Goyenechea E., Holst C., Saris W.H. et al. On behalf of DIOGenes. Effects of different protein content and glycemic index of ad libitum diets on diabetes risk factors in overweight adults: The DIOGenes multicentre, randomised, dietary intervention trial. *Diabetes Metab Res Rev* (2011):705–716. doi: 10.1002/dmrr.1218.
112. Aller E.E., Larsen T.M., Claus H. et al. Weight loss maintenance in overweight subjects on ad libitum diets with high or low protein content and glycemic index: the DIOGENES trial 12-month results. *Int J Obes* (2014):(12):1511–1517.
113. Raben A., Fogelholm M., Feskens E., Westerterp-Plantenga M., Schlicht W. and Brand-Miller J. PREVIEW: PREVention of diabetes through lifestyle Intervention and population studies in Europe and around the World. On behalf of the PREVIEW consortium. *Obes Facts* (2013):6(Suppl. 1):194.
114. Kong A.P., Chan R.S., Nelson E.A. and Chan J.C. Role of low-glycemic index diet in management of childhood obesity. *Obes Rev* (2011):12(7):492–498.
115. Spieth L.E., Harnish J.D., Lenders C.M. et al. A low-glycemic index diet in the treatment of pediatric obesity. *Arch Pediatr Adolesc Med* (2000):154(9):947–951.
116. Ebbeling C.B., Leidig M.M., Sinclair K.B., Hangen J.P. and Ludwig D.S. A reduced-glycemic load diet in the treatment of adolescent obesity. *Arch Pediatr Adolesc Med* (2003):157(8):773–779.
117. Fajcsak Z., Gabor A., Kovacs V., and Martos E. The effects of 6-week low glycemic load diet based on low glycemic index foods in overweight/obese children—Pilot study. *J Am Coll Nutr* (2008):27(1):12–21.
118. Armeno M.L., Krochik A.G., and Mazza C.S. Evaluation of two dietary treatments in obese hyperinsulinemic adolescents. *J Pediatr Endocrinol Metab* (2011):24(9–10):715–722.
119. Mirza N.M., Palmer M.G., Sinclair K.B. et al. Effects of a low glycemic load or a low-fat dietary intervention on body weight in obese Hispanic American children and adolescents: A randomized controlled trial. *Am J Clin Nutr* (2013):97(2):276–285.
120. Papadaki A., Linardakis M., Larsen T.M. et al. On behalf of the DiOGenes Study Group. The effect of protein and glycemic index on children's body composition: the DiOGenes randomized study. *Pediatrics* (2010):126(5):e1143–52.
121. Goran, M.I., Beer, W.H., Wolfe, R.R., Poehlman, E.T., and Young, V.R., Variation in total energy expenditure in young healthy free-living men, *Metabolism* (1993):42:487–496.
122. Prentice, A.M., Black, A.E., Coward, W.A. et al. High levels of energy expenditure in obese women, *Br Med J* (1986):292:983–987.
123. Ravussin, E. and Swinburn, B.A. Pathophysiology of obesity, *Lancet* (1992):340:404–408.
124. Lissner L. Measuring food intake in studies of obesity. *Public Health Nutr* (2002):5(6A):889–892.
125. Niedhammer I., Bugel I., Bonenfant S., Goldberg M., and Leclerc A. Validity of self-reported weight and height in the French GAXEL cohort. *Int J Obes Relat Metab Disord* (2000):24:1111–1118.
126. Roberts R.J. Can self-reported data accurately describe the prevalence of overweight? *J Public Health* (1995):109:275–284.
127. Bendixen H., Holst C., Sørensen T.I.A., Raben A., Bartels E.M., and Astrup A. Major increase in prevalence of overweight and obesity between 1987 and 2001 among Danish adults. *Obes Res* (2004):12:1464–1472.

7 Glycemic Index, Glycemic Load, and Cancer Prevention

Livia S.A. Augustin, Laura Chiavaroli, Stephanie Nishi, Arash Mirrahimi, Cyril W.C. Kendall, and David J.A. Jenkins

CONTENTS

7.1 INTRODUCTION

7.1.1 Background

Cancer is a leading cause of death, accounting for 8.2 million deaths globally in 2012 (Stewart and Wild 2014). Migration studies observed a 20-fold variation in cancer rates across geographical regions, suggesting that environmental causes are central to the etiology of cancer (King et al. 1985, Ziegler et al. 1993, Rastogi et al. 2008). Indeed, approximately one third of cancer deaths are due to the five leading behavioral and dietary risk factors: high body mass index (BMI), low fruit and vegetable intake, lack of physical activity, tobacco use, and alcohol use (Stewart and Wild 2014). It has been estimated that approximately 35% of cancer deaths could be avoided by dietary modifications alone (Doll and Peto 1981, Willett 1995, McCullough and Giovannucci 2004). Dietary factors associated with Western lifestyles, such as high intakes of refined carbohydrates, saturated fat, red meat, and excess energy, are linked to increased cancer rates and cancer mortality (Willett 1995, Santarelli et al. 2008, Kushi et al. 2012, Pan et al. 2012). Among dietary compounds, carbohydrates have been implicated in the etiology of cancer at various sites (Giovannucci 1995, Franceschi et al. 1997, Augustin et al. 2002). Specifically, it has been proposed that the extent of the rise in blood glucose produced by carbohydrates and captured by the glycemic index (GI) may play a differential role in cancer development (Augustin et al. 2002). The GI is a ranking of carbohydrate foods based on their ability to raise blood glucose concentration (Jenkins et al. 1981), and the glycemic load (GL) is the mathematical multiplication of the GI of a food by its available carbohydrate content (without fiber) (Salmeron et al. 1997b). Generally, the slower the rate of carbohydrate absorption, the lower the rise of blood glucose and insulin and the lower the GI value. Compared with low-GI foods, high-GI foods result in larger rises in blood glucose and insulin for the same amount of carbohydrate ingested (Jenkins et al. 1981), resulting in a further metabolic challenge, particularly in the presence of metabolic conditions such as impaired glucose tolerance (Hanefeld et al. 2003). Consuming high- compared with low-GI diets have been shown to increase the risk of developing type 2 diabetes (T2DM) (Salmeron et al. 1997a, 1997b, Barclay et al. 2008, Livesey et al. 2013), cardiovascular disease (CVD) (Liu et al. 2000, Kushi et al. 2012, Mirrahimi et al. 2012), CVD risk factors (Frost et al. 1999, Liu et al. 2001, 2002), and cancer (Augustin et al. 2001, Franceschi et al. 2001, Barclay et al. 2008, Turati et al. 2015a). Hyperglycemia and hyperinsulinemia have been involved in carcinogenesis, and several conditions linked to the disruption of glucose metabolism, including diabetes, obesity, hyperglycemia, hyperinsulinemia, and insulin resistance, may have relevant roles in cancer development (Kaaks and Lukanova 2001, Stocks et al. 2009, Campbell et al. 2012, Bosetti et al. 2012b, Boyle et al. 2013).

7.1.2 Diet and Cancer

Cancer is a degenerative disease that develops over many years in stages: initiation, promotion, and progression. The initiation phase is characterized by an acute damage to the genome. When this damage escapes the endogenous and environmental protective mechanisms, DNA adducts accumulate, and over time, a neoplasm may form. Free radicals generated from dietary metabolic processes generate DNA damage and produce genetic mutations (Ames and Gold 1991). Of all the environmental mechanisms, diet has been proposed to be a large contributor. In 1914, Peyton Rous first observed that food restriction in mice reduced tumor metastasis (Rous 1914), whereas in the 1920s, obesity was found to be associated with greater cancer mortality, and in the 1930s, high consumption of plant food was suggested to be protective in cancer development (Stocks et al. 2009). In 1981, Doll and Peto (1981) attempted to quantify the cancer risk attributable to various environmental causes and estimated that approximately 35% of cancer deaths could be avoided by dietary modifications alone. This seems to hold true even today (Willett 1995, McCullough and Giovannucci 2004). High-fat and high-calorie diets, as well as high consumption of red meat, are linked to increased cancer risk, whereas high vegetable and fruit intake, particularly citrus fruit and vegetables from the Brassica family, are consistently found to be protective against cancer development (Willett 1995, Santarelli et al. 2008, Bosetti et al. 2012a, Kushi et al. 2012, Pan et al. 2012, Turati et al. 2015b). Clinical trials of diet in cancer patients, such as the Women's Intervention Nutrition Study (Chlebowski et al. 2006), found that a low-fat diet reduced breast cancer recurrence by 24%, whereas the combination of low-fat and high-fruit and -vegetable diets in the Women's Healthy Eating and Living trial (Pierce et al. 2007) did not show benefits in breast cancer recurrence or survival after more than 7 years' intervention. The latter result may be partly explained by the recruitment methodology, which included diagnosis within the previous 4 years (Pierce et al. 2007). It is possible that such a diet may be found to be protective if consumed earlier, possibly within 1 year of first cancer diagnosis, as in the Women's Intervention Nutrition Study (Chlebowski et al. 2006).

7.1.3 Glycemia and Cancer

A link between hyperglycemia and cancer had been suspected since the 1800s, and until the 1920s, glycosuria was used as a marker in cancer screening (Freund 1885, Trinkler 1890, Boas 1903, Marble 1934, Ellinger and Landsman 1944). McKeown-Eyssen (1994) and Giovannucci (1995) independently suggested that blood glucose and insulin might be important factors for promoting malignant transformation and tumor growth. Indeed, T2DM, a condition resulting from long-term exposure to high glucose and insulin concentrations, significantly increases cancer risk (Giovannucci et al. 2010, Noto et al. 2013). Furthermore, T2DM increases mortality in cancer patients and reduces disease-free survival compared with those without T2DM (Liu et al. 2012, Ma et al. 2014). In addition, glycated hemoglobin (HbA1c) at diabetes and prediabetes levels has been associated with greater cancer incidence (de Beer and Liebenberg 2014) and mortality, albeit only in women (Joshu et al. 2012). In this study, among women with diabetes, those with good glycemic control (HbA1c $\leq$ 7%) had a 52% lower risk of cancer death than those with poor glycemic control (HbA1c > 7%) (Joshu et al. 2012). Furthermore, hyperglycemia, both fasting and postprandial, and even at concentrations below the diabetes threshold, has been associated with a higher risk of cancer incidence and death, independent of body weight (Jee et al. 2005, Stattin et al. 2007, Stocks et al. 2009) and cancer site (Crawley et al. 2014). A meta-analysis showed that blood glucose concentration greater than 110 mg/dL (6.11 mmol/L), the concentration defined by the World Health Organization as a cut-off for high fasting glucose (impaired glucose tolerance), increased the risk of all cancers by 32% compared with glycemic concentrations less than 110 mg/dL (6.11 mmol/L) (Crawley et al. 2014). These results are supported by those from a 10-year prospective cohort study, in which fasting blood glucose concentration of 140 mg/dL or greater ($\geq$7.8 mmol/L) was associated with significantly higher (23%–29%) death rates from major cancer sites, including colorectum, liver, and pancreas, compared with blood glucose concentration less than 90 mg/dL (<5.0 mmol/L) (Jee et al. 2005). Furthermore, hyperglycemia can enhance cancer progression and promotion (Li et al. 2015), and in a dose–response meta-analysis, it was shown that every 10 mg/dL (0.56 mmol/L) increase in blood glucose concentration corresponded to a 15% increased risk of pancreatic cancer (Liao et al. 2015). On the other hand, reducing hyperglycemia by dietary means (e.g., switching from a high- to a low-GI diet) (Augustin et al. 2001, Barclay et al. 2008, Turati et al. 2015a) or pharmacologically by the use of antihyperglycemic medications (e.g., metformin and acarbose) (Noto et al. 2012, Tseng et al. 2015) has shown benefits in reducing the risk of major cancers.

It is of interest that most cancer cells exhibit increased glucose uptake compared with normal tissue cells (Gillies et al. 2008), and this forms the basis for utilizing 18F-fluorodeoxyglucose-positron emission tomography scans in cancer detection and investigations. In cancer cells, glucose is utilized to produce energy and to build blocks for cellular mitosis. As in nonneoplastic cells, in cancer cells also, energy is produced in the form of ATP. However, in cancer cells, the conversion of glucose into ATP follows a fermentative glycolytic pathway (cellular anaerobic respiration) even in the presence of oxygen, which generates only two ATP molecules. Hence, glucose use in cancer cells is less efficient than that in oxidative phosphorylation (cellular aerobic respiration), which generates 36 ATP molecules, typically seen in nonneoplastic cells of differentiated normal tissue. This phenomenon was termed the Warburg effect by Otto Warburg, who, in 1924, made the initial observations in cancer cells (Warburg 1956). Although the anaerobic glycolytic pathway produces 18-fold less ATPs than aerobic oxidative phosphorylation, it allows the generation of the building blocks (ribose for nucleotide formation, acetyl-CoA for fatty acid production, etc.) necessary for cell proliferation. This fermentative glycolytic pathway also leads to a more acidic environment, which may provide a competing survival and metastatic advantage to cancer cells (e.g., greater spreading capacity), than normal cells, which are unable to survive below a pH of 7.2 (Fais et al. 2014). Indeed, emerging evidence suggests a potential role of antacids in the treatment of cancer cells (Robey et al. 2009, Udelnow et al. 2011). Overall, the Warburg effect may explain why cancer cells are heavy consumers of glucose. The lower amount of ATP molecules produced by cancer cells is indeed sufficient to sustain the energy requirements of the proliferating cells, as long as there is a continuous supply of glucose from the circulation. This process is halted or reduced by starvation (Dunn et al. 1997, Kritchevsky 2003), whereas it may be enhanced in conditions characterized by excess energy exposure (e.g., obesity) or by long-term hyperglycemia (e.g., T2DM). Indeed, both T2DM and obesity increase the risk of cancer development (Kushi et al. 2012, Noto et al. 2013), and antihyperglycemic medications have been shown to reduce cancer risk in people with T2DM (Noto et al. 2012).

7.2 GLYCEMIC INDEX AND CANCER RISK

7.2.1 Background

Several lines of evidence suggest a differential impact of carbohydrates in cancer development, and hence, it was proposed that the nature of the carbohydrates consumed (e.g., the GI) may play a role in carcinogenesis (Augustin et al. 2002). Initially, a difference in cancer risk was noticed with two carbohydrate foods at the opposite end of the GI spectrum—pasta, a low-GI food, and white bread, a high-GI food. These results were confirmed in a later publication of the same dataset, and it was demonstrated that white bread increased the risk of breast and colorectal cancers, whereas pasta was not associated with the risk (Augustin et al. 2013). Indeed, the hypothesis that high-GI foods increased cancer risk more than low-GI foods was tested in case-control studies, and the results suggested a protective role of low-GI foods in the risk of colorectal and breast cancers, with risk reductions ranging from 30% to 80% (Augustin et al. 2001, Franceschi et al. 2001). A recent systematic review and meta-analysis has found that since these initial observations, 79 more studies have been conducted that assessed the association between dietary GI and the risk of cancer at several sites and 81 studies have been conducted that assessed dietary GL (Turati et al. 2015a), which included all epidemiological studies (cohort and case-controls). Overall, Turati et al. (2015a) demonstrated a direct but modest association between dietary GI and GL, which reached significance mainly in colorectal cancer and approached significance in breast cancer. Considering that these latter two neoplasms have a high incidence worldwide, the results of this comprehensive meta-analysis are of significance at the population level. After the meta-analysis by Turati et al. (2015a) two new epidemiological studies have been published on the associations between GI/GL and breast cancer risk: one in Mexican women and one in young premenopausal women in the United States, and both found no significant associations (Amadou et al. 2015, Farvid et al. 2015). As cancer is a general term for a group of more than 100 diseases, specific types of cancers and their association with dietary GI/GL with regard to prevention and management, where evidence is available, will be discussed in the following sections.

7.2.2 Breast Cancer

7.2.2.1 Breast Cancer Background

Breast cancer has one of the five highest cancer incidences and is the second leading cause of cancer mortality in women (World Health Organization 2015b). In part due to the observed increased risk of breast cancer among women with T2DM (Larsson et al. 2007b), there is growing recognition that breast cancer may be promoted by insulin resistance and hyperinsulemia (Frasca et al. 2008). Hence, the role of the GI and GL in breast cancer risk is of interest and has been extensively studied.

7.2.2.2 Glycemic Index, Glycemic Load, and Breast Cancer Prevention

Multiple systematic reviews and meta-analyses discussing GI/GL and breast cancer have been published in the last decade (Barclay et al. 2008, Gnagnarella et al. 2008, Mulholland et al. 2008a, Dong and Qin 2011). A number of studies were subsequently published on this topic, and their results have been considered in more recent systematic reviews and meta-analyses. The meta-analysis of prospective cohort studies by Mullie et al. (2015) involved 20,973 breast cancer cases and 773,971 cohort members and showed that compared with women consuming low-GI/GL dietary patterns, women with high-GI/GL dietary patterns had a small 5%–6% increase in breast cancer risk. Specifically, Mullie et al. (2015) demonstrated that a dietary pattern with a high GI was associated with a relative risk (RR) of 1.05 (95% confidence interval [CI]: 1.00, 1.11), and a high GL was associated with an RR of 1.06 (95% CI: 1.00, 1.13). In the same year, another systematic review and meta-analysis conducted by Turati et al. (2015a) assessed both cohort and case-control studies. Eligible studies presented wide-ranging median GI intakes from 27 to 81 in the lowest-GI categories and from greater than 57 to 100 in the highest-GI categories, and daily GL intakes ranged from 44 to 172 in the lowest-GL category and from 133.7 and above in the highest-GL category (Turati et al. 2015a). The summary RR in relation to breast cancer for the highest versus the lowest category of GI was 1.05 (95% CI: 0.99, 1.11; $p = .0003$) and for the highest versus the lowest category of GL was 1.07 (95% CI: 0.98, 1.16; $p < .001$) (Figures 7.1 and 7.2).

Subgroup analyses indicated that the RRs were higher for cohort than for case-control studies: 1.03 (95% CI: 0.82, 1.31) and 1.05 (95% CI: 1.01, 1.09) for the highest versus the lowest category of GI of the seven case-control studies and the 12 included cohort studies, respectively (Turati et al. 2015a). GL did not show differences, depending on study design. The values for GL were 1.19 (95% CI: 0.87, 1.65) and 1.03 (95% CI: 0.96, 1.10) for 6 case-control studies and 12 cohort studies, respectively (Turati et al. 2015a).

Many studies and meta-analyses have taken menopausal status into consideration. Menopause is related to increasing age, adiposity, and hormonal changes, which have been associated with increased breast cancer risk (American Cancer Society 2015a). Turati et al. (2015a) identified 12 observational studies on a premenopausal population and 14 observational studies on a postmenopausal population, investigating the association between breast cancer risk with GI and GL. For GI, subgroup analysis by menopausal status showed that the RR of the highest (vs. lowest) GI category was 1.09 (95% CI: 0.95, 1.40) and 1.04 (95% CI: 0.96, 1.13) in the premenopausal

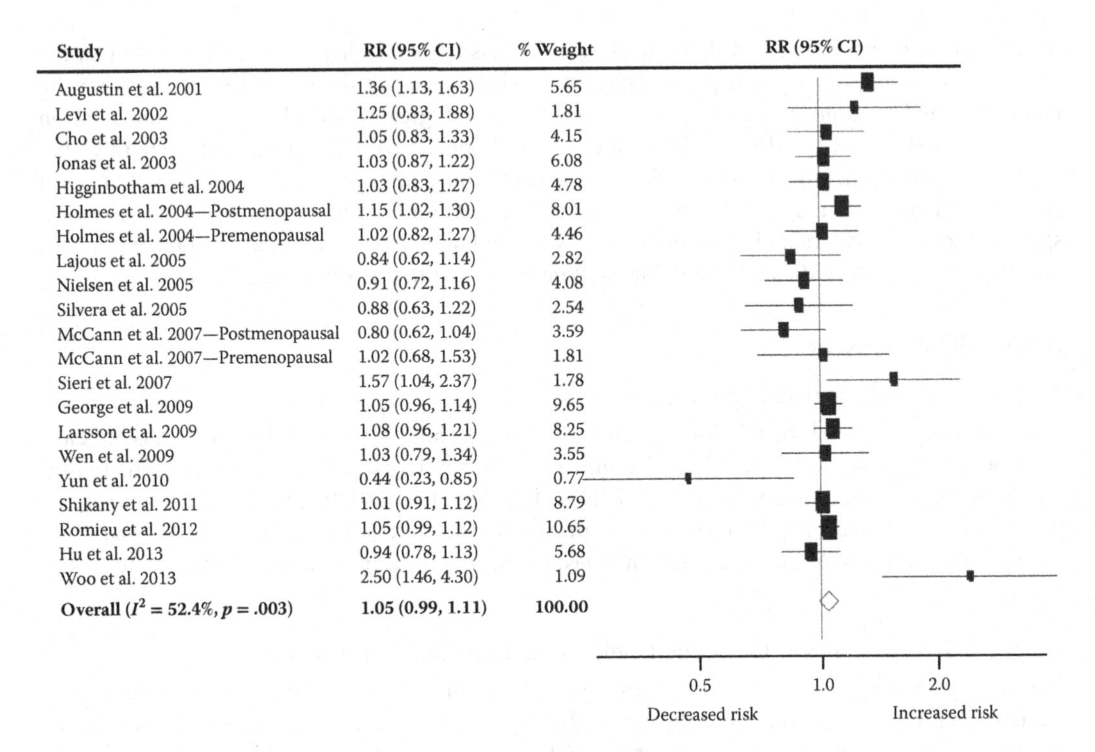

FIGURE 7.1 Meta-analysis of prospective cohort and case-control studies investigating the association between GI and risk of breast cancer. The pooled effect estimate is represented as a diamond. The p-value is for a random-effects model. All data are presented as RRs with 95% confidence intervals. GI, glycemic index; RR, relative risk. (Adapted from Turati, F. et al., *Mol. Nutr. Food Res.*, 59, 1384–1394, 2015a. With permission.)

and postmenopausal subgroups, respectively. For GL, these values were 1.18 (95% CI: 1.00, 1.39) and 1.07 (95% CI: 0.95, 1.20) in the premenopausal and postmenopausal subgroups, respectively (Turati et al. 2015a). Neither subgroup analysis demonstrated a significant effect modification by menopausal status; however, the effect within the premenopausal subgroup for GL was marginally significant for an increased risk in the highest-GL category. Further exploration is warranted to address whether there is a difference within these menopausal subgroups.

Body mass index has been implicated in breast cancer risk (American Cancer Society 2015a); however, subgroup analyses by GI or GL categories in the study by Turati et al. (2015a) did not show any modifying effect of BMI in the associations between GI or GL and breast cancer risk (for GI, RR = 1.16; 95% CI: 0.95, 1.40 for BMIs < 25 kg/m^2 and RR = 0.99; 95% CI: 0.87, 1.13 for BMI ≥ 25 kg/m^2; for GL, RR = 1.14; 95% CI: 0.92, 1.42 for BMIs < 25 kg/m^2 and RR = 0.99; 95% CI: 0.83, 1.18 for BMI ≥ 25 kg/m^2).

Some limitations of these studies that may account for the inconsistent findings include the method of dietary GI and/or GL assessment and residual confounding factors. The majority of studies used food frequency questionnaires to analyze dietary GI and GL, which were not originally designed to assess these dietary traits. In order to determine GI and GL, International GI tables were used, which is a potential limiting factor because dietary GI/GL may not be accurately determined or comparable between studies. Although many studies adjusted for risk factors of breast cancer, not all studies controlled for physical activity (Cho et al. 2003, Sieri et al. 2007, Larsson et al. 2009) and smoking (Cho et al. 2003, Lajous et al. 2008, Larsson et al. 2009), thus this may have resulted in residual confounding factors affecting the study outcomes.

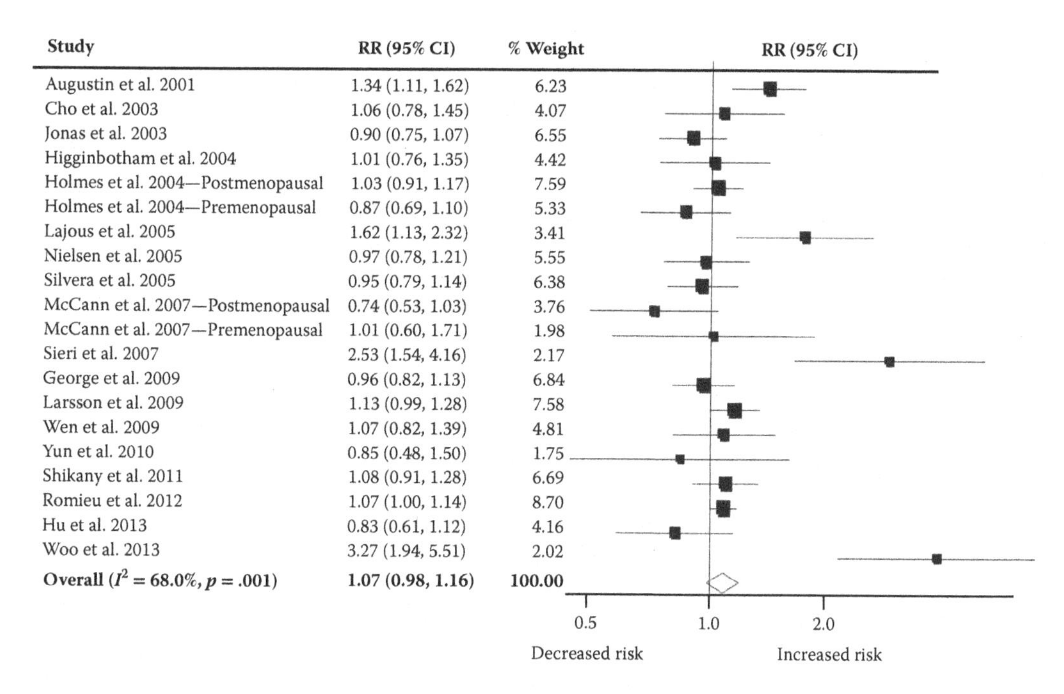

FIGURE 7.2 Meta-analysis of prospective cohort and case-control studies investigating the association between GL and risk of breast cancer. The pooled effect estimate is represented as a diamond. The p-value is for a random-effects model. All data are presented as RRs with 95% confidence intervals. GL, glycemic load; RR, relative risk. (Adapted from Turati, F. et al., *Mol. Nutr. Food Res.*, 59, 1384–1394, 2015a. With permission.)

7.2.2.3 Glycemic Index, Glycemic Load, and Breast Cancer Management

The dietary GI and GL may influence breast cancer survival; however, convincing evidence is lacking. The Health, Eating, Activity, and Lifestyle prospective cohort study investigated the association of GI and GL with breast cancer prognosis among 688 stage I to IIIA breast cancer survivors and showed no association between GI or GL and risk of death from any cause during an average follow-up period of 31 months after diagnosis (Belle et al. 2011). However, this study did not investigate whether the association was different in women with more aggressive cancers. The same study suggested a linear association between GI and mortality which became no longer significant after multivariate adjustments (Belle et al. 2011). Clinical trials that include GI in breast cancer management are currently lacking.

7.2.3 Colorectal Cancer

7.2.3.1 Colorectal Cancer Background

Colorectal cancer is a major cause of morbidity and mortality throughout the world, accounting for more than 9% of cancer incidence globally (Boyle and Langman 2000, World Health Organization 2002, World Cancer Research Fund and American Institute for Cancer Research 2007). Affecting both men and women, it is the third most common cancer worldwide and the fourth most common cause of mortality (World Health Organization 2002, World Cancer Research Fund and American Institute for Cancer Research 2007). Observational studies have indicated that environmental factors, including dietary and lifestyle, may be significant determinants of colorectal cancer risk (Armstrong and Doll 1975, Kolonel 1980, Kono 2004).

Several lines of evidence suggest that insulin resistance may be a factor in the etiology of colorectal cancer. Insulin resistance has been associated with overweight and obesity, low physical activity, and T2DM, all of which are the risk factors for colorectal cancer (Giovannucci 2001, World Cancer Research Fund and American Institute for Cancer Research 2007, Larsson et al. 2007a). Furthermore, epidemiological studies have reported increased colorectal cancer risk with elevated blood glucose concentrations or increased C-peptide levels (Ma et al. 2004, Jee et al. 2005, Pisani 2008, Otani et al. 2007). Dietary carbohydrate intake is the main dietary component affecting insulin secretion and glycemic response (Brand-Miller 2004), but the effect varies depending on the type and amount of carbohydrate consumed. Hence, it is thought that GI and GL may play a role in colorectal cancer prevention and management (Augustin et al. 2002).

7.2.3.2 Glycemic Index, Glycemic Load, and Colorectal Cancer Prevention

Epidemiological studies have investigated the association between dietary GI and GL in relation to colorectal cancer risk; however, results have been inconsistent (Bostick et al. 1994, Chyou et al. 1996, Kato et al. 1997, Terry et al. 2003, Higginbotham et al. 2004a, Michaud et al. 2005, McCarl et al. 2006, Larsson et al. 2007a, Strayer et al. 2007, Kabat et al. 2008, Howarth et al. 2008, Weijenberg et al. 2008, George et al. 2009, Li et al. 2011).

In 2009, a systematic review and meta-analysis looked at GI/GL and risk of digestive tract neoplasms. All 12 cohort and case-control studies in relation to colorectal cancer that met eligibility criteria were conducted in Europe or North America, and the ranges of GI (49–80) and GL (67–210) were wide (Mulholland et al. 2008a). A small but nonsignificant increased risk of colorectal cancer in the highest category of GI was observed (RR 1.15; 95% CI: 0.99, 1.34); however, the authors note that this was largely attributed to case-control study results and was subject to marked heterogeneity ($I^2 = 77\%$; $p < .01$) (Mulholland et al. 2008a). No significant associations were observed between GI and colorectal cancer risk when combining cohort studies (RR 1.04; 95% CI: 0.92, 1.16) (Mulholland et al. 2008a). Mulholland et al. (2008a) indicated subgroup analyses were not performed based on strata of BMI because of variation in cut-points or lack of information provided by the studies. Of the studies that did possess BMI information, there were inconsistent findings, with studies observing associations between GI and GL and colorectal cancer risk among overweight participants as positive (Franceschi et al. 2001, McCarl et al. 2006), neutral (Oh et al. 2004, Larsson et al. 2007a, Kabat et al. 2008, Weijenberg et al. 2008), or inverse (Strayer et al. 2007). Studies included in this meta-analysis, which presented stratified analyses based on diabetes status, also illustrated inconsistent results (McCarl et al. 2006, Weijenberg et al. 2008).

By 2012, an additional three large cohort studies investigating the association between GI or GL and colorectal cancer risk were published (Howarth et al. 2008, George et al. 2009, Li et al. 2011). A systematic review and meta-analysis by Aune et al. (2012a) incorporated these three cohorts, assessing a total of 14 cohort studies, and indicated no association between high-GI (RR 1.07; 95% CI: 0.99, 1.16; $n = 10$ studies) or -GL (RR 1.00; 95% CI: 0.91, 1.10; $n = 12$ studies) diets and colorectal cancer risk.

In 2015, the systematic review and meta-analysis by Turati et al. (2015a), which assessed both cohort and case-control studies, included an additional three studies (Hu et al. 2013, Zelenskiy et al. 2014, Sieri et al. 2015). Their results showed a significant association of the highest (vs. lowest) category of GI with colorectal cancer risk (RR = 1.16; 95% CI: 1.07, 1.25) (Figure 7.3). The summary RR of colorectal cancer and GL was 1.10 (95% CI: 0.97, 1.25) (Turati et al. 2015a) (Figure 7.4). Subgroup analyses indicated that the RR for the highest (versus the lowest) category of GI of the five case-control studies included was 1.30 (95% CI: 1.01, 1.53) and of the 10 cohort studies included was 1.09 (95% CI: 1.01, 1.18) (Turati 2015a). For GL, subgroup analysis of case-control studies showed RR 1.55 (95% CI: 1.25, 1.91; $n = 3$ studies) and analysis of cohort studies showed RR 1.00 (95% CI: 0.91, 1.11; $n = 12$ studies) (Turati 2015a).

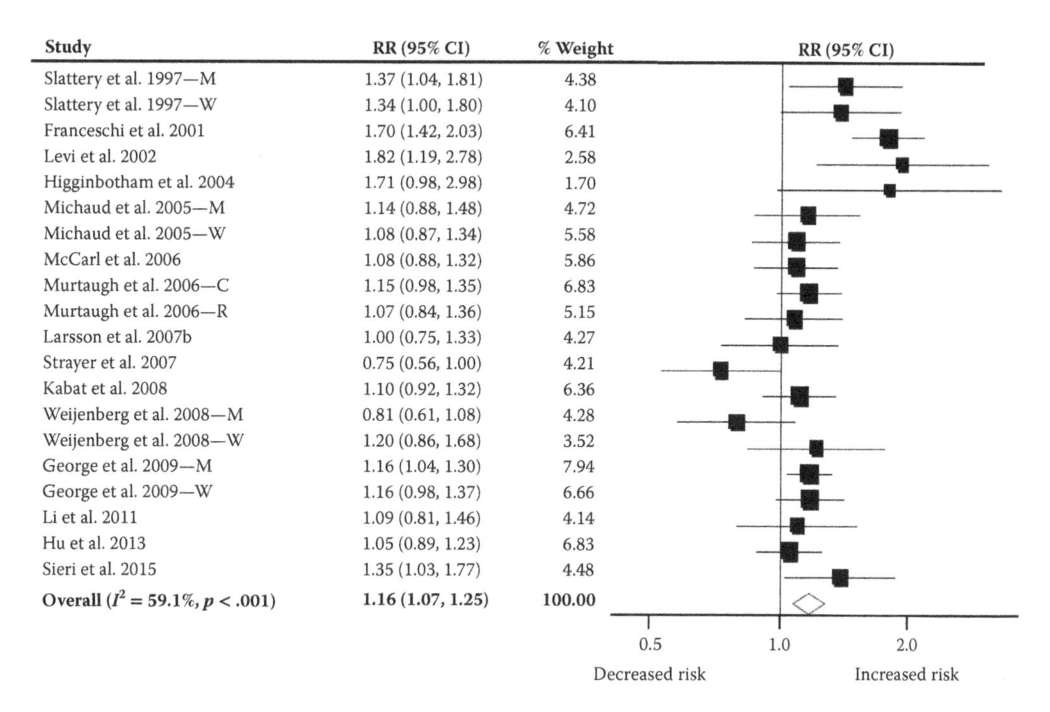

Study	RR (95% CI)	% Weight
Slattery et al. 1997—M	1.37 (1.04, 1.81)	4.38
Slattery et al. 1997—W	1.34 (1.00, 1.80)	4.10
Franceschi et al. 2001	1.70 (1.42, 2.03)	6.41
Levi et al. 2002	1.82 (1.19, 2.78)	2.58
Higginbotham et al. 2004	1.71 (0.98, 2.98)	1.70
Michaud et al. 2005—M	1.14 (0.88, 1.48)	4.72
Michaud et al. 2005—W	1.08 (0.87, 1.34)	5.58
McCarl et al. 2006	1.08 (0.88, 1.32)	5.86
Murtaugh et al. 2006—C	1.15 (0.98, 1.35)	6.83
Murtaugh et al. 2006—R	1.07 (0.84, 1.36)	5.15
Larsson et al. 2007b	1.00 (0.75, 1.33)	4.27
Strayer et al. 2007	0.75 (0.56, 1.00)	4.21
Kabat et al. 2008	1.10 (0.92, 1.32)	6.36
Weijenberg et al. 2008—M	0.81 (0.61, 1.08)	4.28
Weijenberg et al. 2008—W	1.20 (0.86, 1.68)	3.52
George et al. 2009—M	1.16 (1.04, 1.30)	7.94
George et al. 2009—W	1.16 (0.98, 1.37)	6.66
Li et al. 2011	1.09 (0.81, 1.46)	4.14
Hu et al. 2013	1.05 (0.89, 1.23)	6.83
Sieri et al. 2015	1.35 (1.03, 1.77)	4.48
Overall (I^2 = 59.1%, $p < .001$)	**1.16 (1.07, 1.25)**	**100.00**

FIGURE 7.3 Meta-analysis of prospective cohort and case-control studies investigating the association between GI and risk of colorectal cancer. The pooled effect estimate is represented as a diamond. The p-value is for a random-effects model. All data are presented as relative risks with 95% confidence intervals. C, colon; GI, glycemic index; M, men; R, rectum; RR, relative risk; W, women. (Adapted from Turati, F. et al. *Mol. Nutr. Food Res.*, 59, 1384–1394, 2015a. With permission.)

Obesity and overweight are risk factors for colorectal cancer (Centres for Disease Control and Prevention 2014). Hence, Turati et al. (2015a) also conducted subgroup analyses based on BMI. A subgroup analysis of BMI indicated that the RR in the highest-GI category was 1.02 (95% CI: 0.86, 1.21; n = 3 studies) for those with a BMI of less than 25 kg/m^2 and 0.97 (95% CI: 0.77–1.22; n = 3 studies) for those with a BMI of 25 kg/m^2 or more, whereas for GL, these values were 1.07 (95% CI: 0.86, 1.33; n = 4 studies) and 1.13 (95% CI: 0.92, 1.39; n = 4 studies) (Turati et al. 2015a). These results suggest no effect modification of BMI on the association of GI or GL with colorectal cancer risk.

7.2.3.3 Glycemic Index, Glycemic Load, and Colorectal Cancer Management

Very few studies to date have focused on the effect of a low-GI dietary pattern in relation to colorectal cancer recurrence. A prospective cohort derived from participants in the National Cancer Institute-sponsored Cancer and Leukemia Group B was studied by Meyerhardt et al. (2012) to investigate the influence of GL on survival among 1011 stage III colon cancer patients. Dietary information was reported via 131-item semiquantitative food frequency questionnaires conducted over the median 7.3 years of follow-up. Findings demonstrated no significant associations with GI, whereas higher dietary GL was significantly associated with worse disease-free, recurrence-free, and overall survival hazard ratio (HR) 1.79 (95% CI: 1.29, 2.48; $p < .001$). These findings were particularly evident in overweight or obese participants (Meyerhardt et al. 2012). However, this study did not adjust GL for energy intake, and it is possible that the worsening of the patients' health conditions corresponded with preferential intakes of carbohydrates over other macronutrients.

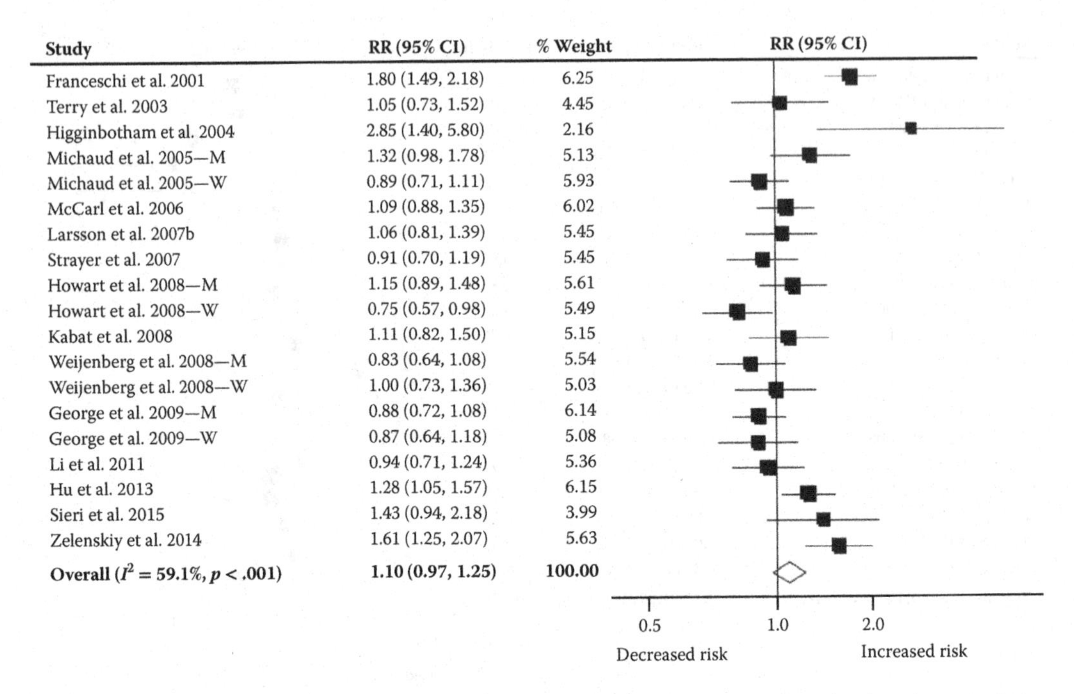

FIGURE 7.4 Meta-analysis of prospective cohort and case-control studies investigating the association between GL and risk of colorectal cancer. The pooled effect estimate is represented as a diamond. The *p*-value is for a random-effects model. All data are presented as relative risks with 95% confidence intervals. GL, glycemic load; M, men; RR, relative risk; W, women. (Adapted from Turati, F. et al., *Mol. Nutr. Food Res.*, 59, 1384–1394, 2015a. With permission.)

7.2.4 Pancreatic Cancer

7.2.4.1 Pancreatic Cancer Background

In 2015, the American Cancer Society estimated the prevalence of pancreatic cancer to be approximately 48,960 people (24,840 men and 24,120 women) in the United States (American Cancer Society 2015c), with pancreatic cancer accounting for approximately 3% of all cancers in the United States and for about 7% of all cancer mortality (American Cancer Society 2015c). Pancreatic cancer has the highest mortality rate of all major cancers. Risk factors for pancreatic cancer include family history of the disease, smoking, age, and diabetes risk factors, including obesity (American Cancer Society 2013). Although relatively little is known about the etiology of pancreatic cancer, there is some evidence that plasma insulin concentration may be relevant (Ekbom and Hunter 2012). Consumption of high-GI diets has been associated with hyperinsulinemia (Byrnes et al. 1995, Holt et al. 1997, Foster-Powell et al. 2002), whereas the consumption of low-GI diets has been associated with lower postprandial insulin rises (Ludwig 2000). Therefore, GI/GL may be associated with pancreatic cancer risk.

7.2.4.2 Glycemic Index, Glycemic Load, and Pancreatic Cancer Prevention

Epidemiological studies on the association between GI and GL on pancreatic cancer risk have been inconsistent. A recent systematic review and meta-analysis of prospective studies by Turati et al. (2015a) identified 10 studies (seven cohorts and three case-control) for GI and found a nonsignificant summary RR of 1.10 (95% CI: 0.99, 1.22) and 11 studies (eight cohorts and three case-control) for GL and found a nonsignificant summary RR of 1.01 (95% CI: 0.85, 1.19). When subgroup analyses by sex were conducted for GI, there was a significant association within the female subgroup of eight studies (summary RR = 1.23; 95% CI: 1.04, 1.46) but not in the four studies in men (summary RR = 1.01; 95% CI: 0.76, 1.34). In addition, in the subgroup analyses by BMI, a significant association with GL and pancreatic cancer was found only in the subgroup with BMI of 25 kg/m^2 or more (summary RR = 1.44; 95% CI: 1.02, 2.03). Interestingly, it has been reported that GI and GL have a significant association with coronary heart disease in women but not in men (Mirrahimi et al. 2012), and specifically in overweight women for GL (Fan et al. 2012). The observed sex differences may be a result of the larger total representation of women compared with men (eight studies vs. four studies). In other words, women may have better reporting of dietary intake and thus result in greater power to detect differences. It could also be that women are more sensitive to glycemic and insulinemic fluctuations because of their lower muscle mass compared with men. In a study investigating two staple carbohydrate foods at the opposite ends of the GI spectrum, white bread and pasta, for their possible associations with colorectal cancer risk, it also found that the direct associations were significant only in women and not in men (Augustin et al. 2013).

A previous systematic review and meta-analysis by Aune et al. (2012b), which only included cohort studies investigating GI/GL and pancreatic cancer risk for a total of more than 1 million participants and approximately 3000 cases, found a nonsignificant summary RR of 1.04 (95% CI: 0.93, 1.17) for GI and a nonsignificant summary RR of 1.01 (95% CI: 0.88, 1.15) for GL. No subgroup differences that modified the association for either GI or GL were found. These results are consistent with previous meta-analyses, which also did not find an association between GI or GL and pancreatic cancer risk based on cohort studies (Barclay et al. 2008, Gnagnarella et al. 2008, Mulholland et al. 2009).

7.2.5 Endometrial Cancer

7.2.5.1 Endometrial Cancer Background

Endometrial cancer is the most common type of uterine cancer. It is the sixth most common cancer in women worldwide and the 12 most common cancer overall (Ferlay et al. 2014). Studies have suggested that polycystic ovary syndrome and insulin resistance, components of metabolic syndrome, may play a role in the pathogenesis of endometrial cancer, possibly via hormonal disruption (Hardiman et al. 2003). This is thought to be influenced by insulin-like growth factor (IGF-1) activity and bioavailable estrogen (Kaaks et al. 2002, Lukanova et al. 2004, Becker et al. 2009). Owing to the potential role of insulin resistance and hyperinsulinemia in the etiology of endometrial cancer, amount and rate of digestion of dietary carbohydrate, specifically GI and GL, are thought to be associated with endometrial risk (Augustin et al. 2003a).

7.2.5.2 Glycemic Index, Glycemic Load, and Endometrial Cancer Prevention

A recent systematic review and meta-analysis by Turati et al. (2015a) identified 10 studies (six cohorts and four case-controls) and found a nonsignificant increased risk of endometrial cancer for highest versus lowest intake category of GI (RR = 1.13; 95% CI: 0.98, 1.32) (Figure 7.5). Interestingly, when the analyses were stratified by BMI (<25 vs. ≥25kg/m^2), both GI subgroups became significant (RR = 1.31; 95% CI: 1.07, 1.62 and RR = 1.26; 95% CI: 1.07, 1.48, respectively). In terms of GL, Turati et al. (2015a) identified 11 studies (seven cohorts and four case-controls) and found a significant increased risk for highest versus lowest intake category of GL (RR = 1.17; 95% CI: 1.00, 1.37) (Figure 7.6), particularly in high-BMI subgroup (RR = 1.34; 95% CI: 1.13, 1.59), whereas significance was lost in the low-BMI subgroup (RR = 1.07; 95% CI: 0.86, 1.34). Similarly, in a 2008 meta-analysis by Mulholland et al. (2008b), which included five observational studies examining GI and GL and endometrial cancer risk, the effect estimates for endometrial cancer showed an increased risk for high GL (RR 1.20; 95% CI: 1.06, 1.37), which

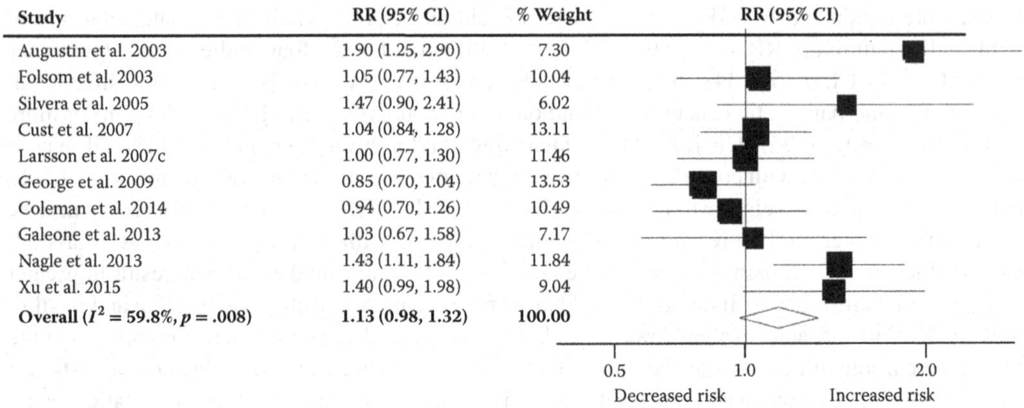

Study	RR (95% CI)	% Weight
Augustin et al. 2003	1.90 (1.25, 2.90)	7.30
Folsom et al. 2003	1.05 (0.77, 1.43)	10.04
Silvera et al. 2005	1.47 (0.90, 2.41)	6.02
Cust et al. 2007	1.04 (0.84, 1.28)	13.11
Larsson et al. 2007c	1.00 (0.77, 1.30)	11.46
George et al. 2009	0.85 (0.70, 1.04)	13.53
Coleman et al. 2014	0.94 (0.70, 1.26)	10.49
Galeone et al. 2013	1.03 (0.67, 1.58)	7.17
Nagle et al. 2013	1.43 (1.11, 1.84)	11.84
Xu et al. 2015	1.40 (0.99, 1.98)	9.04
Overall ($I^2 = 59.8\%, p = .008$)	**1.13 (0.98, 1.32)**	**100.00**

RR (95% CI)
0.5 1.0 2.0
Decreased risk Increased risk

FIGURE 7.5 Meta-analysis of prospective cohort and case-control studies investigating the association between GI and risk of endometrial cancer. The pooled effect estimate is represented as a diamond. The *p*-value is for a random-effects model. All data are presented as relative risks with 95% confidence intervals. GI, glycemic index; M, men; RR, relative risk; W, women. (Adapted from Turati, F. et al., *Mol. Nutr. Food Res.*, 59, 1384–1394, 2015a. With permission.)

Study	RR (95% CI)	% Weight
Augustin et al. 2003	1.90 (0.60, 2.02)	4.61
Folsom et al. 2003	1.24 (0.90, 1.71)	9.48
Silvera et al. 2005	1.36 (1.01, 1.84)	10.08
Cust et al. 2007	1.15 (0.94, 1.41)	12.69
Larsson et al. 2007c	1.15 (0.88, 1.51)	10.86
George et al. 2009	1.25 (0.86, 1.81)	8.37
Cui et al. 2011	1.48 (1.14, 1.92)	11.11
Coleman et al. 2014	0.63 (0.47, 0.85)	10.05
Galeone et al. 2013	1.01 (0.64, 1.60)	6.64
Nagle et al. 2013	1.15 (0.90, 1.47)	11.43
Xu et al. 2015	2.20 (1.21, 4.02)	4.69
Overall ($I^2 = 60.4\%, p = .005$)	**1.17 (1.00, 1.37)**	**100.00**

RR (95% CI)
0.5 1.0 2.0
Decreased risk Increased risk

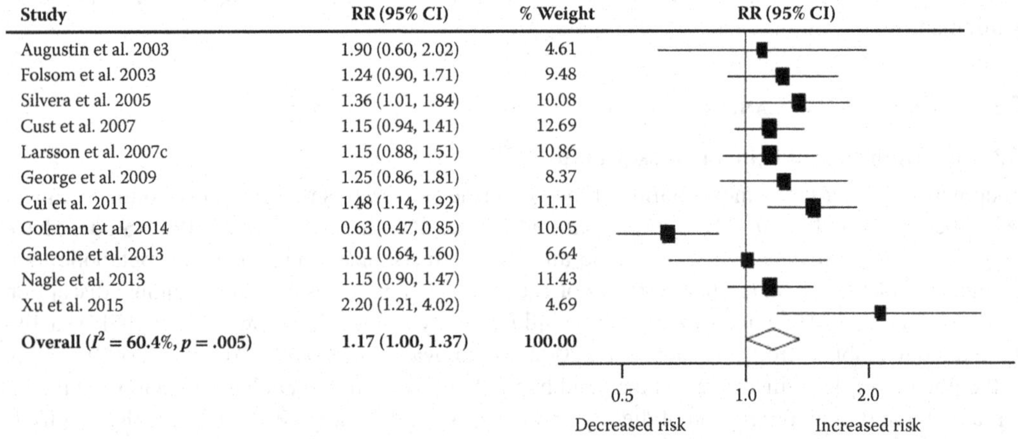

FIGURE 7.6 Meta-analysis of prospective cohort and case-control studies investigating the association between GL and risk of endometrial cancer. The pooled effect estimate is represented as a diamond. The *p*-value is for a random-effects model. All data are presented as relative risks with 95% confidence intervals. GL, glycemic load; M, men; RR, relative risk; W, women. (Adapted from Turati, F. et al., *Mol. Nutr. Food Res.*, 59, 1384–1394, 2015a. With permission.)

was further elevated in obese women (RR 1.54; 95% CI: 1.18, 2.03). However, a linear relationship between BMI and endometrial cancer risk has been previously demonstrated (Jain et al. 2000, Furberg and Thune 2003, Schouten et al. 2004, Friedenreich et al. 2007). In previous systematic reviews and meta-analyses, significant direct associations with endometrial cancer risk were also observed for GL but not for GI (Barclay et al. 2008, Mulholland et al. 2008b, Choi et al. 2012, Galeone et al. 2013, Nagle et al. 2013), whereas in the meta-analysis by Gnagnarella et al. (2008), which included five studies (cohorts and case-controls), both GI and GL were significantly associated with endometrial cancer risk (RR 1.22; 95% CI: 1.01, 1.49 for GI and RR 1.36; 95% CI: 1.14, 1.62 for GL).

7.2.6 Prostate Cancer

7.2.6.1 Prostate Cancer Background

Among men, prostate cancer is one of the top five diagnosed cancers, and it has been estimated that prostate cancer accounts for approximately 14% of all newly diagnosed cancer worldwide (Jemal et al. 2011). According to the World Health Organization, the incidence of prostate cancer in high-income countries is about 10 times higher than that of lower-middle-income countries, suggesting lifestyle role(s) in its etiology (World Health Organization 2015a). Risk factors for prostate cancer include the nonmodifiable factors of age, ethnicity, and family history, in addition to the modifiable factors of physical activity, BMI, hormones, and diet (American Cancer Society 2015d). Similar to other cancers, it has been proposed that high dietary GI and GL may increase prostate cancer risk by increasing insulin concentrations. This is thought to lead to chronic hyperinsulinemia and subsequently influence the IGF axis, synthesis of sex hormone-binding globulin, and circulating testosterone and estrogen levels, all of which may increase prostate cancer risk (Jenkins et al. 1987, Castagnetta et al. 1995, Yu and Rohan 2000, Pollak 2001, Biddinger and Ludwig 2005).

7.2.6.2 Glycemic Index, Glycemic Load, and Prostate Cancer Prevention

The observational studies assessing the association between GI and prostate cancer have demonstrated a fairly consistent lack of association. The recent systematic review and meta-analysis by Turati et al. (2015a) identified three cohort studies and three case-control studies, demonstrating a nonsignificant summary RR of 1.06 (95% CI: 0.96, 1.18). Interestingly, all three cohorts had fairly low variability around the null; however, two case-control studies demonstrated significant increased risk of prostate cancer when comparing the highest with lowest intakes of GI (summary RR for the three case-control studies = 1.34; 95% CI: 1.10, 1.62). Similar results were found for the association with GL (summary RR = 1.04; 95% CI: 0.91, 1.18; summary RR for two case-control studies = 1.36; 95% CI: 1.08, 1.70). These results were confirmed in a systematic review and meta-analysis by Wang et al. (2015), which included the same studies.

7.2.7 Ovarian Cancer

7.2.7.1 Ovarian Cancer Background

According to the National Cancer Institute's Surveillance, Epidemiology, and End Results Program, there were 12.1 new cases of ovarian cancer per 100,000 women per year, based on 2008–2012 data. The five-year survival rate is estimated at 45.6%, whereas the number of deaths was 7.7 per 100,000 women per year (National Cancer Institute 2012a). Few established risk factors for ovarian cancer are considered modifiable. It has been hypothesized that hyperinsulinemia, associated with chronic consumption of a high-GI/GL dietary pattern, may increase the risk of ovarian cancer by lowering the concentrations of IGF-binding protein (IGFBP), thus increasing the bioavailability of IGF-1 (Kalli and Conover 2003, Lukanova and Kaaks 2005).

7.2.7.2 Glycemic Index, Glycemic Load, and Ovarian Cancer Prevention

The few observational studies completed to date have been summarized in a recent systematic review and meta-analysis by Turati et al. (2015a), in which a nonsignificant positive association was found for GI in the five studies identified (two cohorts and three case-controls) (summary RR = 1.11; 95% CI: 0.85, 1.46). Similar results were observed for the association with GL (summary RR = 1.19; 95% CI: 0.85, 1.68). However, three of the studies individually found a significant increased risk with GL, one of which was a cohort study conducted by Silvera et al. (2007). In this cohort, a significant 72% increased risk of ovarian cancer was found with GL by quartiles (HR = 1.72; 95% CI: 1.13, 2.62; p = .011) in more than 49,000 middle-aged (mean age 48 years) Canadian women with normal to overweight BMI (mean BMI 25kg/m^2), who were followed for a mean of 16.4 years. When the data were divided by menopausal status, the magnitude of the association was slightly greater among postmenopausal (HR = 1.89; 95% CI: 0.98, 3.65; $p = .03$) than among premenopausal women (HR = 1.64; 95% CI: 0.95, 2.88; $p = .07$). However, this cohort study did not find an effect of GI (HR = 1.27; 95% CI: 0.65, 2.48; $p = .483$) or of total carbohydrate (HR = 1.30; 95% CI: 0.92, 1.84; $p = .37$) on the risk of ovarian cancer. One of the case-control studies included by Augustin et al. (2003a) was a large study conducted in Italy on 1031 confirmed cases and 2411 controls. In this study, the dietary GI was significantly associated with increased risk of ovarian cancer (OR for highest vs. lowest quartile = 1.7; 95% CI 1.3, 2.1). Similarly, GL (OR = 1.7; 95% CI 1.3, 2.1) and total carbohydrate (OR for highest vs. lowest quartile = 1.8; 95% CI 1.3, 2.4) were also significantly associated with increased risk of ovarian cancer. Similar to what was found by Silvera et al. (2007) the association was stronger in postmenopausal women than in premenopausal women (OR = 1.84; 95% CI: 1.37, 2.48; $p = < .01$ vs. OR = 1.36; 95% CI: 0.90, 2.05; $p = .15$, respectively, for GI, and OR = 1.83; 95% CI: 1.36, 2.46; $p < .01$ vs. OR = 1.39; 95% CI: 0.92, 2.10; $p = .13$, respectively, for GL) (Augustin et al. 2003b). In addition, in the analysis by Augustin et al (2003a), an elevated risk of ovarian cancer was noted in the second quartile for both GI and GL, which did not show a further increase at the third and fourth quartiles, which Silvera et al. (2007) had demonstrated for GL.

7.2.8 Gastric Cancer

7.2.8.1 Gastric Cancer Background

Worldwide, gastric cancer has the fourth highest incidence and is the second leading cause of cancer mortality (Parkin et al. 2005). According to the National Cancer Institute's (2012b) Surveillance, Epidemiology, and End Results Program statistics, the number of new cases of gastric cancer was 7.4 per 100,000 men and women per year, and the number of deaths was 3.4 per 100,000 men and women per year, based on 2008–2012 cases and deaths, whereas the five-year survival was estimated at 29.3% (2005–2011). Dietary factors play a major role in the etiology of gastric cancer (World Cancer Research Fund and American Institute for Cancer Research 2007). Similar to other cancers, diets high in certain types and amount of carbohydrate (dietary patterns with high GI/GL) have been proposed to increase the risk of gastric cancer via hyperinsulinemia, leading to increased IGF (Franciosi et al. 2003, Zhang et al. 2004, Zhao et al. 2005).

7.2.8.2 Glycemic Index, Glycemic Load, and Gastric Cancer Prevention

There are inconsistencies in the few studies that have explored the association between GI and GL and gastric cancer. A recent systematic review and meta-analysis by Turati et al. (2015a), which included six studies (three cohort and three case-controls) on gastric cancer, found that GI was nonsignificantly associated with an increased risk (RR = 1.17; 95% CI: 0.83, 1.66). However, subgroup analyses revealed that there was a significant association between GI and GL and risk of gastric cancer in men (RR = 1.39; 95% CI: 1.00, 1.95, based on two studies, and RR = 1.56; 95% CI: 1.10, 2.20, based on three studies, for GI and GL, respectively) but not in women (RR = 1.42; 95% CI: 0.62, 3.25, based on three studies, and RR = 1.29; 95% CI: 0.53, 3.17, based on four studies). This difference between sex is demonstrated in the cohort study by George et al. (2009) of more than 500,000 Americans who were followed from 1995/1996 to 2003. In this study, GI was found to be significantly associated with gastric cancer in men (RR highest vs. lowest quintile = 1.50; 95% CI: 1.09, 2.08; $p = .020$) but not in women (RR highest vs. lowest quintile = 1.12; 95% CI: 0.64, 1.97; $p = .520$). It should be noted that although the analyses were multivariate RRs and smoking status was included in the model, when the data were stratified by smoking status, the significance of GI in men was lost in nonsmokers, and thus, the authors highlight that high GI may be confounded by other diet and lifestyle factors (George et al. 2009). The only other cohort study in the recent systematic review and meta-analysis identified by Turati et al. (2015a) with regard to gastric cancer is that of Larsson et al. (2006).

In more than 60,000 middle-aged and elderly women from the population-based Swedish mammography cohort, Larsson et al. (2006) found that after up to 18 years of follow-up, there was no association between either GI (HR of highest vs. the lowest quintile = 0.77; 95% CI: 0.46, 1.30; $p = .30$) or GL (HR of highest vs. the lowest quintile = 0.76; 95% CI: 0.46, 1.25; $p = .16$) and risk of gastric cancer. Therefore, the limited evidence presently available does not appear to support a role of GI or GL in altering the risk of gastric cancers in women; however, these may play a role in men. More studies are necessary to understand whether GI or GL contributes to the risk of gastric cancers.

7.2.9 Esophageal Squamous Cell Carcinoma

7.2.9.1 Esophageal Squamous Cell Carcinoma Background

Esophageal cancer, including squamous cell carcinoma, is the eighth most common cancer worldwide and the sixth most common cause of cancer-related mortality (Ferlay et al. 2010). Smoking, alcohol consumption, and some dietary factors are the predominant risk factors that increase the risk for squamous cell carcinoma (Bosetti et al. 2008, Liu et al. 2013, Bagnardi et al. 2015). As with other types of cancers, GI and GL have been implicated as possible etiologic factors. Specifically, high GI and GL may lead to chronic elevations in blood glucose concentrations, whereas hyperglycemia, T2DM, and hyperinsulinemia have been implicated as potential risk factors for some cancers, including cancers of the digestive tract (Mulholland et al. 2009, Neale et al. 2009, Kubo et al. 2010). Furthermore, a high-GI diet may increase cancer risk by modulating the IGF axis (Biddinger and Ludwig 2005, Brand-Miller et al. 2005).

7.2.9.2 Glycemic Index, Glycemic Load, and Esophageal Squamous Cell Carcinoma Prevention

The few observational studies conducted on Esophageal squamous cell carcinoma and GI have demonstrated fairly consistent associations. Nevertheless, in a recent systematic review and meta-analysis by Turati et al. (2015a), which identified one cohort and three case-control studies, the summary RR was nonsignificant, but positive (RR = 1.46; 95% CI: 0.90, 2.38). The results are not as consistent for GL, with a nonsignificant summary RR of 1.25 (95% CI: 0.45, 3.48). In subgroup analyses by sex, there were significant associations for increased risk in men (RR = 1.39; 95% CI: 1.00, 1.95 for GI and RR = 1.56; 95% CI: 1.10, 2.20 for GL).

7.2.10 Liver Cancer

7.2.10.1 Liver Cancer Background

Worldwide, primary liver cancer is the sixth most common cancer morbidity, accounting for more than 700,000 new cases diagnosed each year (Ferlay et al. 2014), and the third leading cause of cancer-related mortality, accounting for more than 600,000 deaths each year (American Cancer Society 2015b). The prevalence of liver cancer is higher in developing than developed countries (American Cancer Society 2015b). The risk of hepatocellular carcinomas (HCC), the major form of primary liver cancer, has been shown to be higher in diabetic populations. The association of diabetes mellitus, insulin resistance, and hyperglycemia with HCC suggests that dietary GI/GL may influence HCC risk.

7.2.10.2 Glycemic Index, Glycemic Load, and Liver Cancer Prevention

The few observational studies on liver cancer have been inconsistent. The recent systematic review and meta-analysis by Turati et al. (2015a) identified three cohorts and one case-control study demonstrating a nonsignificant summary RR of 1.11 (95% CI: 0.80, 1.53) for GI and identified three cohorts and three case-control studies demonstrating a nonsignificant summary RR of 1.10 (95% CI: 0.85, 1.42) for GL.

Two of the cohort studies found that higher dietary GI increased the risk of developing liver cancer, however after stratification by sex the association was significant only in men in one study (George et al. 2009) and only in women only in the other study (Vogtmann et al. 2013). The former cohort was from six U.S. states, whereas the latter was a Chinese cohort from the Shanghai Health Study; thus, further research is required to determine whether there are sex- and ethnicity differences in the associations. In addition, in the former study (George et al. 2009), which demonstrated a significant inverse association between higher dietary GL and liver cancer in women, the association was lost when the analysis was restricted to those who never smoked. Therefore, smoking status may be an important confounding factor or may be indicative of an overall poorer lifestyle.

Some case-control studies that have demonstrated the association between higher dietary GL and increased risk of liver cancer also found that the association was stronger in the presence of hepatitis B virus and/or hepatitis C virus markers (Lagiou et al. 2009, Rossi et al. 2009). However, one of the cohort studies conducted (Vogtmann et al. 2013) stratified results by chronic liver disease and hepatitis status and found no statistically significant trends for men or women with a history of chronic liver disease or hepatitis. However, the significant association in the overall analysis for women persisted in those without a history of chronic liver disease or hepatitis, even after adjustment for all potential confounders. Thus, further exploration into this potential important confounding factor should be considered in future analyses.

7.3 LIMITATIONS

The most recent systematic review and meta-analysis by Turati et al. (2015a) which included all epidemiological studies (cohort and case-controls) and assessed the associations between dietary GI and GL and various cancer types, mainly found direct but modest associations, which reached significance mainly in colorectal cancer and approached significance in breast cancer. Nevertheless, the weak associations found in this meta-analysis may be due to the high heterogeneity between studies and ultimately the different geographical areas reflecting different dietary habits. It is of note that case-control studies tended to show stronger associations than cohort studies and that the greatest number of case-control studies were conducted in Europe (17 of 32, of which only six were conducted in North America), whereas most cohort studies were conducted in North America (12 of 20). The dietary pattern in Europe is characterized by higher carbohydrate intake, with large varieties of both low- and high-GI foods, compared with North America (Favero et al. 1997, Slimani et al. 2002, Wirfalt et al. 2002). This is reflected by the larger GI and GL ranges found in the case-control studies. Smaller GI and GL ranges would preclude finding associations of small magnitude, particularly if the food frequency questionnaire (FFQ) had not been designed to test the GI association (FFQs that combine high- and low-GI foods into one item). Despite these differences, many large cohort studies did find significant direct associations between dietary GI and GL and cancer of the colorectum (Women's Health Study) (Higginbotham et al. 2004b), breast (Hormones and Diet in the Etiology of Breast Cancer and European Prospective Investigation into Cancer and Nutrition studies) (Sieri et al. 2007, Romieu et al. 2012), and endometrium (Canadian National Breast Screening Study and Nurses' Health Study studies) (Silvera et al. 2005, Cui et al. 2011).

It is also possible that the population that can mostly benefit from consuming low-GI diets may be those characterized by high prevalence of overweight and/or obesity. Indeed, the strongest associations of GI or GL have been found in people with higher body weight for both cancer (Franceschi et al. 2001, Coleman et al. 2014) and other chronic diseases (Liu et al. 2000). Owing to the underlying insulin resistance in people who are overweight or obese, the resulting insulin response may be higher for the same dietary GI/GL rank. As known, insulin has growth-promoting and proliferating effects (Kaaks and Lukanova 2001, Giovannucci 2003). It is therefore possible that diets higher in GI/GL may contribute to greater cancer risk by providing a greater rate of fuel and building blocks to cancer cells (see Section 7.1.3) and increasing hyperinsulinemia (Franceschi et al. 2001, Coleman et al. 2014) compared with diets with lower GI/GL.

These mechanisms may also contribute to increased cancer recurrence (Meyerhardt et al. 2012). It is of note that assignment of GI values to items in FFQ may be associated with a number of issues, leading to inconsistencies between studies. Although in most studies, the GI values are obtained from International GI tables (Atkinson et al. 2008), the tables contain many values for apparently similar foods, and it is not clear which values are assigned to which food item. Furthermore, as GI values may be country- or ethnicity-specific and there are no requirements by scientific reviewers and editors alike to publish the GI value assigned to each carbohydrate item in the FFQ, homogeneity between studies is not established. It is also not known how investigators deal with foods that do not have a GI value or how foods with different GI values are combined within one item in the FFQ; for example, how breads are dealt with. This may be done by calculating a weighted GI average based on the frequency of consumption of those foods in the population under study. Correct calculations require nutrition knowledge and particularly a good understanding of the GI concept. Nevertheless, despite this lack of information and potential for measurement error, which may lower the strength of the GI associations, the majority of epidemiological investigations suggest consistency in showing either a protective or a neutral role for low-GI foods in cancer risk.

7.4 POTENTIAL MECHANISMS

It has been hypothesized that the nature of carbohydrates (the GI and GL) consumed may be associated with carcinogenesis (Augustin et al. 2002). Specifically, it has been suggested that dietary GI and GL may influence oxidative stress, as well as the secretion of insulin and IGF, thus playing a role directly in carcinogenesis and indirectly via the development of diabetes and obesity, both of which have been associated with cancer risk (Augustin et al. 2002, Larsson 2007a, Renehan et al. 2008). There has been much speculation that the IGF system plays a role in the association between GI and/or GL and cancer risk; however, there is limited evidence in the literature.

7.4.1 Cancer and Insulin-Like Growth Factor-1

The IGF-1 is a peptide, similar in molecular structure to insulin, produced mainly by the liver in response to growth hormone but can be synthesized by almost any tissue in the body (Olivecrona et al. 1999). It is the primary circulating growth factor in the IGF system, which performs a fundamental role in the regulation of cellular proliferation, differentiation, and apoptosis (Jerome et al. 2003). Specifically, IGF-1 acts to stimulate mitosis and inhibit apoptosis. Thus, it is not only associated with normal cell and systemic body growth but also has been insinuated as a factor in stimulating malignant tumor proliferation (Jerome et al. 2003). It is also important to note that 99% of IGF-1 circulates while bound to 1–6 IGFBPs and is influenced by the effects of IGFBPs, which function to regulate IGF-1 transport between intra- and extravascular spaces and interaction with their receptors (Zapf 1995), to prolong IGF half-life (Stewart and Rotwein 1996), and to prevent excessive cell growth or to promote apoptosis (Rajah et al. 1999).

In relation to breast cancer, there have been inconsistent findings as to whether it is specifically the alteration(s) in IGF-1 and/or IGFBP-3 that is/are related to increased risk. Results of a case-controlled prospective study showed no overall association between plasma IGF-1 concentrations (the authors did not report whether it was free [which refers to the biologically active, unbound form] or total IGF-1 that was analyzed) and the disease risk; however, a positive relationship was observed among premenopausal women (RR = 2.33; 95% CI: 1.06, 5.16; $p = .08$) and it increased to significance at (RR = 2.88; 95% CI: 1.21, 6.85; $p < .05$) when adjusted for plasma IGFBP-3 concentrations (Hankinson et al. 1998). This association was not seen in postmenopausal women (Hankinson et al. 1998). These results are similar to those reported by Li et al. (2001), who found that a high ratio of free IGF-1 to IGFBP-3 was associated with increased risk of breast cancer, with odds ratios for breast cancer patients with high levels of IGF-1 after adjusting for menopausal status and IGFBP-3 being 2.00 for total IGF-1 and 6.31 for free IGF-1.

Conversely, a more recent study showed an association between circulating IGF-1 (not specified whether it was free or bound) and breast cancer risk, which was not altered by adjusting for IGFBP-3 (Endogenous Hormones Breast Cancer Collaborative Group et al. 2010). In this study conducted by the Endogenous Hormones and Breast Cancer Collaborative Group, in which 17 prospective studies were analyzed, IGF-1 was shown to be positively associated with breast cancer risk, where the odds ratio for breast cancer for women in the highest vs. lowest quintile of IGF-1 concentration was 1.28 (95% CI: 1.14–1.44; $p < .0001$) (Endogenous Hormones Breast Cancer Collaborative Group et al. 2010). Again, menopausal status was shown to have an effect, where in premenopausal women, IGF-1 was weakly positively associated with breast cancer risk ($p = .050$), but in postmenopausal women, IGF-1 was significantly positively associated with breast cancer risk ($p = .0002$) (Endogenous Hormones Breast Cancer Collaborative Group et al. 2010). This finding regarding menopausal status in relation to the association between IGF-1 and breast cancer risk is opposite to that reported in the study by Li et al. (2001). Thus, despite the ambiguity as to the effect of menopausal status and whether it is IGF-1 alone or the ratio of IGF-1 to IGFBP-3 that affects breast cancer risk, overall, the majority of studies appear to agree that there is a positive relationship between the IGF system and breast cancer risk.

7.4.2 Dietary Glycemic Index and Glycemic Load and IGF-1

To our knowledge, there have been two studies that assessed the effect of either a low-GI and/or -GL diet on the IGF system. Brand-Miller et al. (2005) were the first to conduct a randomized trial comparing the postprandial responses of IGFs and IGFBP to a low-GI food with high-GI food in 10 healthy young adults. In this trial, a high-GI challenge of an 82 g serving of instant mashed potatoes was compared with a low-GI challenge of a 160 g serving of pearled barley, both providing 50 g of the available carbohydrates and content similar in energy and macronutrient (Brand-Miller et al. 2005). The incremental area under the curve after the low-GI meal (122 + 16 mmol/L/120 min) was significantly lower (40%) than that after the high-GI meal (203 + 23 mmol/L/120 min) (Brand-Miller et al. 2005). Results from this study showed that acutely consuming a low-GI challenge significantly decreased serum IGFBP-1 and increased IGFBP-3 at 4 h ($p < .05$), which suggests that consuming low-GI foods may lead to an environment that is less conducive to tumor growth compared with high-GI foods; however, changes in free and total IGF-1 were nonsignificant (Brand-Miller et al. 2005). After this in 2012, Runchey et al. (2012) assessed the effect of a low-versus high-GL diet on IGF-1 and IGFBP-3 in a randomized, controlled crossover feeding trial of 84 overweight obese and normal weight healthy individuals over two 28-day periods. It is important to note that the difference in GL between the high- and low-GL groups was due to the differences in GI and not the carbohydrate component (the percentage of total energy of carbohydrate was 57% and 59% in the high- and low-GL groups, respectively, whereas the GI was on average 73 and 33 in the high- and low-GL groups, respectively) (Runchey et al. 2012). Findings from this trial showed that the low-GL diet led to 4% lower fasting concentrations of IGF-1 (10.6 ng/mL, $p = .04$) and a 4% lower ratio of IGF-1 to IGFBP-3 (0.24, $p = .01$) compared with the high-GL diet (Runchey et al. 2012). Adiposity did not appear to sway IGF-1 results; however, having a high adiposity and consuming the high-GL diet were found to have a higher ratio of IGF-1 to IGFBP-3 compared with the low-GL diet ($p = .02$) (Runchey et al. 2012). This limited evidence suggests that consuming a low-GL diet (with low-GL designation being attributed to the consumption of low-GI foods) may have implications for influencing the IGF system and hence having an effect on breast cancer risk, in light of the findings by the Endogenous Hormones and Breast Cancer Collaborative Group, Hankinson, and others, as well as by Li and colleagues (Hankinson et al. 1998, Li et al. 2001, Endogenous Hormones Breast Cancer Collaborative Group et al. 2010). Nevertheless, it should be noted that both of the studies done to date, assessing the effect of GI and/or GL on the IGF system, have been conducted in healthy individuals, and therefore, results may not be directly applicable to a population with breast cancer.

7.4.3 Cancer and Oxidative Stress

Damage to DNA by reactive metabolites has been widely accepted as a major cause of cancer (Ames and Gold 1991, Beckman and Ames 1997, Halliwell 2007). Oxidative stress can activate a variety of transcription factors, including NF-κB, AP-1, p53, HIF-1α, PPAR-γ, β-catenin/Wnt, and Nrf2, leading to the expression of more than 500 different genes, including those for growth factors, inflammatory cytokines, chemokines, cell cycle regulatory molecules, and anti-inflammatory molecules (Reuter et al. 2010). Activation of these inflammatory pathways via oxidative damage has been implicated in the initiation, promotion, and progression of a normal cell into a tumor cell (Valko et al. 2007, Reuter et al. 2010).

7.4.4 Dietary Glycemic Index and Glycemic Load and Oxidative Stress

Consumption of high-GI foods have been suggested to increase oxidative stress through the formation of free radicals that are capable of damaging biological molecules and hence initiating abnormal cell growth through gene mutation; however, few studies have examined the relationship between GI, GL, and oxidative stress in humans.

Studies have indicated that hyperglycemia contributes to increased oxidative stress through an incremental generation of reactive oxygen species during the mitochondrial oxidative metabolism of carbohydrates, which depletes antioxidant defenses, for example, by glycation of antioxidant enzymes (Ceriello et al. 1998, Title et al. 2000, Brownlee 2005). Reducing the GI of a meal using acarbose has been shown to significantly reduce markers of oxidative stress in individuals with impaired glucose tolerance (Quagliaro et al. 2005, Inoue et al. 2006, Monnier et al. 2006). Furthermore, studies by Monnier et al. (2006) and Quagliaro et al. (2005) suggested that the greater the amplitude of glucose excursions, the more rapid the rate of oxidative stress, implying that higher-GI foods would increase oxidative stress further by virtue of their greater glycemic fluctuations. Some initial evidence supports this hypothesis because consumption of a low-GI diet for 1 week was associated with an increased plasma total antioxidant capacity compared with a high-GI diet (Botero et al. 2009). Arikawa et al. (2015) recently conducted a study in 306 healthy premenopausal women, assessing F_2-isoprostanes, the markers of oxidative stress. It was shown that plasma F_2-isoprostanes increased with each quartile of GL ($p = .033$) and also increased with each quartile of GI in participants with BMI of 25 or more ($p = .035$) but not in those with BMI less than 25 ($p = .924$) (Arikawa et al. 2015). Thus, in overweight and obese, the GI and GL statuses of the diet were suggested to influence oxidative status.

7.5 CONCLUSIONS AND FUTURE DIRECTIONS

Carbohydrates with a slow absorption rate (e.g., most low-GI foods) have been associated with several health benefits, including improved blood glucose control and reduced insulin demand, inflammatory factors, and blood lipid concentrations, all of which may play important roles in the prevention and management of several chronic diseases, including cancer. On the other hand, high-GI foods result in higher blood glucose concentration and hence greater insulin demand. In an environment characterized by sedentary behavior, overeating, and obesity, higher circulating blood glucose as a result of high-GI food intake could represent a greater burden for an already-stressed metabolism caused by obesity and lack of physical activity. Lowering the GI of foods may therefore be particularly relevant in affluent societies, considering that the metabolic syndrome has a 34% prevalence in the U.S. adult population (Ervin 2009), as it is becoming a health concern in developing countries and represents a major risk factor for CHD, T2DM (Janghorbani et al. 2012), and possibly cancer (Bhandari et al. 2014). Furthermore, a lower dietary GI may be particularly relevant in countries with high consumption of dietary carbohydrates as in the Mediterranean region.

With regard to the prevention of cancer recurrence (secondary prevention), the guidelines for cancer survivors by the American Cancer Society include foremost maintaining healthy body weight, engaging in physical activity, and consuming a healthy diet, which are consistent with guidelines for cancer and heart disease prevention (Kushi et al. 2012). However, there is no mention of carbohydrate quality, beyond whole grains, with regard to longer survival. At present, there is a lack of clinical trials that investigate possible beneficial effects of low-GI diets in secondary cancer prevention. There is a need for clinical trials in which cancer patients are randomized to follow a healthy high- or low-GI diet and those with end points inclusive of cancer recurrence, disease-free survival, response to cancer therapy, incidence of new T2DM and CVD, and management of cardiometabolic risk factors. Nevertheless, when summarizing the mechanistic evidence for linking glycemia to carcinogenesis and the evidence from primary prevention studies, there is a general support for cancer-protecting effects of lower fluctuations of blood glucose and insulin (Rock et al. 2012) and hence potentially for low-GI diets. Considering the longer survival of people diagnosed with cancer and therefore their potential risk of developing or worsening other chronic conditions such as T2DM, where low-GI diets proved largely beneficial, the inclusion in cancer guidelines for a preference of low-GI whole grains and low-GI carbohydrates, in general, could be a sensible decision.

REFERENCES

Amadou, A., J. Degoul, P. Hainaut, V. Chajes, C. Biessy, G. Torres Mejia, I. Huybrechts et al. 2015. Dietary carbohydrate, glycemic index, glycemic load, and breast cancer risk among Mexican women. *Epidemiology* 26(6): 917–924. doi: 10.1097/EDE.0000000000000374.

American Cancer Society. 2013. *Cancer Facts & Figures 2013*. American Cancer Society Inc., Atlanta, GA.

American Cancer Society. 2015a. *Breast Cancer: Causes, Risk Factors and Prevention Topics*. American Cancer Society Inc., Atlanta, GA. http://www.cancer.org/cancer/breastcancer/detailedguide/breast-cancer-risk-factors. (Accessed August 18, 2015.)

American Cancer Society. 2015b. *Liver Cancer*. American Cancer Society Inc., Atlanta, GA. http://www.cancer.org/cancer/livercancer/detailedguide/liver-cancer-what-is-key-statistics. (Accessed January 13, 2015.)

American Cancer Society. 2015c. *Pancreatic Cancer*. American Cancer Society Inc., Atlanta, GA. http://www.cancer.org/cancer/pancreaticcancer/detailedguide/pancreatic-cancer-key-statistics. (Accessed January 9, 2015.)

American Cancer Society. 2015d. *Prostate Cancer*. American Cancer Society Inc., Atlanta, GA. http://www.cancer.org/cancer/prostatecancer/detailedguide/prostate-cancer-risk-factors. (Accessed March 12, 2015.)

Ames, B. N. and L. S. Gold. 1991. Endogenous mutagens and the causes of aging and cancer. *Mutat Res* 250(1–2):3–16.

Arikawa, A. Y., H. E. Jakits, A. Flood, W. Thomas, M. Gross, K. H. Schmitz, and M. S. Kurzer. 2015. Consumption of a high glycemic load but not a high glycemic index diet is marginally associated with oxidative stress in young women. *Nutr Res* 35(1):7–13. doi: 10.1016/j.nutres.2014.10.005.

Armstrong, B. and R. Doll. 1975. Environmental factors and cancer incidence and mortality in different countries, with special reference to dietary practices. *Int J Cancer* 15(4):617–631.

Atkinson, F. S., K. Foster-Powell, and J. C. Brand-Miller. 2008. International tables of glycemic index and glycemic load values: 2008. *Diabetes Care* 31(12):2281–2283. doi: 10.2337/dc08-1239.

Augustin, L. S., L. Dal Maso, C. La Vecchia, M. Parpinel, E. Negri, S. Vaccarella, C. W. Kendall, D. J. Jenkins, and S. Franceschi. 2001. Dietary glycemic index and glycemic load, and breast cancer risk: A case-control study. *Ann Oncol* 12(11):1533–1538.

Augustin, L. S., S. Franceschi, D. J. Jenkins, C. W. Kendall, and C. La Vecchia. 2002. Glycemic index in chronic disease: A review. *Eur J Clin Nutr* 56(11):1049–1071. doi: 10.1038/sj.ejcn.1601454.

Augustin, L. S., S. Gallus, C. Bosetti, F. Levi, E. Negri, S. Franceschi, L. Dal Maso, D. J. Jenkins, C. W. Kendall, and C. La Vecchia. 2003a. Glycemic index and glycemic load in endometrial cancer. *Int J Cancer* 105(3):404–407. doi: 10.1002/ijc.11089.

Augustin, L. S., S. Malerba, A. Lugo, S. Franceschi, R. Talamini, D. Serraino, D. J. Jenkins, and C. La Vecchia. 2013. Associations of bread and pasta with the risk of cancer of the breast and colorectum. *Ann Oncol* 24(12):3094–3099. doi: 10.1093/annonc/mdt383.

Augustin, L. S., J. Polesel, C. Bosetti, C. W. Kendall, C. La Vecchia, M. Parpinel, E. Conti et al. 2003b. Dietary glycemic index, glycemic load and ovarian cancer risk: A case-control study in Italy. *Ann Oncol* 14(1):78–84.

Aune, D., D. S. Chan, R. Lau, R. Vieira, D. C. Greenwood, E. Kampman, and T. Norat. 2012a. Carbohydrates, glycemic index, glycemic load, and colorectal cancer risk: A systematic review and meta-analysis of cohort studies. *Cancer Causes Control* 23(4):521–535. doi: 10.1007/s10552-012-9918-9.

Aune, D., D. S. Chan, A. R. Vieira, D. A. Navarro Rosenblatt, R. Vieira, D. C. Greenwood, J. E. Cade, V. J. Burley, and T. Norat. 2012b. Dietary fructose, carbohydrates, glycemic indices and pancreatic cancer risk: a systematic review and meta-analysis of cohort studies. *Ann Oncol* 23(10):2536–2546. doi: 10.1093/annonc/mds076.

Bagnardi, V., M. Rota, E. Botteri, I. Tramacere, F. Islami, V. Fedirko, L. Scotti et al. 2015. Alcohol consumption and site-specific cancer risk: A comprehensive dose-response meta-analysis. *Br J Cancer* 112(3):580–593. doi: 10.1038/bjc.2014.579.

Barclay, A. W., P. Petocz, J. McMillan-Price, V. M. Flood, T. Prvan, P. Mitchell, and J. C. Brand-Miller. 2008. Glycemic index, glycemic load, and chronic disease risk—a meta-analysis of observational studies. *Am J Clin Nutr* 87(3):627–637.

Becker, S., L. Dossus, and R. Kaaks. 2009. Obesity related hyperinsulinaemia and hyperglycaemia and cancer development. *Arch Physiol Biochem* 115(2):86–96. doi: 10.1080/13813450902878054.

Beckman, K. B. and B. N. Ames. 1997. Oxidative decay of DNA. *J Biol Chem* 272(32):19633–19636.

Belle, F. N., E. Kampman, A. McTiernan, L. Bernstein, K. Baumgartner, R. Baumgartner, A. Ambs, R. Ballard-Barbash, and M. L. Neuhouser. 2011. Dietary fiber, carbohydrates, glycemic index, and glycemic load in relation to breast cancer prognosis in the HEAL cohort. *Cancer Epidemiol Biomarkers Prev* 20(5):890–899. doi: 10.1158/1055-9965.EPI-10-1278.

Bhandari, R., G. A. Kelley, T. A. Hartley, and I. R. Rockett. 2014. Metabolic syndrome is associated with increased breast cancer risk: A systematic review with meta-analysis. *Int J Breast Cancer* 2014:189384. doi: 10.1155/2014/189384.

Biddinger, S. B. and D. S. Ludwig. 2005. The insulin-like growth factor axis: A potential link between glycemic index and cancer. *Am J Clin Nutr* 82(2):277–278.

Boas, J. 1903. Ueber carcinom und diabetes. *Berlin Klin. Wschr* 40:243–247.

Bosetti, C., M. Filomeno, P. Riso, J. Polesel, F. Levi, R. Talamini, M. Montella, E. Negri, S. Franceschi, and C. La Vecchia. 2012a. Cruciferous vegetables and cancer risk in a network of case-control studies. *Ann Oncol* 23(8):2198–2203. doi: 10.1093/annonc/mdr604.

Bosetti, C., S. Gallus, R. Peto, E. Negri, R. Talamini, A. Tavani, S. Franceschi, and C. La Vecchia. 2008. Tobacco smoking, smoking cessation, and cumulative risk of upper aerodigestive tract cancers. *Am J Epidemiol* 167(4):468–473. doi: 10.1093/aje/kwm318.

Bosetti, C., V. Rosato, J. Polesel, F. Levi, R. Talamini, M. Montella, E. Negri et al. 2012b. Diabetes mellitus and cancer risk in a network of case-control studies. *Nutr Cancer* 64(5):643–651. doi: 10.1080/01635581.2012.676141.

Bostick, R. M., J. D. Potter, L. H. Kushi, T. A. Sellers, K. A. Steinmetz, D. R. McKenzie, S. M. Gapstur, and A. R. Folsom. 1994. Sugar, meat, and fat intake, and non-dietary risk factors for colon cancer incidence in Iowa women (United States). *Cancer Causes Control* 5(1):38–52.

Botero, D., C. B. Ebbeling, J. B. Blumberg, J. D. Ribaya-Mercado, M. A. Creager, J. F. Swain, H. A. Feldman, and D. S. Ludwig. 2009. Acute effects of dietary glycemic index on antioxidant capacity in a nutrient-controlled feeding study. *Obesity (Silver Spring)* 17(9):1664–1670. doi: 10.1038/oby.2009.203.

Boyle, P. and J. S. Langman. 2000. ABC of colorectal cancer: Epidemiology. *BMJ* 321(7264):805–808.

Boyle, P., A. Koechlin, C. Pizot, M. Boniol, C. Robertson, P. Mullie, G. Bolli, J. Rosenstock, and P. Autier. 2013. Blood glucose concentrations and breast cancer risk in women without diabetes: A meta-analysis. *Eur J Nutr* 52(5):1533–1540. doi: 10.1007/s00394-012-0460-z.

Brand-Miller, J. C. 2004. Postprandial glycemia, glycemic index, and the prevention of type 2 diabetes. *Am J Clin Nutr* 80(2):243–244.

Brand-Miller, J. C., V. Liu, P. Petocz, and R. C. Baxter. 2005. The glycemic index of foods influences postprandial insulin-like growth factor-binding protein responses in lean young subjects. *Am J Clin Nutr* 82(2):350–354.

Brownlee, M. 2005. The pathobiology of diabetic complications: A unifying mechanism. *Diabetes* 54(6):1615–1625.

Byrnes, S. E., J. C. Miller, and G. S. Denyer. 1995. Amylopectin starch promotes the development of insulin resistance in rats. *J Nutr* 125(6):1430–1437.

Campbell, P. T., C. C. Newton, A. V. Patel, E. J. Jacobs, and S. M. Gapstur. 2012. Diabetes and cause-specific mortality in a prospective cohort of one million U.S. adults. *Diabetes Care* 35(9):1835–1844. doi: 10.2337/dc12-0002.

Castagnetta, L. A., M. D. Miceli, C. M. Sorci, U. Pfeffer, R. Farruggio, G. Oliveri, M. Calabro, and G. Carruba. 1995. Growth of LNCaP human prostate cancer cells is stimulated by estradiol via its own receptor. *Endocrinology* 136(5):2309–2319. doi: 10.1210/endo.136.5.7536668.

Centres for Disease Control and Prevention (CDC). 2014. *Colorectal (Colon) Cancer: What are the Risk Factors for Colorectal Cancer*? http://www.cdc.gov/cancer/colorectal/basic_info/risk_factors.htm. (Accessed December 1, 2014.)

Ceriello, A., N. Bortolotti, A. Crescentini, E. Motz, S. Lizzio, A. Russo, Z. Ezsol, L. Tonutti, and C. Taboga. 1998. Antioxidant defences are reduced during the oral glucose tolerance test in normal and non-insulin-dependent diabetic subjects. *Eur J Clin Invest* 28(4):329–333.

Chlebowski, R. T., G. L. Blackburn, C. A. Thomson, D. W. Nixon, A. Shapiro, M. K. Hoy, M. T. Goodman et al. 2006. Dietary fat reduction and breast cancer outcome: Interim efficacy results from the Women's Intervention Nutrition Study. *J Natl Cancer Inst* 98(24):1767–1776. doi: 10.1093/jnci/djj494.

Cho, E., D. Spiegelman, D. J. Hunter, W. Y. Chen, G. A. Colditz, and W. C. Willett. 2003. Premenopausal dietary carbohydrate, glycemic index, glycemic load, and fiber in relation to risk of breast cancer. *Cancer Epidemiol Biomarkers Prev* 12(11 Pt 1):1153–1158.

Choi, Y., E. Giovannucci, and J. E. Lee. 2012. Glycaemic index and glycaemic load in relation to risk of diabetes-related cancers: A meta-analysis. *Br J Nutr* 108(11):1934–1947. doi: 10.1017/S0007114512003984.

Chyou, P. H., A. M. Nomura, and G. N. Stemmermann. 1996. A prospective study of colon and rectal cancer among Hawaii Japanese men. *Ann Epidemiol* 6(4):276–282.

Coleman, H. G., C. M. Kitahara, L. J. Murray, K. W. Dodd, A. Black, R. Z. Stolzenberg-Solomon, and M. M. Cantwell. 2014. Dietary carbohydrate intake, glycemic index, and glycemic load and endometrial cancer risk: A prospective cohort study. *Am J Epidemiol* 179(1):75–84. doi: 10.1093/aje/kwt222.

Crawley, D. J., L. Holmberg, J. C. Melvin, M. Loda, S. Chowdhury, S. M. Rudman, and M. Van Hemelrijck. 2014. Serum glucose and risk of cancer: A meta-analysis. *BMC Cancer* 14:985. doi: 10.1186/1471-2407-14-985.

Cui, X., B. Rosner, W. C. Willett, and S. E. Hankinson. 2011. Dietary fat, fiber, and carbohydrate intake in relation to risk of endometrial cancer. *Cancer Epidemiol Biomarkers Prev* 20(5):978–989. doi: 10.1158/1055-9965.EPI-10-1089.

de Beer, J. C. and L. Liebenberg. 2014. Does cancer risk increase with HbA1c, independent of diabetes? *Br J Cancer* 110(9):2361–2368. doi: 10.1038/bjc.2014.150.

Doll, R. and R. Peto. 1981. The causes of cancer: Quantitative estimates of avoidable risks of cancer in the United States today. *J Natl Cancer Inst* 66(6):1191–1308.

Dong, J. Y. and L. Q. Qin. 2011. Dietary glycemic index, glycemic load, and risk of breast cancer: Meta-analysis of prospective cohort studies. *Breast Cancer Res Treat* 126(2):287–294. doi: 10.1007/s10549-011-1343-3.

Dunn, S. E., F. W. Kari, J. French, J. R. Leininger, G. Travlos, R. Wilson, and J. C. Barrett. 1997. Dietary restriction reduces insulin-like growth factor I levels, which modulates apoptosis, cell proliferation, and tumor progression in p53-deficient mice. *Cancer Res* 57(21):4667–4672.

Ekbom, A. and D. Hunter. 2012. Pancreatic cancer. In *Cancer Epidemiology*, edited by H. Adami, D. Hunter, and D. Trichopoulos. New York, NY: Oxford University Press.

Ellinger, F. and H. Landsman. 1994. Frequency and course of cancer in diabetics. *NY State J Med* 44:259–265.

Endogenous Hormones Breast Cancer Collaborative Group, T. J. Key, P. N. Appleby, G. K. Reeves, and A. W. Roddam. 2010. Insulin-like growth factor 1 (IGF1), IGF binding protein 3 (IGFBP3), and breast cancer risk: Pooled individual data analysis of 17 prospective studies. *Lancet Oncol* 11(6):530–542. doi: 10.1016/S1470 - 2045(10)70095-4.

Ervin, R. B. 2009. Prevalence of metabolic syndrome among adults 20 years of age and over, by sex, age, race and ethnicity, and body mass index: United States, 2003–2006. *Natl Health Stat Report* (13):1–7.

Fais, S., G. Venturi, and B. Gatenby. 2014. Microenvironmental acidosis in carcinogenesis and metastases: New strategies in prevention and therapy. *Cancer Metastasis Rev* 33(4):1095–1108. doi: 10.1007/s10555-014-9531-3.

Fan, J., Y. Song, Y. Wang, R. Hui, and W. Zhang. 2012. Dietary glycemic index, glycemic load, and risk of coronary heart disease, stroke, and stroke mortality: A systematic review with meta-analysis. *PLoS One* 7(12):e52182. doi: 10.1371/journal.pone.0052182.

Farvid, M. S., A. H. Eliassen, E. Cho, W. Y. Chen, and W. C. Willett. 2015. Adolescent and early adulthood dietary carbohydrate quantity and quality in relation to breast cancer risk. *Cancer Epidemiol Biomarkers Prev* 24(7):1111–1120. doi: 10.1158/1055-9965.EPI-14-1401.

Favero, A., S. Salvini, A. Russo, M. Parpinel, E. Negri, A. Decarli, C. La Vecchia, A. Giacosa, and S. Franceschi. 1997. Sources of macro- and micronutrients in Italian women: Results from a food frequency questionnaire for cancer studies. *Eur J Cancer Prev* 6(3):277–287.

Ferlay, J., D. M. Parkin, and E. Steliarova-Foucher. 2010. Estimates of cancer incidence and mortality in Europe in 2008. *Eur J Cancer* 46(4):765–781. doi: 10.1016/j.ejca.2009.12.014.

Ferlay, J., I. Soerjomataram, M. Ervik, R. Dikshit, S. Eser, C. Mathers, M. Rebelo, D. M. Parkin, D. Forman, and F. Bray. 2014. GLOBOCAN 2012 v1.1, Cancer Incidence and Mortality Worldwide: IARC CancerBase No. 11. International Agency for Research on Cancer. http://globocan.iarc.fr. (Accessed June 16, 2016.)

Foster-Powell, K., S. H. Holt, and J. C. Brand-Miller. 2002. International table of glycemic index and glycemic load values: 2002. *Am J Clin Nutr* 76(1):5–56.

Franceschi, S., L. Dal Maso, L. Augustin, E. Negri, M. Parpinel, P. Boyle, D. J. Jenkins, and C. La Vecchia. 2001. Dietary glycemic load and colorectal cancer risk. *Ann Oncol* 12(2):173–178.

Franceschi, S., A. Favero, C. La Vecchia, E. Negri, E. Conti, M. Montella, A. Giacosa, O. Nanni, and A. Decarli. 1997. Food groups and risk of colorectal cancer in Italy. *Int J Cancer* 72(1):56–61.

Franciosi, C. M., M. G. Piacentini, M. Conti, F. Romano, F. Musco, R. Caprotti, F. Rovelli, and F. Uggeri. 2003. IGF-1 and IGF-1BP3 in gastric adenocarcinoma. Preliminary study. *Hepatogastroenterology* 50(49):297–300.

Frasca, F., G. Pandini, L. Sciacca, V. Pezzino, S. Squatrito, A. Belfiore, and R. Vigneri. 2008. The role of insulin receptors and IGF-I receptors in cancer and other diseases. *Arch Physiol Biochem* 114(1):23–37. doi: 10.1080/13813450801969715.

Freund, E. 1885. Zur diagnose des carcinoms. *Wien Med Blat* 8:268–269.

Friedenreich, C., A. Cust, P. H. Lahmann, K. Steindorf, M. C. Boutron-Ruault, F. Clavel-Chapelon, S. Mesrine et al. 2007. Anthropometric factors and risk of endometrial cancer: The European prospective investigation into cancer and nutrition. *Cancer Causes Control* 18(4):399–413. doi: 10.1007/s10552-006-0113-8.

Frost, G., A. A. Leeds, C. J. Dore, S. Madeiros, S. Brading, and A. Dornhorst. 1999. Glycaemic index as a determinant of serum HDL-cholesterol concentration. *Lancet* 353(9158):1045–1048.

Furberg, A. S. and I. Thune. 2003. Metabolic abnormalities (hypertension, hyperglycemia and overweight), lifestyle (high energy intake and physical inactivity) and endometrial cancer risk in a Norwegian cohort. *Int J Cancer* 104(6):669–676. doi: 10.1002/ijc.10974.

Galeone, C., L. S. Augustin, M. Filomeno, S. Malerba, A. Zucchetto, C. Pelucchi, M. Montella, R. Talamini, S. Franceschi, and C. La Vecchia. 2013. Dietary glycemic index, glycemic load, and the risk of endometrial cancer: a case-control study and meta-analysis. *Eur J Cancer Prev* 22(1):38–45. doi: 10.1097/CEJ.0b013e328354d378.

George, S. M., S. T. Mayne, M. F. Leitzmann, Y. Park, A. Schatzkin, A. Flood, A. Hollenbeck, and A. F. Subar. 2009. Dietary glycemic index, glycemic load, and risk of cancer: A prospective cohort study. *Am J Epidemiol* 169(4):462–472. doi: 10.1093/aje/kwn347.

Gillies, R. J., I. Robey, and R. A. Gatenby. 2008. Causes and consequences of increased glucose metabolism of cancers. *J Nucl Med* 49(Suppl 2):24S–42S. doi: 10.2967/jnumed.107.047258.

Giovannucci, E. 1995. Insulin and colon cancer. *Cancer Causes Control* 6(2):164–179.

Giovannucci, E. 2001. Insulin, insulin-like growth factors and colon cancer: A review of the evidence. *J Nutr* 131(11 Suppl):3109S–3120S.

Giovannucci, E. 2003. Nutrition, insulin, insulin-like growth factors and cancer. *Horm Metab Res* 35(11–12):694–704. doi: 10.1055/s-2004-814147.

Giovannucci, E., D. M. Harlan, M. C. Archer, R. M. Bergenstal, S. M. Gapstur, L. A. Habel, M. Pollak, J. G. Regensteiner, and D. Yee. 2010. Diabetes and cancer: A consensus report. *Diabetes Care* 33(7):1674–1685. doi: 10.2337/dc10-0666.

Gnagnarella, P., S. Gandini, C. La Vecchia, and P. Maisonneuve. 2008. Glycemic index, glycemic load, and cancer risk: a meta-analysis. *Am J Clin Nutr* 87(6):1793–1801.

Halliwell, B. 2007. Oxidative stress and cancer: Have we moved forward? *Biochem J* 401(1):1–11. doi: 10.1042/BJ20061131.

Hanefeld, M., C. Koehler, K. Fuecker, E. Henkel, F. Schaper, T. Temelkova-Kurktschiev, and Atherosclerosis Impaired Glucose Tolerance for, and study Diabetes. 2003. Insulin secretion and insulin sensitivity pattern is different in isolated impaired glucose tolerance and impaired fasting glucose: The risk factor in Impaired Glucose Tolerance for Atherosclerosis and Diabetes study. *Diabetes Care* 26(3):868–874.

Hankinson, S. E., W. C. Willett, G. A. Colditz, D. J. Hunter, D. S. Michaud, B. Deroo, B. Rosner, F. E. Speizer, and M. Pollak. 1998. Circulating concentrations of insulin-like growth factor-I and risk of breast cancer. *Lancet* 351(9113):1393–1396. doi: 10.1016/S0140-6736(97)10384-1.

Hardiman, P., O. C. Pillay, and W. Atiomo. 2003. Polycystic ovary syndrome and endometrial carcinoma. *Lancet* 361(9371):1810–1812.

Higginbotham, S., Z. F. Zhang, I. M. Lee, N. R. Cook, J. E. Buring, and S. Liu. 2004a. Dietary glycemic load and breast cancer risk in the Women's Health Study. *Cancer Epidemiol Biomarkers Prev* 13(1):65–70.

Higginbotham, S., Z. F. Zhang, I. M. Lee, N. R. Cook, E. Giovannucci, J. E. Buring, S. Liu, and Study Women's Health. 2004b. Dietary glycemic load and risk of colorectal cancer in the Women's Health Study. *J Natl Cancer Inst* 96(3):229–233.

Holt, S. H., J. C. Miller, and P. Petocz. 1997. An insulin index of foods: The insulin demand generated by 1000-kJ portions of common foods. *Am J Clin Nutr* 66(5):1264–1276.

Howarth, N. C., S. P. Murphy, L. R. Wilkens, B. E. Henderson, and L. N. Kolonel. 2008. The association of glycemic load and carbohydrate intake with colorectal cancer risk in the Multiethnic Cohort Study. *Am J Clin Nutr* 88(4):1074–1082.

Hu, J., C. La Vecchia, L. S. Augustin, E. Negri, M. de Groh, H. Morrison, and L. Mery. 2013. Glycemic index, glycemic load and cancer risk. *Ann Oncol* 24(1):245–251. doi: 10.1093/annonc/mds235.

Inoue, I., Y. Shinoda, T. Nakano, M. Sassa, S. Goto, T. Awata, T. Komoda, and S. Katayama. 2006. Acarbose ameliorates atherogenecity of low-density lipoprotein in patients with impaired glucose tolerance. *Metabolism* 55(7):946–952. doi: 10.1016/j.metabol.2006.03.002.

Jain, M. G., T. E. Rohan, G. R. Howe, and A. B. Miller. 2000. A cohort study of nutritional factors and endometrial cancer. *Eur J Epidemiol* 16(10):899–905.

Janghorbani, M., M. Dehghani, and M. Salehi-Marzijarani. 2012. Systematic review and meta-analysis of insulin therapy and risk of cancer. *Horm Cancer* 3(4):137–146. doi: 10.1007/s12672-012-0112-z.

Jee, S. H., H. Ohrr, J. W. Sull, J. E. Yun, M. Ji, and J. M. Samet. 2005. Fasting serum glucose level and cancer risk in Korean men and women. *JAMA* 293(2):194–202. doi: 10.1001/jama.293.2.194.

Jemal, A., F. Bray, M. M. Center, J. Ferlay, E. Ward, and D. Forman. 2011. Global cancer statistics. *CA Cancer J Clin* 61(2):69–90. doi: 10.3322/caac.20107.

Jenkins, D. J., T. M. Wolever, G. R. Collier, A. Ocana, A. V. Rao, G. Buckley, Y. Lam, A. Mayer, and L. U. Thompson. 1987. Metabolic effects of a low-glycemic-index diet. *Am J Clin Nutr* 46(6):968–975.

Jenkins, D. J., T. M. Wolever, R. H. Taylor, H. Barker, H. Fielden, J. M. Baldwin, A. C. Bowling, H. C. Newman, A. L. Jenkins, and D. V. Goff. 1981. Glycemic index of foods: A physiological basis for carbohydrate exchange. *Am J Clin Nutr* 34(3):362–366.

Jerome, L., L. Shiry, and B. Leyland-Jones. 2003. Deregulation of the IGF axis in cancer: Epidemiological evidence and potential therapeutic interventions. *Endocr Relat Cancer* 10(4):561–578.

Joshu, C. E., A. E. Prizment, P. J. Dluzniewski, A. Menke, A. R. Folsom, J. Coresh, H. C. Yeh, F. L. Brancati, E. A. Platz, and E. Selvin. 2012. Glycated hemoglobin and cancer incidence and mortality in the Atherosclerosis in Communities (ARIC) Study, 1990 - 2006. *Int J Cancer* 131(7):1667–1677. doi: 10.1002/ijc.27394.

Kaaks, R. and A. Lukanova. 2001. Energy balance and cancer: The role of insulin and insulin-like growth factor-I. *Proc Nutr Soc* 60(1):91–106.

Kaaks, R., A. Lukanova, and M. S. Kurzer. 2002. Obesity, endogenous hormones, and endometrial cancer risk: A synthetic review. *Cancer Epidemiol Biomarkers Prev* 11(12):1531–1543.

Kabat, G. C., J. M. Shikany, S. A. Beresford, B. Caan, M. L. Neuhouser, L. F. Tinker, and T. E. Rohan. 2008. Dietary carbohydrate, glycemic index, and glycemic load in relation to colorectal cancer risk in the Women's Health Initiative. *Cancer Causes Control* 19(10):1291–1298. doi: 10.1007/s10552-008-9200-3.

Kalli, K. R. and C. A. Conover. 2003. The insulin-like growth factor/insulin system in epithelial ovarian cancer. *Front Biosci* 8:d714–d722.

Kato, I., A. Akhmedkhanov, K. Koenig, P. G. Toniolo, R. E. Shore, and E. Riboli. 1997. Prospective study of diet and female colorectal cancer: The New York University Women's Health Study. *Nutr Cancer* 28(3):276–281. doi: 10.1080/01635589709514588.

King, H., J. Y. Li, F. B. Locke, E. S. Pollack, and J. T. Tu. 1985. Patterns of site-specific displacement in cancer mortality among migrants: the Chinese in the United States. *Am J Public Health* 75(3):237–242.

Kolonel, L. N. 1980. Cancer patterns of four ethnic groups in Hawaii. *J Natl Cancer Inst* 65(5):1127–1139.

Kono, S. 2004. Secular trend of colon cancer incidence and mortality in relation to fat and meat intake in Japan. *Eur J Cancer Prev* 13(2):127–132.

Kritchevsky, D. 2003. Diet and cancer: What's next? *J Nutr* 133(11 Suppl 1):3827S–3829S.

Kubo, A., D. A. Corley, C. D. Jensen, and R. Kaur. 2010. Dietary factors and the risks of oesophageal adenocarcinoma and Barrett's oesophagus. *Nutr Res Rev* 23(2):230–246. doi: 10.1017/S0954422410000132.

Kushi, L. H., C. Doyle, M. McCullough, C. L. Rock, W. Demark-Wahnefried, E. V. Bandera, S. Gapstur, A. V. Patel, K. Andrews, T. Gansler, Nutrition American Cancer Society, and Committee Physical Activity Guidelines Advisory. 2012. American Cancer Society Guidelines on nutrition and physical activity for cancer prevention: reducing the risk of cancer with healthy food choices and physical activity. *CA Cancer J Clin* 62(1):30–67. doi: 10.3322/caac.20140.

Lagiou, P., M. Rossi, A. Tzonou, C. Georgila, D. Trichopoulos, and C. La Vecchia. 2009. Glycemic load in relation to hepatocellular carcinoma among patients with chronic hepatitis infection. *Ann Oncol* 20(10):1741–1745. doi: 10.1093/annonc/mdp059.

Lajous, M., M. C. Boutron-Ruault, A. Fabre, F. Clavel-Chapelon, and I. Romieu. 2008. Carbohydrate intake, glycemic index, glycemic load, and risk of postmenopausal breast cancer in a prospective study of French women. *Am J Clin Nutr* 87(5):1384–1391.

Larsson, S. C., L. Bergkvist, and A. Wolk. 2006. Glycemic load, glycemic index and carbohydrate intake in relation to risk of stomach cancer: A prospective study. *Int J Cancer* 118(12):3167–3169. doi: 10.1002/ijc.21753.

Larsson, S. C., L. Bergkvist, and A. Wolk. 2009. Glycemic load, glycemic index and breast cancer risk in a prospective cohort of Swedish women. *Int J Cancer* 125(1):153–157. doi: 10.1002/ijc.24310.

Larsson, S. C., E. Giovannucci, and A. Wolk. 2007a. Dietary carbohydrate, glycemic index, and glycemic load in relation to risk of colorectal cancer in women. *Am J Epidemiol* 165(3):256–261. doi: 10.1093/aje/kwk012.

Larsson, S. C., C. S. Mantzoros, and A. Wolk. 2007b. Diabetes mellitus and risk of breast cancer: A meta-analysis. *Int J Cancer* 121(4):856–862. doi: 10.1002/ijc.22717.

Li, B. D., M. J. Khosravi, H. J. Berkel, A. Diamandi, M. A. Dayton, M. Smith, and H. Yu. 2001. Free insulin-like growth factor-I and breast cancer risk. *Int J Cancer* 91(5):736–739.

Li, H. L., G. Yang, X. O. Shu, Y. B. Xiang, W. H. Chow, B. T. Ji, X. Zhang et al. 2011. Dietary glycemic load and risk of colorectal cancer in Chinese women. *Am J Clin Nutr* 93(1):101–107. doi: 10.3945/ajcn.110.003053.

Li, J., J. Ma, L. Han, Q. Xu, J. Lei, W. Duan, W. Li et al. 2015. Hyperglycemic tumor microenvironment induces perineural invasion in pancreatic cancer. *Cancer Biol Ther* 16(6):912–921. doi: 10.1080/15384047.2015.1040952.

Liao, W. C., Y. K. Tu, M. S. Wu, J. T. Lin, H. P. Wang, and K. L. Chien. 2015. Blood glucose concentration and risk of pancreatic cancer: Systematic review and dose-response meta-analysis. *BMJ* 349:g7371. doi: 10.1136/bmj.g7371.

Liu, X., J. Ji, K. Sundquist, J. Sundquist, and K. Hemminki. 2012. Mortality causes in cancer patients with type 2 diabetes mellitus. *Eur J Cancer Prev* 21(3):300–306. doi: 10.1097/CEJ.0b013e32834c9cd9.

Liu, S., J. E. Manson, J. E. Buring, M. J. Stampfer, W. C. Willett, and P. M. Ridker. 2002. Relation between a diet with a high glycemic load and plasma concentrations of high-sensitivity C-reactive protein in middle-aged women. *Am J Clin Nutr* 75(3):492–498.

Liu, S., J. E. Manson, M. J. Stampfer, M. D. Holmes, F. B. Hu, S. E. Hankinson, and W. C. Willett. 2001. Dietary glycemic load assessed by food-frequency questionnaire in relation to plasma high-density-lipoprotein cholesterol and fasting plasma triacylglycerols in postmenopausal women. *Am J Clin Nutr* 73(3):560–566.

Liu, J., J. Wang, Y. Leng, and C. Lv. 2013. Intake of fruit and vegetables and risk of esophageal squamous cell carcinoma: A meta-analysis of observational studies. *Int J Cancer* 133(2):473–485. doi: 10.1002/ijc.28024.

Liu, S., W. C. Willett, M. J. Stampfer, F. B. Hu, M. Franz, L. Sampson, C. H. Hennekens, and J. E. Manson. 2000. A prospective study of dietary glycemic load, carbohydrate intake, and risk of coronary heart disease in US women. *Am J Clin Nutr* 71(6):1455–1461.

Livesey, G., R. Taylor, H. Livesey, and S. Liu. 2013. Is there a dose-response relation of dietary glycemic load to risk of type 2 diabetes? Meta-analysis of prospective cohort studies. *Am J Clin Nutr* 97(3):584–596. doi: 10.3945/ajcn.112.041467.

Ludwig, D. S. 2000. Dietary glycemic index and obesity. *J Nutr* 130(2S Suppl):280S–283S.

Lukanova, A. and R. Kaaks. 2005. Endogenous hormones and ovarian cancer: Epidemiology and current hypotheses. *Cancer Epidemiol Biomarkers Prev* 14(1):98–107.

Lukanova, A., A. Zeleniuch-Jacquotte, E. Lundin, A. Micheli, A. A. Arslan, S. Rinaldi, P. Muti et al. 2004. Prediagnostic levels of C-peptide, IGF-I, IGFBP-1, -2 and -3 and risk of endometrial cancer. *Int J Cancer* 108(2):262–268. doi: 10.1002/ijc.11544.

Ma, F. J., Z. B. Liu, L. Qu, S. Hao, G. Y. Liu, J. Wu, and Z. M. Shao. 2014. Impact of type 2 diabetes mellitus on the prognosis of early stage triple-negative breast cancer in People's Republic of China. *Onco Targets Ther* 7:2147–2154. doi: 10.2147/OTT.S71095.

Ma, J., E. Giovannucci, M. Pollak, A. Leavitt, Y. Tao, J. M. Gaziano, and M. J. Stampfer. 2004. A prospective study of plasma C-peptide and colorectal cancer risk in men. *J Natl Cancer Inst* 96(7):546–553.

Marble, A. 1934. Diabetes and cancer. *N Engl J Med* 211:339–349.

McCarl, M., L. Harnack, P. J. Limburg, K. E. Anderson, and A. R. Folsom. 2006. Incidence of colorectal cancer in relation to glycemic index and load in a cohort of women. *Cancer Epidemiol Biomarkers Prev* 15(5):892–896. doi: 10.1158/1055-9965.EPI-05-0700.

McCullough, M. L. and E. L. Giovannucci. 2004. Diet and cancer prevention. *Oncogene* 23 (38):6349–6364. doi: 10.1038/sj.onc.1207716.

McKeown-Eyssen, G. 1994. Epidemiology of colorectal cancer revisited: Are serum triglycerides and/or plasma glucose associated with risk? *Cancer Epidemiol Biomarkers Prev* 3(8):687–695.

Meyerhardt, J. A., K. Sato, D. Niedzwiecki, C. Ye, L. B. Saltz, R. J. Mayer, R. B. Mowat et al. 2012. Dietary glycemic load and cancer recurrence and survival in patients with stage III colon cancer: Findings from CALGB 89803. *J Natl Cancer Inst* 104(22):1702–1711. doi: 10.1093/jnci/djs399.

Michaud, D. S., C. S. Fuchs, S. Liu, W. C. Willett, G. A. Colditz, and E. Giovannucci. 2005. Dietary glycemic load, carbohydrate, sugar, and colorectal cancer risk in men and women. *Cancer Epidemiol Biomarkers Prev* 14(1):138–147.

Mirrahimi, A., R. J. de Souza, L. Chiavaroli, J. L. Sievenpiper, J. Beyene, A. J. Hanley, L. S. Augustin, C. W. Kendall, and D. J. Jenkins. 2012. Associations of glycemic index and load with coronary heart disease events: A systematic review and meta-analysis of prospective cohorts. *J Am Heart Assoc* 1(5):e000752. doi: 10.1161/JAHA.112.000752.

Monnier, L., E. Mas, C. Ginet, F. Michel, L. Villon, J. P. Cristol, and C. Colette. 2006. Activation of oxidative stress by acute glucose fluctuations compared with sustained chronic hyperglycemia in patients with type 2 diabetes. *JAMA* 295(14):1681–1687. doi: 10.1001/jama.295.14.1681.

Mulholland, H. G., L. J. Murray, C. R. Cardwell, and M. M. Cantwell. 2008a. Dietary glycaemic index, glycaemic load and breast cancer risk: A systematic review and meta-analysis. *Br J Cancer* 99(7):1170–1175. doi: 10.1038/sj.bjc.6604618.

Mulholland, H. G., L. J. Murray, C. R. Cardwell, and M. M. Cantwell. 2008b. Dietary glycaemic index, glycaemic load and endometrial and ovarian cancer risk: A systematic review and meta-analysis. *Br J Cancer* 99(3):434–441. doi: 10.1038/sj.bjc.6604496.

Mulholland, H. G., L. J. Murray, C. R. Cardwell, and M. M. Cantwell. 2009. Glycemic index, glycemic load, and risk of digestive tract neoplasms: A systematic review and meta-analysis. *Am J Clin Nutr* 89(2):568–576. doi: 10.3945/ajcn.2008.26823.

Mullie, P., A. Koechlin, M. Boniol, P. Autier, and P. Boyle. 2015. Relation between breast cancer and high glycemic index or glycemic load: A meta-analysis of prospective cohort studies. *Crit Rev Food Sci Nutr.* doi: 10.1080/10408398.2012.718723.

Nagle, C. M., C. M. Olsen, T. I. Ibiebele, A. B. Spurdle, P. M. Webb, Group Australian National Endometrial Cancer Study, and Group Australian Ovarian Cancer Study. 2013. Glycemic index, glycemic load and endometrial cancer risk: Results from the Australian National Endometrial Cancer study and an updated systematic review and meta-analysis. *Eur J Nutr* 52(2):705–715. doi: 10.1007/s00394-012-0376-7.

National Cancer Institute. 2012a. SEER Stat Fact Sheets: Ovary Cancer. National Cancer Institute: Surveillance, Epidemiology, and End Results Program. http://seer.cancer.gov/statfacts/html/ovary.html. (Accessed June 16, 2016.)

National Cancer Institute. 2012b. SEER Stat Fact Sheets: Stomach Cancer. National Cancer Institute: Surveillance, Epidemiology, and End Results Program. http://seer.cancer.gov/statfacts/html/stomach.html. (Accessed June 16, 2016.)

Neale, R. E., J. D. Doecke, N. Pandeya, S. Sadeghi, A. C. Green, P. M. Webb, D. C. Whiteman, and Study Australian Cancer. 2009. Does type 2 diabetes influence the risk of oesophageal adenocarcinoma? *Br J Cancer* 100(5):795–798. doi: 10.1038/sj.bjc.6604908.

Noto, H., A. Goto, T. Tsujimoto, and M. Noda. 2012. Cancer risk in diabetic patients treated with metformin: a systematic review and meta-analysis. *PLoS One* 7(3):e33411. doi: 10.1371/journal.pone.0033411.

Noto, H., A. Goto, T. Tsujimoto, K. Osame, and M. Noda. 2013. Latest insights into the risk of cancer in diabetes. *J Diabetes Investig* 4(3):225–232. doi: 10.1111/jdi.12068.

Oh, K., W. C. Willett, C. S. Fuchs, and E. L. Giovannucci. 2004. Glycemic index, glycemic load, and carbohydrate intake in relation to risk of distal colorectal adenoma in women. *Cancer Epidemiol Biomarkers Prev* 13(7):1192–1198.

Olivecrona, H., A. Hilding, C. Ekstrom, H. Barle, B. Nyberg, C. Moller, P. J. Delhanty et al. 1999. Acute and short-term effects of growth hormone on insulin-like growth factors and their binding proteins: Serum levels and hepatic messenger ribonucleic acid responses in humans. *J Clin Endocrinol Metab* 84(2):553–560. doi: 10.1210/jcem.84.2.5466.

Otani, T., M. Iwasaki, S. Sasazuki, M. Inoue, S. Tsugane, and Group Japan Public Health Center-based Prospective Study. 2007. Plasma C-peptide, insulin-like growth factor-I, insulin-like growth factor binding proteins and risk of colorectal cancer in a nested case-control study: The Japan public health center-based prospective study. *Int J Cancer* 120(9):2007–2012. doi: 10.1002/ijc.22556.

Pan, A., Q. Sun, A. M. Bernstein, M. B. Schulze, J. E. Manson, M. J. Stampfer, W. C. Willett, and F. B. Hu. 2012. Red meat consumption and mortality: Results from 2 prospective cohort studies. *Arch Intern Med* 172(7):555–563. doi: 10.1001/archinternmed.2011.2287.

Parkin, D. M., F. Bray, J. Ferlay, and P. Pisani. 2005. Global cancer statistics, 2002. *CA Cancer J Clin* 55(2):74–108.

Pierce, J. P., L. Natarajan, B. J. Caan, B. A. Parker, E. R. Greenberg, S. W. Flatt, C. L. Rock et al. 2007. Influence of a diet very high in vegetables, fruit, and fiber and low in fat on prognosis following treatment for breast cancer: The Women's Healthy Eating and Living (WHEL) randomized trial. *JAMA* 298(3):289–298. doi: 10.1001/jama.298.3.289.

Pisani, P. 2008. Hyper-insulinaemia and cancer, meta-analyses of epidemiological studies. *Arch Physiol Biochem* 114(1):63–70. doi: 10.1080/13813450801954451.

Pollak, M. 2001. Insulin-like growth factors and prostate cancer. *Epidemiol Rev* 23(1):59–66.

Quagliaro, L., L. Piconi, R. Assaloni, R. Da Ros, A. Maier, G. Zuodar, and A. Ceriello. 2005. Intermittent high glucose enhances ICAM-1, VCAM-1 and E-selectin expression in human umbilical vein endothelial cells in culture: The distinct role of protein kinase C and mitochondrial superoxide production. *Atherosclerosis* 183(2):259–267. doi: 10.1016/j.atherosclerosis.2005.03.015.

Rajah, R., A. Khare, P. D. Lee, and P. Cohen. 1999. Insulin-like growth factor-binding protein-3 is partially responsible for high-serum-induced apoptosis in PC-3 prostate cancer cells. *J Endocrinol* 163(3):487–494.

Rastogi, T., S. Devesa, P. Mangtani, A. Mathew, N. Cooper, R. Kao, and R. Sinha. 2008. Cancer incidence rates among South Asians in four geographic regions: India, Singapore, UK and US. *Int J Epidemiol* 37(1):147–160. doi: 10.1093/ije/dym219.

Renehan, A. G., M. Tyson, M. Egger, R. F. Heller, and M. Zwahlen. 2008. Body-mass index and incidence of cancer: A systematic review and meta-analysis of prospective observational studies. *Lancet* 371(9612):569–578. doi: 10.1016/S0140-6736(08)60269-X.

Reuter, S., S. C. Gupta, M. M. Chaturvedi, and B. B. Aggarwal. 2010. Oxidative stress, inflammation, and cancer: how are they linked? *Free Radic Biol Med* 49(11):1603–1616. doi: 10.1016/j.freeradbiomed.2010.09.006.

Robey, I. F., B. K. Baggett, N. D. Kirkpatrick, D. J. Roe, J. Dosescu, B. F. Sloane, A. I. Hashim et al. 2009. Bicarbonate increases tumor pH and inhibits spontaneous metastases. *Cancer Res* 69(6):2260–2268. doi: 10.1158/0008-5472.CAN-07-5575.

Rock, C. L., C. Doyle, W. Demark-Wahnefried, J. Meyerhardt, K. S. Courneya, A. L. Schwartz, E. V. Bandera et al. 2012. Nutrition and physical activity guidelines for cancer survivors. *CA Cancer J Clin* 62(4):243–274. doi: 10.3322/caac.21142.

Romieu, I., P. Ferrari, S. Rinaldi, N. Slimani, M. Jenab, A. Olsen, A. Tjonneland, K. Overvad et al. 2012. Dietary glycemic index and glycemic load and breast cancer risk in the European Prospective Investigation into Cancer and Nutrition (EPIC). *Am J Clin Nutr* 96(2):345–355. doi: 10.3945/ajcn.111.026724.

Rossi, M., L. Lipworth, L. D. Maso, R. Talamini, M. Montella, J. Polesel, J. K. McLaughlin et al. 2009. Dietary glycemic load and hepatocellular carcinoma with or without chronic hepatitis infection. *Ann Oncol* 20(10):1736–1740. doi: 10.1093/annonc/mdp058.

Rous, P. 1914. The influence of diet on transplanted and spontaneous mouse tumors. *J Exp Med* 20(5):433–451.

Runchey, S. S., M. N. Pollak, L. M. Valsta, G. D. Coronado, Y. Schwarz, K. L. Breymeyer, C. Wang, C. Y. Wang, J. W. Lampe, and M. L. Neuhouser. 2012. Glycemic load effect on fasting and post-prandial serum glucose, insulin, IGF-1 and IGFBP-3 in a randomized, controlled feeding study. *Eur J Clin Nutr* 66(10):1146–1152. doi: 10.1038/ejcn.2012.107.

Salmeron, J., A. Ascherio, E. B. Rimm, G. A. Colditz, D. Spiegelman, D. J. Jenkins, M. J. Stampfer, A. L. Wing, and W. C. Willett. 1997a. Dietary fiber, glycemic load, and risk of NIDDM in men. *Diabetes Care* 20(4):545–550.

Salmeron, J., J. E. Manson, M. J. Stampfer, G. A. Colditz, A. L. Wing, and W. C. Willett. 1997. Dietary fiber, glycemic load, and risk of non-insulin-dependent diabetes mellitus in women. *JAMA* 277(6):472–477.

Santarelli, R. L., F. Pierre, and D. E. Corpet. 2008. Processed meat and colorectal cancer: A review of epidemiologic and experimental evidence. *Nutr Cancer* 60(2):131–144. doi: 10.1080/01635580701684872.

Schouten, L. J., R. A. Goldbohm, and P. A. van den Brandt. 2004. Anthropometry, physical activity, and endometrial cancer risk: Results from the Netherlands Cohort Study. *J Natl Cancer Inst* 96(21):1635–1638. doi: 10.1093/jnci/djh291.

Sieri, S., V. Krogh, C. Agnoli, F. Ricceri, D. Palli, G. Masala, S. Panico et al. 2015. Dietary glycemic index and glycemic load and risk of colorectal cancer: Results from the EPIC-Italy study. *Int J Cancer* 136(12):2923–2931. doi: 10.1002/ijc.29341.

Sieri, S., V. Pala, F. Brighenti, N. Pellegrini, P. Muti, A. Micheli, A. Evangelista et al. 2007. Dietary glycemic index, glycemic load, and the risk of breast cancer in an Italian prospective cohort study. *Am J Clin Nutr* 86(4):1160–1166.

Silvera, S. A., M. Jain, G. R. Howe, A. B. Miller, and T. E. Rohan. 2007. Glycaemic index, glycaemic load and ovarian cancer risk: A prospective cohort study. *Public Health Nutr* 10(10):1076–1081. doi: 10.1017/S1368980007696360.

Silvera, S. A., T. E. Rohan, M. Jain, P. D. Terry, G. R. Howe, and A. B. Miller. 2005. Glycaemic index, glycaemic load and risk of endometrial cancer: A prospective cohort study. *Public Health Nutr* 8(7):912–919.

Slimani, N., M. Fahey, A. A. Welch, E. Wirfalt, C. Stripp, E. Bergstrom, J. Linseisen et al. 2002. Diversity of dietary patterns observed in the European Prospective Investigation into Cancer and Nutrition (EPIC) project. *Public Health Nutr* 5(6B):1311–1328. doi: 10.1079/PHN2002407.

Stattin, P., O. Bjor, P. Ferrari, A. Lukanova, P. Lenner, B. Lindahl, G. Hallmans, and R. Kaaks. 2007. Prospective study of hyperglycemia and cancer risk. *Diabetes Care* 30(3):561–567. doi: 10.2337/dc06-0922.

Stewart, B. W. and C. P. Wild (eds). 2014. International Agency for Research on Cancer. *World Cancer Report 2014*. Lyon, France.

Stewart, C. E. and P. Rotwein. 1996. Growth, differentiation, and survival: Multiple physiological functions for insulin-like growth factors. *Physiol Rev* 76(4):1005–1026.

Stocks, T., K. Rapp, T. Bjorge, J. Manjer, H. Ulmer, R. Selmer, A. Lukanova et al. 2009. Blood glucose and risk of incident and fatal cancer in the metabolic syndrome and cancer project (me-can): Analysis of six prospective cohorts. *PLoS Med* 6(12):e1000201. doi: 10.1371/journal.pmed.1000201.

Strayer, L., D. R. Jacobs, Jr., C. Schairer, A. Schatzkin, and A. Flood. 2007. Dietary carbohydrate, glycemic index, and glycemic load and the risk of colorectal cancer in the BCDDP cohort. *Cancer Causes Control* 18(8):853–863. doi: 10.1007/s10552-007-9030-8.

Terry, P. D., M. Jain, A. B. Miller, G. R. Howe, and T. E. Rohan. 2003. Glycemic load, carbohydrate intake, and risk of colorectal cancer in women: A prospective cohort study. *J Natl Cancer Inst* 95(12):914–916.

Title, L. M., P. M. Cummings, K. Giddens, and B. A. Nassar. 2000. Oral glucose loading acutely attenuates endothelium-dependent vasodilation in healthy adults without diabetes: An effect prevented by vitamins C and E. *J Am Coll Cardiol* 36(7):2185–2191.

Trinkler, N. 1890. Ueber die diagnostische Verwertung des Gehaltes an Zucker und reducirender Substanz im Blute vom Menschen bei verschiedenen Krankheiten. *Zbl. Med. Wissen* 28:498–499.

Tseng, Y. H., Y. T. Tsan, W. C. Chan, W. H. Sheu, and P. C. Chen. 2015. Use of an alpha-glucosidase inhibitor and the risk of colorectal cancer in patients with diabetes: A nationwide, population-based cohort study. *Diabetes Care*. doi: 10.2337/dc15-0563.

Turati, F., C. Galeone, S. Gandini, L. S. Augustin, D. J. Jenkins, C. Pelucchi, and C. La Vecchia. 2015a. High glycemic index and glycemic load are associated with moderately increased cancer risk. *Mol Nutr Food Res* 59(7):1384–1394. doi: 10.1002/mnfr.201400594.

Turati, F., M. Rossi, C. Pelucchi, F. Levi, and C. La Vecchia. 2015b. Fruit and vegetables and cancer risk: A review of southern European studies. *Br J Nutr* 113(Suppl 2):S102–S110. doi: 10.1017/S0007114515000148.

Udelnow, A., A. Kreyes, S. Ellinger, K. Landfester, P. Walther, T. Klapperstueck, J. Wohlrab, D. Henne-Bruns, U. Knippschild, and P. Wurl. 2011. Omeprazole inhibits proliferation and modulates autophagy in pancreatic cancer cells. *PLoS One* 6(5):e20143. doi: 10.1371/journal.pone.0020143.

Valko, M., D. Leibfritz, J. Moncol, M. T. Cronin, M. Mazur, and J. Telser. 2007. Free radicals and antioxidants in normal physiological functions and human disease. *Int J Biochem Cell Biol* 39(1):44–84. doi: 10.1016/j.biocel.2006.07.001.

Vogtmann, E., H. L. Li, X. O. Shu, W. H. Chow, B. T. Ji, H. Cai, J. Gao et al. 2013. Dietary glycemic load, glycemic index, and carbohydrates on the risk of primary liver cancer among Chinese women and men. *Ann Oncol* 24(1):238–244. doi: 10.1093/annonc/mds287.

Wang, R. J., J. E. Tang, Y. Chen, and J. G. Gao. 2015. Dietary fiber, whole grains, carbohydrate, glycemic index, and glycemic load in relation to risk of prostate cancer. *Onco Targets Ther* 8:2415–2426. doi: 10.2147/OTT.S88528.

Warburg, O. 1956. On respiratory impairment in cancer cells. *Science* 124(3215):269–270.

Weijenberg, M. P., P. F. Mullie, H. A. Brants, M. M. Heinen, R. A. Goldbohm, and P. A. van den Brandt. 2008. Dietary glycemic load, glycemic index and colorectal cancer risk: Results from the Netherlands Cohort Study. *Int J Cancer* 122(3):620–629. doi: 10.1002/ijc.23110.

Willett, W. C. 1995. Diet, nutrition, and avoidable cancer. *Environ Health Perspect* 103(Suppl 8):165–170.

Wirfalt, E., A. McTaggart, V. Pala, B. Gullberg, G. Frasca, S. Panico, H. B. Bueno-de-Mesquita et al. 2002. Food sources of carbohydrates in a European cohort of adults. *Public Health Nutr* 5(6B):1197–1215. doi: 10.1079/PHN2002399.

World Cancer Research Fund and American Institute for Cancer Research. 2007. *Food, Nutrition, Physical Activity, and the Prevention of Cancer: A Global Perspective*. Washington, DC: American Institute for Cancer Research.

World Health Organization. 2002. *Cancer Incidence in Five Continents*. Lyon: The World Health Organization and The International Agency for Research on Cancer.

World Health Organization. 2015a. *Cancer Mortality and Morbidity*. http://www.who.int/gho/ncd/mortality_morbidity/cancer_text/en/. (Accessed June 16, 2016.)

World Health Organization. 2015b. *Cancer*. http://www.who.int/mediacentre/factsheets/fs297/en/. (Accessed June 16, 2016.)

Yu, H. and T. Rohan. 2000. Role of the insulin-like growth factor family in cancer development and progression. *J Natl Cancer Inst* 92(18):1472–1489.

Zapf, J. 1995. Physiological role of the insulin-like growth factor binding proteins. *Eur J Endocrinol* 132(6):645–654.

Zelenskiy, S., C. L. Thompson, T. C. Tucker, and L. Li. 2014. High dietary glycemic load is associated with increased risk of colon cancer. *Nutr Cancer* 66(3):362–368. doi: 10.1080/01635581.2014.884231.

Zhang, Z. W., P. V. Newcomb, M. Moorghen, J. Gupta, R. Feakins, P. Savage, A. Hollowood, D. Alderson, and J. M. Holly. 2004. Insulin-like growth factor binding protein-3: Relationship to the development of gastric pre-malignancy and gastric adenocarcinoma (United Kingdom). *Cancer Causes Control* 15(2):211–218. doi: 10.1023/B:CACO.0000019510.96285.e9.

Zhao, M. D., X. M. Hu, D. J. Sun, Q. Zhang, Y. H. Zhang, and W. Meng. 2005. Expression of some tumor associated factors in human carcinogenesis and development of gastric carcinoma. *World J Gastroenterol* 11(21):3217–3221.

Ziegler, R. G., R. N. Hoover, M. C. Pike, A. Hildesheim, A. M. Nomura, D. W. West, A. H. Wu-Williams et al. 1993. Migration patterns and breast cancer risk in Asian-American women. *J Natl Cancer Inst* 85(22):1819–1827.

World Health Organization [illegible] The World Health Organization [illegible]
and the [illegible]

[illegible]

[illegible]

[illegible]

[illegible]

[illegible]

[illegible]

[illegible]

Zhang [illegible]

8 Manipulating Dietary Glycemic Index as a Means of Improving Exercise and Sports Performance

Lars McNaughton, David Bentley, and S. Andy Sparks

CONTENTS

8.1 INTRODUCTION

Research in the 1980s showed that exercise capacity could be significantly improved by ingesting carbohydrate (CHO) (Coyle et al. 1983). Since then, a plethora of research has investigated the optimal type, amount, and timing of CHO to maximize endurance performance as well as to optimize adaptation to resistance training (Stellingwerff and Cox 2014). The early 1980s also saw the introduction of the concept of the glycemic index (GI) as a means of classifying CHO types based on blood glucose concentration following consumption (Jenkins et al. 1981). However, it was not until the early 1990s that different GI meals ingested before exercise, were investigated for their role on exercise performance (Thomas et al. 1991). It was proposed that the contrasting exchange lists for CHO might influence the metabolic response and exercise performance outcomes to diets of different GI. However, CHO feeding before, during, and after exercise performance is now generally accepted as a means of improving or recovering from such performance. While high-GI (HGI) meals are also now widely used in the recovery from exercise, the role of HGI compared to low GI (LGI) foods in sports nutrition is still under debate. Taken together, the reviews of Burke et al. (1996), Siu and Wong (2004), Wright (2005), and more recently Donaldson et al. (2010), O'Reilly et al. (2010), and Mondazzi and Arcelli (2009), provide a comprehensive overview of the first 16 years of research in this area. The aim of this chapter is to provide an up-to-date summary and practical application of the evidence regarding GI and exercise performance and the recovery process.

As discussed in Chapter 1, the GI was first introduced on the basis of work with diabetic patients suggesting that CHO exchange lists for CHOs used by them did not sufficiently reflect the physiological effect of CHO on the actual blood glucose and insulin response (Jenkins et al. 1981). In essence, the GI classifies CHO-rich foods based on their postprandial blood glucose response when compared to a reference glucose meal.

The GI of a food can be influenced by the physical and chemical characteristics of the food (Foster-Powell et al. 2002), and although an individual's glycemic response can be highly vary (Venn and Green 2007), most participant characteristics such as age, sex, body mass index, and ethnicity are not believed to influence GI (Wolever et al. 2003). However, there is some evidence to suggest an interaction between the glycemic response to fast or slowly digestible CHO foods, gender, and training status. Several studies have found a difference in the glycemic response between trained and sedentary men (Jackson 2007; Mettler et al. 2006, 2007), whereas others have found no difference in the glycemic response using trained and sedentary women (Mettler et al. 2008) or a mixed-gender group (Kim et al. 2008; Trompers et al. 2010). Therefore, since different foods are quickly or slowly digested and absorbed, and will be rated as HGI or LGI foods, the rationale for the manipulation of GI in meals consumed before, during, and after exercise is clear. If the GI of CHO influences the rate at which CHO elicits a blood glucose/insulin response, it seems plausible that feeding CHOs of differing GI before, during, and after exercise will influence sport performance and recovery. Despite the fact that the first research on GI and sport performance was carried out some 25 years ago (Thomas et al. 1991), there is still much indecision and a paucity of data about the benefits of consuming HGI and LGI CHO to improve exercise performance.

8.2 PRE-EXERCISE CARBOHYDRATE CONSUMPTION

The use of CHO as an ergogenic aid to improve sport and exercise performance has received a considerable amount of attention in the literature because the potential of glucose ingestion to enhance exercise performance was first investigated in the classic Boston Marathon studies of the 1920s (Levine et al. 1924; Gordon et al. 1925). The development of the muscle biopsy technique for the measurement of muscle glycogen stores was the main catalyst in the further focus on the importance of CHO for exercise performance (Bergström et al. 1967). In the same year, the observations of Ahlborg et al. (1967) showed that the manipulation of the absolute amounts of CHO content of the diet had an impact on subsequent exercise capacity. Thereafter, Alborg and Felig (1977) and Costill et al. (1977) were instrumental in determining that blood glucose concentrations were reduced at the start of exercise even when CHO was ingested in the final hour before the initiation of activity. Evidence of a concomitant accelerated muscle glycogenolysis (muscle glycogen breakdown) led to the suggestion that ingestion of CHO in this brief period before exercise might be detrimental to performance (Jeukendrup and Killer 2010), but the research in this area is equivocal to say the least. This finding was further supported by the work of Foster et al. (1979), who reported reduced time to exhaustion (TTE) during cycling at 80% VO_{2max} following a glucose load compared to water. It has been suggested that a hypoglycemic rebound effect is associated with the observed performance decrement when CHO is consumed proximal to the initiation of exercise (Jentjens et al. 2003). However, other studies have revealed that hypoglycaemia is not common, and the incidence of this can be reduced when CHO is consumed during a warm-up period before exercise (Brouns et al. 1989; Moseley et al. 2003).

8.2.1 METABOLIC RESPONSES TO PRE-EXERCISE LGI AND HGI MEALS

Following the work of Jenkins et al. (1981), on classifying CHOs according to the rate of glucose release, interest in the provision of food or meals with potentially reduced postprandial, pre-exercise insulin, and glucose responses (i.e., low GI meals) has been an area of sport and exercise nutrition research that attracted some considerable attention (Table 8.1). The first study to deliberately

TABLE 8.1
Key Glycemic Index Interventions and Exercise Performance

		Exercise Protocol		Ingestion Time	Responses	
Publication	**Participants**	**Design (GI)**	**Category**		**Metabolic**	**Performance**
Thomas et al. (1991)	Endurance-trained male cyclists ($n = 8$)	Cycling exercise at 65%–70% VO_{2max} until volitional exhaustion. LGI (29) versus HGI (98 and 100) single foods and drinks.	TTE	1 h pre-exercise	Plasma FFA was highest after water followed by LGI, glucose, and HGI. From 45 to 60 post ingestion, plasma lactate was higher in HGI than LGI trial and remained higher throughout the period of exercise.	20 min (%) improved TTE in LGI.
Febbraio and Stewart (1996)	Endurance-trained males ($n = 6$)	2 h cycling at 70% VO_{2peak} followed by 15 min total work done performance trial. LGI (29) versus HGI (80).	Submax. fixed duration + FDWD	45 min pre-exercise	Increased blood glucose 15 min post ingestion in HGI. Increased insulin response in the postprandial, pre-exercise period. Lower plasma FFA throughout submax. exercise in HGI. No differences in rates of muscle glycogenolysis.	No difference in total work done.
DeMarco et al. (1999).	Endurance-trained male cyclists ($n = 10$)	2 h at 70% VO_{2max} followed by TTE at 100% VO_{2max}. LGI (36) versus HGI (69.3) meals.	Submax. fixed duration + TTE at 100% VO_{2max}	30 min pre-exercise	Increased postprandial insulin and glucose in HGI. Elevated CHO oxidation during submax. exercise in HGI. Higher post submax. exercise glucose in LGI.	59% increase in TTE in LGI.
Stannard et al. (2000).	Endurance-trained male cyclists ($n = 10$)	Incremental cycling 3 min work bouts LGI (41) pasta versus HGI (100) glucose drink.	Incremental TTE	65 min pre-exercise	Elevated postprandial glucose in HGI. Lower plasma lactate at low intensities in LGI. Lower glucose at higher intensities in HGI.	No difference in TTE.
Febbraio et al. (2000)	Endurance-trained males ($n = 8$)	120 min cycling at 70% VO_{2peak} Followed by 30 min total work done performance test. LGI (~52) versus HGI (~80).	Submax. fixed duration + FDWD	30 min pre-exercise	Reduced postprandial and during exercise plasma FFA in HGI. Glucose rebound in HGI. Higher glycogen use in HGI reflected in elevated rate and total CHO oxidation.	No difference in total work done.
Sparks et al. (1998)	Endurance-trained male triathletes ($n = 8$)	50 min at 67%VO_{2max} followed by a 15 min total work done performance trial. LGI (29) versus HGI (80) foods.	Submax. fixed duration + FDWD	45 min pre-exercise	Increased postprandial plasma glucose in HGI. Lower glucose in HGI until 30 min into exercise. Increased insulin response in HGI. Reduced FFA concentrations at the start and end of exercise in LGI. Increase CHO oxidation in HGI.	No difference in total work done.

(Continued)

TABLE 8.1 (*Continued*)
Key Glycemic Index Interventions and Exercise Performance

		Exercise Protocol		Ingestion Time	Responses	
Publication	**Participants**	**Design (GI)**	**Category**		**Metabolic**	**Performance**
Wee et al. (2005)	Trained male recreational runners ($n = 7$)	30 min treadmill running at 71% VO_{2max} following LGI (36) versus HGI (80) meals.	Submax. fixed duration	3 h pre-exercise	Increased glucose and insulin responses in the postprandial period following HGI. A 15% increase in muscle glycogen pre-exercise following HGI, but no change with LGI. Glycogen sparing during exercise in LGI.	Not assessed.
Wu and Williams (2006)	Recreational male runners ($n = 8$)	Treadmill running to exhaustion at 70% $VO_{2max.}$ LGI (37) versus HGI (77) meals.	TTE	3 h pre-exercise	Increased glucose and insulin in postprandial period with HGI. Elevated fat oxidation during exercise in LGI.	6.8% increase in TTE with LGI.
Backhouse et al. (2007)	Healthy females ($n = 6$)	60 min treadmill walk with 5% gradient at 50% VO_{2peak}. Medium GI (51) versus HGI (77) meals.	Energy expended	3 h pre-exercise	Elevated insulin postprandial response not different between meals. Reduced glucose in first 15 min of exercise in HGI. No differences in substrate oxidation rates.	Not assessed.
Chen et al. (2008)	Trained runners ($n = 8$)	60 min treadmill run preload at 70% VO_{2max} followed by 10 km TT. LGI/LGL (40/42) HGI/HGL (79/82) HGI/LGL (78/44).	Submax. fixed duration + TT	2 h pre-exercise	Greater postprandial glucose and insulin responses in HGI/HGL. Lower CHO and elevated fat oxidation in the LGL trials.	No differences between meals.
Wong et al. (2008)	Endurance-trained male runners ($n = 8$)	5 km preload running at 70% VO_{2max} followed by 16 km TT LGI (37) versus HGI (77) meal.	TT	2 h pre-exercise	Increased postprandial glucose concentration in HGI. Higher glucose concentration during exercise in LGI. Elevated glycerol in latter half of TT in LGI.	2.8% improvement in TT performance time with LGI.
Wong et al. (2009)	Endurance-trained male runners ($n = 9$)	5 km preload running at 70% VO_{2max} followed by 16 km TT. LGI (36) vs. HGI (83) meal. Ingestion of 6.6% CHO solution during exercise.	TT	3 h pre-exercise	Greater postprandial pre- exercise glucose and insulin response in HGI. Smaller glucose elevations during exercise in LGI. No differences in fat or CHO oxidation rates.	No differences between foods.

(Continued)

TABLE 8.1 (*Continued*)
Key Glycemic Index Interventions and Exercise Performance

		Exercise Protocol		Ingestion Time	Responses	
Publication	**Participants**	**Design (GI)**	**Category**		**Metabolic**	**Performance**
Moore et al. (2009)	Endurance-trained male cyclists ($n = 8$)	40 km TT following either a LGI (30) or HGI (72) meal.	TT	45 min pre-exercise	Increased pre-exercise glucose in HGI. Increased post exercise glucose in LGI. Higher CHO oxidation rates during the TT in LGI.	3.2% improvement in TT performance time with LGI.
Little et al. (2009)	Trained intermittent sport athletes and distance runners ($n = 7$)	Intermittent 90 min treadmill soccer simulation protocol followed by 5 × 1 min repeated sprints with 2.5 min recovery in final 15 min of protocol following LGI (29) food versus HGI (81) meal additional ingestion after 45 min of exercise.	Game simulation + repeated sprint performance test	3 h pre-exercise	Increased postprandial blood glucose with HGI. No difference in substrate oxidation between meals. No difference in blood glucose during exercise.	No differences between foods.
Little et al. (2010)	Varsity soccer players ($n = 8$), club level soccer players ($n = 5$), and middle distance runners ($n = 3$) (Total $n = 16$)	Intermittent 90 min treadmill soccer simulation protocol followed by 5 × 1 min repeated sprints with 2.5 min recovery in final 15 min of protocol. LGI (26) versus HGI (76) foods.	Game simulation + repeated sprint performance test	2 h pre-exercise	Increased postprandial blood glucose with HGI, but no differences in insulin response. No main effect of GI in substrate oxidation during exercise.	No difference between meals.
Hulton et al. (2012)	Recreational soccer players ($n = 9$)	Intermittent 90 min treadmill soccer simulation protocol followed by 1 km TT. LGI (44) versus HGI (80) meals.	Game simulation + TT	3.5 h pre-exercise	Increased FFA in LGI during exercise. Increased post exercise ketone concentration. No differences in oxidation rates during protocol.	No difference between meals.

Note: HGI, High glycemic index; LGI, Low glycemic index; HGL, High glycemic load; LGL, Low glycemic load; FFA, Free fatty acids; TTE, Time to Exhaustion; TT, Time Trial; FDWD, Fixed duration work done.

TABLE 8.2
Key Glycemic Index Recovery Interventions and Exercise Performance.

		Exercise Protocol		Ingestion Time	Responses	
Publication	Participants	Design (GI)	Category		Metabolic	Performance
Burke et al. (1993)	Well-trained cyclists ($n = 5$)	120 min cycling at 75% VO_{2max} followed by four 30 s sprints. 24 h recovery diets of 10g.kg^{-1} LGI versus HGI	Glycogen depletion cycling.	24 h post-cycling recovery diet.	Increased glucose and insulin responses in HGI. Increased muscle glycogen resynthesis with the HGI diet.	Not assessed
Stevenson et al. (2005a)	Trained recreational runners ($n = 8$)	90 min run at 70% VO_{2max} followed by breakfast and a further recovery meal 2 h later. LGI (35) versus HGI (70) meals.	Glycogen depletion running.	Breakfast 30 min post 90 min of exercise + 2nd meal 2 h post exercise.	Postprandial glucose elevated in HGI. No difference between meals on post breakfast insulin response. Higher insulin following 2nd meal in HGI. No differences in recovery substrate oxidation rates.	Not assessed
Stevenson et al. (2005b)	Trained recreational runners ($n = 9$)	90 min running at 70% VO_{2max}. Then 24 h recovery with 8 g.kg^{-1} LGI (35) or HGI (70) diet followed by a TTE run.	Glycogen depletion running—then TTE run.	24 h post run recovery diet.	Increased fatty acid availability and fat oxidation in TTE trial with LGI. Higher post-exercise plasma glucose in HGI.	12.4% improvement in running TTE with LGI
Erith et al. (2006)	Trained semi-pro soccer players ($n = 7$)	90 min intermittent running test. Then 22 h recovery with 8 g.kg^{-1} LGI (35) or HGI (70) diet followed by 75 min intermittent running test then sprint + jog TTE.	Glycogen depletion intermittent running—then TTE.	22 h post run recovery diet.	No differences in metabolic responses to exercise as a result of diet.	No differences between diets
Bennett et al. (2012)	Trained soccer players ($n = 14$: 10M + 4F)	2 intermittent 90 min treadmill protocols separated by recovery period. Followed by sprint performance test. LGI (36) versus HGI (75) meals	5 × 1 min sprint distance covered following intermittent exercise.	Immediate ingestion following first 90 min protocol, 3 h pre second 90 min protocol.	Higher postprandial glucose and insulin in HGI. Lower CHO oxidation during start of first exercise bout LGI. Higher lactate and lower glucose at end of 2nd exercise bout in HGI.	No differences between meals
Brown et al. (2013)	Endurance trained male cyclists ($n = 7$)	2 min bouts of cycling at 90% WR_{max}. With 2 min recovery bouts at 50% WR_{max}—to exhaustion. 3 h recovery then 5 km TT. LGI (40) versus HGI (72) meal.	Glycogen depletion cycling + TT.	Immediate ingestion following depletion protocol, 3 h pre-TT.	Elevated insulin postprandial response to HGI. No difference in glucose response between meals. 30 min postprandial elevation in FFA in LGI. Increased CHO oxidation during recovery in HGI.	No differences between meals

investigate the effects of LGI and HGI ingestion before exercise was conducted by Thomas et al. (1991). These authors used eight endurance-trained cyclists who were provided with either an LGI food (lentils) and LGI water as drink or an HGI food (potatoes) and HGI drink (glucose solution), 1 h before the start of a TTE trial at 65%–75% VO_{2max}. The main finding was a 20-min improvement in TTE following the ingestion of the LGI meal. Thomas et al. (1991) also observed increased post-prandial and exercise plasma lactate concentrations following HGI ingestion, along with reduced plasma free fatty acid (FFA) concentrations. Furthermore, at the termination of exercise, blood glucose concentrations were higher in the LGI trials, leading to the suggestion that LGI foods consumed an hour before exercise provided a potential performance advantage over their HGI counterparts. Subsequent studies, however, have had varying degrees of success in the replication of these findings. Febbraio and Stewart (1996) used a longer submaximal exercise protocol of 120 min during which six endurance-trained males cycled at 70% VO_{2peak} following LGI, HGI, or a control meal ingested 45 min before exercise. Exercise performance was assessed using a 15-min fixed duration work done trial (FDWD), but no differences in total work output were observed. Despite metabolic perturbances following the meal conditions, again there were no effects on the rate of glycogenolysis. Wee et al. (1999) also used a similar TTE protocol to that of Thomas et al. (1991) in active male and female participants. This was the first study manipulating the GI of pre-exercise meals that used an ingestion period of 3 h before the start of exercise; however, while observing mild hypoglycemic rebound during the first 20 min of the exercise bout along with concurrent reductions in serum FFA and plasma glycerol with the HGI meal, they found no significant performance effects between meals.

Some of the main reasons for the equivocal findings of studies manipulating pre-exercise meal GI relate to the wide variety of exercise and performance protocols that are used. The most common experimental exercise protocols typically use submaximal TTE trials where participants cycle at a fixed and standardized exercise intensity until fatigue (Thomas et al., 1991; Wu and Williams 2006), a submaximal fixed duration exercise bout followed by either a TTE (DeMarco et al. 1999) or a fixed duration total work done trial (Febbraio and Stewart 1996; Febbraio et al. 2000; Sparks et al. 1998). Less commonly used protocols include incremental TTE (Stannard et al. 2000) and fixed duration submaximal exercise with no performance trial (Wee et al. 2005; Backhouse et al. 2007). In studies of endurance performance, researchers have focused on more ecologically valid indicators of performance such as running (Wong et al. 2008, 2009), cycling (Moore et al. 2009), and time trials (TT) where performance level is determined by the duration an athlete takes to complete a set distance. Subsequent sections of this chapter will focus on recent studies that have investigated the effects of different GI foods on endurance and intermittent exercise and will attempt to evaluate the key findings for the development of recommendations and future directions of research in this area.

After the ingestion of pre-exercise meals containing CHO of different GIs, a consistently observed response of an increase in glucose availability (Figure 8.1a) and insulin concentration has been reported (Figure 8.1b). In the initial few minutes, an increase in plasma insulin has been shown to occur (Febbraio and Stewart 1996; DeMarco et al. 1999; Sparks et al. 1998; Wee et al. 2005; Wu and Williams, 2006; Wong et al. 2009), reaching a peak between 15 and 30 min post ingestion (Febbraio et al. 2000; Wee et al. 2005). Typically, these peaks occur at the same time irrespective of the GI of the meal, but with a lower magnitude following LGI compared to HGI CHO ingestion in most studies (Febbraio and Stewart 1996, DeMarco et al. 1999; Sparks et al. 1998; Wee et al. 2005; Wu and Williams 2006; Wong et al. 2009), but not all (Backhouse et al. 2007). In this post-prandial situation, there is an increased CHO availability that is associated with the reduction in the rate of lipolysis via insulin-mediated suppression of hormone-sensitive lipase (Watt 2009). These responses are key considerations in the timings of the ingestion periods before the start of exercise, especially if CHO is not going to be consumed during the exercise bout, because the increased insulin response associated with HGI meals has the potential to induce hypoglycemic rebound, especially if the ingestion time is less than 3 h before the start of exercise (Febbraio et al. 2000).

Many studies also use vague terminology in the description of their populations and rarely use appropriate criteria to categorize participants (De Pauw et al. 2013). Differences in training status may be a key consideration in the metabolic responses to LGI and HGI meals. Studies investigating the glycemic response to different GI meals have reported disparities between trained and untrained males (Mettler et al. 2006). The reason for these differences is likely to be a result of the increased cellular uptake of glucose in the postprandial resting period via GLUT-4 transporters, which proliferate following endurance exercise training (Richter and Hargreaves 2013) and result in enhanced insulin sensitivity (Tsao et al. 1996). Interestingly, such observations have not been seen between varying training status levels in females (Mettler et al. 2007, 2008) or in mixed-gender populations (Trompers et al. 2010). This may be a result of the associated variation in the glycemic response of participants to the same foods, which may vary by up to 60% rather than the variation of the GI relative to a reference food, which only varies by approximately 5% (Wolever et al., 1990). Given that the vast majority of studies have used trained or well-trained male participants, it is possible that the recommendations of the studies would not be appropriate for recreational or less well-trained individuals. Hence in practice, athletes should try foods of different GIs in order to establish which type of CHO is most effective for their performance, as the within-individual difference in glycemic response is only approximately 25% (see Chapter 3).

8.3 EXERCISE ADAPTATIONS FOLLOWING LGI AND HGI MEAL INGESTION

8.3.1 Endurance Exercise

The main physiological and metabolic responses during submaximal prolonged exercise following the ingestion of meals of varying GIs have been widely documented. Typically, following the ingestion of a HGI meal or food, there is an increase in the availability of blood glucose followed by insulin release (Figure 8.1). In some instances, this may lead to a hypoglycemic rebound response at the start of exercise, especially if the ingestion period is 1 h but less than 3 h before the exercise bout (Thomas et al. 1991; Backhouse et al. 2007). This is likely to lead to reduced blood glucose concentrations during the first 15–30 min of prolonged exercise (Febbraio and Stewart 1996; Febbraio et al. 2000). However, Wong et al. (2008) have shown that this is may not be detrimental to exercise performance (Figure 8.2). During exercise following an HGI meal 3 h before, increased glucose availability was associated with reduced rates of lipolysis and reductions in plasma FFA, leading to lower fat oxidation rates compared to LGI ingestion or continued fasting (Wu and Williams 2006). Such disturbances to substrate availability are frequently reported postprandially, but are less likely to be observed during running or cycling TT performance studies, such as time to complete 10 km running or 40 km cycling (Wong et al. 2009), but are more likely to be responsible for performance alterations in TTE studies (Wu and Williams 2006).

Despite the absence of clear acute performance advantages, the prolonged use of LGI pre-exercise meals may provide some potentially advantageous training adaptations, but this has not yet been investigated. Previously, Morton et al. (2009) have shown that exercise training in combination with lower absolute dietary CHO content is associated with enhanced skeletal muscle oxidative enzyme activity. More recently, Bartlett et al. (2013) have also demonstrated that following exercise in conditions of reduced CHO restriction results in greater increases in p53 phosphorylation, a key regulator of mitochondrial biogenesis. This is a potentially desirable training response for both athletes and clinical populations, because p53 mediated mitochondrial biogenesis improves skeletal muscle function and may reduce the severity of many metabolic disorders associated with inactivity (Bartlett et al. 2014a). At present, it is unclear whether LGI meals before exercise induce similar responses (albeit likely to be somewhat blunted), while maintaining blood glucose during exercise (Gulve 2008).

What is clear is that the acute provision of exogenous CHO during exercise reduces lipolysis (Coyle et al. 1997; Horowitz et al. 1999) and may also reduce the expression of genes responsible for improving the fat oxidative capacity of skeletal muscle (Civitarese et al. 2005). At present, there

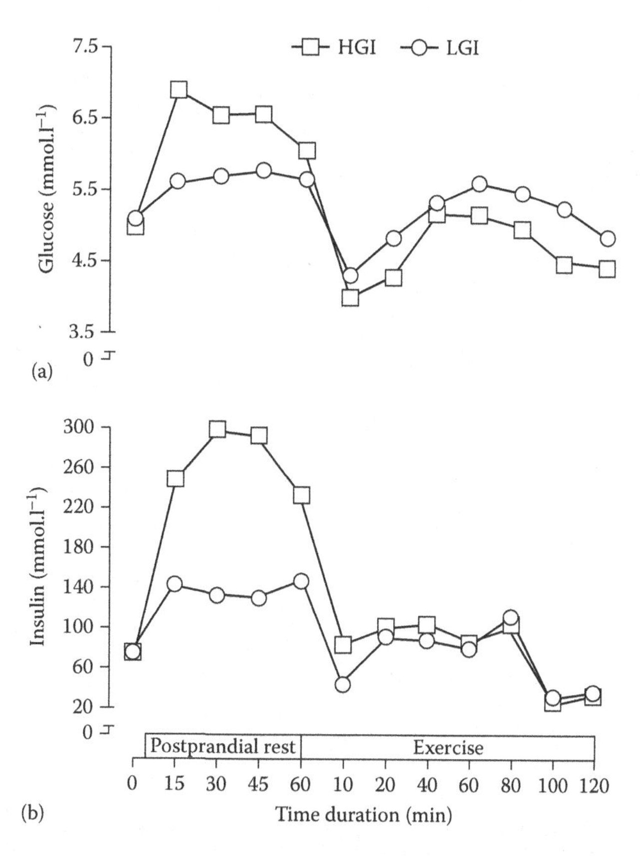

FIGURE 8.1 Typical plasma glucose (a), and insulin (b) concentrations at rest and during submaximal exercise following the ingestion of a high-glycemic index (HGI) and low-glycemic index (LGI), meals. (Data represent typical mean responses calculated from Thomas, DE. et al., *Int. J. Sports Med.*, 12:180–186, 1991; Febbraio, MA., Stewart, KL. *J. Appl. Physiol.*, 81:1115–1120, 1996; Sparks, MJ. et al., *Med. Sci. Sports Exerc.*, 30:844–849,1998; DeMarco, HM. et al., *Med. Sci. Sports Exerc.*, 31:164–170, 1999. With Permission.)

is only one study that has investigated the provision of foods of different GIs during endurance exercise (Earnest et al. 2004). This study used trained male cyclists that were required to complete 64 km TTs during which either a 15 g placebo, an LGI (35), or an HGI (100) gel were consumed every 16 km of the TT. TT performance in the LGI and HGI conditions provided a significant performance advantage over the placebo, but there were no significant differences between the two GI gels. Unfortunately, this study did not measure substrate oxidation during the exercise bout, but did show that exogenous CHO lowered blood glucose concentrations in the HGI trial. Increased exogenous glucose availability may ultimately lead to reduced glucose concentrations, because cellular uptake of glucose (and therefore the rate of disappearance) is elevated by upregulated CHO metabolism during exercise (Jeukendrup and Killer, 2010). While there is little available data on GI use during exercise, it seems reasonable to suggest that simply the provision of some CHO during exercise is likely to reduce fat metabolism, and for there to be no real performance advantage between CHO with different GIs. The current advice for individuals considering exogenous CHO provision during exercise is, therefore, that food and liquids should contain different CHO molecules (glucose, fructose, sucrose, galactose, and maltodextrins), as these have been shown to increase exogenous CHO substrate metabolism and improve exercise performance (Jeukendrup 2010). This is because the current literature appears to suggest that the GI nature of the CHO is much less important. However, the timing and amount of such intake should be based upon the event duration as these are defining factors in providing a performance advantage (Rowlands et al. 2012).

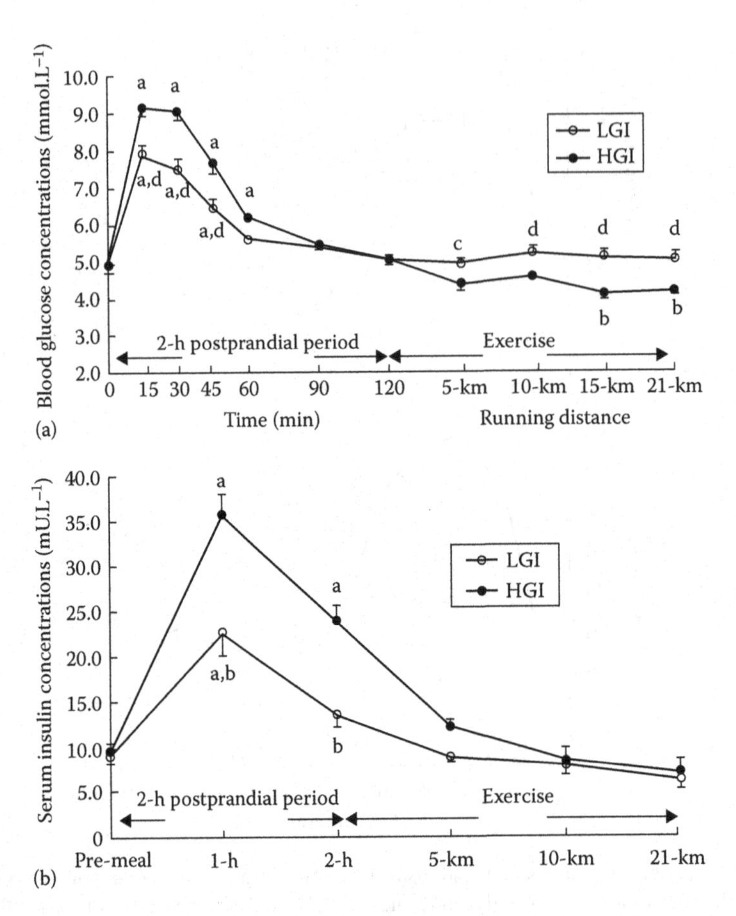

FIGURE 8.2 Blood glucose (a) and serum insulin (b) concentrations during a 2 h postprandial period and during a 21 km treadmill running performance trial following low glycemic index (LGI) and high glycemic index (HGI) meals. Values are means ± SE. (a): $^{a}p < .01$ versus pre-meal; $^{b}p < .01$ versus 120 min; $^{c}p < .05$ versus HGI; $^{d}p < .01$ versus HGI. (b): $^{a}p < .01$ versus pre-meal; $^{b}p < .01$ versus HGI. (From Wong, SHS. et al., *Eur. J. Sport Sci.*, 8, 1:23–33, 2008; Copyright European College of Sport Science, reprinted by permission of Taylor & Francis Group, www.tandfonline.com on behalf of European College of Sport Science. With Permission.)

8.3.2 Intermittent Exercise

Intermittent, high-intensity exercise is a common requirement in team sport environments (Bangsbo et al., 2006) as well as during periods in individual sports. Single bouts of all out activity ranging from 6 to 30 s have been shown to result in elevated rates of glycogenolysis (Nevill et al. 1989; Esbjörnsson et al. 1999). Pioneering studies, as well as more contemporary investigations involving repeated bouts of brief high intensity exercise simulating the competitive requirements of team sports, have also shown considerably higher rates of glycogen depletion compared to continuous submaximal exercise (Essen 1978; Kustrup et al. 2006). Hence, dietary manipulation before intermittent high-intensity exercise may influence performance and adaptations subsequent to this type of exercise.

Few studies have considered pre-exercise GI manipulations for potential performance improvements in intermittent sports, such as team sports, as well as exercise training bouts where demands might differ over the course of a training session. To date, there have only been three well-controlled studies that have prescribed pre-exercise meals of varying GIs before the performance of intermittent exercise (Little et al. 2009, 2010; Hulton et al. 2012). Each of these studies used a laboratory treadmill based soccer simulation protocol lasting 90 min with a 15 min half-time rest period. In each case, postprandial blood glucose was elevated following the HGI food or meal, but this did not result in differences in the substrate oxidation rates during the exercise protocols, despite elevations in FFA following an LGI meal (Hulton et al. 2012). Indeed, Hulton et al. (2012) were the only investigators to compare two isocaloric meals that differed in GI, whereas the other studies compared an LGI single food with an HGI meal. On completion of the game simulation in these studies, participants either completed a repeated sprint performance test (Little et al. 2009, 2010) or a 1 km self-paced TT (Hulton et al. 2012) as a postgame performance measure. Despite obvious methodological differences, different ingestion periods (ranging from 2 to 3.5 h pre-exercise), as well as diverse participant populations, none of these studies observed any differences in performance between the ingestion conditions, suggesting that while there are some metabolic alterations following an LGI or an HGI pre-exercise meal, consideration of the GI of a pre-match meal is unimportant. What is yet to be investigated are the effects of pre-exercise GI meal manipulation before intermittent exercise during which exogenous CHO is ingested, a practice that is likely to occur during competitive athletic situations. Intermittent activities have also been considered by some other investigators, but with a focus on the use of GI manipulations as a recovery strategy (Erith et al. 2006; Bennett et al., 2012), and thus these will be discussed in Section 8.4.

8.4 GI AND POST-EXERCISE RECOVERY

At present, only a small selection of studies have directly investigated the effect of GI meal manipulations with a specific focus on their efficacy for recovery from exercise bouts. These studies have scrutinized recovery from both high-intensity intermittent exercise (Erith et al., 2006; Bennett et al., 2012), prolonged exercise (Stevenson et al. 2005a, 2005b), and cycling TT performance following glycogen depletion and subsequent recovery (Brown et al. 2013). The primary focus of meal provision following prolonged or intense exercise is the replacement of nutrients to aid glycogen resynthesis (Millard-Stafford et al. 2008), replace fluids, promote skeletal muscle adaptations (Jensen and Richter 2012), and reduce immunosuppression (Bartlett et al. 2014b). The use of a high-CHO meal post exercise has been previously shown to be key in these processes. Burke et al. (1993) were one of the first groups to investigate the effect of GI meals as a recovery strategy from glycogen depleting exercise. They showed that the provision of HGI meals containing 10 g.kg body mass $(BM)^{-1}$ CHO provided improved glycogen resynthesis compared to a LGI meal containing the same total CHO 24 h after ingestion. The same research group also investigated the use of two eating strategies that were designed to provide the same total CHO in the 24 h recovery period (10 g.kg BM^{-1}), but found that there was no difference between a more frequent eating pattern (~0.67 g.kg BM^{-1} per feeding × $16.d^{-1}$—a *nibbling approach*) compared to less frequent larger meals (2.5 g.kg BM^{-1} per feeding × $4.d^{-1}$—a *gorging* approach). More recently, Stevenson et al. (2005a) investigated the metabolic responses in the recovery period following glycogen depleting running at 70% VO_{2max}. when either LGI or HGI post-exercise isocaloric breakfasts and lunches were provided. Following the first meal, there were no differences in the glycemic responses, but following the lunch (provided 2 h after exercise), a significantly elevated insulin response was observed in the HGI trial. This may indicate that the GI of the meal ingested immediately after exercise is less important than the provision of some CHO, but later in recovery, HGI meals may facilitate greater glycogen resynthesis, a finding consistent with Chen et al. (2008) and the earlier work of Burke et al. (1993). Erith et al. (2006) examined the effects of HGI and LGI recovery diets on subsequent exercise capacity during intermittent high-intensity running. Seven male soccer players undertook the Loughborough Intermittent Shuttle Test (LIST), which involved two runs separated by a recovery period of 22 h. They found no differences between trials in time to fatigue or for sprint performance and distance covered.

The recovery from single exercise bouts is clearly important, but when exercise is performed on successive days either during a multiday event or in repeated training bouts, adequate glycogen resynthesis is critical to ensure that exercise of a similar intensity can be performed (Costill and Miller 1980). Stevenson et al. (2005b) have subsequently shown that running TTE at 70% VO_{2max} is improved following a 24 h-LGI recovery diet, which was provided after glycogen depleting exercise the previous day. Interestingly, the LGI diet also increased markers of fat oxidation and reduced the pre-exercise subjective ratings of hunger before the TTE trial after an overnight fast. Indeed, these metabolic responses have also been observed following an intermittent glycogen depleting protocol in endurance trained cyclists (Brown et al. 2013). In this instance, a 5 km TT was used as a performance criteria 3 h after the ingestion of macronutrient matched LGI (40) versus HGI (72) meals. Interestingly, this study did not provide isocaloric meals and only provided approximately 2 g.kg BM^{-1} CHO as a glycogen repletion strategy but showed no performance differences between strategies.

8.5 GLYCEMIC LOAD

A relatively new and novel concept in the area of sports nutrition has been the use of the glycemic load (GL—O'Reilly et al., 2010). This concept (the mathematical product of the GI of a food and its carbohydrate content) was first introduced by Harvard researchers in 1997 (Salmeron et al. 1997a, 1997b). It suggests that exercise performance is affected by the overall glycemic effect of the diet, and not simply by the amount of carbohydrate consumed. In other words, we need to consider the quantity and quality (nature or source) of carbohydrate, and how these affect the overall GI. Needless to say, the concept has not at this time, been widely used in the area of sport and exercise performance nutrition, but has been used more widely in the exercise and chronic disease literature (Brand-Miller 2003; Barclay et al. 2008). Coaches, athletes, and researchers can find the necessary data for both GI and GL in the International Table of Glycemic Index and Glycemic Load Values: 2008 (Atkinson et al. 2008).

8.6 RECOMMENDATIONS FOR FUTURE RESEARCH

Future research should consider the daily nutritional practices that athletes use, as well as their training regime, since often, the type of training and competition dictates dietary strategies. Sports nutritionists, for example, could closely track an individual athlete and directly monitor his/her nutritional intake and exercise regimes. Furthermore, more work needs to be carried out to examine the specific individual variability in glycemic response, and its effects on other physiological factors, for example, the hormonal response. Finally, the concept of the GL, which takes into account both CHO quality and quantity and may be a better predictor of glycemic response than the GI alone (Scaglioni et al. 2004; O'Reilly et al. 2010), also needs further investigation in an exercise setting.

8.7 PRACTICAL RECOMMENDATIONS

1. Most studies suggest that consuming LGI CHO before endurance exercise results in a favorable metabolic profile during exercise, but only some report an enhancement in performance (Moore et al. 2010). However, there are no studies that have suggested or found there to be a negative effect of performance. Since the strategy is unlikely to have a detrimental effect, athletes should practice using such LGI CHO diets in training and other less important competitions to see whether they are effective for them.
2. On the basis of research findings, athletes should be aware of their individual response to their pre-competition meal based on training experience. Practical matters will dictate their use of HGI or LGI meals during the exercise session, based on availability.

3. The consumption of CHO during exercise is common practice, and many athletes opt to consume HGI CHO. It has been shown (Wong et al. 2009) that if a large amount (>1.5 g $CHO.kg^{-1}$ BM) of CHO is ingested during exercise, the GI of the pre-exercise meal is irrelevant, and hence, has no significant impact on performance. Athletes are encouraged to let individual preference guide their selection of CHO while giving consideration primarily to the length and intensity of each competition, type of training, or exercise regime.
4. Research has suggested that consuming an HGI CHO meal/food during recovery increases muscle glycogen synthesis post-exercise, which may be important to athletes who have a limited recovery time between sessions. However, when recovery periods are longer, LGI foods (and liquids) may be included without any negative impact on glycogen re-synthesis and benefits in terms of muscle protein synthesis.

8.8 CONCLUSIONS

Between individuals of equal athletic ability, nutrition may be the key factor in success. Optimizing dietary strategies before, during, and after exercise may provide athletes with the winning advantage. However, the role GI plays in the complex area of enhancing endurance performance is inconclusive and such strategies should be applied on an individual basis for each athlete.

REFERENCES

Ahlborg, BG., Bergström, J., Brohult, L., Ekelund, G., Hultman, E. (1967). Human muscle glycogen content and capacity for prolonged exercise after different diets. *Foersvarsmedicin*, 3:85–99.

Alborg, G., Felig, P. (1977). Substrate utilization during prolonged exercise preceded by ingestion of glucose. *Am. J. Physiol.*, 233:E188–E194.

Atkinson, FS., Foster-Powell, K., Brand-Miller, JC. (2008). International tables of glycemic index and glycemic load values: 2008. *Diabetes Care,* 31(12):2281–2283.

Backhouse, SH., Williams, C., Stevenson, E., Nute, M. (2007). Effects of the glycemic index of breakfast on metabolic responses to brisk walking in females. *Eur. J. Clin. Nutr.,* 61:590–596.

Bangsbo, J., Mohr, M., Krustrup, P. (2006). Physical and metabolic demands of training and match-play in the elite football player. *J. Sports Sci.,* 24:665–674.

Barclay, AW., Petocz, P., McMillan-Price, J., Flood, VM., Prvan, T.,Mitchell, P., Brand-Miller, JC. (2008). Glycemic index, glycemic load, and chronic disease risk—A meta-analysis of observational studies. *Am. J. Clin. Nutr.*, 87:627–637.

Bartlett, JD., Close, GL., Drust, B., Morton, JP. (2014a). The emerging role of p53 in exercise metabolism. *Sports Med.*, 44(3):303–309. doi: 10.1007/s40279-013-0127-9.

Bartlett, JD., Hawley, JA., Morton, JP. (2014b). Carbohydrate availability and exercise training adaptation: Too much of a good thing? *Eur. J. Sport Sci.,* 15(1):3–12.

Bartlett, JD., Louhelainen, J., Iqbal, Z., Cochran, AJ., Gibala, MJ., Gregson, W., Close, GL., Drust, B., Morton, JP. (2013). Reduced carbohydrate availability enhances exercise-induced p53 signaling in human skeletal muscle: Implications for mitochondrial biogenesis. *Am. J. Physiol. Regul. Integr. Comp. Physiol.,* 304(6):R450–R458. doi: 10.1152/ajpregu.00498.2012.

Bennett, CB., Chilibeck, PD., Barss, T., Vatanparast, H., Vandenberg, A., Zello, GA. (2012). Metabolism and performance during extended high-intensity intermittent exercise after consumption of low- and high-glycaemic index pre-exercise meals. *Br. J. Nutr.*, 108(Suppl. 1):S81–S90. doi: 10.1017/S0007114512000840.

Bergström, J., Hermansen, L., Hultman, E., Saltin, B. (1967). Diet, muscle glycogen and physical performance. *Acta Physiol. Scand.,* 71(2–3):140–150.

Brand-Miller, JC. (2003). Glycemic load and chronic disease. *Nutr. Rev.,* 61:S49–S55.

Brouns. F., Rehrer, NJ., Saris, WHM., Beckers, E., Menheere, P., ten Hoor, F. (1989). Effect of carbohydrate intake during warming up on the regulation of blood glucose during exercise. *Int. J. Sports Med.,* 10:S568–S575.

Brown, LJS., Midgley, AW., Vince, RV., Madden, LA., McNaughton, LR. (2013). High versus low glycemic index 3-h recovery diets following glycogen-depleting exercise has no effect on subsequent 5-km cycling time trial performance. *J. Sci. Med. Sport.,* 6(5):450–454. doi: 10.1016/j.jsams.2012.10.006.

Burke, LM., Collier, GR., Davis, PG., Fricker, PA., Sanigorski, AJ., Hargreaves, M. (1996). Muscle glycogen storage after prolonged exercise: Effect of the frequency of carbohydrate feedings. *Am. J. Clin. Nutr.,* 64:115–119.

Burke, LM., Collier, GR., Hargreaves, M. (1993). Muscle glycogen storage after prolonged exercise: Effect of the glycemic index of carbohydrate feedings. *J. Appl. Physiol.,* 75(2):1019–1023.

Chen, YJ., Wong, SH., Xu, X., Hao, X., Wong, CK., Lam, CW. (2008). Effects of CHO loading patterns on running performance. *Int. J. Sports Med.*, 29(7):598–606.

Civitarese, AE., Hesselink, MK., Russell, AP., Ravussin, E., Schrauwen, P. (2005). Glucose ingestion during exercise blunts exercise-induced gene expression of skeletal muscle fat oxidative genes. *Am. J. Physiol. Endocrinol. Metab.,* 289(6):E1023–E1029.

Costill, DL., Coyle, E., Dalshy, G., Evans, W., Fink, W., Hoopes, D. (1977). Effects of elevated plasma FFA and insulin on muscle glycogen usage during exercise. *J. Appl. Physiol.,* 43:695–699.

Costill, DL., Miller, JM. (1980). Nutrition for endurance sport: Carbohydrate and fluid balance. *Int. J. Sports Med.*, 1:2–14.

Coyle, EF., Hagberg, JM., Hurley, BF., Martin, WH., Ehsani, AA., Holloszy, JO. (1983). Carbohydrate feeding during prolonged strenuous exercise can delay fatigue. *J. Appl. Physiol.,* 55(1):230–235.

Coyle, EF., Jeukendrup, AE., Wagenmakers, AJ., Saris, WH. (1997). Fatty acid oxidation is directly regulated by carbohydrate metabolism during exercise. *Am. J. Physiol.*, 273(2 Pt1):E268–E275.

De Pauw, K., Roelands, B., Cheung, SS., De Geus, B., Rietjens, G., Meeusen, R. (2013). Guidelines to classify subject groups in sport-science research. *Int. J. Sports Physiol. Perform.*, 8(2):111–122.

DeMarco, HM., Sucher, KP., Cisar, CJ., Butterfield, GE. (1999). Pre-exercise carbohydrate meals: Application of glycemic index. *Med. Sci. Sports Exerc.,* 31(1):164–170.

Donaldson, CM., Perry, TL., Rose, MC. (2010). Glycemic index and endurance performance. *Int. J. Sports Nutr. Exerc. Metab.,* 20:154–165.

Earnest, CP., Lancaster, SL., Rasmussen, CJ., Kerksick, CM., Lucia, A., Greenwood, MC., Almada, AL., Cowan, PA., Kreider, RB. (2004). Low vs. high glycemic index carbohydrate get ingestion during simulated 64-km cycling time trial performance. *J. Strength. Cond. Res.*, 18(3):466–472.

Erith, S., Williams, C., Stevenson, E., Chamberlain, S., Crews, P., Rushbury, I. (2006). The effect of high carbohydrate meals with different glycemic indices on recovery of performance during prolonged intermittent high-intensity shuttle running. *Int. J. Sport. Nutr. Exerc. Metab.*, 16(4):393–404.

Esbjörnsson-Liljedahl, M., Sundberg, CJ., Norman, B., Jansson, E. (1999). Metabolic response in type I and type II muscle fibers during a 30-s cycle sprint in men and women. *J. Appl. Physiol.,* 87(4):1326–1332.

Essen, B. (1978). Glycogen depletion of different fibre types in human skeletal muscle during intermittent and continuous exercise. *Acta Physiol. Scand.,* 103(4):446–455.

Febbraio, MA., Keenan, J., Angus, DJ., Campbell, SE., Garnham, AP. (2000). Preexercise carbohydrate ingestion, glucose kinetics, and muscle glycogen use: Effect of the glycemic index. *J Appl. Physiol.*, 89:1845–1851.

Febbraio, MA., Stewart, KL. (1996). CHO feeding before prolonged exercise: Effect of glycemic index on muscle glycogenolysis and exercise performance. *J. Appl. Physiol.*, 81:1115–1120.

Foster, C., Costill, DL., Fink, WJ. (1979). Effects of pre-exercise feedings on endurance performance. *Med. Sci. Sports Exerc.*, 11:1–5.

Foster-Powell, K., Holt, SH., Brand-Miller, JC. (2002). International table of glycemic index and glycemic load values: 2002. *Am. J. Clin. Nutr.,* 76(1):5–56.

Gordon, B., Kohn, SA., Levine, SA., Matton, M., de Scriver, WM., Whiting, WB. (1925). Sugar content of the blood in runners following a marathon race. With especial reference to the prevention of hypoglycemia: Further observations. *JAMA.*, 85:508–509.

Gulve, EA. (2008). Exercise and glycemic control in diabetes: Benefits, challenges, and adjustments to pharmacotherapy. *Phys. Ther.*, 88(11):1297–1321.

Horowitz, JF., Mora-Rodriguez, R., Byerley, LO., Coyle, EF. (1999). Substrate metabolism when subjects are fed carbohydrate during exercise. *Am. J. Physiol.*, 276(5 Pt 1):E828–E835.

Hulton, AT., Gregson, W., MacLaren, D., Doran, DA. (2012). Effects of GI meals on intermittent exercise. *Int. J. Sports Med.*, 33:756–762.

Jackson, AC. (2007). Glycemic response to fast and slow digestible carbohydrate in high and low aerobic fitness men. Master's thesis, Ohio University. Retrieved from http://www.ohiolink.edu/etd/view.cgi?acc_num=ohiou1194542916. (Accessed June 16, 2016.)

Jentjens, RL., Cale, C., Gutch, C., Jeukendrup, AE. (2003). Effects of pre-exercise ingestion of differing amounts of carbohydrate on subsequent metabolism and cycling performance. *Eur. J. Appl. Physiol.,* 88:444–452.

Jenkins, DJ., Wolever, TM., Taylor, RH., Barker, H., Fielden, H., Baldwin, JM., Bowling, AC., Newman., HC., Jenkins, AL., Goff, DV. (1981). Glycemic index of foods: A physiological basis for carbohydrate exchange. *Am. J. Clin. Nutr.*, 34:362–366.

Jensen, TE., Richter, EA. (2012). Regulation of glucose and glycogen metabolism during and after exercise. *J. Physiol.*, 590(Pt 5):1069–1076.

Jeukendrup, AE. (2010). Carbohydrate and exercise performance: The role of multiple transportable carbohydrates. *Curr. Opin. Clin. Nutr. Metab. Care*, 13(4):452–457.

Jeukendrup, AE., Killer, SC. (2010). The myths surrounding pre-exercise carbohydrate feeding. *Ann. Nutr. Metab.*, 57(Suppl. 2):18–25.

Kim, Y., Hertzler, SR., Byrne, HK., Mattern, CO. (2008). Raisins are a low to moderate glycemic index food with a correspondingly low insulin index. *Nutr. Res. (New York)*, 28(5):304–308.

Krustrup, P., Mohr, M., Steensberg, A., Bencke, J., Kiaer, M., Bangsbo, J. (2006). Muscle and blood metabolites during a soccer game: implications for sprint performance. *Med. Sci. Sports Exerc.*, 38:1–10.

Levine, SA., Gordon, B., Derick, CL. (1924). Some changes in the chemical constituents of the blood following a marathon race. With special reference to the development of hypoglycemia. *JAMA*, 82:1778–1779.

Little, JP., Chilibeck, PD., Ciona, D., Vandenberg, A., Zello, GA. (2009). *Int. J. Sports Physiol. Perform*, 4:367–380.

Little, JP., Chilibeck, PD., Ciona, D., Forbes, S., Rees, H., Vandenberg, A., Zello, GA. (2010). Effect of low- and high glycemic-index meals on metabolism and performance during high-intensity, intermittent exercise. *Int. J. Sports Nutr. Exerc. Metab.*, 20:447–456.

Mettler, S., Lamprecht-Rusca, F., Stoffel-Kurt, N., Wenk, C., Colombani, PC. (2007). The influence of the subjects' training state on the glycemic index. *Eur. J. Clin. Nutr.*, 61(1):19–24.

Mettler, S., Vaucher, P., Weingartner, PM., Wenk, C., Colombani, PC. (2008). Regular endurance training does not influence the glycemic index determination in women. *J. Am. Coll. Nutr.*, 27(2):321–325.

Mettler, S., Wenk, C., Colombani, PC. (2006). Influence of training status on glycemic index. *Int. J. Vit. Nutr. Res.*, 76(1):39–44.

Millard-Stafford, M., Childers, WL., Conger, SA., Kampfer, AJ., Rahnert, JA. (2008). Recovery nutrition: Timing and composition after endurance exercise. *Curr. Sports Med. Rep.*, 7(4):193–201.

Mondazzi, L., Arcelli, E. (2009). Glycemic index in sport nutrition. *J. Am. Coll. Nutr.*, 28(Suppl. 4):455S–463S.

Moore, LJS., Midgley, AW., Thomas, G., Thurlow, S., McNaughton, LR. (2009). The effects of low- and high-glycemic index meals on time trial performance. *Int. J. Sports Physiol. Perform.*, 4(3):331–334.

Moore, LJS., Midgley, AW., Thurlow, S., Thomas, G., Mc Naughton, LR. (2010). Effect of the glycaemic index of a pre-exercise meal on metabolism and cycling time trial performance. *J. Sci. Med. Sports*, 13:182–188.

Morton, JP., Croft, L., Bartlett, JD., MacLaren, DPM., Reilly, T., Evans, L., McArdle, A., Drust, B. (2009). Reduced carbohydrate availability does not modulate training-induced heat shock protein adaptations but does upregulate oxidative enzyme activity in human skeletal muscle. *J. Appl. Physiol.*, 106(5):1513–1521.

Moseley, L., Lancaster, GI., Jeukendrup, AE. (2003). Effects of timing of pre-exercise ingestion of carbohydrate on subsequent metabolism and cycling performance. *Eur. J. Appl. Physiol.*, 88:453–458.

Nevill, ME., Boobis, LH., Brooks, S., Williams., C. (1989). Effect of training on muscle metabolism during treadmill sprinting. *J. Appl. Physiol.*, 67(6):2376–2382.

O'Reilly, J., Stephen HS. Wong, SHS., Chen, Y. (2010). Glycaemic index, glycaemic load and exercise performance. *Sports Med.*, 40:27–39.

Richter, EA., Hargreaves, M. (2013). Exercise, GLUT4, and skeletal muscle glucose uptake. *Physiol. Rev.*, 93:993–1017.

Rowlands, DS., Swift, M., Ros, M., Green, JG. (2012). Composite versus single transportable carbohydrate solution enhances race and laboratory cycling performance. *Appl. Physiol. Nutr. Metab.*, 37(3):425–436. doi: 10.1139/h2012-013.

Salmeron, J., Ascherio, A., Rimm, E. et al. (1997a). Dietary fiber, glycemic load, and risk of NIDDM in men. *Diabetes Care*, 20:545–550.

Salmeron, J., Manson, J., Stampfer, M., Colditz, G., Wing, A., Willett, W. (1997b). Dietary fiber, glycemic load, and risk of non-insulin-dependent diabetes mellitus in women. *JAMA*, 277:472–477.

Scaglioni, S., Stival, G., Giovannini, M. (2004). Dietary glycaemic load, overall glycaemic index, and serum insulin concentrations in healthy schoolchildren. *Am. J. Clin. Nutr.*, 79(2):339–340.

Siu, PM., Wong, SHS. (2004). Use of the glycemic index: Effects on feeding patterns and exercise performance. *J. Physiol. Anthropol. Appl. Human Sci.*, 23(1):1–6.

Sparks, MJ., Selig, SS., Febbraio, MA. (1998). Pre-exercise carbohydrate ingestion: Effect of the glycemic index on endurance exercise performance. *Med. Sci. Sports Exerc.*, 30(6):844–849.

Stannard, SR., Thompson, MW., Brand Miller, JC. (2000). The effect of glycemic index on plasma glucose and lactate levels during incremental exercise. *Int. J. Sports Nutr. Exerc. Metab.*, 10:51–61.
Stellingwerff, T., Cox, GR. (2014). Systematic review: Carbohydrate supplementation on exercise performance or capacity of varying durations. *Appl. Physiol. Nutr. Metab.*, 39:998–1011.
Stephen, HS., Wong, SHS., Siu, PM., Lok, A., Chen, YJ., Morris, J., Lam, CW. (2008). Effect of the glycaemic index of pre-exercise carbohydrate meals on running performance. *Eur. J. Sport Sci.*, 8(1):23–33.
Stevenson, E., Williams, C., Biscoe, H. (2005a). The metabolic responses to high carbohydrate meals with different glycemic indices consumed during recovery from prolonged strenuous exercise. *Int. J. Sports Nutr. Exerc. Metab.*, 15:291–307.
Stevenson, E., Williams, C., McComb, G., Oram, C. (2005b). Improved recovery from prolonged exercise following the consumption of low glycemic index carbohydrate meals. *Int. J. Sports Nutr. Exerc. Metab.*, 15:333–349.
Thomas, DE., Brotherhood, JR., Brand, JC. (1991). Carbohydrate feeding before exercise: Effect of glycemic index. *Int. J. Sports Med.*, 12:180–186.
Trompers, W., Perry, TL., Rose, MC., Rehrer, NJ. (2010). Glycemic and insulinemic response to selected snack bars in trained versus sedentary individuals. *Int. J. Sports Nutr. Exerc. Metab.*, 20:27–33.
Tsao, TS., Burcelin, R., Katz, EB., Huang, L., Charron, MJ. (1996). Enhanced insulin action due to targeted GLUT4 overexpression exclusively in muscle. *Diabetes*, 45:28–36.
Venn, BJ., Green, TJ. (2007). Glycemic index and glycemic load: Measurement issues and their effect on diet–disease relationships. *Eur. J. Clin. Nutr.,* 61(Suppl. 1):S122–S131.
Watt, MJ. (2009). Triglyceride lipases alter fuel metabolism and mitochondrial gene expression. *Appl. Physiol. Nutr. Metab.*, 34(3):340–347. doi: 10.1139/H09-019.
Wee, SL., Williams, C., Gray, S., Horabin, J. (1999). Influence of high and low glycemic index meals on endurance running capacity. *Med. Sci. Sports Exerc.*, 31(3):393–399.
Wee, SL., Williams, C., Tsintzas, K., Boobis, L. (2005). Ingestion of a high glycemic-index meal increases muscle glycogen storage at rest but augments its utilisation during subsequent exercise. *J. Appl. Physiol.*, 99:707–714.
Wolever, TM., Jenkins, DJ., Vuksan, V., Josse, RG., Wong, GS., Jenkins, AL. (1990). Glycemic index of foods in individual subjects. *Diabetes Care*, 13(2):126–132.
Wolever, TM., Vorster, HH., Bjorck, I., Brand-Miller, J., Brighenti, F., Mann, JI., Xiaomei, W. (2003). Determination of the glycaemic index of foods: interlaboratory study. *Eu. J. Clin. Nutr.,* 57(3):475–482.
Wong, SHS., Chan, OW., Chen, YJ., Hu, HL., Lam, CW., Chung, PK. (2009). Effect of preexercise glycemic-index meal on running when CHO-electrolyte solution is consumed during exercise. *Int. J. Sports Nutr. Exerc. Metab.*, 19:222–242.
Wong, SHS., Siu, PM., Lok, A., Chen, YJ., Morris, J., Lam, CW. (2008). Effect of the glycemic index of pre-exercise carbohydrate meals on running performance. *Eur. J. Sport Sci.*, 8(1):23–33.
Wright, H. (2005). The glycaemic index and sports nutrition. *S. Afr. J. Clin. Nutr.,* 18(3):222–228.
Wu, CL., Williams, C. (2006). A low glycemic index meal before exercise improves endurance running capacity in men. *Int. J. Sports Nutr. Exerc. Metab.*, 16:510–527.

9 Dietary Glycemic Index Manipulation to Improve Cognitive Functioning

Is It Possible?

Elena Philippou and Marios Constantinou

CONTENTS

9.1 INTRODUCTION

9.1.1 The Role of Carbohydrates in Cognitive Function (CF)

The brain relies on carbohydrates, and in particular glucose, as its main energy source, which is indeed essential for its functioning (Amiel 1994). Difficult tasks requiring intensive cognitive resources have been shown to result in a measurable decline in peripheral blood glucose concentration in human studies suggested to be due to increased neural energy expenditure (Reivich and Alavi 1983; Donohoe and Benton 1999; Scholey et al. 2006). In animals, it has been shown that at a high cognitive load, the glucose demand of the hippocampus exceeds supply, whereas exogenous glucose supply enhances performance (McNay et al. 2000). This is also supported by a number of human studies that have shown that glucose consumption compared to placebo or breakfast omission enhances cognitive performance both in healthy participants and in participants with memory deficits and those with poor glucose regulation (Smith et al. 1994; Korol and Gold 1998).

The optimal glucose dose for enhancing verbal episodic memory, relative to placebo in elderly participants, was found to be 25 g, or a blood glucose concentration of approximately 8–10 mmol/L (144–180 mg/dL) (Parsons and Gold 1992), whereas in healthy young women, the optimal glucose dosage was found to be 300 mg/kg body weight (Messier et al. 1998).

It is worth noting that the glucose-enhancing effect on memory is more consistent in healthy elderly participants (Manning et al. 1997) and in patients with Alzheimer's disease (Manning et al. 1993) who present with memory decline (Meneilly et al. 1993) than in healthy young participants. In the latter group, glucose reliably facilitates memory when the cognitive demand of the task is high or under conditions of divided attention (Smith et al. 2011). In addition, it is now well established that poor glucose regulation is a risk factor for impaired cognitive functioning (CF), as shown in patients with diabetes mellitus (DM) and in people with poor glucose regulation. A systematic review on this issue concluded that poor glucose tolerance affects cognitive performance, with some cognitive domains being more sensitive than others (Lamport et al. 2009). The evidence is stronger although not entirely consistent for cognitive functions such as verbal memory, working memory, vigilance, and attention, which appear to be the most vulnerable ones in the case of brain impairment, and also the most susceptible to hyperglycemia and insulin resistance (Lamport et al. 2009). On the contrary, although repeated episodes of hypoglycaemia observed in insulin-treated diabetic patients were thought to cause cognitive dysfunction in patients with diabetes (Kodl and Seaquist 2008), this was not supported by the Diabetes Control and Complications Trial (Austin and Deary 1999) or its 18-year follow up (Jacobson et al. 2007). Thus, the parameters of glucose tolerance that are most strongly associated with cognition still remain to be determined (Lamport et al. 2009).

Normally, glucose would not be consumed as part of the normal diet in its pure form, but instead it is obtained from carbohydrate (CHO)-containing foods that are then broken down to glucose, supplying the brain and other organs with the necessary energy. A number of studies investigated the hypothesis that the rate of glucose release would affect CF using the CHO classification of the glycemic index (GI) or using the composite of GI and food's CHO content—glycemic load (GL). The effect of the diet's GL on cognitive performance has been previously critically evaluated, reaching the conclusion that the data, at the time, was insufficient to support an effect of GL on short-term cognitive performance because the findings of the available studies were inconsistent (Gilsenan et al. 2009). It should be noted, however, that this review included a study where the meals varied in macronutrient content (Nabb and Benton 2006), and a study where the GL was reduced by manipulating the CHO content of the meal, not the GI of the meal (Benton et al. 2007) and thus confounding the conclusions. To establish whether the "quality" (i.e., diet GI), rather than the quantity of CHO consumed, affects CF, a review of studies where diet GI, rather than the amount of CHO consumed is manipulated, would be required, and we have recently published such a systematic review (Philippou and Constantinou 2014). This chapter aims to critically review the evidence, including any research published since our last review (Philippou and Constantinou 2014), linking dietary GI with CF, as well as the evidence linking dietary GL and CF and subsequently offer practical recommendations on the use of CHO manipulation to enhance CF. Such findings could assist in the provision of nutritional recommendations for both children and adults aiming to enhance their CF with potential influence on studying, working, and performing everyday activities more efficiently and effectively.

9.1.2 Domains of CF Assessed

There are quite a few cognitive constructs that have been assessed to decipher the relationship between CHO consumption and CF. A number of neuropsychological tests, which are regularly employed in cognitive assessments, are sensitive to even small deviations in CF. In addition, cognitive functions such as processing speed, immediate-short-and-long-term recall, vigilance and concentration, working memory, and alternating attention, are functions that tend to be the most sensitive to cognitive decline. Therefore, studies often assess these areas in an attempt to link glucose or CHO consumption to CF (see, e.g., in Micha et al. 2010, 2011; Brindal et al. 2012).

9.1.3 Assessment of CF

The aforementioned cognitive constructs are briefly discussed in order for the reader to fully comprehend what these tests are attempting to measure.

Processing speed is usually measured with reaction time tests. The reaction time of individuals after the presentation of a stimulus (e.g., a sound or a picture or a puzzle) is recorded.

Immediate and short-term recall measures uniformly present the individual with verbal or pictorial (sometimes tactile, as well) stimuli that are to be recalled either immediately following the presentation (0 min following the presentation) of the stimuli or after a short period (e.g., 2–7 min). If the recall of the material is asked following more than 20 min after the presentation of the material, then the long-term recall is assessed. Verbal material is usually composed of lists of words, whereas pictorial material is usually composed of shapes or abstract designs.

Vigilance (the state of remaining mentally active during a period) and concentration are also two areas that are assessed. These cognitive domains could be assessed with tests that present continuous stimuli for long periods, and the participant is asked to remain as accurate as possible on a given task throughout the assessment period.

Working memory is the transient mental store of information that is used to arrive at the solution of a computational problem, mental reasoning task, and/or until the information should be used. For example, working memory is needed to keep a mathematical problem in our minds for a few seconds before arriving at the answer. The processing of information of course depends not only on the store of new information but also on the combination of this information with already existing mental "data" or abilities. A test that is sometimes used is the serial sevens or serial nines, where the individual is asked to count backward starting from 100 and each time subtracting seven or nine. This task is thought to use working memory (and vigilance to some extent), as it requires the transient mental store of some information in order to arrive to the next answer (e.g., remembering 93 in order to compute and arrive to 86 after subtracting 7).

Alternating attention or attention switching is the ability of an individual to alternate (switch) between competing stimuli whose importance alternates (switches). Tasks that measure this cognitive construct may ask the individual, for example, to alternate between numbers and letters in sequencing tasks.

There are of course numerous cognitive constructs, which could be measured in a research study given the variables measured or the variables affecting the outcome of a study. The main cognitive areas of focus in general, however, are concentration, memory/recall, processing speed, and other executive functioning measures.

9.2 DIET GI OR GL AND COGNITION

A number of research studies have been conducted to assess the effect of varying diet GI or GL on CF, and these are summarized in Tables 9.1 and 9.2, respectively. In the following sections, the characteristics of these studies, with regard to participants, design, and cognitive function assessment are described, followed by a discussion of their main findings.

TABLE 9.1
Studies Assessing the Effect of Altering Dietary Glycemic Index (GI) on Cognitive Functioning (CF)

	Source	Sample	Study Design	CHO Intervention	GI and GL of Intervention (Based on Glucose)	Timing of Blood Glucose Sampling	Timing of Cognitive Function Tests	Assessed Cognitive Function/Domain	Cognitive Function Tests Used	Outcomes/Findings and Comments
1	Kaplan et al. 2000	20 elderly $M = 10$ 60–82 years	Repeated-measures cross-over Blinded to placebo and glucose	50 g CHO provided as: glucose drink or instant mashed potatoes (HGI) or barley (LGI) or placebo (sweetened water)	Glucose: 100 Potatoes: 83 Barley: 25 Placebo: 0	0, 15, 60, 105 min after breakfast	15, 60, 105 min	1. Verbal recall and learning 2. Prose memory 3. Attention, mental flexibility, graphomotor, and visual spatial skills 4. Sustained attention	1. Self-developed test as word list recall 2. Wechsler memory scale—Third edition 3. Trail making test A & B 4. Self-developed attention test	No differences in performance were observed. Worse performance by individuals with poorer glucose regulation. Poor β cell function individuals were most sensitive to the cognitive-enhancing effects of CHOs.
2	Micha et al. 2010	60 children $M = 24$ 11–14 years	Participants were categorized into four groups based on GI and GL of their breakfast	Breakfast and snacks eaten on study day categorized as: LGI, HGL; HGI, HGL; LGI, LGL; HGI, LGL *Note*: LGI, HGL was 32% higher in energy than HGI, HGL breakfast	GI: < or > 61 GL: < or > 27	105, 149 min after breakfast	90 min	1. Verbal fluency 2. Immediate verbal recall 3. Alternating attention, selective attention, and impulsivity 4. Visual reasoning and nonverbal intelligence 5. Visual attention 6. Sustained attention 7. Delayed verbal recall 8. State psychological assessment	1. Word generation task 2. Immediate word recall 3. Strool test 4. Matrices 5. Number search 6. Serial sevens 7. Delayed word recall 8. Profile of mood states bipolar form (POMS-BI)	HGI: Better short-term memory. HGL: Better inductive reasoning. LGI and HGL: Better vigilance, sustained attention, and inductive reasoning LGI and HGL: Associated with the two CF tasks that were reported to be most difficult—mentally demanding for the participants. An LGI, HGL breakfast could selectively facilitate mentally demanding CF tasks. GI may be differentially associated with different domains.
3	Papanikolaou et al. 2006	21 type 2 diabetic $M = 10$ 65 ± 7.29 years	Within-individual	50 g CHO: Pasta (LGI) or white bread (HGI) or water	LGI: GI: 43 GL: 22 HGI: GI: 73 GL: 37[a]	−5, 15, 62, 100, 138 min after breakfast	15, 62, 100 min (digit span, Trail-making, and test of everyday attention: between 62 and 100 min)	1. Verbal recall 2. Prose memory 3. Learning and retrieving verbal information 4. Immediate recall, immediate attention, and working memory 5. Sustained and selective attention	1. Hopkins verbal learning test—revised 2. Wechsler memory scales (revised and third edition) 3. Verbal paired associates 4. Digit span 5. Test of everyday attention	Worse working memory, executive function, and auditory selective attention following HGI than LGI breakfast. No differences for sustained attention. An LGI meal relative to an HGI meal generally resulted in better cognitive performance in the postprandial period in participants, particularly in those with the greatest food-induced elevations in BG.

(Continued)

TABLE 9.1 (*Continued*)
Studies Assessing the Effect of Altering Dietary Glycemic Index (GI) on Cognitive Functioning (CF)

	Source	Sample	Study Design	CHO Intervention	GI and GL of Intervention (Based on Glucose)	Timing of Blood Glucose Sampling	Timing of Cognitive Function Tests	Assessed Cognitive Function/Domain	Cognitive Function Tests Used	Outcomes/Findings and Comments
4	Ingwersen et al. 2007	64 children $M = 26$ 6–11 years	Cross-over	35 g of HGI or LGI cereal with milk *Note*: Differed in energy, protein, CHO, fat, and fiber	LGI: 42 HGI: 77 GL: Not provided Calc as: LGI: GL: 7, HGI: GL: 23	Not done	−30, 10, 70, 130 min	Speed of attention (reaction times in attending to stimuli) Memory (reaction times in recalling and recognition and immediate and delayed recall) Accuracy of attention (accuracy of responses) Working memory	Cognitive drug research (CDR) computerized assessment battery	A significant decline in accuracy of attention (reflecting ability to sustain attention) 2 h after the HGI cereal compared with the LGI cereal. Better secondary memory performance (reflecting ability to store, hold, and retrieve information) following the LGI than the HGI meal. No effect of GI on speed of attention, speed of memory and working memory.
5	Benton et al. 2003	106 students All female Mean age: 21 years, 1 min Rat study: not included	Random allocation to one of two breakfasts (between-subject)	Two breakfasts differing in type of CHO (SAG vs. RAG)	Diet 1: GI: 42.3 Diet 2: GI: 65.9	0, 20, 50, 80, 140, 200 and 230 min	30, 90, 150 and 210 min	Word recall in different time intervals	Self-developed memory test	Recall of more concrete words at 210 min after the LGI meal, but not earlier. Better memory throughout the morning for abstract words after the LGI breakfast.
6	Lamport et al. 2011	14 participants All male 19–28 years	WS LGI and HGI evening meals and HGI standard breakfast	Evening meals: HGI: white bread, banana, and lucozade. LGI: Pasta, pear, and apple juice. HGI breakfast: White bread and lucozade	Evening meals: HGI: GI: 72 GL: 96 LGI: GI: 47 GL: 63 Breakfast GI: 75 GL: 106	Evening meal: 30, 45, 60, 75, 90 Breakfast: −15, 0, 15, 30, 45, 60, 75	−15, 30 min	1. Recall of visually presented words 2. Alternating attention 3. Visual recognition memory	1. Visual verbal learning test (VVLT) 2. Attention switching test 3. Word recognition test	The HGI evening meal was associated with a non-significant trend for better verbal recall the following morning and a trend for better word recognition after but not before the breakfast. No differences in attention. Note that the above were non-statistically significant.

(*Continued*)

TABLE 9.1 (*Continued*)
Studies Assessing the Effect of Altering Dietary Glycemic Index (GI) on Cognitive Functioning (CF)

	Source	Sample	Study Design	CHO Intervention	GI and GL of Intervention (Based on Glucose)	Timing of Blood Glucose Sampling	Timing of Cognitive Function Tests	Assessed Cognitive Function/Domain	Cognitive Function Tests Used	Outcomes/Findings and Comments
7	Smith and Foster 2008	38 adolescents *M* = 18 15.6 ± 0.9 years	BS	LGI breakfast: 30 g all-bran with milk. HGI breakfast: 30 g cornflakes with milk. Breakfasts differed in composition.	LGI: 30 HGI: 77	−10, 10, 50 and 90 min	CVLT: 20, 60, 100 min Bond–Lader scale: −10, 10, 50, 90 min	1. Verbal recall 2. Psychological state	1. California verbal learning 2. Bond–Lader questionnaire	No differences in CVLT, blood glucose concentration or alertness, calmness, feeling contend, and satiety. HGI group remembered significant more items after the long delay relative to the short delay and remembered significantly more items than the LGI group after the long delay. The HGI breakfast was associated with reduced forgetting of previously encoded verbal episodic memory materials under conditions of *divided attention*. May be related to a more rapid supply of glucose to the bloodstream. *Note*: No differences in BG conc between the two meals.
8	Mahoney et al. 2005 Note: GI was not the primary aim of the study	Exp 1: 30 students *M* = 15 9–11 years Exp 2: 30 students *M* = 15 6–8 years	WS	Breakfast: Oatmeal (LGI) or ready-to-eat (HGI) cereal with milk or no breakfast. *Note*: Diff in nutrient composition (CHO, fiber and protein).	NA	Not done	75 min after start of breakfast Visual attention: 75, 95, 125 min	1. Spatial recall and learning 2. Immediate recall, Immediate attention, and working memory 3. Visual spatial perception 4. Visual attention and vigilance and auditory attention 5. Prose memory 6. Psychological state	1. Self-developed spatial map test 2. Digit span test 3. Rey complex figure test (RCFT) 4. Continuous performance test (CPT) 5. Self-developed prose memory test 6. Mini questionnaire (Likert scale)	Exp 1: Better performance in short term memory task after consuming LGI breakfast compared to HGI breakfast or no breakfast. Exp 2: Better performance on a short-term memory task and an auditory attention task after consuming LGI breakfast than HGI breakfast. Younger children may be affected more by breakfast composition. Greater benefits in girls than boys from LGI meal, but reason unclear.

(*Continued*)

TABLE 9.1 (*Continued*)
Studies Assessing the Effect of Altering Dietary Glycemic Index (GI) on Cognitive Functioning (CF)

	Source	Sample	Study Design	CHO Intervention	GI and GL of Intervention (Based on Glucose)	Timing of Blood Glucose Sampling	Timing of Cognitive Function Tests	Assessed Cognitive Function/Domain	Cognitive Function Tests Used	Outcomes/Findings and Comments
9	Nilsson et al. 2012	40 adults $M = 12$ 49–71 years	WS	HGI: White wheat bread (WWB) LGI: Guar gum enriched WWB (G-WWB) Aim of G-WWB: low, sustained BG for 240 min post consumption	WWB (ref): GI: 100 G-WWB: GI: 45 Glucose (ref) WWB GI: 70 G-WWB GI: 32 (own calculations)	0, 15, 30, 45, 60, 90, 120, 150 min after a 50 g glucose drink to assess gluco-regulation	WM: 90, 135, 180, 225 min SA: 75, 120, 165, 210 min	1. Working memory 2. Selective attention and reaction time	1. Reading sentences (self-developed test) 2. Picture test (computerized self-developed test)	SA test: Significant better performance at 120 min and between 75 and 235 min (late postprandial period) following the LGI than HGI meal. No significant differences between breakfast in reaction time or in the WM tests. Superior performance in participants with better glucoregulation. Superior performance in the SA test in participants with better than worse glucoregulation after the WWB test. *Comment*: Significant improvements after LGI meal predominantly occurred in the late postprandial period.
10	Cooper et al. 2012	41 $M = 18$ 12–14 years	WS	Provided 1.5 g/kg body mass available CHO. Matched for energy, protein and fat. HGI: cornflakes, white bread, margarine, milk LGI: muesli, milk, apple	HGI: GI: 72 GL: 54 LGI GI: 48 GL: 36	0, 15, 30, 60, 90, 120 min	30, 120 min	1. Alternating Attention, selective attention, and impulsivity 2. Working memory and information processing speed 3. Attention and response times	1. Stroop Test 2. Sternberg Paradigm 3. Flanker Task	The LGI breakfast enhanced cognitive function in adolescents, when compared to both the HGI breakfast and breakfast omission. For all three cognitive function tests, the LGI breakfast enhanced both response times and accuracy later in the morning when compared with the HGI breakfast or breakfast omission, particularly on the more cognitively demanding levels of the tests. Higher BG concentrations enhance response times, but this is to the detriment of accuracy (speed-accuracy trade-off).

(*Continued*)

TABLE 9.1 (*Continued*)
Studies Assessing the Effect of Altering Dietary Glycemic Index (GI) on Cognitive Functioning (CF)

	Source	Sample	Study Design	CHO Intervention	GI and GL of Intervention (Based on Glucose)	Timing of Blood Glucose Sampling	Timing of Cognitive Function Tests	Assessed Cognitive Function/Domain	Cognitive Function Tests Used	Outcomes/Findings and Comments
11	Micha et al. 2011	74 children $M = 37$ 11–14 years	Matched, random allocation to high-GL or low-GL group. Each group was given a HGI and LGI breakfast	1. LGI, HGL 2. HGI, HGL 3. LGI, LGL 4. HGI, LGL Varied amounts of muesli, cornflakes, milk, apple juice and sugar	1. GI: 48 GL: 41 2. GI: 61 GL: 55 3. GI: 48 GL: 21 4. GI: 61 GL: 28	0, 90 min (Salivary cortisol also assessed at same times)	0, 90 min	1. Verbal fluency 2. Immediate verbal recall 3. Alternating attention, selective attention, and impulsivity 4. Visual reasoning and nonverbal intelligence 5. Visual attention 6. Sustained attention 7. Delayed verbal recall 8. State psychological assessment	1. Word generation task 2. Immediate word recall 3. Stroop test 4. Matrices 5. Number search 6. Serial sevens 7. Delayed word recall 8. Profile of mood states bipolar form (POMS-BI)	LGI meals: Better performance on the word generation task. HGI meals: Better performance on the Stroop (in the high GL meals only), speed of information processing and serial sevens task. HGI meals increased cortisol concentration both before and after the CF tests. A LGI, HGL breakfast meal improved learning, possibly through its effects on glucose and cortisol concentrations. HGL and LGI meals decrease fatigue and increase alertness.

Source: Adapted from Philippou, E. and Constantinou, M., *Adv. Nutr.* 5, 119–130, 2014. With permission.

[a] GI and GL were obtained from data provided by Dr. Yianni Papanikolaou, Kunin-Lunenfeld Applied Research Unit, Baycrest, Toronto, ON, Canada (pers. comm.).

BS, between-subject; CF, cognitive functioning; CHO, carbohydrate; CVLT, Modified California Verbal Learning Test; LT, long-term; RAG, rapidly available glucose; SAG, slowly available glucose; ST, short term; WS, within-subject.

TABLE 9.2
Studies Assessing the Effect of Altering Dietary Glycemic Load (GL) on Cognitive Functioning (CF)

Source	Sample	Study Design	CHO Intervention	GI and GL of Intervention (Based on Glucose)	Timing of Blood Glucose Sampling	Timing of Cognitive Function Tests	Assessed Cognitive Function /Domain	Cognitive Function Tests Used	Outcomes/ Findings and Comments
Lamport et al. 2013	14 (12 males) Type 2 DM, 10 (4 males) with NGT (controls), 45–77 years Ethnicity: White British/North American	Counter-balanced, randomized, crossover, 2 × 3 mixed design. Between groups factor: diabetes status Within groups factor: b/fast type	1. Low GL breakfast: seeded bread, margarine, yoghurt and water. 2. High GL breakfast: glucose drink. 3. Water breakfast. Breakfasts matched for weight.	GI: LGL: 32 HGL: 95 GL: LGL: 12 HGL: 71 Water: 0	0, 15, 30, 60, 90, 120, 150, 180 min	Session 1: 30 min after b/fast Session 2: 120 min after b/fast	1. Verbal memory and delayed memory 2. Visuospatial memory and learning 3. Delayed memory 4. Psycho-motor skill 5. Executive function	1a. Visual verbal learning test (VVLT) (a visual analogue of the Rey auditory-verbal learning test [RAVLT]). 1b. Paragraph recall using the Wechsler Memory scale—revised. 2a. Visual spatial learning test (VSLT) (3 trials). 2b. Corsi block tapping test. 3. Delayed VVLT, paragraph and VSLT recall 30 min after initial presentation. 4. Grooved peg board (manual dexterity assessment). 5. Tower of Hanoi (planning ability assessment).	Type 2 DM was associated with cognitive impairment across all cognitive domains as evidenced by fewer correct responses and slower reaction times. No differences were observed between the NGT and type 2 diabetes groups following the LGL or HGL b/fasts at sessions 1 or 2. Only one main effect of b/fast showing that psychomotor skill was better following the LGL b/fast. Small sample size of the non-diabetic group—potentially lack of statistical power to detect an interaction between diabetes status and b/fast GL. Small sample, patients in the early stages of type 2 DM thus results may not be representative to all type 2 DM pts. Possible issues with b/fasts: small amount of energy provided by b/fasts (307 kcal), different form of b/fasts (solid vs. beverage), variation in macronutrients, habitual b/fast consumption not recorded.

(Continued)

TABLE 9.2 (*Continued*)
Studies Assessing the Effect of Altering Dietary Glycemic Load (GL) on Cognitive Functioning (CF)

Source	Sample	Study Design	CHO Intervention	GI and GL of Intervention (Based on Glucose)	Timing of Blood Glucose Sampling	Timing of Cognitive Function Tests	Assessed Cognitive Function /Domain	Cognitive Function Tests Used	Outcomes/ Findings and Comments
Lamport et al. 2014a	65 pre-menopausal females 30–50 years, NGT: $n = 47$, IGT: $n = 18$ Each participant belonged to one of four groups: 1. NGT/LWC ($n = 25$), 2. NGT/HWC ($n = 22$), 3. IGT/LWC (n = 9) or IGT/HWC ($n = 9$)	Counter-balanced, randomized, crossover, 2 × 2 × 3 mixed design. Between groups factors: glucose tolerance (NGT and IGT) and waist circumference (high and low). Within groups factor: breakfast (water, LGL and HGL)	Same as Lamport et al. 2013	Same as Lamport et al. 2013	Same as Lamport et al. 2013	Same as Lamport et al. 2013	Same as Lamport et al. 2013	Same as Lamport et al. 2013.	IGT in healthy middle-aged females was associated with impairment in a range of cognitive domains compared to healthy controls. The majority of cognitive outcomes showed no main effect of b/fast. During test session 2, the IGT/HWC (high risk) group demonstrated significantly poorer immediate verbal memory and delayed spatial memory than all other groups and this impairment was attenuated by the consumption of the LGL b/fast. Caution with generalizing findings since population was only white British females. Same issues with b/fasts as in Lamport et al. (2013).

(*Continued*)

TABLE 9.2 (*Continued*)
Studies Assessing the Effect of Altering Dietary Glycemic Load (GL) on Cognitive Functioning (CF)

Source	Sample	Study Design	CHO Intervention	GI and GL of Intervention (Based on Glucose)	Timing of Blood Glucose Sampling	Timing of Cognitive Function Tests	Assessed Cognitive Function /Domain	Cognitive Function Tests Used	Outcomes/ Findings and Comments
Lamport et al. 2014b	Combination of 2 studies with same design: Lamport et al. (2013, 2014a)	Counter-balanced, randomized, crossover, mixed design.	Same as Lamport et al. 2013	Same as Lamport et al. 2013	Same as Lamport et al. 2013	Same as Lamport et al. 2013	1. Verbal memory (familiarity) 2. Battery of cognitive function tests discussed in same as Lamport et al. 2013 and 2014a 3. Source monitoring test performed 30 min later (recollection)	1. Visual verbal learning test (visual analogue of the Rey auditory-verbal learning test). 2. Same as Lamport et al., 2013. 3. Source monitoring test based on three lists of words (lists A and B previously seen, list C: new words) that had to be correctly identified by pressing keys labeled 1, 2, or 3 corresponding to word lists A, B, and C.	No effect of b/fast GL manipulations on source monitoring retrieval processes. No effects of GL on either recollection or familiarity. No cognitive benefit since no differences between breakfast or water consumption. Type 2 DM and IGT were association with source monitoring recollection deficits compared to NGT. Possible mechanisms: hippocampal impairments but these are accounted for by underlying deleterious mechanisms but not circulating peripheral glucose. Same issues with b/fasts as in Lamport et al. (2013).

(*Continued*)

TABLE 9.2 (*Continued*)
Studies Assessing the Effect of Altering Dietary Glycemic Load (GL) on Cognitive Functioning (CF)

Source	Sample	Study Design	CHO Intervention	GI and GL of Intervention (Based on Glucose)	Timing of Blood Glucose Sampling	Timing of Cognitive Function Tests	Assessed Cognitive Function /Domain	Cognitive Function Tests Used	Outcomes/ Findings and Comments
Power et al. 2014	$n = 208$ (Males: 94) community-dwelling elderly 64–93 years	Cross-sectional study of diet and cognitive capacity.	No intervention. FFQ used to collect dietary data.	GL per 2000 kcal based on analysis of FFQ. Mean (SD) GL: Males: 146.78 (20.15) Females: 142.42 (18.34)	N/A	N/A (test completed once)	Orientation to time and place, naming, repeating, writing, copying, instantaneous recall, short-term memory, backward spelling	Mini-Mental State Examination. Range of MMSE score: 0–30 Mild cognitive impairment: MMSE ≤ 24.	Subjects with mild cognitive impairment consumed a higher GL diet compared to those with normal cognitive function. An individual who consumed a high GL diet had a 4.5-fold increased chance of being cognitively impaired compared to individuals who consumed a low GL diet. Issues: MMSE assesses global cognitive function and may not be sensitive enough to subtle changes caused by diet. Study was able to carefully control for several confounders but information on others such as physical activity were not collected. Cohort was self-selected

(*Continued*)

TABLE 9.2 (*Continued*)
Studies Assessing the Effect of Altering Dietary Glycemic Load (GL) on Cognitive Functioning (CF)

Source	Sample	Study Design	CHO Intervention	GI and GL of Intervention (Based on Glucose)	Timing of Blood Glucose Sampling	Timing of Cognitive Function Tests	Assessed Cognitive Function /Domain	Cognitive Function Tests Used	Outcomes/ Findings and Comments
Benton et al. 2007	19 children, (males: 9) 6 years, 10 m	WS	Three experimental meals with similar energy content, differing in GL High GL, Medium GL, Low GL	GL based on amount of consumed meals: HGL: 17.86 (SD: 8.85) MGL: 12.09 (4.13) LGL: 2.85 (2.97)	N/A	Varied between 110 and 210 min post b/fast	1. Classroom behavior 2. Memory 3. Reaction to frustration 4. Ability to sustain attention	1. Secret 30 min recording of class and analysis of behavior of each child. 2. Recall of Objects test of the British Ability Scale 3. A television video game adjusting the condition to make the task difficult and recording responses to failure. 4. Paradigm of Shakow.	Consumption of a low GL meal resulted in better scores on measures of memory, ability to sustain attention, likelihood of frustration and spending time on task while in the classroom. Some of the effects were short-lived and did not survive negative experiences such as frustration. The three b/fasts were significantly different in fat and protein apart from CHO.

(Continued)

TABLE 9.2 (*Continued*)
Studies Assessing the Effect of Altering Dietary Glycemic Load (GL) on Cognitive Functioning (CF)

Source	Sample	Study Design	CHO Intervention	GI and GL of Intervention (Based on Glucose)	Timing of Blood Glucose Sampling	Timing of Cognitive Function Tests	Assessed Cognitive Function /Domain	Cognitive Function Tests Used	Outcomes/ Findings and Comments
Brindal et al. 2012	39 children, 11.6 ± 0.7years	Three-way, repeated measures crossover	Three isocaloric b/fasts: HGL, MGL, LGL	GI: HGL: 67 MGL: 54 LGL: 48 GL: HGL: 33 MGL: 24 LGL: 18	0–200 min after meals. Measured by Med-tronic MiniMed Continuous Glucose Monitoring System. Extracellular glucose measured every 10 s, average of values stored in memory every 5 min.	0, 1 h, 2 h, 3 h after b/fast (20 min required to complete tests each time)	1. Speed of processing 2. Short-term memory 3. Working memory 4. Perceptual speed 5. Attention switching 6. Inspection time	1. Composite measure of the responses to three reaction times a simple reaction time, a two-choice reaction time and an odd-man-out reaction time. 2. Computerized word memory task, based on the Rey auditory verbal learning test. 3. Digitspan backward task from the Weschler intelligence scale for children. 4. Finding *A*s task: participants were given a list of words and asked to strikeout as many words containing an *A* as possible in 60 s. 5. Participant was required to respond as accurately and quickly as possible to the stimulus, by applying one of two simple rules that participants had to switch between on every second trial. 6. Measured using a Windows-based program requiring participants to make a simple, perceptually based decision.	Breakfast GL did not significantly alter changes in cognitive function. Test meals varied in GL by manipulating dairy content. Blood glucose concentration fell to below baseline within 90 min for all test meals. Pronounced differences in protein content between the meals.

(*Continued*)

TABLE 9.2 (*Continued*)
Studies Assessing the Effect of Altering Dietary Glycemic Load (GL) on Cognitive Functioning (CF)

Source	Sample	Study Design	CHO Intervention	GI and GL of Intervention (Based on Glucose)	Timing of Blood Glucose Sampling	Timing of Cognitive Function Tests	Assessed Cognitive Function /Domain	Cognitive Function Tests Used	Outcomes/ Findings and Comments
Brindal et al. 2013	40 children, 11.6 (SE: 0.13) year	Three-way, repeated measures crossover	Three beverages: Very HGL (VHGL): pure glucose, HGL: half milk, half glucose, LGL: pure milk	GI: VHGL:100 HGL: 84 LGL: 27 GL: VHGL: 65 HGL: 35 LGL: 5	Same as Brindal et al. 2012	Same as Brindal et al. 2012	Same as Brindal et al. 2012	Same as Brindal et al. 2012.	No significant effects of test drink on any of the cognitive domains assessed. Girls only responded better to the LGL drink with regard to short-term memory. Drinks varied in protein and fat content (apart from being different in CHO content). The difference in responses between boys and girls may be related to gender variations in energy requirements. In the study, the same-sized energy preload was used in all children.

NGT, normal glucose tolerance.

9.2.1 Characteristics of Studies Assessing the Effect of Dietary GI on CF

The effect of GI on CF was assessed in populations of various ages, ranging from children (Mahoney et al. 2005; Ingwersen et al. 2007) or adolescents (Smith and Foster 2008; Micha et al. 2010, 2011; Cooper et al. 2012), young adults (Benton et al. 2003; Lamport et al. 2011), middle-aged to elderly (Nilsson et al. 2012), or only elderly (Kaplan et al. 2000; Papanikolaou et al. 2006), and the study populations were mostly healthy except in one study where the participants had Type 2 diabetes (Papanikolaou et al. 2006). Assessment of CF took place in the morning following an overnight fast and the provision of a breakfast meal/drink varying in GI. A within-subjects' design was employed by most studies in that participants consumed either the LGI or the HGI meal/drink on different occasions (Kaplan et al. 2000; Mahoney et al. 2005; Papanikolaou et al. 2006; Ingwersen et al. 2007; Lamport et al. 2011; Cooper et al. 2012; Nilsson et al. 2012), whereas in some studies, each participant consumed only one of the two breakfasts varying in GI (between-subjects' design) (Benton et al. 2003; Smith and Foster 2008; Micha et al. 2011). Another method employed was to assess the effect of diet GI on CF following categorization of the participants into one of four groups based on their own breakfast GI and GL (Micha et al. 2010), whereas in the Lamport et al. (2011) study, the evening meals, rather than the breakfast, were manipulated to examine the second meal effect—whether the GI of the previous meal affected CF the following morning both before and after a standardized HGI breakfast.

9.2.2 Characteristics of Studies Assessing the Effect of Dietary GL on CF

Fewer studies assessed the impact of altering diet GL rather than GI on CF as can be seen in Table 9.2. As with the studies assessing GI, the age range also varied, ranging from children (Benton et al. 2007; Brindal et al. 2012, 2013) to adult women (30–77 years) (Lamport et al. 2013, 2014a, b) and elderly adults (64–93 years) (Power et al. 2014). As with the studies assessing GI on CF, most research was conducted in healthy populations, but research in people with Type 2 diabetes (Lamport et al. 2013) and impaired glucose tolerance (IGT) (Lamport et al. 2014a) has also been carried out. CF was also assessed in the morning and most studies employed a within-subjects' design, with the exception of a cross-sectional study of diet and CF, which examined the association between dietary patterns, dietary GL, and cognition using a validated 147-item semi-quantitative food frequency questionnaire (FFQ) (Power et al. 2014).

9.2.3 Meal Interventions

The nutritional composition of the meals was not reported in all studies (Micha et al. 2010; Lamport et al. 2011; Nilsson et al. 2012), while in most of the rest of the studies, the composition of the meals provided to the two groups was not matched, mainly because of differences in the amounts of fiber and protein between the meals. An exception was the study by Cooper et al. (2012), in which both the HGI and LGI meals contained 1.5 g/kg body mass available CHO and were matched for energy, protein, and fat content. In the studies assessing GL and cognition by Lamport et al. (2013, 2014a, b), the three breakfasts (LGL, HGL, and water) were matched for weight, whereas the LGL and HGL meals were isocaloric. Nevertheless, other than this, since the LGL meal consisted of toast and yoghurt and the HGL meal consisted of a glucose drink, the LGL and HGL breakfasts differed in form and consistency (meal vs. drink) and in macronutrients and fiber content.

It should also be noted that in all the discussed studies, there was no attempt, with the exception of one investigation (Micha et al. 2011), to blind the participants or the investigators with regard to the GI/GL of the meal provided, although concealment of randomization was not done in any study.

9.2.4 Assessment of CF

Assessment of CF was carried out using a variety of tests, and with the exception of two studies, which used only one type of assessment (Benton et al. 2003; Power et al. 2014), a battery of tests—a number of different assessments (2–8 tests)—were employed. In some studies, the utilized CF tests were subscales of larger known cognitive assessment tools, such as the Wechsler memory scale-IV (WMS-IV; Wechsler 2009), trial making test A & B (TMT A & B; Tombaugh 2004), and Hopkins verbal learning test (HVLT; Benedict et al. 1998). In some other studies, however, self-developed instruments were administered for assessing several neuropsychological/cognitive functions, such as memory (verbal recall, prose memory, working memory, and visual recognition memory), attention (sustained and selective attention, speed of attention, visual attention, and attention switching), learning (learning and retrieving verbal information and information processing skill), reasoning and intelligence (mental flexibility, verbal fluency, visual reasoning, graphomotor and visual spatial skills, and nonverbal intelligence). Psychopathology was also a domain assessed by some self-developed instruments. Benton et al. (2007), in addition to assessing memory and attention, also recorded classroom behavior by filming children un-obtrusively for 30 min and analyzing each child's behavior and their reaction to frustration every 10 s.

There was no consistency among studies in the timing of the administration of tests, specifically the timing between food intake and cognitive assessment; in most studies, CF was assessed at least three times starting before breakfast and up to 210 min following the provision of a meal (postprandially). Some studies, however, assessed CF only once (Micha et al. 2010) or only twice (Lamport et al. 2011; Micha et al. 2011; Cooper et al. 2012).

9.2.5 Findings of Studies Assessing GI and Cognition in Children

Research findings are not consistent with regard to the effects of diet GI on CF in children (refer to Table 9.1 for a summary of the studies). In Micha et al. (2010), who studied adolescents aged 11–14 years, the LGI and HGL breakfast was associated with better performance in the two most mentally demanding assessments of CF, specifically speed of information processing and serial sevens task (see Section 9.1.3); although the HGI breakfast was associated with better short-term memory, and the HGL breakfast with better inductive reasoning, leading the authors to conclude that GI "may be differentially associated with different domains" (Micha et al. 2010). In a study by the same investigators on similar-aged children (Micha et al. 2011), LGI meals resulted in a better performance on the word generation task, but in contrast to their previous findings, the authors found that HGI meals lead to better performance on the speed of information processing and serial sevens task, although the LGI HGL meal improved learning (Micha et al. 2011).

In the Ingwersen et al. (2007) study, the results were also mixed because there was a significant decline in attention 2 h following consumption of the HGI cereal and better verbal recall following the LGI than the HGI meal. However, the breakfast GI had no effect on cognitive processing speed in measures of attention, memory, and working memory. Similarly, in the Mohoney et al. (2005) study, there was an improved performance in a short-term memory task and a verbal auditory attention task after the LGI compared to the HGI breakfast; however, for unclear reasons, girls benefited more than boys from the LGI meal. Cooper et al.'s findings (2012) also favored the LGI meal because it appeared to enhance CF via the improvement of both response times and accuracy in cognitive tasks, in comparison to the HGI meal and breakfast omission. In contrast, Smith and Foster (2008) found that the HGI group recalled significantly more after a long delay compared to the LGI group, and the HGI breakfast was associated with reduced memory decay of previously learned materials under conditions of divided attention.

9.2.6 Findings of Studies Assessing GI and Cognition in Adults

As with the studies in children, there was a lot of variation in the findings of the studies assessing GI and cognition in adults (summary shown in Table 9.1). No differences in performance in four different cognitive function tests were found following consumption of meals of different GI in elderly adults (Kaplan et al. 2000). A study assessing whether the GI of the evening meal had any effects on CF the following morning also found no differences between the HGI and LGI meals, although a statistical trend favoring the HGI evening meal was observed (Lamport et al. 2011). On the other hand, the results by Benton et al. (2003) who studied young females, favored the LGI meals since verbal recall of abstract words appeared improved throughout the morning after the LGI breakfast, while more concrete words could be recalled in the late postprandial phase (210 min) following consumption of the LGI meal. Nilsson et al. (2009) also showed that performance was better in the late postprandial period following consumption of a LGI than a HGI meal but only in selective attention. In the latter study, no significant differences were observed in cognitive reaction time or working memory. Finally, in the study by Papanikolaou et al. (2006), which was the only one performed in adults diagnosed with Type 2 diabetes, (as opposed to healthy participants), the results also favored the LGI breakfast, as general CF was better in the postprandial period following the consumption of the LGI than the HGI meal.

9.2.7 Findings of Studies Assessing GL and Cognition in Children

As shown in Table 9.2, the results of studies assessing GL and CF in children were contradictory. In the Benton et al. (2007) study, consumption of an LGL breakfast was associated with more favorable results in behavior and cognition. In this study, the LGL meal resulted in significantly more time spent on task compared to the medium or HGL meal, while with regard to reaction to frustration when performing a difficult task, performance was poorer in those consuming the HGL meal, and GL negatively predicted performance. With regard to memory, it was found that better immediate but not delayed memory was significantly associated with GL, and the lower the GL, the better the memory scores. Moreover, more lapses in attention were displayed by those who consumed more CHO, less fat, and a greater GL. Nevertheless, no effect of the type of meal was seen with behaviors such as time spent looking around the room or time spent talking, fidgeting, or being out of seat. Thus, in this group of children, the findings favored the LGL meal, although the variation in macronutrients other than CHO between the three types of breakfast confounded the findings, and it was actually shown that the amount of fat also correlated with performance. As the authors noted, however, GL should not be considered in isolation, given the role played by fat, protein, and fiber in the rate at which glucose is released. It is true that one of the most important criticisms against assessing a diet's GL instead of GI is that the former is affected mostly by the amount rather than the type of CHO (i.e., GI) (Brand-Miller et al. 2003b). In reality, a meal's GL could be lowered both by reducing the CHO content (and in effect increasing the other macronutrients, these being fat and protein) and by choosing foods of lower GI, but the metabolic effects in each of these scenarios would be different. Moreover, caution should be taken when attempting to lower a meal's GL by reducing the CHO content to very low amounts because this may result in an unbalanced diet with potentially detrimental health effects.

Contradicting Benton et al.'s (2007) findings, Brindal et al. (2012), in a study assessing the effects of isocaloric breakfast meals differing in GL on cognitive performance of children aged 10–12 years, did not find any significant effects of breakfast GL on changes in cognitive performance for any of the cognitive tasks assessed (speed of processing, working memory, short-term memory, perceptual speed or attention switching, and inspection time). Another study by the same researchers (Brindal et al. 2013) using beverages differing in GL in the same group of children also found no effect of GL on cognition with the exception of an effect on short-term memory in girls only, who seemed to respond more favorably to the LGL drink compared to HGL drinks. The authors note that this may be due to gender variations in energy requirements. The reasons for inconsistent findings between studies are not clear but possible factors are discussed in Section 9.4.

9.2.8 Findings of Studies Assessing GL and Cognition in Adults

Studies of GL and CF in adults showed that there was limited evidence for LGL meals or diets being more beneficial to females at risk of diabetes and possibly to elderly adults (summary shown in Table 9.2), but further research is warranted to confirm such findings.

In the study by Lamport et al. (2013), it was shown that type 2 diabetes was associated with impairments in all cognitive functions examined compared to adults with normal glucose tolerance (NGT), although varying breakfast GL did not impact cognitive performance in either type 2 diabetes or NGT participants. Similarly, in a second study by the same group of investigators (Lamport et al. 2014a), impaired glucose tolerance (IGT) was associated with impairment of verbal and spatial memory and psychomotor function relative to NGT, and increased waist circumference (WC) was associated with impairment of verbal memory and executive function in comparison to low WC. The LGL breakfast attenuated the verbal memory impairment in the IGT/high WC group (high-risk group) relative to the HGL breakfast or water used as control. Thus, in type 2 diabetes, there was no evidence that acute manipulation of breakfast GL could benefit cognitive function (Lamport et al. 2013), and in females with abnormal glucose tolerance and increased WC—abnormalities usually preceding type 2 diabetes—there is limited evidence that acute consumption of an LGL breakfast is potentially more beneficial with regard to cognitive function compared to an HGL breakfast or no breakfast, something that needs to be further investigated (Lamport et al. 2014a). Lamport et al. (2014b) also studied the effects of the same acute GL breakfast manipulations at 30 and 120 min in the same two populations following breakfast on simple word recognition (familiarity) and complex source monitoring (recollection). Both type 2 diabetes and IGT were associated with significant source monitoring recollection deficits but not impairments in familiarity, suggestive of impairments of the hippocampus, which, nevertheless, as in the previous studies, were not attenuated by the breakfast GL manipulations. Thus, in all three studies, it could be speculated that the impairments seen in type 2 diabetes and IGT could be accounted by the underlying metabolic and physiological mechanisms, the discussion of which is outside of the scope of this chapter, and not circulating peripheral glucose obtained from external sources that is food intake. What was not examined, however, in the above studies but was suggested by previous authors, are the metabolic responses to the HGL meal in the very late postprandial phase—200 min post consumption (Nilsson et al. 2012)—at which point, the hyperglycemia induced by the HGL meal would be expected to result in increased concentration of insulin, cortisol, free fatty acids as well as oxidative stress and inflammatory markers (Ludwig 2002) with potentially detrimental effects on cognitive function. This possibility renders further study since as suggested by Lamport et al. (2011) in the second meal effect study, the metabolic effects of food intake on cognition influence outcomes even during the following day.

Power et al. (2014) in a cross-sectional study examining the association between dietary patterns, dietary GL, and cognition using a FFQ found that for every one unit increase in GL, the mean number of MMSE errors increased by 1%, and that subjects with a mild cognitive impairment consumed a higher GL diet compared to those with normal cognitive function. Additionally, using a model adjusted for various confounders, it was found that an individual who consumed a high GL diet had a four-and-a-half fold increased chance of being cognitively impaired compared to one who consumed a low GL diet. As noted by the authors, the variation in the MMSE explained by GL was higher than (or roughly equivalent to) that explained by variables known to affect cognitive function such as age, hypertension, diabetes, and nutritional status. Nevertheless, since the MMSE assesses global cognitive function, it may not be sensitive enough to pick up specific or subtle cognitive deficits related to diet.

9.3 SUMMARY OF FINDINGS OF STUDIES ASSESSING THE EFFECT OF GI/GL ON CF

The results of studies assessing the effect of diet GI and GL on CF are inconsistent, with some showing benefits toward either the LGI/LGL or the HGI/HGL meal, others not finding any differences between the meals and yet others showing a positive or negative effect on performance on only one or some cognitive domain(s) after the consumption of one of the two meals. Nevertheless, at the time of writing this chapter, there was some, although limited, evidence for low GL meals or diets being more beneficial to females at risk of diabetes and possibly to elderly adults, but further research is warranted to confirm the findings.

9.4 CONTRASTING OUTCOMES

The inconsistencies between research findings could be because of the small number of existing relevant studies and the many methodological differences between studies (e.g., type of design, meal composition, and types and timing of cognitive function tests). At the same time, the presence of many confounding factors (e.g., age and glucose tolerance) may not have allowed for a larger consensus in the findings.

With regard to age, it is known that children are more susceptible to glucose provision than adults. This is because per gram of weight, a child's brain tissue uses more glucose than that of an adult but also since compared to adults, children's brains are relatively bigger and more active per unit weight. These factors may result in children being more responsive to glucose provision than adults (Chugani 1998). This may partly explain why the findings of the studies in children and adults differed since if, for children, the *amount* rather than the *type* of glucose is more important, then the cognitive domains that required a quick release of glucose would be more likely to benefit from HGI (and/or HGL meals), whereas if testing was carried out at a late postprandial period, then the LGI (i.e., slowly released meal) and HGL (i.e., the meal containing most glucose) would most likely be more beneficial because these meals would provide the brain with most available glucose. This points out to the necessity of a better understanding of the impact of CHO manipulation on different cognitive domains because it is clear that they are not all affected in the same way. One way to achieve this would be to concentrate more on testing one specific cognitive domain using different cognitive instruments rather than testing many domains in the same study. Such approach could decipher the most sensitive cognitive assessment instruments for assessing the impact of the quality of the consumed CHO (the reader is referred to Section 9.6 for a detailed discussion of recommendations for future research and research design).

The inconsistencies in the findings might also be due to the differences in meal composition. For example, in some studies (e.g., Micha et al. 2010, 2011), the energy content of the meals was significantly different, with the LGI, HGL breakfast having the highest energy content of all meals, which was almost double that of the HGI, LGL breakfast. Thus, as the authors themselves point out the differences in GL cannot be differentiated. However, at least for these two studies, the energy and macronutrient composition of HGI and LGI meals was similar within the same GL group and thus any GI effects could be differentiated from energy and macronutrient content differences. Nevertheless, the fact that in some studies such as those by Lamport et al. (2013, 2014a, b), the LGL and HGL breakfasts differed in form and consistency (meal vs. drink), in addition to macronutrients and fiber content, may have also affected the outcomes. It is recommended that in all studies, there is an account of not only the meal's GI and GL but also its energy and macronutrient content.

Another factor that might have affected the studies' outcomes may be the individual differences between the participants' usual breakfast GI and GL. At present, it is not clear if the consumption of meals under experimental conditions has a different impact on the individual when the experimental meal is of similar GI to the one they usually consume (at breakfast) as opposed to a meal with a higher or a lower GI than their regular one. The effect of breakfast consumption *per se*, irrespective of GI, on the cognitive function of individuals who usually skip this meal is also not known. These parameters are important and should be taken into consideration in future studies, given that meal composition may have an impact on factors such as fullness, bloating, satiety, meal rating, or even mood that subsequently affects motivation and arousal and thus test performance (Micha et al. 2010). A different experimental approach could have been to test (in the same participants) meals with a similar GI, GL, and total energy content as a way to determine the extent by which the above confounders (e.g., fullness) contribute to the inconsistency in the findings. In addition to the previous factors, the timing of testing is equally crucial and could also explain some of the inconsistencies between studies because timing in the reported studies varied.

With regard to adult studies, there are additional reasons that might have contributed to the observed inconsistencies. The first is the variation in the participants' age while the second is the participants' blood glucose regulation and the interaction with age. Cognition (Brayne and Calloway, 1988) and perhaps glucose tolerance (Lamport et al. 2009) are affected by age. As shown in a review by Lamport et al. (2009), individuals with poor glucose tolerance are benefited more by glucose consumption compared to those with better glucoregulation. Moreover, in studies of older adults, glucose is more beneficial irrespective of their glucose tolerance but older better glucoregulators are more likely to benefit from glucose consumption than younger ones (Awad et al. 2002; Messier et al. 2003; Lamport et al. 2009). On the other hand, in individuals with good cognition and good glucose tolerance, glucose consumption could hamper performance (Kaplan et al. 2000). Irrespective of age though, the cognitive benefits of glucose consumption increase with worsening glucose tolerance (Lamport et al. 2009). These factors are important because in the studies discussed in this chapter, the age range was very wide, and although the majority of studies included healthy participants, glucose tolerance was not necessarily assessed before enrolment. Additionally, even in the study with type 2 diabetic participants, there seems to be a wide variation in glucose tolerance since some of the participants were on oral hypoglycemic agents and some were controlled by diet alone (Papanikolaou et al. 2006). Although the question under discussion is how the rate of glucose release rather than glucose provision itself affects cognitive function, it is possible that the differences between the participants with regard to their glucose tolerance might have affected their cognitive function.

In addition, another issues that complicates the extraction of conclusions is the wide inter-study methodological variability, for example, in study design (between- or within-subject design), timing of testing, cognitive domain being examined, number and type of cognitive tests used, meals provided and timing of blood samples collected. Additionally, studies, with the exception of Lamport et al. (2011), did not control for the previous evening meal, known to affect the glycemic response the next morning (Wolever et al. 1988; Granfeldt et al. 2006). Moreover, none of the studies refer to restricting physical activity the previous day, which is important since exercise increases glucose muscle uptake (Malkova et al. 2000), and again could influence the glycemic response to the meals. Of course, the fact that with the exception of one study (Micha et al. 2011), the subjects and the investigators were not blinded to the meal GI, and that concealment to randomization was not done in any study, are other limitations. Although owing to the nature of the intervention in nutrition studies—the provision of meals—concealment and blinding may not always be possible; this is indeed a source of bias. To minimize bias and improve research design, a list of recommendations for future research and research design is provided in Section 9.6.

9.5 POSSIBLE MECHANISMS EXPLAINING THE EFFECT OF DIET GI ON COGNITIVE FUNCTION

Even though the findings of the studies were inconsistent, there are many possible mechanisms that might explain why altering the diet GI/GL may affect cognition, although these are thought to be complex, and they have not been fully elucidated yet. A review of the relationship of cognitive performance with postprandial metabolic changes after ingestion of different macronutrients, referred to three targets with direct or indirect influences on CF, these being energy supply to nerve cells, neurotransmitter and hormone modulations, and activation or deactivation of the nervous system (Fischer et al. 2001). As is known, the brain is very sensitive to changes in nutrient supply; nevertheless, it has been suggested that it is not the "amount" of glucose but the blood glucose "concentration" following glucose delivery that is the most relevant factor in determining the glucose memory-enhancement effect (Parsons and Gold 1992; Smith et al. 2011). Thus, a potential mechanism in favor of the LGI as opposed to the HGI meal could be the more constant postprandial blood glucose concentration associated with the ingestion of the first type of meal. On the other hand, consumption of an HGI meal leads to a rapid increase in plasma glucose concentration followed by a concomitant high insulin response resulting in a rapid blood glucose disposal, which may cause the blood glucose concentration to decrease to below the fasting concentration in the later postprandial period (Ludwig, 2002). In support of this are the findings of studies showing that the changes in blood glucose concentration rather than the absolute levels are critical for a modulation of cognitive function (Owens and Benton 1994). Moreover, studies examining the effect of GI on cognitive function have shown that significant improvements occur in the late (rather than early) postprandial phase (Benton et al. 2003; Nilsson et al. 2012), presumably because of the more stable glucose (and insulin) profile resulting after consumption of the LGI meal.

With regard to hormone modulations, a potential hormone that might affect cognitive function both through short- and long-term mechanisms is insulin. It has already been proven that the more stable postprandial glucose profile characteristic of a LGI meal is beneficial to whole body insulin sensitivity (Rizkalla et al. 2004). It is also known that the brain contains insulin receptors with important roles in cognitive function that are affected by insulin resistance (Banks et al. 2012). As mentioned above, individuals with type 2 diabetes and also those with glucose regulation abnormalities have a higher risk of Alzheimer's disease and cognitive dysfunction (Lamport et al. 2009). It may be possible that a LGI diet results in a better cognitive function in the long term through improvements in insulin sensitivity. In support of this hypothesis is the fact that a LGI diet has been shown to improve glucose tolerance and reduce HbA1c and fructosamine concentrations in diabetic patients (Brand-Miller et al. 2003a); important findings with regard to cognition since, among others, both hypo- and hyperglycemia as well as insulin resistance and poor glucose regulation are implicated as possible mechanisms in cognitive dysfunction (Kodl and Seaquist 2008). Moreover, in patients with type 1 diabetes, a better glycemic control was related to an improved cognitive performance as shown in the 18-year follow up of the Diabetes Control and Complications Trial, where the performance on cognitive function tests of those patients with a time weighted mean HbA1c of $<7.4\%$ was better than those with an HbA1c of 8.8% (Jacobson et al. 2007). Thus, the diet's GI could potentially influence cognitive function both in the short term—through the variation in the rate of glucose release—and in the long term through its effects on the mechanisms linking glucose regulation and cognition.

Another hormone that has been explored as a potential mechanism linking GI and cognition is cortisol (Micha et al. 2011). Although, a difference in GI and GL would not normally be expected to affect cortisol concentration, it has been found that an HGI meal resulted in higher cortisol concentration both before and after the CF tests, suggesting that LGI meals may be associated with a reduced response to stressful stimuli (Micha et al. 2011). It was argued that the lower blood glucose concentration following consumption of a LGI meal could result in lower activation of the hypothalamic-pituitary-adrenal axis and thus lower cortisol concentrations. The outcome was that the participants were feeling less stressed or nervous before carrying out the CF tests that ultimately improved their performance on memory tests. On the other hand, the HGI meal caused an increase in cortisol concentration and the resulting nervousness is thought to have led to a better performance on vigilance tasks—how quickly the participants could process information. It would be interesting to further explore the role of this hormone; for example, in a recent study, greater cortisol responses during a test were related to enhanced memory in children 2 weeks later (Quas et al. 2011). The contradicting findings might be due to the CF being assessed and the type of tests used to assess it. For example, in the Cooper et al. study (2012), the higher blood glucose concentrations after the ingestion of an HGI meal enhanced response times on the one hand, but resulted in a detrimental effect on accuracy on the other, thus "possibly causing a speed-accuracy trade-off" (Cooper et al. 2012). If stress hormones were indeed involved in this study, the findings might be explained by the large body of evidence showing that stress enhances memory for information that is directly related to the cause of the stress at the expense of memory for unrelated, peripheral details (Deffenbacher et al. 2004). It is clear that further studies are needed in order to shed more light on stress hormones as a possible mechanism with regard to diet GI and cognition.

9.6 RECOMMENDATIONS FOR FUTURE RESEARCH AND RESEARCH DESIGN

As discussed in this chapter, there are many inconsistencies in the research findings and still a number of unanswered questions. Apart from doing more research to unravel the short-term effect of altering diet GI on CF and exploring the possible mechanisms, a very under-studied research area is the long-term effect of varying GI on CF, especially in people with IGT or type 2 diabetes who are more prone to experience a decline in CF. There should also be an attempt to identify specific mechanisms that might link diet GI and cognition, such as hormonal or inflammatory pathways. In addition, it is recommended that future studies aim to employ more consistent methodologies and try to eliminate all potential aforementioned confounders; the most important being meal composition, type and timing of cognitive function tests, and participants studied. In this way, it would be possible to both compare the findings of different studies and understand how CF is (if at all significantly) affected by manipulation of dietary CHOs. Ultimately, this will allow for the setting of recommendations on this issue and potentially the development of food products aiming to enhance CF. In addition, the authors believe that it is imperative that future studies employ some of the following recommendations when designing a study on the effect of diet GI on cognitive function:

1. Utilize cognitive/neuropsychological instruments that are standardized and normed in the studied population, so that the conclusions drawn are more confident and reliable as well as easily comparable to the greater population.
2. Utilize cognitive/neuropsychological instruments with high specificity and sensitivity that are known to detect even small, but significant for everyday functioning, variations in cognition. For example, the Trail Making Test, particularly the second part of the test (B), is very sensitive to even small declines in cognition. Another example is a short battery of cognitive tests (which includes a variation of the Trail Making Test) called Montreal Cognitive Assessment (MoCA) (Nasreddine et al. 2005), which is used for detecting small cognitive declines in adults.
3. Concentrate on testing one specific domain using different appropriate (see above) instruments rather than assessing many domains with the aim of examining the effect of diet GI on the particular domain.
4. Ensure that the composition of the HGI and LGI meals used for testing is as closely matched as possible for energy, macronutrients, and fiber to reduce the effect of confounding.
5. Manipulate a meal's GL by altering the individual meal components' GI rather than just or mainly by reducing the meal's CHO content. This could be done, for example, by exchanging brown bread with seeded bread, a breakfast cereal with a high GI with one having a low GI instead of using two slices of bread in the high GL breakfast and one in the low GL breakfast (i.e., just reducing the amount of CHO).
6. Ensure that standardized conditions are adhered to on the day before the test day. In particular, the participants should not engage in heavy exercise, should not consume alcohol, and should consume the same evening meal before each of the test days if the study has a within-subject design.
7. Take into account the subjects' usual breakfast composition and size since factors such as fullness, bloating, satiety, and meal rating, as well as whether the subjects usually consume breakfast, might be confounding to the study's findings.
8. Ensure that other potentially confounding factors such as glucose tolerance and medication that affects glucose regulation are taken into account as part of the inclusion/exclusion criteria and that these are sufficiently assessed. Aim for, as far as possible, a homogeneous population.

9.7 CONCLUSION AND SUGGESTED CLINICAL PRACTICE

Although there are a number of possible mechanisms to support the hypothesis that a low GI meal or diet may be more beneficial compared to a high-GI meal/diet on cognitive function, at present, the available evidence is not consistent enough to allow drawing any definitive conclusions with regard to the effect of diet GI or GL on CF. There is some evidence that low GL meals are more beneficial than high GL to females at risk of diabetes and possibly to elderly adults; however, further research is warranted to confirm the findings.

Based on this evidence and general healthy eating recommendations, the authors make the following recommendations to be used by people in practice:

1. Ensure that you always consume breakfast especially before participating in cognitively demanding activities such as reading, learning, writing, and memorizing information in settings such as school, work, or exams.
2. Ensure that your breakfast is based on carbohydrates and prefer low as opposed to high-GI foods such as seeded bread, muesli, or traditional oats that will be served with protein-containing foods, for example, dairy products.
3. Have regular meals and snacks throughout the day, always ensuring that they contain carbohydrates, which should preferably be low in GI.
4. Consume a healthy balanced diet and achieve and sustain a healthy body weight throughout life.
5. If you are insulin-resistant, overweight or obese, have an increased WC (i.e., visceral obesity), polycystic ovary syndrome or a family history of diabetes, consume mainly low GI CHOs as the basis of your meals and snacks such as seeded breads, traditional oats, pulses and legumes, sweet potatoes, bulgur wheat, and quinoa.
6. If you have DM (type 1 or type 2), try to control your blood glucose as advised by your health professional (through medication if needed, nutrition and exercise) and have regular check-ups, aiming to avoid both hypo- and hyperglycemia. It is recommended to consult a dietitian for advice on the consumption of a healthy, balanced, low GI diet.
7. Do not cut carbohydrate-containing foods from your diet, for example, by following diets that exclude carbohydrate, as this could be detrimental to your CF.

REFERENCES

Amiel, S.A. (1994). Nutrition of the brain: Macronutrient supply. *Proc. Nutr. Soc.* 53, 401–405.

Austin, E.J. and Deary, I.J. (1999). Effects of repeated hypoglycemia on cognitive function: A psychometrically validated reanalysis of the diabetes control and complications trial data. *Diabetes Care.* 22, 1273–1277.

Awad, N., Gagnon, M., Desrochers, A., Tsiakas, M., and Messier, C. (2002). Impact of peripheral glucoregulation on memory. *Behav. Neurosci.* 116, 691–702.

Banks, W.A., Owen, J.B., and Erickson, M.A. (2012). Insulin in the brain: There and back again. *Pharmacol. Ther.* 136, 82–93.

Benedict, R.H.B., Schretlen, D., Groninger, L., and Brandt, J. (1998). Hopkins verbal learning test-revised: normative data and analysis of inter-form and test-retest reliability. *Clin. Neuropsychol.* 12, 43–55.

Benton, D., Maconie, A., and Williams, C. (2007). The influence of the glycaemic load of breakfast on the behaviour of children in school. *Physiol. Behav.* 92, 717–724.

Benton, D., Ruffin, M.-P., Lassel, T.N.S., Messaoudi, M., Vinoy, S., Desor, D., and Lang, V. (2003). The delivery rate of dietary carbohydrates affects cognitive performance in both rats and humans. *Psychopharmacology* 166, 86–90.

Brand-Miller, J., Hayne, S., Petocz, P., and Colagiuri, S. (2003a). Low-glycemic index diets in the management of diabetes: A meta-analysis of randomized controlled trials. *Diabetes Care.* 26, 2261–2267.

Brand-Miller, J.C., Holt, S.H.A., and Petocz, P. (2003b). Reply to R. Mendosa. *Am. J. Clin. Nutr.* 77, 994–995.

Brayne, C. and Calloway, P. (1988). Normal ageing, impaired cognitive function, and senile dementia of the alzheimer's type: A continuum. *Lancet.* 331, 1265–1267.

Brindal, E., Baird, D., Danthiir, V., Wilson, C., Bowen, J., Slater, A., and Noakes, M. (2012). Ingesting breakfast meals of different glycaemic load does not alter cognition and satiety in children. *Eur. J Clin. Nutr.* 66, 1166–1171.

Brindal, E., Baird, D., Slater, A., Danthiir, V., Wilson, C., Bowen, J., and Noakes, M. (2013). The effect of beverages varying in glycaemic load on postprandial glucose responses, appetite and cognition in 10–12-year-old school children. *Br. J Nutr.* 110, 529–537.

Chugani, H.T. (1998). A critical period of brain development: Studies of cerebral glucose utilization with PET. *Prev. Med.* 27, 184–188.

Cooper, S.B., Bandelow, S., Nute, M.L., Morris, J.G., and Nevill, M.E. (2012). Breakfast glycaemic index and cognitive function in adolescent school children. *Br. J. Nutr.* 107, 1823–1832.

Deffenbacher, K.A., Bornstein, B.H., Penrod, S.D., and McGorty, E.K. (2004). A meta-analytic review of the effects of high stress on eyewitness memory. *Law Hum. Behav.* 28, 687–706.

Donohoe, R.T. and Benton, D. (1999). Cognitive functioning is susceptible to the level of blood glucose. *Psychopharmacology (Berl).* 145, 378–385.

Fischer, K., Colombani, P.C., Langhans, W., and Wenk, C. (2001). Cognitive performance and its relationship with postprandial metabolic changes after ingestion of different macronutrients in the morning. *Br. J. Nutr.* 85, 393–405.

Gilsenan, M.B., de Bruin, E.A., and Dye, L. (2009). The influence of carbohydrate on cognitive performance: A critical evaluation from the perspective of glycaemic load. *Br. J. Nutr.* 101, 941–949.

Granfeldt, Y., Wu, X., and Bjorck, I. (2006). Determination of glycaemic index; some methodological aspects related to the analysis of carbohydrate load and characteristics of the previous evening meal. *Eur. J. Clin. Nutr.* 60, 104–112.

Ingwersen, J., Defeyter, M.A., Kennedy, D.O., Wesnes, K.A., and Scholey, A.B. (2007). A low glycaemic index breakfast cereal preferentially prevents children's cognitive performance from declining throughout the morning. *Appetite.* 49, 240–244.

Jacobson, A.M., Musen, G., Ryan, C.M., Silvers, N., Cleary, P., Waberski, B., Burwood, A. et al. (2007). Long-term effect of diabetes and its treatment on cognitive function. *N. Engl. J. Med.* 356, 1842–1852.

Kaplan, R.J., Greenwood, C.E., Winocur, G., and Wolever, T.M. (2000). Cognitive performance is associated with glucose regulation in healthy elderly persons and can be enhanced with glucose and dietary carbohydrates. *Am. J. Clin. Nutr.* 72, 825–836.

Kodl, C.T. and Seaquist, E.R. (2008). Cognitive dysfunction and diabetes mellitus. *Endocr. Rev.* 29, 494–511.

Korol, D.L. and Gold, P.E. (1998). Glucose, memory, and aging. *Am. J. Clin. Nutr.* 67, 764S–771S.

Lamport, D.J., Chadwick, H.K., Dye, L., Mansfield, M.W., and Lawton, C.L. (2014a). A low glycaemic load breakfast can attenuate cognitive impairments observed in middle aged obese females with impaired glucose tolerance. *Nutr. Metab Cardiovasc. Dis.* 24, 1128–1136.

Lamport, D.J., Dye, L., Mansfield, M.W., and Lawton, C.L. (2013). Acute glycaemic load breakfast manipulations do not attenuate cognitive impairments in adults with type 2 diabetes. *Clin. Nutr.* 32, 265–272.

Lamport, D.J., Hoyle, E., Lawton, C.L., Mansfield, M.W., and Dye, L. (2011). Evidence for a second meal cognitive effect: Glycaemic responses to high and low glycaemic index evening meals are associated with cognition the following morning. *Nutr. Neurosci.* 14, 66–71.

Lamport, D.J., Lawton, C.L., Mansfield, M.W., and Dye, L. (2009). Impairments in glucose tolerance can have a negative impact on cognitive function: a systematic research review. *Neurosci. Biobehav. Rev.* 33, 394–413.

Lamport, D.J., Lawton, C.L., Mansfield, M.W., Moulin, C.A., and Dye, L. (2014b). Type 2 diabetes and impaired glucose tolerance are associated with word memory source monitoring recollection deficits but not simple recognition familiarity deficits following water, low glycaemic load, and high glycaemic load breakfasts. *Physiol. Behav.* 124, 54–60.

Ludwig, D.S. (2002). The glycemic index: Physiological mechanisms relating to obesity, diabetes, and cardiovascular disease. *JAMA.* 287, 2414–2423.

Mahoney, C.R., Taylor, H.A., Kanarek, R.B., and Samuel, P. (2005). Effect of breakfast composition on cognitive processes in elementary school children. *Physiol. Behav.* 85, 635–645.

Malkova, D., Evans, R.D., Frayn, K.N., Humphreys, S.M., Jones, P.R., and Hardman, A.E. (2000). Prior exercise and postprandial substrate extraction across the human leg. *Am. J. Physiol. Endocrinol. Metab.* 279, E1020–E1028.

Manning, C.A., Parsons, M.W., Cotter, E.M., and Gold, P.E. (1997). Glucose effects on declarative and nondeclarative memory in healthy elderly and young adults. *Psychobiol.* 25, 103–108.

Manning, C.A., Ragozzino, M.E., and Gold, P.E. (1993). Glucose enhancement of memory in patients with probable senile dementia of the Alzheimer's type. *Neurobiol. Aging.* 14, 523–528.

McNay, E.C., Fries, T.M., and Gold, P.E. (2000). Decreases in rat extracellular hippocampal glucose concentration associated with cognitive demand during a spatial task. *Proc. Natl. Acad. Sci. U. S. A.* 97, 2881–2885.

Meneilly, G.S., Dawson, K., and Tessier, D. (1993). Alterations in glucose metabolism in the elderly patient with diabetes. *Diabetes Care.* 16, 1241–1248.

Messier, C., Pierre, J., Desrochers, A., and Gravel, M. (1998). Dose-dependent action of glucose on memory processes in women: Effect on serial position and recall priority. *Brain. Res. Cogn. Brain. Res.* 7, 221–233.

Messier, C., Tsiakas, M., Gagnon, M., Desrochers, A., and Awad, N. (2003). Effect of age and glucoregulation on cognitive performance. *Neurobiol. Aging.* 24, 985–1003.

Micha, R., Rogers, P.J., and Nelson, M. (2010). The glycaemic potency of breakfast and cognitive function in school children. *Eur. J. Clin. Nutr.* 64, 948–957.

Micha, R., Rogers, P.J., and Nelson, M. (2011). Glycaemic index and glycaemic load of breakfast predict cognitive function and mood in school children: A randomised controlled trial. *Br. J. Nutr.* 106, 1552–1561.

Nabb, B. and Benton D. (2006). The influence on cognition of the interaction between the macro-nutrient content of breakfast and glucose tolerance. *Physiol. Behav.* 87, 16–23.

Nasreddine, Z.S., Phillips, N.A., Bedirian, V., Charbonneau, S., Whitehead, V., Collin, I., Cummings, J.L., and Chertkow, H. (2005). The montreal cognitive assessment, MoCA: A brief screening tool for mild cognitive impairment. *J. Am. Geriatr. Soc.* 53, 695–699.

Nilsson, A., Radeborg, K., and Bjorck, I. (2009). Effects of differences in postprandial glycaemia on cognitive functions in healthy middle-aged subjects. *Eur. J. Clin. Nutr.* 63, 113–120.

Nilsson, A., Radeborg, K., and Bjorck, I. (2012). Effects on cognitive performance of modulating the postprandial blood glucose profile at breakfast. *Eur. J. Clin. Nutr.* 66, 1039–1043.

Owens, D.S. and Benton, D. (1994). The impact of raising blood glucose on reaction times. *Neuropsychobiology.* 30, 106–113.

Papanikolaou, Y., Palmer, H., Binns, M.A., Jenkins, D.J., and Greenwood, C.E. (2006). Better cognitive performance following a low-glycaemic-index compared with a high-glycaemic-index carbohydrate meal in adults with type 2 diabetes. *Diabetologia* 49, 855–862.

Parsons, M.W. and Gold, P.E. (1992). Glucose enhancement of memory in elderly humans: An inverted-U dose-response curve. *Neurobiol. Aging.* 13, 401–404.

Philippou, E. and Constantinou, M. (2014). The influence of glycemic index on cognitive functioning: A systematic review of the evidence. *Adv. Nutr.* 5, 119–130.

Power, S.E., O'Connor, E.M., Ross, R.P., Stanton, C., O'Toole, P.W., Fitzgerald, G.F., and Jeffery, I.B. (2014). Dietary glycaemic load associated with cognitive performance in elderly subjects. *Eur. J Nutr.* 54, 557–568.

Quas, J.A., Yim, I.S., Edelstein, R.S., Cahill, L., and Rush, E.B. (2011). The role of cortisol reactivity in children's and adults' memory of a prior stressful experience. *Dev. Psychobiol.* 53, 166–174.

Reivich, M. and Alavi, A. (1983). Positron emission tomographic studies of local cerebral glucose metabolism in humans in physiological and pathophysiological conditions. *Adv. Metab Disord.* 10, 135–176.

Rizkalla, S.W., Taghrid, L., Laromiguiere, M., Huet, D., Boillot, J., Rigoir, A., Elgrably, F., and Slama, G. (2004). Improved plasma glucose control, whole-body glucose utilization, and lipid profile on a low-glycemic index diet in type 2 diabetic men: A randomized controlled trial. *Diabetes Care.* 27, 1866–1872.

Scholey, A.B., Laing, S., and Kennedy, D.O. (2006). Blood glucose changes and memory: Effects of manipulating emotionality and mental effort. *Biol. Psychol.* 71, 12–19.

Smith, A., Kendrick, A., Maben, A., and Salmon, J. (1994). Effects of breakfast and caffeine on cognitive performance, mood and cardiovascular functioning. *Appetite* 22, 39–55.

Smith, M.A. and Foster, J.K. (2008). The impact of a high versus a low glycaemic index breakfast cereal meal on verbal episodic memory in healthy adolescents. *Nutr. Neurosci.* 11, 219–227.

Smith, M.A., Riby, L.M., van Eekelen, A.M., and Foster, J.K. (2011). Glucose enhancement of human memory: A comprehensive research review of the glucose memory facilitation effect. *Neurosci. Biobehav. Rev.* 35, 770–783.

Tombaugh, T.N.T.N. (2004). Trail making test A and B: normative data stratified by age and education. *Arch. Clin. Neuropsychol.* 19, 203–214.

Wechsler, D. (2009). *Wechsler Memory Scale-Fourth Edition.* San Antonio, TX: Pearson.

Wolever, T.M., Jenkins, D.J., Ocana, A.M., Rao, V.A., and Collier, G.R. (1988). Second-meal effect: Low-glycemic-index foods eaten at dinner improve subsequent breakfast glycemic response. *Am. J. Clin. Nutr.* 48, 1041–1047.

10 Glycemic Index and Women's Health

Dietary GI in Management of Polycystic Ovary Syndrome and during Pregnancy

Kate Marsh

CONTENTS

10.1 INTRODUCTION

As previous chapters have discussed, modifying the glycemic index (GI) of the diet can have several health benefits, which are relevant to women at all ages and stages of life. However, two areas where the GI of a woman's diet takes on particular importance are in the management of polycystic ovary syndrome (PCOS) and during pregnancy. The impact of dietary GI on blood glucose and insulin concentrations in both PCOS and pregnancy is one of the most significant aspects of dietary modification in both cases. This chapter discusses the nutritional management of PCOS and pregnancy, presenting the current evidence and effects of manipulating dietary GI in these situations.

10.2 DIETARY GI IN THE MANAGEMENT OF PCOS

10.2.1 Overview

PCOS is the most common endocrine disorder in women, affecting up to 21% of women of reproductive age, although the prevalence varies widely depending on the population studied, ethnicity, and diagnostic criteria used (Knochenhauer et al. 1998, Diamanti-Kandarakis et al. 1999, Asuncion et al. 2000, Azziz et al. 2004, March et al. 2010, Yildiz et al. 2012). Once thought of as predominantly a fertility problem, it is now recognized that PCOS is a metabolic disorder with significant health consequences. A large proportion of women with PCOS have significant metabolic risks resulting from underlying insulin resistance, and are at increased risk of cardiometabolic disease, including impaired glucose tolerance (IGT), type 2 diabetes (T2DM), metabolic syndrome (MetS), and adverse cardiovascular risks factors (Teede et al. 2010). Although these risks are seen in all women with PCOS, the risk are higher in those who are overweight or obese (Lim et al. 2013). It has been estimated that the identification and management of PCOS costs the U.S. Healthcare system $4 billion annually (Azziz et al. 2005).

Classic features of the syndrome include menstrual abnormalities (dysfunctional uterine bleeding, oligomenorrhoea, or amenorrhoea), anovulation, infertility, and hyperandrogenism (resulting in hirsutism, acne, and accelerated scalp hair loss). However, there is some disagreement regarding the diagnosis of PCOS, with three different diagnostic criteria currently used, summarized in Table 10.1 (Zawadski and Dunaif 1992, Rotterdam ESHRE Sponsored PCOS consensus workshop group 2004, Azziz et al. 2009). All three criteria rely on the exclusion of other etiologies such as congenital adrenal hyperplasia, androgen-secreting tumors, and Cushing's syndrome.

10.2.2 PCOS, Insulin Resistance, and Associated Health Risks

Insulin resistance, with compensatory hyperinsulinaemia, has been identified as a key component in the pathophysiology of PCOS in both lean and obese women, with 50%–70% of these women estimated to have some degree of insulin resistance (Legro et al. 2004, Teede et al. 2007). A recent study found that women with PCOS were significantly more insulin resistant than BMI-matched controls and that insulin resistance was present in 75% of lean PCOS and 95% of overweight PCOS women, compared to 62% of overweight controls (Stepto et al. 2013). As discussed earlier, this underlying insulin resistance contributes to the increased cardiometabolic risks seen in women with PCOS, including IGT, T2DM, and MetS (Figure 10.1).

10.2.3 Management of PCOS

Treatment of PCOS aims to normalize hyperandrogenaemia and its associated hirsutism and acne, improve menstrual cyclicity and reproductive function, and must address the increased metabolic risks associated with this condition. Detailed discussion of the management of PCOS is beyond

TABLE 10.1
Diagnostic Criteria for PCOS

NIH (1990)	Rotterdam (2003)	Androgen Excess Society (2006)
Hyperandrogenism + chronic anovulation	Two of the following: Hyperandrogenism Chronic anovulation Polycystic ovaries	Hyperandrogenism + chronic anovulation or polycystic ovaries

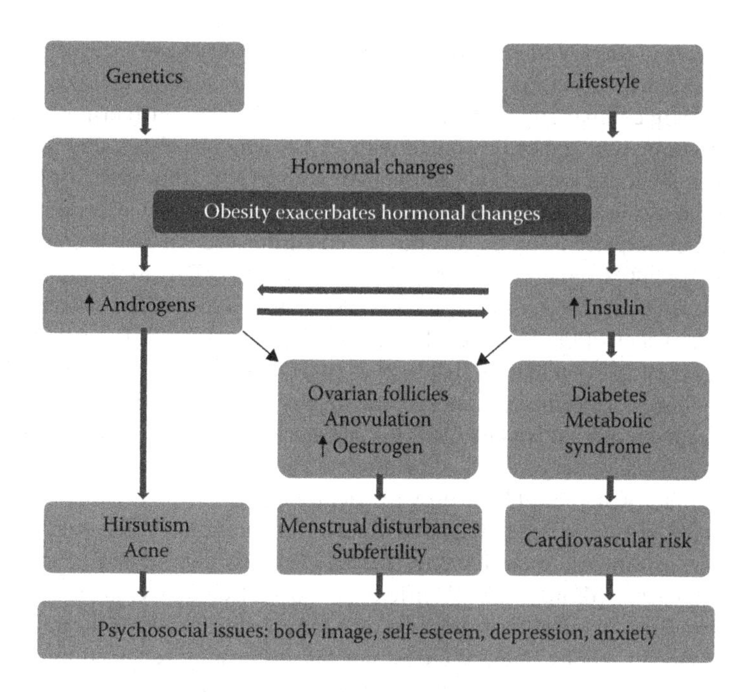

FIGURE 10.1 The aetiological, hormonal, and clinical features of polycystic ovary syndrome. (Reproduced from Teede, H. J. et al., *Med. J. Aust.*, 195, S65–S112, 2011. With permission.)

the scope of this chapter but may involve lifestyle modification in conjunction with pharmacological (including oral contraceptives, insulin sensitizers, anti-androgens, and ovulation induction), cosmetic (including waxing, electrolysis, and laser treatment), and surgical (including laproscopic and bariatric surgery) treatment where required (Teede et al. 2011, Legro et al. 2013). However, lifestyle modification, including diet and physical activity, is recommended as the first line of treatment for women with PCOS and should always accompany any medical interventions (Teede et al. 2011).

10.2.4 Dietary Management of PCOS and the Role of GI

Dietary intervention and weight loss has been shown to have significant benefits in the management of PCOS, improving body composition, hyperandrogenism (and associated symptoms), and insulin resistance in these women (Moran et al. 2011, Haqq et al. 2014a, 2014b). In overweight and obese women with PCOS, a modest weight loss of 5%–10% of weight through lifestyle modification results in reproductive and metabolic improvements (Moran et al. 2009). This includes a reduction in hyperandrogenism, improved menstrual regularity and ovulation, and improvements in fasting insulin, glucose, and glucose tolerance.

Despite the proven benefits of dietary intervention, the role of dietary composition, versus energy restriction and weight loss, is not as clear. Only a handful of well-controlled studies are available, and a recent systematic review of five studies found only subtle differences between the diets studied (Moran et al. 2013a). Greater weight loss was achieved with a monounsaturated fat-enriched diet, improved menstrual regularity with a low GI diet, greater reductions in insulin resistance, fibrinogen, total, and HDL-cholesterol with a low-carbohydrate or low GI diet, improved quality of life with a low GI diet, and improved depression and self-esteem with a high protein diet, while a high-carbohydrate diet resulted in an increased free androgen index. In the majority of studies, improvements in metabolic and psychological measures were seen with weight loss, regardless of dietary composition (Moran et al. 2013a).

Most of the studies of dietary intervention in women with PCOS have focused on energy restriction rather than dietary composition *per se*, yet the weight loss seen in most of these studies has been relatively small in comparison to the other outcomes achieved. Furthermore, while the prevalence of insulin resistance is higher in women with PCOS who are obese, and weight loss clearly improves outcomes for these women, not all women with PCOS who have insulin resistance are overweight or obese. Several studies have demonstrated a higher incidence of insulin resistance, beta-cell dysfunction, impaired glucose tolerance and cardiovascular risk factors in women with PCOS of normal weight (Chang et al. 1983, Jialal et al. 1987, Dunaif et al. 1989, Dunaif and Finegood 1996, Dereli et al. 2003, Orio et al. 2004, Svendsen et al. 2008, Cussons et al. 2009, Lee et al. 2009, Rajendran et al. 2009, Macut et al. 2011, Kurdoglu et al. 2012, Blair et al. 2013, Flannery et al. 2013, Sprung et al. 2014), a finding that implies that dietary management of PCOS needs to go beyond just weight loss. Furthermore, in most of the dietary studies in women with PCOS, improvements in metabolic and reproductive outcomes have been closely related to improvements in insulin sensitivity, suggesting that dietary modification designed to improve insulin resistance may produce benefits greater than those achieved by energy restriction alone.

Reducing dietary glycemic load (GL) can reduce postprandial glucose concentrations and the resulting hyperinsulinemia that characterizes PCOS. This can be achieved by either reducing GI or reducing carbohydrate intake. While both types of dietary change will reduce insulin concentrations, resulting in short-term benefits, the long-term impact of these changes is likely to be quite different. If carbohydrate intake is reduced, it must be replaced by either fat or protein, and both of these strategies have potential problems for women with PCOS. Diets high in saturated fat can worsen insulin resistance (Rivellese et al. 2002, Riccardi et al. 2004, Haag and Dippenaar 2005, Riserus 2008), and high intakes of animal protein, particularly red meat, are associated with an increased risk of T2DM (Aune et al. 2009, Pan et al. 2011, 2013, Feskens et al. 2013), GDM (Zhang et al. 2006b, Bowers et al. 2011, Bao et al. 2013), MetS (Pereira et al. 2002, Azadbakht and Esmaillzadeh 2009, Babio et al. 2012, de Oliveira Otto et al. 2012), CHD (Bernstein et al. 2010, Pan et al. 2012), and stroke (Bernstein et al. 2012, Kaluza et al. 2012). Although not specifically in women with PCOS, a combined analysis of the Nurses' Health Study (NHS) and Health Professionals Follow-up Study (HPFS) found that a higher animal-based low-carbohydrate intake was associated with a 23% higher all-cause mortality, 14% higher cardiovascular mortality, and 28% higher cancer mortality comparing extreme deciles of intake (Fung et al. 2010). A recent systematic review similarly found an increased risk of mortality with low carbohydrate diets (Noto et al. 2013). Furthermore, while low carbohydrate diets result in an immediate lowering of blood glucose levels, long-term ingestion of such diets results in an increase in hepatic glucose production and a reduction in peripheral glucose utilization, a state of insulin resistance (Colagiuri and Brand Miller 2002).

There is also little evidence for the benefits of lower carbohydrate (LC) diets in women with PCOS. A systematic review and meta-analysis of 15 studies found no significant benefits of an LC diet for improving ovulation rates, conception, hyperandrogenemia, glucose and insulin concentrations, insulin resistance, or satiety hormones, all of which improved with weight loss, with no effect of dietary composition (Frary et al. 2014). In most studies, weight loss was also achieved independent of dietary composition, but in three studies, an additional 1%–5% weight loss was achieved with an LC diet. While dropout rates were high in general (ranging from 18% to 54%), the LC diet resulted in a 10%–20% higher dropout rate compared to other interventions, suggesting that this type of eating plan may be harder to sustain.

Low GI diets, on the other hand, have been found to lower fasting insulin and inflammatory markers (Schwingshackl and Hoffmann 2013), reduce fasting blood glucose, glycated proteins and insulin sensitivity (Livesey et al. 2008), result in greater weight loss and improved lipid profiles (Thomas et al. 2007), and reduce the risk of T2DM (Barclay et al. 2008, Dong et al. 2011, Greenwood et al. 2013) and CHD (Barclay et al. 2008). Particularly relevant to women with PCOS, diets with a low GI/GL have been found to improve acne, primarily as a result of increased sex hormone binding globulin levels following a reduction in insulin resistance, whereas high GL diets can worsen acne (Smith et al. 2007a, 2007b, 2008).

Despite the potential benefits of a low GI diet in this population, only a few studies have investigated the use of low GI diets in women with PCOS. Marsh et al. (2010) compared a low GI and conventional healthy diet in 99 women with PCOS and found that the low GI diet resulted in a greater improvement in insulin sensitivity measured by insulin sensitivity index (ISI) derived from the oral glucose tolerance test (OGTT) (ISI–OGTT) (2.2 ± 0.7 vs. 0.7 ± 0.6; $p = .03$) and regularity of menstrual cycles (95% vs. 63%; $p = .03$) (Marsh et al. 2010). Serum fibrinogen levels were also reduced to a greater extent on the low GI diet. Barr et al. (2013) similarly demonstrated improvements in insulin sensitivity with a low GI isocaloric diet in 21 women with PCOS despite no significant changes in weight or body composition (Barr et al. 2013). They also observed a decrease in nonesterified fatty acid (NEFA) concentration following the 12-week intervention. However the study was not randomized or controlled and the participants also reduced their intake of saturated fat, which may also have contributed to improvements in insulin sensitivity.

A low GL high protein (HP) hypocaloric diet was found to improve insulin sensitivity in women with PCOS compared to a conventional diet, despite similar weight loss in both groups over 12 weeks (Mehrabani et al. 2012). The low GL HP diet also improved high sensitivity C-reactive protein (hsCRP) concentration to a greater extent. Finally, a low GI vegan diet led to significantly greater weight loss at 3 months but not 6 months compared to a low-calorie diet in a pilot study of 18 overweight women with PCOS (Turner-McGrievy et al. 2014). In these two studies, however, it was not possible to separate the effect of dietary GI/GL from the other dietary modifications made in the intervention groups.

A recent study investigating the Dietary Approaches to Stop Hypertension (DASH) diet in 48 overweight and obese women with PCOS who were randomized to the DASH diet or a control diet for 8 weeks, found that the DASH diet group experienced significantly greater reductions in body weight, BMI, waist circumference (WC), fasting insulin, homeostatic model assessment—insulin resistance (HOMA-IR), triglycerides, very-low-density lipoprotein (VLDL) cholesterol, and hs-CRP levels and improved markers of oxidative stress (Asemi et al. 2013, 2014) compared to the control group. The DASH diet is rich in fruit, vegetables, whole grains, and low fat dairy foods and low in saturated fats, cholesterol, refined grains, and sweets, so likely to be lower GI. Both diets contained 52% carbohydrate, 18% protein, and 30% total fat. However, the GI of the diets was not reported and like the previous studies, the results cannot be attributed only to the differences in GI between the two diets.

Several studies have assessed the GI of the habitual diets of women with PCOS. Douglas et al. (2006) found no significant difference in total intake of high-GI foods between PCOS and controls although women with PCOS did eat more white bread and potatoes, foods which typically have a high GI. Barr et al. (2011) found that mean dietary GI in women with PCOS (54.6) was similar to the average dietary GI reported by women in the general UK population but higher than that recommended to reduce long-term disease risk. They also observed that obese women with PCOS had a higher dietary GI than lean women with PCOS (55.7 vs. 53.8) (Barr et al. 2011). Moran et al. (2013b), on the other hand, found that Australian women with PCOS reported a lower dietary GI (50.3) and better overall dietary intake (increased diet quality and micronutrient intake and lower saturated fat intake) compared to non-PCOS women. These differences may relate to the different population groups, sample sizes, methods of dietary assessment, time since diagnosis, and exposure of the women in these studies to dietary education, particularly with respect to GI.

10.2.5 Conclusion

It is well accepted that the first line of treatment for PCOS is lifestyle modification, of which diet plays a primary role. Although the main focus should be weight management (weight loss in those who are overweight, and prevention of weight gain in all women with PCOS), dietary composition is also important. While more research is needed, limited evidence in women with PCOS in addition to a significant body of evidence in other populations, including those with diabetes, suggests that women with PCOS are likely to benefit from adopting a lower GI diet, in conjunction with energy restriction for those who are overweight.

10.3 DIETARY GI IN PREGNANCY

10.3.1 Overview

An increasing awareness of the link between periconceptual and *in utero* nutrition and the impact on a child's subsequent development of adult obesity and metabolic disease has highlighted the important role that nutrition plays during preconception and pregnancy (Lillycrop 2011, Lillycrop and Burdge 2011, Osborne-Majnik et al. 2013).

While there are many aspects of nutrition that are important in pregnancy, GI has gained considerable interest in recent years, because of its influence on maternal glucose concentration and the resulting impact on pregnancy outcomes. Several studies have now investigated the impact of low GI dietary interventions during pregnancy on outcomes including birth weight, risk of birth defects, gestational weight gain (GWG), and the development and management of gestational diabetes (GDM).

10.3.2 Importance of Blood Glucose Concentration in Pregnancy

Maternal blood glucose concentration is directly correlated with fetal growth, meaning that consistent high or low blood glucose concentrations during pregnancy can result in an infant who is large-for-gestational age (LGA) or small-for-gestational age (SGA), respectively. Both LGA and SGA babies are at risk of future metabolic disease.

While the risks of elevated blood glucose concentrations associated with GDM are well accepted, more recent evidence from the hyperglycemia and adverse pregnancy outcomes (HAPOs) study shows a continuous association between maternal glucose concentration and adverse pregnancy outcomes, with adverse outcomes occurring at levels below the previous criteria for diagnosis of GDM (Metzger et al. 2008). These findings have led to new diagnostic criteria for GDM (Table 10.2) proposed in 2010 by the International Association of Diabetes and Pregnancy Groups (IADPSG), which have now been adopted in many countries (International Association of Diabetes Pregnancy Study Groups [IADPSG] Consensus Panel 2010) and by the World Health Organization (WHO 2013).

These diagnostic criteria were defined by IADPSG on the basis of an odds ratio of 1.75 for adverse neonatal outcomes compared with mean values. However, the findings from HAPO, of a

TABLE 10.2
Diagnostic Criteria for Gestational Diabetes

Gestational Diabetes Mellitus Should Be Diagnosed at Any Time in Pregnancy If One or More of the Following Criteria Are Met

	Mg/dL	Mmol/L
Fasting plasma glucose	92–125	5.1–6.9
1 h plasma glucose following a 75 g glucose load	≥ 180	≥ 10.0
2 h plasma glucose following a 75 g glucose load	153–199	8.5–11.0

Source: WHO (World Health Organization) (2013). *Diagnostic Criteria and Classification of Hyperglycaemia First Detected in Pregnancy*. Geneva, Switzerland, World Health Organization.

continuous relationship between glycemia and adverse outcomes, highlight the importance of optimizing the maternal glucose environment during pregnancy.

10.3.3 Importance of Weight Management in Pregnancy

Worldwide obesity has almost doubled since 1980. In 2008, 35% of adults aged 20 years and over were overweight and 11% were obese (WHO 2014). Of these, nearly 3000 million women were obese. In the United States, more than half of pregnant women are overweight or obese (26.0% overweight and 27.6% obese in 2011) (Centers for Disease Control & Prevention 2012). This has increased significantly, from 29.7% of women being overweight or obese prior to conception in 1983, to 53.7% in 2011 (Centers for Disease Control & Prevention 2012). Rates of GWG are also increasing. In the United States almost half (48%) of pregnant women gained excess weight (based on the IOM recommendations) in 2011, an increase from 37% in 1988 (Centers for Disease Control & Prevention 2012).

Obesity in pregnancy is associated with adverse maternal and infant outcomes (American Congress of Obstetricians and Gynecologists [ACOG] 2013). In the mother, obesity increases the risks of miscarriage, GDM, hypertension and pre-eclampsia, thromoboembolism, infection, caesarian section and traumatic delivery. For the infant, there is a higher risk of stillbirth, shoulder dystocia, preterm delivery, neonatal death, and congenital abnormalities. Maternal obesity also increases the future risk of obesity and metabolic disorders in the child.

A recent systematic review and meta-analysis found significant associations between pre-pregnancy overweight and obesity, and the risk of fetal macrosomia (OR 1.67; 95% CI 1.42–1.97; and OR 3.23; 95% CI 2.39–4.37 for overweight and obesity, respectively), high birthweight (OR 1.53; 95% CI 1.44–1.63; and OR 2.00; 95% CI 1.84–2.18), and large for gestational age (LGA) (OR 1.53; 95% CI 1.44–1.63; and OR 2.08; 95% CI 1.95–2.23) (Yu et al. 2013). The risk of subsequent offspring overweight/obesity was two- to threefold higher (OR 1.95; 95% CI 1.77–2.13; and OR 3.06; 95% CI 2.68–3.49). Furthermore, a recent observational study of 1,857,822 live single births in Sweden found that maternal overweight and obesity are associated with increased risks of infant mortality (Johansson et al. 2014). Compared to women of normal weight, those who were overweight (BMI 25.0–29.9) or with grade 1 obesity (BMI 30.0–34.9) had a modest increase in the risk of infant mortality (adjusted odds ratios 1.25 [95% CI 1.16–1.35] and 1.37 [95% CI 1.22–1.53], respectively). Obesity grade 2 (BMI 35.0–39.9) and grade 3 were associated with more than twice the risk (adjusted odds ratios 2.11 [95% CI 1.79–2.49] and 2.44 [95% CI 1.88–3.17]).

Independent of pregravid BMI, excess GWG is also associated with adverse pregnancy outcomes (Institute of Medicine [United States] and National Research Council [United States] Committee to Reexamine IOM Pregnancy Weight Guidelines 2009). Women who gain excess weight are at a higher risk of pregnancy-related hypertension (including pre-eclampsia), GDM, complications during labor and delivery and unsuccessful breastfeeding. They are also at greater risk of postpartum weight retention and subsequent maternal obesity (Institute of Medicine [United States] and National Research Council [United States] Committee to Reexamine IOM Pregnancy Weight Guidelines 2009). In infants, excess GWG is associated with increased birthweight and risk of being LGA as well as an increased risk of future obesity and associated cardiometabolic disorders (Institute of Medicine [United States] and National Research Council [United States] Committee to Reexamine IOM Pregnancy Weight Guidelines 2009).

Knowledge of the risk of both pregravid overweight and obesity, and excess GWG formed the basis of the new Institute of Medicine (IOM) guidelines for weight gain during pregnancy, which recommend different weight gain targets according to pre-pregnancy BMI (Table 10.3) (Institute of Medicine [United States] and National Research Council [United States] Committee to Reexamine IOM Pregnancy Weight Guidelines 2009).

However, despite these recommendations and the well-documented risks of excess GWG, U.S. statistics show that the number of women who gain excess weight in pregnancy (according to the

TABLE 10.3
Recommendations for Total and Rate of Weight Gain during Pregnancy

	Total Weight Gain		Rates of Weight Gain 2nd and 3rd Trimester	
Pre-pregnancy BMI	**Range (kg)**	**Range (lb)**	**Mean (range) (kg/week)**	**Mean (range) (lb/week)**
Under weight (< 18.5kg/m²)	12.5–18.0	28–40	0.51 (0.44–0.58)	1.0 (1.0–1.3)
Normal weight (18.5–24.9 kg/m²)	11.5–16.0	25–35	0.42 (0.35–0.50)	1.0 (0.8–1)
Overweight (25–29.9 kg/m²)	7.0–11.5	15–25	0.28 (0.23–0.33)	0.6 (0.5–0.7)
Obese (≥ 30 kg/m²)	5.0–9.0	11–20	0.22 (0.17–0.27)	0.5 (0.4–0.6)

IOM guidelines) continues to increase, with almost half (48%) of pregnant women gaining excess weight in 2011 (Centers for Disease Control & Prevention 2012). A large U.S. population based study of 570,672 women aged 18–40 years with a singleton full-term live-birth between 2004 and 2007 similarly found that 41.6% of women began pregnancy as overweight and obese and 51.2% gained excess weight during pregnancy, resulting in a higher risk of an LGA infant (Park et al. 2011).

10.3.4 GI and Weight Management

Research suggests that low GI diets may assist with weight management through effects on satiety and fuel partitioning. A 2007 Cochrane review concluded that low GI diets lead to greater weight loss and reductions in fat mass and BMI (Thomas et al. 2007). More recently, the Diogenes (diet, obesity, and genes) study found that a low GI, moderately higher protein diet led to better weight maintenance following weight loss compared to higher GI and lower protein diets (Larsen et al. 2010).

Several studies have demonstrated reduced GWG in women following a low GI diet. The ROLO study (Randomized cOntrol trial of LOw glycemic index diet to prevent macrosomia in euglycemic women) randomized 800 women who were in their second pregnancy and did not have diabetes but had previously delivered a large baby (>4 kg) to no dietary intervention (control) or a low GI diet from early pregnancy. Women assigned to the low GI intervention gained significantly less weight than the control group (mean difference −1.3 kg, 95% CI −2.4 to −0.2; $p = .01$) and were less likely to exceed the IOM GWG recommendations (38% vs. 48%; $p = .01$) (Walsh et al. 2012). The intervention group had a lower dietary GI in the second and third trimester and a significant reduction in the consumption of food groups with known high-GI values (McGowan et al. 2013).

In the Danish National Birth Cohort, dietary GL was positively associated with GWG, a relationship that was seen in both normal weight and overweight women but not those who were underweight (Knudsen et al. 2013). There was also a positive association between postpartum weight retention (PPWR) and GL in overweight and obese but not normal weight and underweight women. Mean weight gain was 1.13 kg (95% CI 0.48–1.79) in the overweight women and 1.29 kg (95% CI 0.22–2.80) in the obese women, comparing the highest to lowest quintiles of dietary GL. In the pregnancy, infection, and nutrition (PIN) study, however, there was no relationship between dietary GL and GWG after controlling for confounding factors (Deierlein et al. 2008). They did, however, observe a positive relationship between pregravid BMI and dietary GL.

The UK Pregnancies Better Eating and Activity Trial (UPBEAT) found that a behavioural intervention which included advice on reducing dietary GI resulted in reduced gestational weight gain and maternal sum-of-skinfold thicknesses. However the intervention group were also encouraged to make other dietary changes, including reducing saturated fat intake, and to increase physical activity (Poston et al.).

10.3.5 GI and Birth Defects

High glucose concentrations during pregnancy are implicated as one of the causes of birth defects, including neural tube defects (NTDs). In the early stages of pregnancy, the embryo has no beta cells and is unable to secrete insulin or regulate their own glucose levels. Experimental studies in animal models have confirmed that markedly elevated glucose concentrations contribute to the development of congenital anomalies. Although the precise mechanisms are unclear, it has been suggested that hyperglycemia can lead to the generation of free oxygen radicals, embryonic yolk sac vascular impairment, and alterations in the levels of embryonic membrane lipids, including arachidonic acid, prostaglandins, and myo-inositol (Sadler et al. 1988, Reece and Eriksson 1996, Reece et al. 1996, 1998).

A large case-control study investigating the impact of maternal periconceptional dietary intakes of sucrose, glucose, fructose, and foods with a higher GI, within the National Birth Defects Prevention Study, found a positive relationship between maternal dietary GI and having a baby with an NTD (OR 1.86, 95% CI 1.29–2.70 comparing the highest vs. lowest quartiles) (Shaw et al. 2003). In women with a high BMI (>29), those with a higher GI diet had more than a fourfold risk of having a baby with an NTD (OR 4.05; 95% CI 1.04–15.73 for all NTDs and 5.62; 95% CI 1.14–27.61 for Spina Bifida). These findings remained after excluding the mothers with a history of diabetes (type 1, type 2, or GDM). In a further analysis, the authors found a relationship between NTDs and dietary GI in women who were not taking multivitamin and mineral supplements in the 3 months prior to pregnancy, but not in those who were (Carmichael et al. 2009). However, a subsequent study in a larger number of women failed to find an association between dietary GI and the risk of NTDs (Shaw et al. 2008). The authors comment that use of a shorter food frequency questionnaire (FFQ) in the latter study is one possible explanation for the differences since this tool may not have the level of detail required to accurately assess GI.

An investigation of the association between dietary GI and a wide range of birth defects in the National Birth Defects Prevention Study found a significant association between a high dietary GI and risk of a number of birth defects, including encephalocele (OR 2.68, 95% CI 1.13–6.30), diaphragmatic hernia (OR 2.58, 95% CI 1.06–6.27), small intestinal atresia/stenosis (OR 2.97, 1.59–5.56), duodenal atresia/stenosis (OR 2.48, 95% CI 1.21–5.07), and atrial septal defect (OR 1.37, 95% CI 1.01–1.85) after adjustment for confounding factors (Parker et al. 2012). Comparing the highest and lowest quartiles of intake, they also found a significant association with cleft lip with cleft palate, and anorectal atresia/stenosis. Similar to previous studies, the combination of a high-GI diet and maternal obesity increased these risks further.

In the Boston University Slone Epidemiology Birth Defects Study, a high dietary GI was associated with amniotic band defects (adjusted OR 3.0, 95% CI 1.1–8.1), while a high dietary GL was associated with anorectal defects (adjusted OR 2.4, 95% CI 1.1–4.9) in women without diabetes (Yazdy et al. 2011). The same study also found a positive association between dietary GI (OR 1.5; 95% CI 1.1–2.0) and GL (OR 1.8; 95% CI 0.8–4.0) and risk of NTDs (Yazdy et al. 2010).

10.3.6 GI and Birthweight

While dietary GI has the potential to impact birthweight via effects on maternal glycemia, studies investigating the effect of a low GI diet on birthweight have revealed mixed findings.

The first study to investigate this relationship randomized 12 healthy pregnant women to a low GI or high-GI diet and found that those following the higher GI diet had babies with a higher birthweight and fat mass compared to the low GI group (Clapp 1997). A subsequent study of 70 healthy pregnant women randomized to a low GI or conventional high fiber diet for the second and third trimesters of pregnancy found that those following the low GI diet gave birth to babies with a significantly lower birthweight, birthweight centile, and ponderal index (a measure of obesity in newborns) (Moses et al. 2006). They were also 10 times less likely to deliver a LGA baby (3% vs. 33%, $p = .01$). More women in the low GI group gave birth to a SGA baby; however, the difference between the groups was not significant.

In the ROLO study (trial of a low GI index diet to prevent macrosomia in euglycemic women); however, no reduction in LGA babies was seen with a low GI dietary intervention in women at risk of fetal macrosomia (Walsh et al. 2012). Birthweight, birthweight centile, and ponderal index were similar in the low GI and control groups and 51% of women in both groups delivered a LGA baby. Similarly, the Pregnancy and Glycemic Index Outcomes (PREGGIOs) study found no difference in birthweight, birthweight percentile, or ponderal index with a low GI diet or conventional healthy diet (Moses et al. 2014). Again, women in both groups had a similar proportion of LGA and SGA babies. The UPBEAT trial, a behavioural intervention incorporating low GI dietary advice in obese women, also found no differences in the incidence of LGA or SGA infants. A secondary analysis of the ROLO study, however, found a low GI diet to be associated with lower neonatal central adiposity (Horan et al. 2014) and thigh circumference (Donnelly et al. 2014b). There were no differences between the low GI and control groups for other measure of neonatal anthropometry including head, chest, abdominal, or mid-upper arm circumferences, or any skinfold measurements (Donnelly et al. 2014).

Two Australian studies have also failed to show a relationship between dietary GI and fetal growth. In the first study, 63 women diagnosed with GDM were randomized to a low GI diet or conventional high fiber diet at 28–32 weeks gestation (Moses et al. 2009). Birth centile and ponderal index were similar in the two groups and there was no significant difference between the number of LGA and SGA babies. Similarly, in a study of 99 women diagnosed with GDM at 20–32 weeks gestation, a low GI diet resulted in a similar birthweight and birthweight centile and ponderal index compared to a high fiber moderate GI diet (Louie et al. 2011). There was no significant difference between the groups in prevalence of fetal macrosomia, or delivery of LGA or SGA babies.

In the Danish National Birth Cohort, birth weight increased by 36 g from the lowest to highest quintiles of dietary GL and the risk of having an LGA baby was increased by 14% (OR 1.14, 95% CI 1.03–1.25) in the group with the highest GL (Knudsen et al. 2013). There was no increase in risk of an SGA baby associated with dietary GL and in underweight women the risk of an SGA baby was lowest in those with a lower GL. In contrast, an earlier prospective study in urban low income women found that those with a lower dietary GI had a reduced infant birthweight and a higher risk of delivering an SGA baby (Scholl et al. 2004). However, the women with the lowest quintile of dietary GI also had higher intakes of sucrose, and it has been suggested that overall poor diet quality may have explained this association (Louie et al. 2010). Subsequent intervention studies have failed to show a higher risk of SGA babies in pregnant women consuming a low GI diet (Moses et al. 2006, 2009, Louie et al. 2011).

10.3.7 GI and Other Pregnancy Outcomes

In the National Birth Defects Prevention Study, a high-GI diet was found to be associated with a higher risk of preterm delivery (Carmichael et al. 2013). Consistent with this, in a trial of 46 overweight and obese women randomly assigned to a low GI or low fat diet, gestational duration was longer (39.3 vs. 37.9 weeks; $p = .05$) (Rhodes et al. 2010). With the exclusion of planned caesarean deliveries, there were significantly fewer preterm births (≤38 weeks) in the low GI group (5% vs. 53%; $p = .002$). In contrast, a Mexican study of 107 women with GDM or T2DM found a higher risk of premature birth in those randomized to the low GI diet (multivariate RR: 4.74, 95% CI: 1.08–20.84, $p = .03$) (Perichart-Perera et al. 2012).

A U.S. study demonstrated improved cardiovascular risk factors in overweight and obese pregnant women following a low GI diet, who had smaller increases in TG and total cholesterol, and a greater decrease in CRP compared to the low fat group (Rhodes et al. 2010). A recent study of

Chinese women with GDM similarly showed improved lipids (smaller increases in TC and TG and a smaller decrease in HDL) with a low GL dietary intervention compared to general dietary advice (Ma et al. 2014). Although not investigated in the study, this improvement in lipids may be attributed to improvements in insulin sensitivity with the lower GI diet. In the ROLO study, a low GI diet reduced the increase in insulin resistance typically seen from early pregnancy to 28 weeks gestation although had no effect on markers of inflammation or leptin (Walsh et al. 2014).

A recent study of 428 mother-offspring pairs found that dietary GI, but not GL, at 30 weeks gestation, was associated with markers of metabolic syndrome in the offspring at age 20 years (Danielsen et al. 2013). Significant associations were found between dietary GI in pregnancy and HOMA-IR, fasting insulin, and leptin in the young adult offspring, after adjustment for multiple confounding factors.

10.3.8 GI and GDM

Considering that low GI diets have been shown to improve insulin sensitivity, lower postprandial glucose levels and reduce the risk of type 2 diabetes, it is plausible that adopting a healthy low GI diet early in pregnancy might reduce the risk of developing GDM. To date, however, there is insufficient research to demonstrate this. In the Nurses' Health Study II (NHS-II), pre-pregnancy dietary GL was positively associated with risk of developing GDM (Zhang et al. 2006a). The multivariate relative risk (RR) for the highest versus lowest quintiles was 1.61 (95% CI 1.02–2.53). Women who had a high dietary GL and low-cereal fiber intake were more than twice as likely to develop GDM (RR 2.15; 95% CI 1.04–4.29). On the other hand, a smaller study failed to find an association between dietary GL in early pregnancy and the risk of developing GDM (Radesky et al. 2008).

The UPBEAT study found no differences in the development of GDM in obese women were randomised to a behavioural intervention incorporating low GI dietary advice or a control group (25% of the intervention versus 26% of the control group developed GDM).

Most of the research investigating the role of low GI diets in GDM has looked at pregnancy outcomes in women already diagnosed with GDM and the findings have been mixed. In a trial of 63 women with GDM randomly assigned to receive a low GI or conventional high fiber higher GI diet, there was a significant reduction in the number of women requiring insulin on the low GI diet (29% vs. 59%; $p = .023$) (Moses et al. 2009). Furthermore, of those in the high-GI group who met the criteria to commence insulin, almost half (9 out of 19 women) were able to avoid insulin by changing to a low GI diet. However, subsequent studies (discussed below) have been unable to replicate this finding.

A pilot study of 43 women with GDM randomized to a low GI or control diet, failed to show a difference in insulin requirements between the groups (Grant et al. 2011). Fasting and mean postprandial glucose levels were reduced to a similar extent in both groups, although women in the low GI group had fewer postprandial blood glucose levels above the target range (25.9% vs. 30.3%; $p = .003$) (Grant et al. 2011). Louie et al. (2011) in a trial comparing a low GI and conventional high fiber, moderate GI diet in 99 women with GDM, also found no significant differences in insulin treatment between the two groups (53% vs. 65%; $p = .251$) (Louie et al. 2011). A study of 107 Mexican women with GDM ($n = 52$) or T2DM ($n = 55$) similarly found no differences in insulin treatment comparing a diet based on the ADA nutrition practice guidelines for GDM with either low GI carbohydrate or any type of carbohydrate (Perichart-Perera et al. 2012). More recently, Afaghi et al. (2014) found that the combination of a low GI diet and additional fiber (from 15 g wheat bran) resulted in significant reduction in the need for insulin compared to a low GI diet alone (38.9% vs. 76.9%) (Afaghi et al. 2013). In a study of 95 Chinese women with GDM, an intensive low GL dietary intervention resulted in a significantly greater reduction in fasting and 2 h postprandial glucose than individualized general dietary advice (Ma et al. 2014). Only three women in the study required insulin, one in the low GL diet group and two in the control group.

A recent systematic review and meta-analysis of randomized clinical trials of dietary intervention in women with GDM concluded that a low GI diet was associated with less frequent insulin use (RR 0.77; 95% CI 0.60–0.99; $p = .039$) and lower birth weight (WMD −161.9 g; 95% CI −246.4 to −77.4; $p = .000$) compared to control diets (Viana et al. 2014). In contrast, low energy and low carbohydrate diets had no significant impact on maternal or newborn outcomes.

In fact, several studies have shown no benefits of a LC diet in pregnancy, and there is some evidence for benefits of a higher carbohydrate intake. A Spanish study that randomized 152 women with GDM to a lower CHO (40%) versus control (55% CHO) diet found no differences in pregnancy outcomes or insulin requirements (Moreno-Castilla et al. 2013). Previous studies have found improved glucose tolerance, less weight gain, and reduced insulin needs with diets high in unrefined carbohydrate and fiber (Ney et al. 1982, Nolan 1984). One study found a lower risk of newborn macrosomia in women with GDM consuming a higher carbohydrate intake (>210 g/day) (Romon et al. 2001).

10.3.9 Practical Tips on Dietary GI in Women with GDM

Below are given some practical tips on how dietary GI can be lowered during pregnancy in women with GDM.

Practical tips for a low GI diet for women with GDM:

1. Spread carbohydrate intake evenly over the day, with regular meals and snacks.
2. Aim for 30–45 g carbohydrate at meals (i.e., 2–3 portions) (1 portion = 1 slice of bread, 1/3 of cup of legumes) and 15–30 g at snacks (providing a minimum of 175 g carbohydrate/day).
3. Choose lower GI breakfast cereals, such as traditional or steel-cut rolled oats, and dense wholegrain and seeded breads.
4. At meals, choose low GI whole grains (e.g., barley, quinoa, freekeh, low GI brown rice, wholegrain pasta, and dense wholegrain breads) and legumes as the carbohydrate portion of meals.
5. Balance the carbohydrate at meals with a portion of lean protein and a large serving of non-starchy vegetables and salads.
6. Choose lower GI, nutrient dense mid-meal snacks, including lower GI varieties of fresh fruit, natural yoghurt with berries, low GI-dried fruits with nuts, wholegrain bread, or toast with natural nut spread, low GI whole grain crackers with cheese and tomato, yoghurt or legume-based dips with vegetable crudites, or a fruit smoothie (milk, yoghurt, and fruit).

10.3.10 GI and Postpartum Diet

Nutrition and weight management are important not only before and during pregnancy but also post-partum. Pregnancy is recognized as a high risk period for weight gain and excess weight retention is becoming increasingly common, particularly for women who gain excess weight during pregnancy. A large U.S. population-based study found that 51.2% of women gained excess weight compared to the IOM 2009 recommendations and this was greater (56%) in women who were overweight or obese prior to pregnancy (Park et al. 2011). In women who developed GDM in pregnancy, there is an increased risk of developing type 2 diabetes so ongoing dietary and lifestyle modification is encouraged to reduce this risk. Dietary interventions to assist with postpartum weight management and reducing diabetes risk are therefore important.

In the ROLO study significantly greater weight loss from pre-pregnancy to 3 months postpartum was seen in the low GI diet versus the control group (1.3 vs. 0.1 kg, $p = .022$) (Horan et al. 2014a). Similarly, a study of 77 Asian women with previous GDM found that after 6 months, women randomized to a low GI diet had significantly greater reductions in weight, BMI and WHR compared to those following a conventional healthy diet and significantly more women in the low GI group lost at least 5% of weight (33% vs. 8%; $p = .01$) (Shyam et al. 2013). The low GI group also experienced greater improvements in glucose tolerance, and women with higher baseline fasting insulin levels experienced greater reductions in 2 h postload glucose levels on the lower GI diet.

10.3.11 Conclusion

Although more research is needed, it appears that a low GI diet may have a number of benefits during pregnancy, with little risk of harm. Specifically, a low GI diet may help to reduce the risk of excess GWG, lower the risk of birth defects, assist in the management of gestational diabetes, and help with postpartum weight management. Importantly, a low GI diet appears safe in pregnancy and is consistent with general healthy eating recommendations for preconception, pregnancy, and beyond. In contrast, there is some evidence of risks associated with other dietary interventions to lower blood glucose levels in pregnancy. Low carbohydrate diets high in animal protein have been associated with impaired glucose metabolism, elevated blood pressure, and hypercortisolemia in adult offspring (Shiell et al. 2000, 2001, Herrick et al. 2003, Reynolds et al. 2007). Diets high in red meat have also been associated with an increased risk of GDM (Zhang et al. 2006b, Bao et al. 2013). A low carbohydrate diet with high intakes of protein and fat from animal sources (typical of most LC diets) has also been associated with an increased risk of GDM although the same risk was not seen with higher intakes of protein and fat from plant sources (Bao et al. 2014).

REFERENCES

Afaghi, A., L. Ghanei, and A. Ziaee (2013). Effect of low glycemic load diet with and without wheat bran on glucose control in gestational diabetes mellitus: A randomized trial. *Indian J Endocrinol Metab.* **17**(4):689–692. doi: 610.4103/2230-8210.113762.

American Congress of Obstetricians and Gynecologists (ACOG) (2013). Obesity in Pregnancy (Committee Opinion No. 549). Retrieved December 4, 2014, from http://www.acog.org/Resources-And-Publications/Committee-Opinions/Committee-on-Obstetric-Practice/Obesity-in-Pregnancy.

Asemi, Z., M. Samimi, Z. Tabassi, H. Shakeri, S. S. Sabihi, and A. Esmaillzadeh (2014). Effects of DASH diet on lipid profiles and biomarkers of oxidative stress in overweight and obese women with polycystic ovary syndrome: A randomized clinical trial. *Nutrition.* **30**(11–12):1287–1293. doi: 1210.1016/j.nut.2014.1203.1008. Epub 2014 Mar 1215.

Asemi, Z., Z. Tabassi, M. Samimi, T. Fahiminejad, and A. Esmaillzadeh (2013). Favourable effects of the Dietary Approaches to Stop Hypertension diet on glucose tolerance and lipid profiles in gestational diabetes: A randomised clinical trial. *Br J Nutr.* **109**(11):2024–2030. doi: 2010.1017/S0007114512004242. Epub 0007114512002012 Nov 0007114512004213.

Asuncion, M., R. M. Calvo, J. L. San Millan, J. Sancho, S. Avila, and H. F. Escobar-Morreale (2000). A prospective study of the prevalence of the polycystic ovary syndrome in unselected Caucasian women from Spain. *J Clin Endocrinol Metab.* **85**(7):2434–2438.

Aune, D., G. Ursin, and M. B. Veierod (2009). Meat consumption and the risk of type 2 diabetes: A systematic review and meta-analysis of cohort studies. *Diabetologia.* **7**:7.

Azadbakht, L. and A. Esmaillzadeh (2009). Red meat intake is associated with metabolic syndrome and the plasma C-reactive protein concentration in women. *J Nutr.* **139**(2):335–339. doi: 310.3945/jn.3108.096297. Epub 092008 Dec 096211.

Azziz, R., E. Carmina, D. Dewailly, E. Diamanti-Kandarakis, H. F. Escobar-Morreale, W. Futterweit, O. E. Janssen et al. (2009). The Androgen Excess and PCOS Society criteria for the polycystic ovary syndrome: The complete task force report. *Fertil Steril.* **91**(2):456–488. doi: 410.1016/j.fertnstert.2008.1006.1035. Epub 2008 Oct 1023.

Azziz, R., C. Marin, L. Hoq, E. Badamgarav, and P. Song (2005). Health care-related economic burden of the polycystic ovary syndrome during the reproductive life span. *J Clin Endocrinol Metab.* **90**(8):4650–4658. Epub 2005 Jun 4658.

Azziz, R., K. S. Woods, R. Reyna, T. J. Key, E. S. Knochenhauer, and B. O. Yildiz (2004). The prevalence and features of the polycystic ovary syndrome in an unselected population. *J Clin Endocrinol Metab.* **89**(6):2745–2749.

Babio, N., M. Sorli, M. Bullo, J. Basora, N. Ibarrola-Jurado, J. Fernandez-Ballart, M. A. Martinez-Gonzalez, L. Serra-Majem, R. Gonzalez-Perez, and J. Salas-Salvado (2012). Association between red meat consumption and metabolic syndrome in a Mediterranean population at high cardiovascular risk: Cross-sectional and 1-year follow-up assessment. *Nutr Metab Cardiovasc Dis.* **22**(3):200–207. doi: 210.1016/j.numecd.2010.1006.1011. Epub 2010 Sep 1028.

Bao, W., K. Bowers, D. K. Tobias, F. B. Hu, and C. Zhang (2013). Prepregnancy dietary protein intake, major dietary protein sources, and the risk of gestational diabetes mellitus: A prospective cohort study. *Diabetes Care.* **36**(7):2001–2008. doi: 2010.2337/dc2012–2018. Epub 2013 Feb 2001.

Bao, W., K. Bowers, D. K. Tobias, S. F. Olsen, J. Chavarro, A. Vaag, M. Kiely, and C. Zhang (2014). Prepregnancy low-carbohydrate dietary pattern and risk of gestational diabetes mellitus: A prospective cohort study. *Am J Clin Nutr.* **99**(6):1378–1384.

Barclay, A. W., P. Petocz, J. McMillan-Price, V. M. Flood, T. Prvan, P. Mitchell, and J. C. Brand-Miller (2008). Glycemic index, glycemic load, and chronic disease risk—a meta-analysis of observational studies. *Am J Clin Nutr.* **87**(3):627–637.

Barr, S., K. Hart, S. Reeves, K. Sharp, and Y. M. Jeanes (2011). Habitual dietary intake, eating pattern and physical activity of women with polycystic ovary syndrome. *Eur J Clin Nutr.* **65**(10):1126–1132. doi: 1110.1038/ejcn.2011.1181. Epub 2011 Jun 1121.

Barr, S., S. Reeves, K. Sharp, and Y. M. Jeanes (2013). An isocaloric low glycemic index diet improves insulin sensitivity in women with polycystic ovary syndrome. *J Acad Nutr Diet.* **113**(11):1523–1531. doi: 1510.1016/j.jand.2013.1506.1347. Epub 2013 Aug 1530.

Bernstein, A. M., A. Pan, K. M. Rexrode, M. Stampfer, F. B. Hu, D. Mozaffarian, and W. C. Willett (2012). Dietary protein sources and the risk of stroke in men and women. *Stroke.* **43**(3):637–644. doi: 610.1161/STROKEAHA.1111.633404. Epub 632011 Dec 633429.

Bernstein, A. M., Q. Sun, F. B. Hu, M. J. Stampfer, J. E. Manson, and W. C. Willett (2010). Major dietary protein sources and risk of coronary heart disease in women. *Circulation.* **122**(9):876–883. Epub 2010 Aug 2016.

Blair, S. A., T. Kyaw-Tun, I. S. Young, N. A. Phelan, J. Gibney, and J. McEneny (2013). Oxidative stress and inflammation in lean and obese subjects with polycystic ovary syndrome. *J Reprod Med.* **58**(3–4):107–114.

Bowers, K., E. Yeung, M. A. Williams, L. Qi, D. K. Tobias, F. B. Hu, and C. Zhang (2011). A prospective study of prepregnancy dietary iron intake and risk for gestational diabetes mellitus. *Diabetes Care.* **34**(7):1557–1563.

Carmichael, S. L., J. S. Witte, and G. M. Shaw (2009). Nutrient pathways and neural tube defects: A semi-Bayesian hierarchical analysis. *Epidemiology.* **20**(1):67–73. doi: 10.1097/EDE.1090b1013e31818f36375.

Carmichael, S. L., W. Yang, and G. M. Shaw (2013). Maternal dietary nutrient intake and risk of preterm delivery. *Am J Perinatol.* **30**(7):579–588. doi: 510.1055/s-0032-1329686. Epub 1322012 Dec 1329683.

Centers for Disease Control & Prevention (2012). Pediatric & Pregnancy Nutrition Surveillance System 2011. Retrieved December 8, 2014, from http://www.cdc.gov/pednss/pnss_tables/tables_health_indicators.htm.

Chang, R. J., R. M. Nakamura, H. L. Judd, and S. A. Kaplan (1983). Insulin resistance in nonobese patients with polycystic ovarian disease. *J Clin Endocrinol Metab.* **57**(2):356–359.

Clapp, J. F. (1997). Diet, exercise, and feto-placental growth. *Arch Gynecol Obstet.* **260**(1–4):101–108.

Colagiuri, S. and J. Brand Miller (2002). The "carnivore connection"—evolutionary aspects of insulin resistance. *Eur J Clin Nutr.* **56**(Suppl 1):S30–S35.

Cussons, A. J., G. F. Watts, and B. G. Stuckey (2009). Dissociation of endothelial function and arterial stiffness in nonobese women with polycystic ovary syndrome (PCOS). *Clin Endocrinol (Oxf).* **71**(6):808–814. doi: 810.1111/j.1365-2265.2009.03598.x. Epub 02009 Mar 03528.

Danielsen, I., C. Granstrom, T. Haldorsson, D. Rytter, B. Hammer Bech, T. B. Henriksen, A. A. Vaag, and S. F. Olsen (2013). Dietary glycemic index during pregnancy is associated with biomarkers of the metabolic syndrome in offspring at age 20 years. *PLoS One.* **8**(5):e64887. doi: 64810.61371/journal.pone.0064887. Print 0062013.

de Oliveira Otto, M. C., A. Alonso, D. H. Lee, G. L. Delclos, A. G. Bertoni, R. Jiang, J. A. Lima, E. Symanski, D. R. Jacobs, Jr., and J. A. Nettleton (2012). Dietary intakes of zinc and heme iron from red meat, but not from other sources, are associated with greater risk of metabolic syndrome and cardiovascular disease. *J Nutr.* **142**(3):526–533. doi: 510.3945/jn.3111.149781. Epub 142012 Jan 149718.

Deierlein, A. L., A. M. Siega-Riz, and A. Herring (2008). Dietary energy density but not glycemic load is associated with gestational weight gain. *Am J Clin Nutr.* **88**(3):693–699.

Dereli, D., G. Ozgen, F. Buyukkececi, E. Guney, and C. Yilmaz (2003). Platelet dysfunction in lean women with polycystic ovary syndrome and association with insulin sensitivity. *J Clin Endocrinol Metab.* **88**(5):2263–2268.

Diamanti-Kandarakis, E., C. R. Kouli, A. T. Bergiele, F. A. Filandra, T. C. Tsianateli, G. G. Spina, E. D. Zapanti, and M. I. Bartzis (1999). A survey of the polycystic ovary syndrome in the Greek island of Lesbos: Hormonal and metabolic profile. *J Clin Endocrinol Metab.* **84**(11):4006–4011.

Dong, J. Y., L. Zhang, Y. H. Zhang, and L. Q. Qin (2011). Dietary glycaemic index and glycaemic load in relation to the risk of type 2 diabetes: A meta-analysis of prospective cohort studies. *Br J Nutr.* **106**(11): 1649–1654. doi: 1610.1017/S000711451100540X. Epub 000711451102011 Sep 000711451100529.

Donnelly, J. M., J. M. Walsh, J. Byrne, E. J. Molloy, and F. M. McAuliffe (2014). Impact of maternal diet on neonatal anthropometry: A randomized controlled trial. *Pediatr Obes.* **20**(10):2047–6310.

Douglas, C. C., L. E. Norris, R. A. Oster, B. E. Darnell, R. Azziz, and B. A. Gower (2006). Difference in dietary intake between women with polycystic ovary syndrome and healthy controls. *Fertil Steril.* **86**(2): 411–417. Epub 2006 Jun 2008.

Dunaif, A. and D. T. Finegood (1996). Beta-cell dysfunction independent of obesity and glucose intolerance in the polycystic ovary syndrome. *J Clin Endocrinol Metab.* **81**(3):942–947.

Dunaif, A., K. R. Segal, W. Futterweit, and A. Dobrjansky (1989). Profound peripheral insulin resistance, independent of obesity, in polycystic ovary syndrome. *Diabetes.* **38**(9):1165–1174.

Feskens, E. J., D. Sluik, and G. J. van Woudenbergh (2013). Meat consumption, diabetes, and its complications. *Curr Diab Rep.* **13**(2):298–306. doi: 210.1007/s11892-11013-10365-11890.

Flannery, C. A., B. Rackow, X. Cong, E. Duran, D. J. Selen, and T. S. Burgert (2013). Polycystic ovary syndrome in adolescence: Impaired glucose tolerance occurs across the spectrum of BMI. *Pediatr Diabetes.* **14**(1):42–49. doi: 10.1111/j.1399-5448.2012.00902.x. Epub 02012 Aug 00928.

Frary, J. M., K. P. Bjerre, D. Glintborg, and P. Ravn (2014). The effect of dietary carbohydrates in women with polycystic ovary syndrome. *Minerva Endocrinol.* **10**:10.

Fung, T. T., R. M. van Dam, S. E. Hankinson, M. Stampfer, W. C. Willett, and F. B. Hu (2010). Low-carbohydrate diets and all-cause and cause-specific mortality: Two cohort studies. *Ann Intern Med.* **153**(5):289–298.

Grant, S. M., T. M. Wolever, D. L. O'Connor, R. Nisenbaum, and R. G. Josse (2011). Effect of a low glycaemic index diet on blood glucose in women with gestational hyperglycaemia. *Diabetes Res Clin Pract.* **91**(1):15–22. doi: 10.1016/j.diabres.2010.1009.1002. Epub 2010 Nov 1020.

Greenwood, D. C., D. E. Threapleton, C. E. Evans, C. L. Cleghorn, C. Nykjaer, C. Woodhead, and V. J. Burley (2013). Glycemic index, glycemic load, carbohydrates, and type 2 diabetes: Systematic review and dose-response meta-analysis of prospective studies. *Diabetes Care.* **36**(12):4166–4171. doi: 4110.2337/dc4113-0325.

Haag, M. and N. G. Dippenaar (2005). Dietary fats, fatty acids and insulin resistance: Short review of a multifaceted connection. *Med Sci Monit.* **11**(12):RA359–RA367. Epub 2005 Nov 2024.

Haqq, L., J. McFarlane, G. Dieberg, and N. Smart (2014a). The effect of lifestyle intervention on body composition, glycaemic control and cardio-respiratory fitness in women with polycystic ovarian syndrome: A systematic review and meta-analysis. *Int J Sport Nutr Exerc Metab.* **25**:25.

Haqq, L., J. McFarlane, G. Dieberg, and N. Smart (2014b). Effect of lifestyle intervention on the reproductive endocrine profile in women with polycystic ovarian syndrome: A systematic review and meta-analysis. *Endocr Connect.* **3**(1):36–46. doi: 10.1530/EC-1514-0010. Print 2014.

Herrick, K., D. I. Phillips, S. Haselden, A. W. Shiell, M. Campbell-Brown, and K. M. Godfrey (2003). Maternal consumption of a high-meat, low-carbohydrate diet in late pregnancy: Relation to adult cortisol concentrations in the offspring. *J Clin Endocrinol Metab.* **88**(8):3554–3560.

Horan, M. K., C. A. McGowan, E. R. Gibney, J. M. Donnelly, and F. M. McAuliffe (2014a). Maternal diet and weight at 3 months postpartum following a pregnancy intervention with a low glycaemic index diet: Results from the ROLO randomised control trial. *Nutrients.* **6**(7):2946–2955. doi: 2910.3390/nu6072946.

Horan, M. K., C. A. McGowan, E. R. Gibney, J. M. Donnelly, and F. M. McAuliffe (2014b). Maternal low glycaemic index diet, fat intake and postprandial glucose influences neonatal adiposity—secondary analysis from the ROLO study. *Nutr J.* **13**(1):78. doi: 10.1186/1475-2891-1113-1178.

Institute of Medicine (US) and National Research Council (US) Committee to Reexamine IOM Pregnancy Weight Guidelines (2009). *Weight Gain During Pregnancy: Reexamining the Guidelines.* Washington, DC: The National Academies Press.

International Association of Diabetes Pregnancy Study Groups (IADPSG) Consensus Panel (2010). International association of diabetes and pregnancy study groups recommendations on the diagnosis and classification of hyperglycemia in pregnancy. *Diabetes Care.* **33**(3):676–682.

Jialal, I., P. Naiker, K. Reddi, J. Moodley, and S. M. Joubert (1987). Evidence for insulin resistance in nonobese patients with polycystic ovarian disease. *J Clin Endocrinol Metab.* **64**(5):1066–1069.

Johansson, S., E. Villamor, M. Altman, A.-K. E. Bonamy, F. Granath, and S. Cnattingius (2014). Maternal overweight and obesity in early pregnancy and risk of infant mortality: A population based cohort study in Sweden.

Kaluza, J., A. Wolk, and S. C. Larsson (2012). Red meat consumption and risk of stroke: A meta-analysis of prospective studies. *Stroke.* **43**(10):2556–2560. Epub 2012 Jul 2531.

Knochenhauer, E. S., T. J. Key, M. Kahsar-Miller, W. Waggoner, L. R. Boots, and R. Azziz (1998). Prevalence of the polycystic ovary syndrome in unselected black and white women of the southeastern United States: A prospective study. *J Clin Endocrinol Metab.* **83**(9):3078–3082.

Knudsen, V. K., B. L. Heitmann, T. I. Halldorsson, T. I. Sorensen, and S. F. Olsen (2013). Maternal dietary glycaemic load during pregnancy and gestational weight gain, birth weight and postpartum weight retention: A study within the Danish National Birth Cohort. *Br J Nutr.* **109**(8):1471–1478. doi: 1410.1017/S0007114512003443. Epub 0007114512002012 Aug 0007114512003421.

Kurdoglu, Z., H. Ozkol, Y. Tuluce, and I. Koyuncu (2012). Oxidative status and its relation with insulin resistance in young non-obese women with polycystic ovary syndrome. *J Endocrinol Invest.* **35**(3):317–321. doi: 310.3275/7682. Epub 2011 Apr 3226.

Larsen, T. M., S. M. Dalskov, M. van Baak, S. A. Jebb, A. Papadaki, A. F. Pfeiffer, J. A. Martinez et al. (2010). Diets with high or low protein content and glycemic index for weight-loss maintenance. *N Engl J Med.* **363**(22):2102–2113. doi: 2110.1056/NEJMoa1007137.

Lee, H., J. Y. Oh, Y. A. Sung, H. Chung, and W. Y. Cho (2009). The prevalence and risk factors for glucose intolerance in young Korean women with polycystic ovary syndrome. *Endocrine.* **36**(2):326–332. doi: 310.1007/s12020-12009-19226-12027. Epub 12009 Aug 12014.

Legro, R. S., S. A. Arslanian, D. A. Ehrmann, K. M. Hoeger, M. H. Murad, R. Pasquali, and C. K. Welt (2013). Diagnosis and treatment of polycystic ovary syndrome: An Endocrine Society clinical practice guideline. *J Clin Endocrinol Metab.* **98**(12):4565–4592. doi: 4510.1210/jc.2013-2350. Epub 2013 Oct 4522.

Legro, R. S., V. D. Castracane, and R. P. Kauffman (2004). Detecting insulin resistance in polycystic ovary syndrome: Purposes and pitfalls. *Obstet Gynecol Surv.* **59**(2):141–154.

Lillycrop, K. A. (2011). Effect of maternal diet on the epigenome: Implications for human metabolic disease. *Proc Nutr Soc.* **70**(1):64–72.

Lillycrop, K. A. and G. C. Burdge (2011). The effect of nutrition during early life on the epigenetic regulation of transcription and implications for human diseases. *J Nutrigenet Nutrigenomics.* **4**(5):248–260. doi: 210.1159/000334857. Epub 000332012 Feb 000334822.

Lim, S. S., R. J. Norman, M. J. Davies, and L. J. Moran (2013). The effect of obesity on polycystic ovary syndrome: A systematic review and meta-analysis. *Obes Rev.* **14**(2):95–109. doi: 110.1111/j.1467-1789X.2012.01053.x. Epub 02012 Oct 01031.

Livesey, G., R. Taylor, T. Hulshof, and J. Howlett (2008). Glycemic response and health—A systematic review and meta-analysis: Relations between dietary glycemic properties and health outcomes. *Am J Clin Nutr.* **87**(1):258S–268S.

Louie, J. C., J. C. Brand-Miller, T. P. Markovic, G. P. Ross, and R. G. Moses (2010). Glycemic index and pregnancy: A systematic literature review. *J Nutr Metab.* **2010:**282464. doi: 10.1155/2010/282464. Epub 282011 Jan 282462.

Louie, J. C., T. P. Markovic, N. Perera, D. Foote, P. Petocz, G. P. Ross, and J. C. Brand-Miller (2011). A randomized controlled trial investigating the effects of a low-glycemic index diet on pregnancy outcomes in gestational diabetes mellitus. *Diabetes Care.* **34**(11):2341–2346. doi: 2310.2337/dc2311-0985. Epub 2011 Sep 2346.

Ma, W.-J., Z.-H. Huang, B.-X. Huang, B.-H. Qi, Y.-J. Zhang, B.-X. Xiao, Y.-H. Li, L. Chen, and H.-L. Zhu (2014). Intensive low-glycaemic-load dietary intervention for the management of glycaemia and serum lipids among women with gestational diabetes: A randomized control trial. *Public Health Nutr.* (FirstView):1–8:1506–1513.

Macut, D., T. Simic, A. Lissounov, M. Pljesa-Ercegovac, I. Bozic, T. Djukic, J. Bjekic-Macut et al. (2011). Insulin resistance in non-obese women with polycystic ovary syndrome: Relation to byproducts of oxidative stress. *Exp Clin Endocrinol Diabetes.* **119**(7):451–455. doi: 410.1055/s-0031-1279740. Epub 1272011 Jun 1279710.

March, W. A., V. M. Moore, K. J. Willson, D. I. Phillips, R. J. Norman, and M. J. Davies (2010). The prevalence of polycystic ovary syndrome in a community sample assessed under contrasting diagnostic criteria. *Hum Reprod.* **25**(2):544–551. doi: 510.1093/humrep/dep1399. Epub 2009 Nov 1012.

Marsh, K. A., K. S. Steinbeck, F. S. Atkinson, P. Petocz, and J. C. Brand-Miller (2010). Effect of a low glycemic index compared with a conventional healthy diet on polycystic ovary syndrome. *Am J Clin Nutr.* **92**(1):83–92. doi: 10.3945/ajcn.2010.29261. Epub 22010 May 29219.

McGowan, C. A., J. M. Walsh, J. Byrne, S. Curran, and F. M. McAuliffe (2013). The influence of a low glycemic index dietary intervention on maternal dietary intake, glycemic index and gestational weight gain during pregnancy: A randomized controlled trial. *Nutr J.* **12**(1):140. doi: 110.1186/1475-2891-1112-1140.

Mehrabani, H. H., S. Salehpour, Z. Amiri, S. J. Farahani, B. J. Meyer, and F. Tahbaz (2012). Beneficial effects of a high-protein, low-glycemic-load hypocaloric diet in overweight and obese women with polycystic ovary syndrome: A randomized controlled intervention study. *J Am Coll Nutr.* **31**(2):117–125.

Metzger, B. E., L. P. Lowe, and HAPO Study Cooperative Research Group (2008). Hyperglycemia and adverse pregnancy outcomes. *N Engl J Med.* **358**(19):1991–2002.

Moran, L. J., S. K. Hutchison, R. J. Norman, and H. J. Teede (2011). Lifestyle changes in women with polycystic ovary syndrome. *Cochrane Database Syst Rev.* (7):CD007506. doi: 007510.001002/14651858.CD14007506.pub14651853.

Moran, L. J., H. Ko, M. Misso, K. Marsh, M. Noakes, M. Talbot, M. Frearson, M. Thondan, N. Stepto, and H. J. Teede (2013a). Dietary composition in the treatment of polycystic ovary syndrome: A systematic review to inform evidence-based guidelines. *J Acad Nutr Diet.* **113**(4):520–545. doi: 510.1016/j.jand.2012.1011.1018. Epub 2013 Feb 1016.

Moran, L. J., R. Pasquali, H. J. Teede, K. M. Hoeger, and R. J. Norman (2009). Treatment of obesity in polycystic ovary syndrome: A position statement of the Androgen Excess and Polycystic Ovary Syndrome Society. *Fertil Steril.* **92**(6):1966–1982. doi: 1910.1016/j.fertnstert.2008.1909.1018. Epub 2008 Dec 1964.

Moran, L. J., S. Ranasinha, S. Zoungas, S. A. McNaughton, W. J. Brown, and H. J. Teede (2013b). The contribution of diet, physical activity and sedentary behaviour to body mass index in women with and without polycystic ovary syndrome. *Hum Reprod.* **28**(8):2276–2283. doi: 2210.1093/humrep/det2256. Epub 2013 Jun 2215.

Moreno-Castilla, C., M. Hernandez, M. Bergua, M. C. Alvarez, M. A. Arce, K. Rodriguez, M. Martinez-Alonso et al. (2013). Low-carbohydrate diet for the treatment of gestational diabetes mellitus: A randomized controlled trial. *Diabetes Care.* **36**(8):2233–2238. doi: 2210.2337/dc2212-2714. Epub 2013 Apr 2235.

Moses, R. G., M. Barker, M. Winter, P. Petocz, and J. C. Brand-Miller (2009). Can a low-glycemic index diet reduce the need for insulin in gestational diabetes mellitus? A randomized trial. *Diabetes Care.* **32**(6):996–1000. doi: 1010.2337/dc1009-0007. Epub 2009 Mar 1011.

Moses, R. G., S. A. Casey, E. G. Quinn, J. M. Cleary, L. C. Tapsell, M. Milosavljevic, P. Petocz, and J. C. Brand-Miller (2014). Pregnancy and glycemic index outcomes study: Effects of low glycemic index compared with conventional dietary advice on selected pregnancy outcomes. *Am J Clin Nutr.* **99**(3):517–523. doi: 510.3945/ajcn.3113.074138. Epub 072013 Dec 074118.

Moses, R. G., M. Luebcke, W. S. Davis, K. J. Coleman, L. C. Tapsell, P. Petocz, and J. C. Brand-Miller (2006). Effect of a low-glycemic-index diet during pregnancy on obstetric outcomes. *Am J Clin Nutr.* **84**(4):807–812.

Ney, D., D. R. Hollingsworth, and L. Cousins (1982). Decreased insulin requirement and improved control of diabetes in pregnant women given a high-carbohydrate, high-fiber, low-fat diet. *Diabetes Care.* **5**(5):529–533.

Nolan, C. J. (1984). Improved glucose tolerance in gestational diabetic women on a low fat, high unrefined carbohydrate diet. *Aust N Z J Obstet Gynaecol.* **24**(3):174–177.

Noto, H., A. Goto, T. Tsujimoto, and M. Noda (2013). Low-carbohydrate diets and all-cause mortality: A systematic review and meta-analysis of observational studies. *PLoS One.* **8**(1):e55030. doi: 55010.51371/journal.pone.0055030. Epub 0052013 Jan 0055025.

Orio, F., Jr., S. Palomba, T. Cascella, B. De Simone, S. Di Biase, T. Russo, D. Labella, F. Zullo, G. Lombardi, and A. Colao (2004). Early impairment of endothelial structure and function in young normal-weight women with polycystic ovary syndrome. *J Clin Endocrinol Metab.* **89**(9):4588–4593.

Osborne-Majnik, A., Q. Fu, and R. H. Lane (2013). Epigenetic mechanisms in fetal origins of health and disease. *Clin Obstet Gynecol.* **56**(3):622–632. doi: 610.1097/GRF.1090b1013e31829cb31899a.

Pan, A., Q. Sun, A. M. Bernstein, J. E. Manson, W. C. Willett, and F. B. Hu (2013). Changes in red meat consumption and subsequent risk of type 2 diabetes mellitus: Three cohorts of US men and women. *JAMA Intern Med.* **173**(14):1328–1335. doi: 1310.1001/jamainternmed.2013.6633.

Pan, A., Q. Sun, A. M. Bernstein, M. B. Schulze, J. E. Manson, M. J. Stampfer, W. C. Willett, and F. B. Hu (2012). Red meat consumption and mortality: Results from 2 prospective cohort studies. *Arch Intern Med.* **172**(7):555–563. doi: 510.1001/archinternmed.2011.2287. Epub 2012 Mar 1012.

Pan, A., Q. Sun, A. M. Bernstein, M. B. Schulze, J. E. Manson, W. C. Willett, and F. B. Hu (2011). Red meat consumption and risk of type 2 diabetes: 3 cohorts of US adults and an updated meta-analysis. *Am J Clin Nutr.* **94**(4):1088–1096. doi: 1010.3945/ajcn.1111.018978. Epub 012011 Aug 018910.

Park, S., W. M. Sappenfield, C. Bish, H. Salihu, D. Goodman, and D. M. Bensyl (2011). Assessment of the Institute of Medicine recommendations for weight gain during pregnancy: Florida, 2004–2007. *Matern Child Health J.* **15**(3):289–301. doi: 210.1007/s10995-10010-10596-10995.

Parker, S. E., M. M. Werler, G. M. Shaw, M. Anderka, and M. M. Yazdy (2012). Dietary glycemic index and the risk of birth defects. *Am J Epidemiol.* **176**(12):1110–1120. doi: 1110.1093/aje/kws1201. Epub 2012 Nov 1121.

Pereira, M. A., D. R. Jacobs, Jr., L. Van Horn, M. L. Slattery, A. I. Kartashov, and D. S. Ludwig (2002). Dairy consumption, obesity, and the insulin resistance syndrome in young adults: The CARDIA Study. *JAMA.* **287**(16):2081–2089.

Perichart-Perera, O., M. Balas-Nakash, A. Rodriguez-Cano, J. Legorreta-Legorreta, A. Parra-Covarrubias, and F. Vadillo-Ortega (2012). Low glycemic index carbohydrates versus all types of carbohydrates for treating diabetes in pregnancy: A randomized clinical trial to evaluate the effect of glycemic control. *Int J Endocrinol.* **2012**:296017. doi: 10.1155/2012/296017. Epub 292012 Nov 296029.

Radesky, J. S., E. Oken, S. L. Rifas-Shiman, K. P. Kleinman, J. W. Rich-Edwards, and M. W. Gillman (2008). Diet during early pregnancy and development of gestational diabetes. *Paediatr Perinat Epidemiol.* **22**(1):47–59. doi: 10.1111/j.1365-3016.2007.00899.x.

Rajendran, S., S. R. Willoughby, W. P. Chan, E. A. Liberts, T. Heresztyn, M. Saha, M. S. Marber, R. J. Norman, and J. D. Horowitz (2009). Polycystic ovary syndrome is associated with severe platelet and endothelial dysfunction in both obese and lean subjects. *Atherosclerosis.* **204**(2):509–514. doi: 510.1016/j.atherosclerosis.2008.1009.1010. Epub 2008 Sep 1017.

Reece, E. A. and U. J. Eriksson (1996). The pathogenesis of diabetes-associated congenital malformations. *Obstet Gynecol Clin North Am.* **23**(1):29–45.

Reece, E. A., C. J. Homko, and Y.-K. Wu (1996). Multifactorial basis of the syndrome of diabetic embryopathy. *Teratology.* **54**(4):171–182.

Reece, E. A., C. J. Homko, Y.-K. Wu, and A. Wiznitzer (1998). The role of free radicals and membrane lipids in diabetes-induced congenital malformations. *J Soc Gynecol Investig.* **5**(4):178–187.

Reynolds, R. M., K. M. Godfrey, M. Barker, C. Osmond, and D. I. Phillips (2007). Stress responsiveness in adult life: influence of mother's diet in late pregnancy. *J Clin Endocrinol Metab.* **92**(6):2208–2210. Epub 2007 Mar 2206.

Rhodes, E. T., D. B. Pawlak, T. C. Takoudes, C. B. Ebbeling, H. A. Feldman, M. M. Lovesky, E. A. Cooke, M. M. Leidig, and D. S. Ludwig (2010). Effects of a low-glycemic load diet in overweight and obese pregnant women: A pilot randomized controlled trial. *Am J Clin Nutr.* **92**(6):1306–1315. doi: 1310.3945/ajcn.2010.30130. Epub 32010 Oct 30120.

Riccardi, G., R. Giacco, and A. A. Rivellese (2004). Dietary fat, insulin sensitivity and the metabolic syndrome. *Clin Nutr.* **23**(4):447–456.

Riserus, U. (2008). Fatty acids and insulin sensitivity. *Curr Opin Clin Nutr Metab Care.* **11**(2):100–105. doi: 110.1097/MCO.1090b1013e3282f52708.

Rivellese, A. A., C. De Natale, and S. Lilli (2002). Type of dietary fat and insulin resistance. *Ann N Y Acad Sci.* **967**:329–335.

Romon, M., M. C. Nuttens, A. Vambergue, O. Verier-Mine, S. Biausque, C. Lemaire, P. Fontaine, J. L. Salomez, and R. Beuscart (2001). Higher carbohydrate intake is associated with decreased incidence of newborn macrosomia in women with gestational diabetes. *J Am Diet Assoc.* **101**(8):897–902.

Rotterdam ESHRE/ASRM-Sponsored PCOS consensus workshop group (2004). Revised 2003 consensus on diagnostic criteria and long-term health risks related to polycystic ovary syndrome (PCOS). *Hum Reprod.* **19**(1):41–47.

Sadler, T. W., E. S. Hunter, 3rd, W. Balkan, and W. E. Horton, Jr. (1988). Effects of maternal diabetes on embryogenesis. *Am J Perinatol.* **5**(4):319–326.

Scholl, T. O., X. Chen, C. S. Khoo, and C. Lenders (2004). The dietary glycemic index during pregnancy: Influence on infant birth weight, fetal growth, and biomarkers of carbohydrate metabolism. *Am J Epidemiol.* **159**(5):467–474.

Schwingshackl, L. and G. Hoffmann (2013). Long-term effects of low glycemic index/load vs. high glycemic index/load diets on parameters of obesity and obesity-associated risks: A systematic review and meta-analysis. *Nutr Metab Cardiovasc Dis.* **23**(8):699–706. doi: 610.1016/j.numecd.2013.1004.1008. Epub 2013 Jun 1017.

Shaw, G. M., S. L. Carmichael, C. Laurent, and A. M. Siega-Riz (2008). Periconceptional glycaemic load and intake of sugars and their association with neural tube defects in offspring. *Paediatr Perinat Epidemiol.* **22**(6):514–519. doi: 510.1111/j.1365-3016.2008.00964.x.

Shaw, G. M., T. Quach, V. Nelson, S. L. Carmichael, D. M. Schaffer, S. Selvin, and W. Yang (2003). Neural tube defects associated with maternal periconceptional dietary intake of simple sugars and glycemic index. *Am J Clin Nutr.* **78**(5):972–978.

Shiell, A. W., D. M. Campbell, M. H. Hall, and D. J. Barker (2000). Diet in late pregnancy and glucose-insulin metabolism of the offspring 40 years later. *BJOG.* **107**(7):890–895.

Shiell, A. W., M. Campbell-Brown, S. Haselden, S. Robinson, K. M. Godfrey, and D. J. Barker (2001). High-meat, low-carbohydrate diet in pregnancy: Relation to adult blood pressure in the offspring. *Hypertension.* **38**(6):1282–1288.

Shyam, S., F. Arshad, R. Abdul Ghani, N. A. Wahab, N. S. Safii, M. Y. Nisak, K. Chinna, and N. A. Kamaruddin (2013). Low glycaemic index diets improve glucose tolerance and body weight in women with previous history of gestational diabetes: A six months randomized trial. *Nutr J.* **12**:68. doi: 10.1186/1475-2891-1112-1168.

Smith, R. N., N. J. Mann, A. Braue, H. Makelainen, and G. A. Varigos (2007a). The effect of a high-protein, low glycemic-load diet versus a conventional, high glycemic-load diet on biochemical parameters associated with acne vulgaris: A randomized, investigator-masked, controlled trial. *J Am Acad Dermatol.* **57**(2):247–256. Epub 2007 Apr 2019.

Smith, R. N., N. J. Mann, A. Braue, H. Makelainen, and G. A. Varigos (2007b). A low-glycemic-load diet improves symptoms in acne vulgaris patients: A randomized controlled trial. *Am J Clin Nutr.* **86**(1):107–115.

Smith, R., N. Mann, H. Makelainen, J. Roper, A. Braue, and G. Varigos (2008). A pilot study to determine the short-term effects of a low glycemic load diet on hormonal markers of acne: A nonrandomized, parallel, controlled feeding trial. *Mol Nutr Food Res.* **52**(6):718–726.

Sprung, V. S., H. Jones, C. J. Pugh, N. F. Aziz, C. Daousi, G. J. Kemp, D. J. Green, N. T. Cable, and D. J. Cuthbertson (2014). Endothelial dysfunction in hyperandrogenic polycystic ovary syndrome is not explained by either obesity or ectopic fat deposition. *Clin Sci (Lond).* **126**(1):67–74. doi: 10.1042/CS20130186.

Stepto, N. K., S. Cassar, A. E. Joham, S. K. Hutchison, C. L. Harrison, R. F. Goldstein, and H. J. Teede (2013). Women with polycystic ovary syndrome have intrinsic insulin resistance on euglycaemic-hyperinsulaemic clamp. *Hum Reprod.* **28**(3):777–784. doi: 710.1093/humrep/des1463. Epub 2013 Jan 1012.

Svendsen, P. F., L. Nilas, K. Norgaard, J. E. Jensen, and S. Madsbad (2008). Obesity, body composition and metabolic disturbances in polycystic ovary syndrome. *Hum Reprod.* **23**(9):2113–2121. doi: 2110.1093/humrep/den2211. Epub 2008 Jun 2112.

Teede, H., A. Deeks, and L. Moran (2010). Polycystic ovary syndrome: A complex condition with psychological, reproductive and metabolic manifestations that impacts on health across the lifespan. *BMC Med.* **8**:41. doi: 10.1186/1741-7015-1188-1141.

Teede, H., S. Hutchison, and S. Zoungas (2007). The management of insulin resistance in polycystic ovary syndrome. *Trends Endocrinol Metab.* **18**:273–279.

Teede, H. J., M. L. Misso, A. A. Deeks, L. J. Moran, B. G. Stuckey, J. L. Wong, R. J. Norman, and M. F. Costello (2011). Assessment and management of polycystic ovary syndrome: Summary of an evidence-based guideline. *Med J Aust.* **195**(6):S65–S112.

Thomas, D. E., E. J. Elliott, and L. Baur (2007). Low glycaemic index or low glycaemic load diets for overweight and obesity. *Cochrane Database Syst Rev.* (3):CD005105. doi:10.1002/14651858.CD005105.pub2.

Turner-McGrievy, G. M., C. R. Davidson, E. E. Wingard, and D. L. Billings (2014). Low glycemic index vegan or low-calorie weight loss diets for women with polycystic ovary syndrome: A randomized controlled feasibility study. *Nutr Res.* **34**(6):552–558. doi: 510.1016/j.nutres.2014.1004.1011. Epub 2014 Apr 1024.

Viana, L. V., J. L. Gross, and M. J. Azevedo (2014). Dietary intervention in patients with gestational diabetes mellitus: A systematic review and meta-analysis of randomized clinical trials on maternal and newborn outcomes. *Diabetes Care.* **37**(12):3345–3355.

Walsh, J. M., R. M. Mahony, M. Culliton, M. E. Foley, and F. M. McAuliffe (2014). Impact of a low glycemic index diet in pregnancy on markers of maternal and fetal metabolism and inflammation. *Reprod Sci.* **18**:18.

Walsh, J. M., C. A. McGowan, R. Mahony, M. E. Foley, and F. M. McAuliffe (2012). Low glycaemic index diet in pregnancy to prevent macrosomia (ROLO study): Randomised control trial. *BMJ.* **345**:e5605. doi: 10.1136/bmj.e5605.

WHO (World Health Organization) (2013). *Diagnostic Criteria and Classification of Hyperglycaemia First Detected in Pregnancy.* Geneva, Switzerland: World Health Organisation.

WHO (World Health Organization) (2014). Overweight and Obesity (Fact Sheet). Retrieved December 4, 2014, from http://www.who.int/mediacentre/factsheets/fs311/en/.

Yazdy, M. M., S. Liu, A. A. Mitchell, and M. M. Werler (2010). Maternal dietary glycemic intake and the risk of neural tube defects. *Am J Epidemiol.* **171**(4):407–414. doi: 410.1093/aje/kwp1395. Epub 2009 Dec 1030.

Yazdy, M. M., A. A. Mitchell, S. Liu, and M. M. Werler (2011). Maternal dietary glycaemic intake during pregnancy and the risk of birth defects. *Paediatr Perinat Epidemiol.* **25**(4):340–346. doi: 310.1111/j.1365-3016.2011.01198.x. Epub 02011 Apr 01124.

Yildiz, B. O., G. Bozdag, Z. Yapici, I. Esinler, and H. Yarali (2012). Prevalence, phenotype and cardiometabolic risk of polycystic ovary syndrome under different diagnostic criteria. *Hum Reprod.* **27**(10):3067–3073. doi: 3010.1093/humrep/des3232. Epub 2012 Jul 3069.

Yu, Z., S. Han, J. Zhu, X. Sun, C. Ji, and X. Guo (2013). Pre-pregnancy body mass index in relation to infant birth weight and offspring overweight/obesity: A systematic review and meta-analysis. *PLoS One.* **8**(4):e61627. doi: 61610.61371/journal.pone.0061627. Print 0062013.

Zawadski, J. and A. Dunaif (1992). Diagnostic criteria for polycystic ovary syndrome: Towards a rational approach. In: Dunaif, A., J. Givens, F. Haseltine, and G. Merriam. *Polycystic Ovary Syndrome (Current Issues in Endocrinology and Metabolism).* Boston: Blackwell Scientific Publications.

Zhang, C., S. Liu, C. G. Solomon, and F. B. Hu (2006a). Dietary fiber intake, dietary glycemic load, and the risk for gestational diabetes mellitus. *Diabetes Care.* **29**(10):2223–2230.

Zhang, C., M. B. Schulze, C. G. Solomon, and F. B. Hu (2006b). A prospective study of dietary patterns, meat intake and the risk of gestational diabetes mellitus. *Diabetologia.* **49**(11):2604–2613.

11 Glycemic Index and Eye Health
*Dietary Hyperglycemia and Metabolic Retinal Diseases**

Chung-Jung Chiu, Min-Lee Chang, and Allen Taylor

CONTENTS

11.1 INTRODUCTION

Glucose is the most important energy source for the human body. The nutrient has a broad spectrum of physiological effects, and a precise regulation of glucose metabolism is required to maintain health and avoid diseases. The blood glucose concentration (glycemia) reflects the combined effects of dietary carbohydrate uptake, delivery to the blood, production, cellular uptake, and utilization, and is tightly regulated by a homeostatic regulatory system (Jenkins et al. 2002; Ludwig 2002). Among those determinants for glucose metabolism, diet-induced glycemia results in the greatest daily variation (Giugliano et al. 2008). Therefore, it is not surprising that the glycemic index (GI) has been related to many disorders, such as diabetes and cardiovascular disease (CVD). The GI is a kinetic measure of glucose appearance in blood after consuming a carbohydrate-containing food. The dietary GI is a weighted sum of the GIs for all the foods in a diet. Interestingly, recent evidence shows that the dietary GI is related to an increased risk for several major age-related diseases,

* Any opinions, findings, conclusions, or recommendations expressed in this publication are those of the authors and do not necessarily reflect the views or policies of the U.S. Department of Agriculture, nor does mention of trade names, commercial products, or organizations imply endorsement by the U.S. Government.

including atherosclerosis and age-related macular degeneration (AMD) in nondiabetic populations (Balkau et al. 1998; Chiu et al. 2006a; 2007a; 2007b; 2009a; 2009b; Kaushik et al. 2008). In addition, accumulating evidence implies that glucose homeostasis and carbohydrate nutrition play an important role in human aging as well as in disease pathogenesis, and it is proposed that the pathophysiological effects of hyperglycemia that are operative in diabetes also affect nondiabetic people on aging (Brownlee 1995). However, the effects may vary due to subtle "pathophysiological" mechanistic differences as well as differences in composition, structure, homeostatic systems, microenvironment, and function between metabolically different tissues (Brownlee 1995; Chiu et al. 2005; 2006b; 2010).

The retina is the most metabolically active tissue in the human body (Cohen and Noell 1965). Therefore, it is not surprising that glucose homeostasis in the retina plays an important role in retinal health and disease. For example, in people with diabetes, failure to regulate blood glucose leads to diabetic retinopathy (DR), which is the most common microvascular diabetic complication (Fong et al. 2004). Although the detailed pathogenesis of DR is not completely understood, it is believed that hyperglycemia is the major cause of this disease (Diabetes Control and Complications Trial Research Group 1993a; U.K. Prospective Diabetes Study Group 1998). Interestingly, although the pathologic lesions in the retina and other vascular beds differ between diabetic and nondiabetic age-related lesions, similar damages are observed in people with diabetes and in nondiabetics with AMD. This may be due to differences in the time at which the lesions occur, the extent and duration of hyperglycemic exposure (Table 11.1). There seems to be an extensive overlap between etiology for GI-related pathogenesis of diabetes, CVD, DR, and AMD (Figure 11.1).

TABLE 11.1
Comparison of Characteristics between Age-Related Macular Degeneration and Diabetic Retinopathy

	Age-Related Macular Degeneration	Diabetic Retinopathy
Population affected	Elders over 60s	Type I and II diabetic patients
Incidence	The 10-year incidence: 1. Early age-related maculopathy: 12.1% 2. Late age-related maculopathy: 2.1%	
Prevalence	1.47% in the U.S. population 40 years and older	12.7–75.1% in diabetic patients
Blindness	Over 420,000 cases per year in the United States	Over 10,000 cases per year in the United States
Risk factors	1. Older age 2. Caucasian race 3. Female gender 4. Genetic factors (family history) 5. Smoking 6. Obesity 7. Hypertension 8. Cataract surgery 9. Diet	1. Poor blood glucose control 2. Hypertension
Involved blood vessels	Choroidal circulation	Retinal circulation
Primary retinal area involved	Macula in the outer retina: RPE, Bruch's membrane, photoreceptors	Inner retina: Retinal endothelium, pericytes, basement membrane
Early stage lesions	Drusen, pigment abnormality	Cotton wool spots

(Continued)

TABLE 11.1 (*Continued*)
Comparison of Characteristics between Age-Related Macular Degeneration and Diabetic Retinopathy

	Age-Related Macular Degeneration	Diabetic Retinopathy
Advanced lesions	1. Geographic atrophy (GA) 2. Choroidal neovascularization (CNV)	1. Proliferative diabetic retinopathy (PDR; retinal neovascularization [RNV]; most common sight-threatening lesion in type I diabetes) 2. Diabetic macular edema (DME; breakdown of the blood retinal barrier (iBRB); primary cause of poor visual acuity in type 2 diabetes)
Prevention	AREDS formulation (high-dose formulation of antioxidants and zinc) delays and possibly prevents intermediate AMD from progression to advanced AMD in people with: 1. Intermediate AMD in one or both eyes Or 2. Advanced AMD (dry or wet) in one eye but not the other eye	Consistent blood glucose control
Treatment	1. Laser surgery (neovascularization) 2. Photodynamic therapy (Verteporfin; neovascularization) 3. Anti-VEGF therapy (such as Lucentis®, Avastin®, and Macugen®; neovascularization)	1. Argon-laser photocoagulation (for early stages of PDR) 2. Panretinal photocoagulation (also called scatter laser treatment; for PDR) 3. Intravitreal Triamcinolone acetonide (for DME) 4. Vitrectomy (for late stages of PDR)

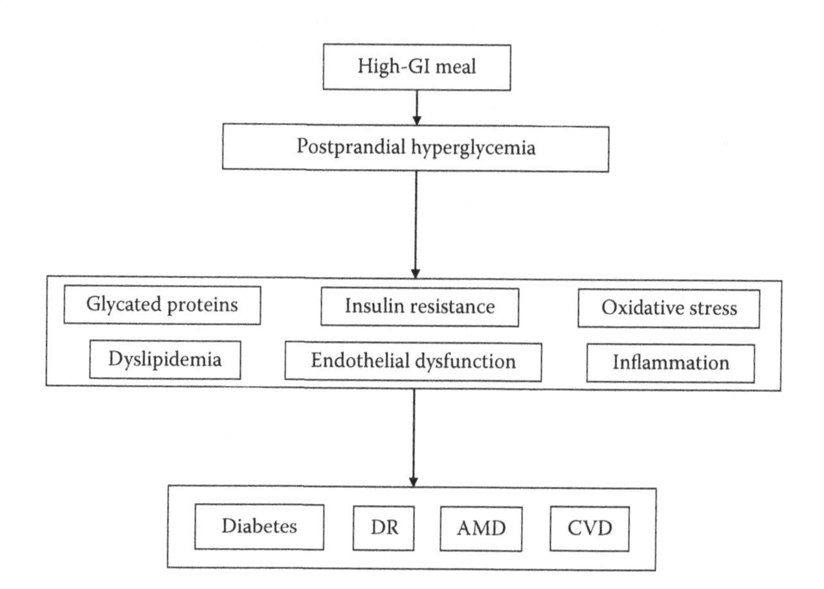

FIGURE 11.1 Adverse metabolic events relating high-GI diets to diabetes and cardiovascular disease.

Although the concept of the GI was introduced almost three decades ago, only recently was the GI related to retinal health (Chiu et al. 2006a). This chapter begins with a brief review of the epidemiological evidence for the associations between the GI and AMD followed by several plausible mechanisms, including our novel hyperglycemic hypoxia-inducible factor (HIF) pathway (Chiu and Taylor 2011; Chang et al. 2014), which may link hyperglycemia to retinal pathology, with emphasis on AMD and DR.

11.2 GI AND AMD

Overall, the GI is a better measure than carbohydrate quantity for the associations between carbohydrate foods and the related diseases (Table 11.2). Observational studies indicate that a low-GI diet is associated with a reduced risk for AMD, but no human intervention study has been conducted. This is a conundrum because an intervention study evaluating the effect of the GI on clinical outcomes of AMD would be difficult to execute as feeding people high-GI diets for prolonged periods would be unethical and the study would be very costly. Furthermore, currently there are no surrogate endpoints for AMD after a short-term intervention. However, observational epidemiological studies support findings that lowering the GI reduces the risk for the progression of both early and late AMDs and a robust animal-feeding data base is available to corroborate the findings (Uchiki et al. 2011).

11.2.1 Epidemiologic Evidence Relating GI to AMD

Recent epidemiological studies have consistently found positive relationships between the GI and AMD in nondiabetic people (Figure 11.2) (Chiu et al. 2006a; 2007; Kaushik 2008). The first study published in 2006 was a case-control study of the Nutrition and Vision Project (NVP) of the Nurses'

TABLE 11.2
Current Evidence-Based Evaluation of the Impact of Quantity (g/d) and Glycemic Index (GI) of Carbohydrate Foods on the Risk for Diabetes, Cardiovascular Disease, and Age-Related Macular Degeneration in Humans

	Overall Association	
	GI	Quantity
Diabetes		
Epidemiological observations	+	±
Intervention studies	?	±[a]
Cardiovascular disease		
Epidemiological observations	+	±
Intervention studies	±[a]	±[a]
Age-related macular degeneration		
Epidemiological observations	+	No
Intervention studies	?	?

[a] Using intermediate risk factors, such as HbA1c and blood pressure, as the endpoints (surrogate endpoints).

+: Positive association.

±: Uncertain association.

No: No association.

?: Unknown.

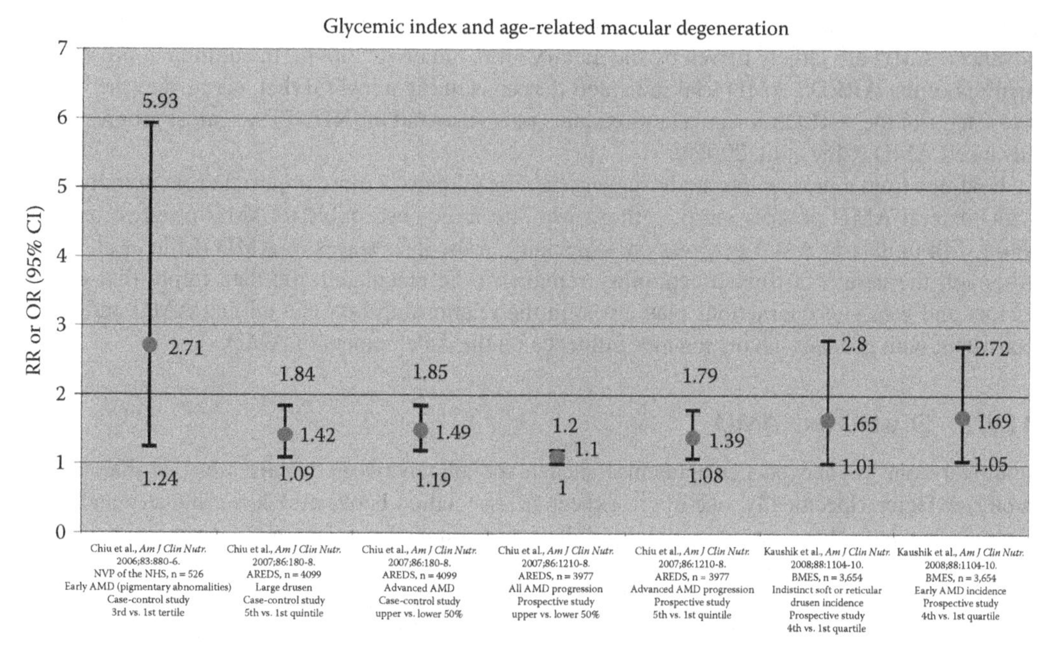

FIGURE 11.2 Studies relating GI to AMD indicate that consuming a low-GI diet is associated with lower risk for both early and advanced AMD.

Health Study (NHS) (Chiu et al. 2006a). The study found that women in the third tertile of the dietary GI, compared with those in the first tertile, had an ~2.7-fold risk for early AMD, mainly pigment abnormalities (Chiu et al. 2006a). The findings were replicated and extended in a much larger American cohort, the Age-Related Eye Disease Study (AREDS) (Chiu et al. 2007). In that case-control study, a diet in the highest quintile of the dietary GI compared with a diet in the lowest quintile was associated with an over 40% increased risk for large drusen (early AMD). When comparing the upper 50% with the lower 50% of the dietary GI, an almost 50% increased risk for advanced AMD was noted. Using these data, the prevalent population attributable fraction of advanced AMD for the high dietary GI was estimated to be 20%. In other words, one in five of the existing cases of advanced AMD would have been eliminated if the AREDS participants consumed diets with a dietary GI below the median. The positive relationship between the GI and AMD was further strengthened in a prospective study that followed the AREDS subjects for up to 8 years (mean = 5.4 years) (Chiu et al. 2007). The multivariate-adjusted risk of progression was significantly higher (hazard ratio = 1.10; 95% CI: 1.00, 1.20; $P = 0.047$) in the upper 50% of the dietary GI than in the lower 50%. We also estimate the incident population attributable fraction for advanced AMD to be 7.8 during the follow-up period, that is, 7.8% of new advanced AMD cases would be prevented in 5 years if people consumed a low GI diet. This could save over 100,000 cases of AMD-related blindness in the United States in 5 years. Even more attractive is that the benefit can be achieved by a minor dietary change, such as by daily substituting as little as five slices of white bread (GI = 70) by whole grain bread (GI = 55) (Chiu et al. 2009a). The GI–AMD relationship was further confirmed in a 10-year follow-up in the Australia Blue Mountains Eye Study (BMES) (Kaushik et al. 2008). After multivariate adjustment, a higher dietary GI was associated with a 77% increased risk of early AMD comparing the fourth with the first quartiles of the dietary GI (95% CI: 1.13, 2.78; P for trend = 0.03).

Importantly, consuming lower GI diets appears to provide additional ophthalmic benefit to that gained from currently known dietary factors. The analysis of a compound score summarizing dietary intakes of antioxidants (including vitamins C and E, and lutein/zeaxanthin), zinc, omega-3 fatty acids (including docosahexaenoic acid [DHA] and eicosapentaenoic acid [EPA]), and the dietary GI suggested that the associations between the compound score and risk for drusen and advanced AMD are largely driven by the dietary GI (Chiu et al. 2009b). In addition, a prospective analysis of the AREDS AMD trial indicated that consuming a low-GI diet augmented the protective effects of the AREDS formula (antioxidants plus zinc) and of DHA/EPA against progression to advanced AMD (Chiu et al. 2009b).

Findings from a prospective study suggest that the GI plays a more important role in individuals with bilateral AMD progression (i.e., those who are more susceptible to AMD progression) than those with unilateral AMD progression, especially in the later stages of AMD (Chiu et al. 2007). Although the nature of this susceptibility remains to be elucidated, the data imply that genetic factors and gene–GI interactions play a role in the relationship between GI and AMD and this is consistent with genetics having a major influence on the development of AMD.

11.2.2 Diabetes and AMD

Intuitively, one might expect an epidemiological association between two diseases that share a common risk factor. Specifically, one might expect an association between risk for diabetes and AMD because they both share consuming high-GI diets as a common risk factor. However, epidemiological data regarding the association between diabetes and AMD have been inconsistent. Some studies found a positive association (Age-Related Eye Disease Study Research Group 2005; Klein et al. 1992, 1997; Leske et al. 2006; Mitchell and Wang 1999; Topouzis et al. 2009), while others did not (Delcourt et al. 2001; Eye Disease Case-Control Study Group 1992; Fraser-Bell et al. 2008; Goldberg et al. 1988; Hyman et al. 2000; Smith et al. 2001; Tomany et al. 2004). But even in studies that found a positive association, the association with specific types of late AMD (neovascular AMD or geographic atrophy [GA]) was inconsistent. Some found an association between diabetes and neovascular AMD (Age-Related Eye Disease Study Research Group 2005; Klein et al. 1992, 1997; Topouzis et al. 2009), while others found an association with GA (Mitchell and Wang 1999; Tomany et al. 2004). None of these studies found an association between diabetes and early AMD.

In the Beaver Dam Eye Study (BDES), in persons older than 75 years, diabetes was found to be associated with neovascular AMD, but not with GA (Klein et al. 1992). Further stratification analysis in the BDES data revealed that the association was only in men but not in women; the relative risk (RR) of neovascular AMD was 10.2 (95% CI: 2.4, 43.7) for men, but only 1.1 (95% CI: 0.4, 3.0) for women. However, in contrast, in the Women's Health Initiative Sight Exam Ancillary study, a history of diabetes was associated with a 2.5-fold increased risk for neovascular AMD but not with either early AMD or GA in these women (Klein et al. 1997). Positive associations between diabetes and neovascular AMD have also been identified by the AREDS and the EUREYE study (Age-Related Eye Disease Study Research Group 2005; Topouzis et al. 2009). In the AREDS, a history of diabetes was associated with the increased risk for incident neovascular AMD (odds ratio [OR] = 1.88) but not for GA in persons at risk of developing advanced AMD in one eye. In the EUREYE study, subjects with neovascular AMD compared with controls had increased odds for diabetes (OR = 1.81; 95% CI: 1.10, 2.98).

Impressively, the BMES reported that diabetes was significantly associated with the prevalence of GA (OR = 4.0; 95% CI: 1.6, 10.3), but no association was found for either neovascular AMD or early AMD (Mitchell and Wang 1999). In the 5- and 10-year incidence studies in the same cohort, diabetes was also related to the increased risk of incident GA (RR = 8.3 and 3.9, respectively) but not to neovascular AMD (Tomany et al. 2004).

In a cohort study of a black population in Barbados, a diabetes history was associated with a 2.7-fold increased risk of incident advanced AMD. However, a subtype analysis of advanced AMD was not performed (Leske et al. 2006). As with the other studies, diabetes history was not associated with early AMD in this study.

Surprisingly, in the BDES, diabetes at baseline was associated with a decreased risk of incident reticular drusen (Klein et al. 2008). Reticular drusen has been reported to be associated with a high risk of progression to neovascular AMD (Smith et al. 2006).

In a recent meta-analysis of 24 manuscripts involving 27 study populations (Chen et al. 2014), the pooled ORs for the risk of neovascular AMD were 1.10 (95% CI, 0.96–1.26), 1.48 (95% CI, 1.44–1.51), and 1.15 (95% CI, 1.11–1.21) from 7 cohort, 9 cross-sectional, and 11 case-control studies, respectively. No obvious divergence existed among different ethnic groups. The authors concluded that diabetes is a risk factor for AMD, stronger for late AMD than earlier stages. However, it was noted that most of the included studies only adjusted for age and sex, and, therefore, they cannot rule out confounding as a potential explanation for the association. The association between diabetes and AMD remains controversial.

11.3 MECHANISMS RELATING HYPERGLYCEMIA TO DR AND AMD

In the following section, the potential underlying mechanisms for GI–disease associations with emphasis on DR and AMD will be discussed. The section will begin with a brief review of the hyperglycemia-related pathologies for DR and AMD, followed by a discussion of the potential molecular pathological mechanisms. Five well-developed hyperglycemic mechanisms are described, including four glycolysis-associated pathways and one mitochondria-associated pathway. However, these hyperglycemic pathways can only explain the pathogenesis under normoxic conditions, that is, normal levels of oxygen in tissue or blood. Therefore, we also propose a novel hyperglycemic HIF pathway to explain the hyperglycemic pathology under low oxygen tension. Interestingly, our recent experimental data suggest that this novel hyperglycemic HIF pathway may be responsible for the pathogenesis under both normoxic and hypoxic conditions. Finally, we also discuss the relationships among the six pathways.

It is useful to mention here that all of the six hyperglycemic pathways could lead to a common intracellular or extracellular insult, oxidative stress. This is consistent with trial data indicating a benefit of antioxidant intake to AMD (Age-Related Eye Disease Study Research Group 2001) as well as with recent epidemiological data that show that a diet high in antioxidants and low in GI brings an additional benefit compared with a diet high in antioxidants or low in GI alone (Chiu et al. 2009a; 2009b).

It should be noted that, although there are major phenotypic differences between DR and AMD (Table 11.1), current evidence suggests that both diseases can be considered metabolic diseases.

11.3.1 Hyperglycemic Pathology of DR

Hyperglycemia has long been recognized as the critical factor in the development of DR (Kohner et al. 1998; 2001; Madsen-Bouterse and Kowluru 2008; The Diabetes Control and Complications Trial Research Group 1993b; 2000; UK Prospective Diabetes Study (UKPDS) Group 1991). The large variations in the prevalence and incidence of DR among different studies are mainly attributable to the difference in the extent of blood glucose control across the different study cohorts (Williams et al. 2004). Prolonged exposure to high glucose causes both acute and chronic, reversible and irreversible changes in cellular metabolism as well as the modification of many macromolecules. However, long before disease pathology is detectable, the cells of the inner blood–retinal barrier (iBRB) start to respond to this hyperglycemic environment by altering their metabolism. The iBRB consists of the basement membrane, and the fusion of membranes between retinal endothelial cells forms tight junctional complexes to help stop the outward flow of circulating proteins (Harhaj and Antonetti 2004). The main pathological feature of very early stage DR is a hyperglycemia-associated iBRB breakdown (Engerman and Kern 1986). The iBRB breakdown begins with the loss of tight junctions between adjacent microvascular endothelial cells. This allows macromolecules to seep out. As the barrier breakdown proceeds, the basement membrane of the capillaries thickens and the capillaries become rigid. This could interfere with the ability of the basement membranes to bind various growth factors (Frank 2004).

Therefore, DR is considered as a retinal microvascular complication of diabetes. It primarily affects the inner retinal circulation, which receives 20%–30% of the blood that flows to the retina through the central retinal artery to nourish the inner neural retina. The retinal capillary wall is surrounded by a connective tissue sheath-the basement membrane. A single layer of the retinal microvascular cells, including pericytes and endothelial cells lies on this membrane (Lorenzi and Gerhardinger 2001). The pericytes are a type of smooth muscle cell. They directly contact the endothelial cells, providing support to the capillaries, and help regulate the endothelial cells. These functions are critical for the development of a proper retinal network, and by cooperating with other retinal cells like astrocytes and Müller cells, pericytes appear protective for retinal endothelial cells under hyperglycemic conditions. Importantly, DR is characterized by pericyte loss followed by increased vascular permeability and progressive vascular occlusion.

Loss of pericytes results in empty, balloon-like spaces on the wall of the retinal capillary. In response to these lesions, endothelial cells try to repair the damaged vessel by proliferation on the inner vessel wall. At this stage, the disease remains clinically nondetectable. However, as the pathology progresses, it results in capillary occlusion and the appearance of small hemorrhages and yellow deposits (hard exudates), followed by the complete loss of all cellular elements from the retinal microvessels (acellular capillaries) and the development of abnormally dilated capillaries around the margins of areas with no capillary blood flow (ischemia). These microaneurysms are the earliest clinically observable lesion of DR. This leads to nonproliferative DR and often progresses into diabetic macular edema (DME). If the disease becomes more severe, the nonproliferative retinopathy may progress to pre-proliferative retinopathy. The ischemia and hypoxia due to preproliferative retinopathy eventually lead to retinal neovascularization (RNV), which is the hallmark of proliferative retinopathy (D'Amico 1994). These newly formed blood capillaries are fragile and tend to hemorrhage. They can also extend into the vitreous of the eye, and their fibrous proliferation on the retina could scar the vitreous body leading to traction retinal detachment, and ultimately to blindness (D'Amico 1994; Frank 2004; Madsen-Bouterse and Kowluru 2008; Singh and Stewart 2009).

11.3.2 Hyperglycemia-Related Pathology in AMD

In contrast with DR, the first indication of AMD is observed in the outer retina, primarily involving the retinal pigment epithelium (RPE) and associated tissues (Table 11.1) (Glenn and Stitt 2009). The RPE lays on a basal lamina, known as Bruch's membrane, and together they form the outer blood–retinal barrier (oBRB). The oBRB separates the retina from the choroidal plexus. The choroidal circulation receives 65%–85% of the blood that flows to the retina through choroidal arteries and is vital for the maintenance of the outer retina (particularly the photoreceptors, which have no direct blood supply) (Henkind 1981; Henkind and Walsh 1980). In addition to the high blood flow into the outer retina, a very high density of mitochondria and lysosomes in RPE also indicates a high metabolic activity. The RPE serves as the headquarters in outer retinal metabolism; it oxygenates and nurtures the outer retina and is also responsible for processing metabolic waste generated from the visual cycle. The high energy requirements of the RPE stem from requirements for metabolism including proteolytic burden, because every night each RPE must digest the outer 10% of the photoreceptor discs that are shed by 30 photoreceptors. In fact, the RPE has the highest proteolytic burden in the body (Young and Bok 1969).

In both the RPE and the photoreceptor inner segments, there are large numbers of mitochondria indicative of the involvement of the tricarboxylic acid (TCA) cycle (also known as citric acid cycle or Kreb's cycle) in energy provision (Kaur et al. 2008). Glucose is the major fuel for energy metabolism in retina and about 60% of blood glucose entering the retina appears to be supplied to RPE (Coffe et al. 2006; Foulds 1990). The high blood flow in the choroid secures an adequate supply of oxygen and glucose to this most energy-demanding tissue in the human body-the retinal photoreceptors and the RPE. It has been shown that RPE exhibits a high saturation level of glucose transport and high rates of oxygen consumption (Miceli et al. 1990; To et al. 1998; Vilchis and Salceda 1996). Indeed, blood flow in the choroid is the highest of any tissue in the body in terms of blood flow per unit mass of tissue (Wilson et al. 1973). The RPE also provides a major transport pathway for the exchange of metabolites and ions between the choroidal blood supply and the neural retina to maintain a normal function of the photoreceptor cells (Pascuzzo et al. 1980; Strauss 2005; Zadunaisky and Degnan 1976). All of these functions indicate that the RPE plays a central role in the health of the outer retina. Therefore, it is not surprising that disorders induced by hyperglycemia in the RPE are associated with the development of AMD.

Tissue aging is associated with a progressive decline in the cellular and physiological function, due in part to diminished capacity to respond to stress, such as hyperglycemia (Beckman and Ames 1998; Pawlak et al. 2008; Szweda et al. 2003). Cellular manifestations of aging include increased chemical damage to proteins, accumulation of intracellular and/or extracellular deposits, and decreased efficiency of antioxidant defenses (Uchiki et al. 2011). These processes are pronounced in long-lived postmitotically differentiated cells, such as RPE (Boulton et al. 2004; Grune et al. 2004; Louie et al. 2002; Terman et al. 2007; Zhang et al. 2008b).

The accumulation of heterogeneous debris within the RPE–Bruch's membrane–choriocapillaris complex is a major histopathologic hallmark of aging and AMD. A range of age-related macular changes have been described in the RPE and underlying Bruch's membrane. It appears that as the function of RPE is compromised during aging or by stress, retinal deposits and drusen, the early stage of maculopathy, and more advanced lesions begin to develop (Uchiki et al. 2011). For example, damage to the metabolic waste processing machinery in the RPE, such as lysosomes and microsomal glutathione S transferase 1, has been related to aging retina (Maeda et al. 2005). This may result in or accelerate the formation of lipofuscin, basal lamina deposits (BLDs), and drusen. Some of their precursors are generated from phagocytosed but insufficiently degraded photoreceptor outer segments that are not well degraded by the RPE. Eventually, they accumulate extracellularly between the RPE and Bruch's membrane (Boulton et al. 1994; Ishibashi et al. 1986a; 1986b; Rakoczy et al. 1996). Carbohydrates have been found to be important components in drusen and BLDs and play an important role in the pathogenesis of AMD (Hageman et al. 2001). Drusen and, to a lesser extent, BLD have deleterious effects on the RPE function, and the accumulation of lipofuscin with age in RPE also has a direct influence on outer retinal integrity (Boulton and Marshall 1986; Johnson et al. 2003; Sarks et al. 1999).

Drusen are commonly seen in people over 60 years old without vision loss but a significant proportion of them will progress to the late stage of AMD, including GA and choroidal neovascularization (CNV), which often result in severe vision loss.

In addition to drusen deposition during aging, there are changes in the chemical composition, physical structure, and hydrodynamics of Bruch's membrane (Cherepanoff et al. 2009; Moore and Clover 2001; Moore et al. 1995; Sarks et al. 1999; Stitt 2005). Such abnormalities are also important in the development of AMD (Anderson et al. 2010; Hageman et al. 2001; Johnson et al. 2003).

11.3.3 Hypothesized Mechanisms Relating Dietary Hyperglycemia to AMD and DR

In aerobic cellular respiration, glucose is metabolized through three major sequential steps: (1) glycolytic pathway, (2) TCA cycle (also known as citric acid cycle or Kreb's cycle), and (3) electron transport chain (ETC). Under normal glucose concentration (euglycemia, left panel in Figure 11.3a), glucose generates energy (i.e., adenosine triphosphate [ATP]) for normal physiological needs, ideally, without inducing deleterious side reactions. However, under hyperglycemic conditions that exceed the physiological needs (right panel in Figure 11.3a), the glycolytic pathway may induce four adverse side pathways to relieve the influx of excess glucose. The four glycolysis-related hyperglycemic pathways include: (1) intracellular production of AGE precursors, (2) increased flux through the polyol pathway, (3) protein kinase C (PKC) activation, and (4) increased hexosamine pathway activity. Each of these will be discussed below. Under normoxic conditions (normal oxygen tension), the TCA cycle will induce an abnormally high mitochondrial membrane potential. This will further induce the ETC to reduce O_2 into superoxide (O_2^-; mitochondria-derived reactive oxygen species [ROS]), which in turn will generate intracellular and even extracellular oxidative stress (Brownlee 2001, 2005).

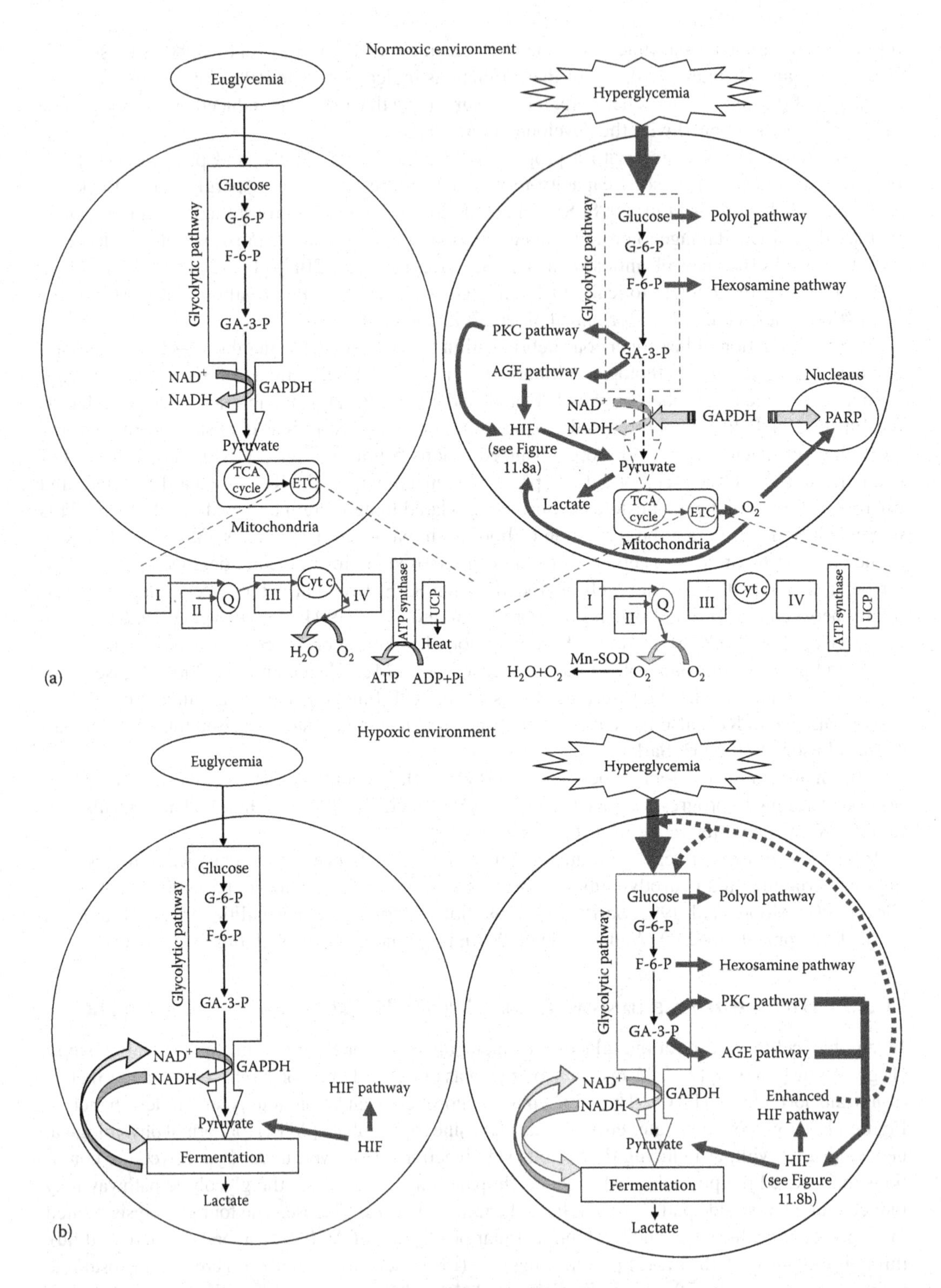

FIGURE 11.3 Cellular responses to euglycemia (normal glycemia) and hyperglycemia under normoxia (a) and hypoxia (b).

Figure 11.3a shows glucose metabolism in euglycemia versus hyperglycemia under normoxic conditions. Compared with euglycemia, hyperglycemia induces mitochondria-derived superoxide (O_2^-) and four glycolysis-related pathways (see Sections 11.3.3.1 through 11.3.3.4), including polyol, hexosamine, AGE, and PKC pathways, and excess cytosolic HIF. The left panel in Figure 11.3a demonstrates normal aerobic respiration in a euglycemic condition. After glycolysis, the glucose metabolite, pyruvate, is produced. Pyruvate enters the mitochondria to generate ATP and water (H_2O). The right panel in Figure 11.3a demonstrates that hyperglycemia drives glycolysis to generate the four adverse side pathways noted above (also see Sections 11.3.3.1 through 11.3.3.4). Also, driven by hyperglycemia, the ETC is obstructed in coenzyme Q by an abnormally high mitochondrial membrane potential and generates superoxide (O_2^-), which may activate PARP, a DNA repair enzyme that needs GAPDH as a cofactor and is only found in the nucleus. This gives rise to the decrease of cytosol GAPDH and further exacerbates of the four glycolysis-associated pathways induced by hyperglycemia. The mechanism underlying the movement of GAPDH from the cytosol to the nucleus under high glucose conditions involves the E3 Ub ligase siah-1, which facilitates hyperglycemia-induced GAPDH nuclear translocation via formation of a complex with GAPDH. Furthermore, because hyperglycemic AGEs, PKC, and mitochondrial ROS may give rise to the overexpression and decreased degradation of HIF, the excess HIF proteins may switch pyruvate metabolism from transformation through the TCA cycle and oxidative phosphorylation in the ETC to conversion to lactate in the cytoplasm (also see Section 11.3.3.6 for more details). Remarkably, PKC can also be activated through hyperglycemic polyol pathway (see Section 11.3.3.2) and hyperglycemic hexosamine pathway (see Section 11.3.3.4). The cell may defend against superoxide using the mitochondrial isoform of superoxide dismutase (Mn-SOD). This enzyme degrades the oxygen-free radical to hydrogen peroxide, which is then converted to H_2O and O_2 by other enzymes.

Figure 11.3b shows glucose metabolism in euglycemia versus hyperglycemia under hypoxic conditions. In euglycemia, HIF pathway is turned on by hypoxia-activated HIF. Under hyperglycemic conditions, the HIF pathway is enhanced by hyperglycemia-induced AGE and PKC pathways. The left panel in Figure 11.3b indicates the HIF is activated and induces two aspects of the cellular responses, including switching glucose metabolism and turning on HIF pathway. Cytosolic HIF switches glucose metabolism from aerobic respiration to fermentation, the end product of which is lactate. The HIF pathway activated by hypoxia-activated HIF may induce a range of deleterious effects. However, when hypoxia coincides with hyperglycemia (right panel of Figure 11.3b), which results in the formation of AGEs and activation of PKC during glycolysis; HIF pathway is further enhanced by hyperglycemia. Remarkably, PKC can also be activated through hyperglycemic polyol pathway (see Section 11.3.3.2) and hyperglycemic hexosamine pathway (see Section 11.3.3.4). Furthermore, in adaptation of lower efficiency of ATP generation from fermentation, the activations of some HIF-inducible genes in HIF pathway may increase glucose uptake and upregulate glycolysis pathway (also see Section 11.3.3.6). Therefore, in hyperglycemic, hypoxic conditions HIF pathway may further deteriorate the four glycolysis-associated pathways.

It has been shown that inhibition of some of these hyperglycemia-related pathways can protect against multiple or specific microvascular complications in diabetic animal models, including retinopathy. For example, studies using the transketolase activator "benfotiamine" indicate that it can inhibit a common convergent pathway and effectively prevent retinopathy in diabetic animals by inhibiting activation of PKC βII, alterations in hemodynamics, flux through the polyol and hexosamine pathways, and AGE formation (Hammes et al. 2003). Furthermore, Brownlee suggests that under hyperglycemic states the overproduction of ROS can also, indirectly, accelerate the four glycolysis-related pathways by blocking the downstream flow of glycolysis (Figure 11.3a) (Brownlee 2001; 2005; Nishikawa and Araki 2008; Nishikawa et al. 2000).

The relative importance of the four glycolysis-related hyperglycemic pathways may vary with the types of tissue in the body (Brownlee 2001). In the retina, some suggested that the polyol pathway, which is upstream of glycolysis, is more important (Diederen et al. 2006; Ola et al. 2006), while others assign priority to the downstream pathways (Ido and Williamson 1997; Nyengaard et al. 2004; Williamson et al. 1993). The discrepancy may arise from the different experimental conditions used. It is likely that the relative importance of the four glycolysis-related hyperglycemic pathways may also vary with the stages of disease progression.

The discussion above focused on the hyperglycemic pathogenesis under normoxia. However, glucose metabolism also depends on the homeostasis of oxygen. Hypoxia is a condition defined as lower oxygen tension (oxygen partial pressure) relative to that observed at sea level (normoxia). Hypoxia is encountered to different degrees in various tissues and arises as a direct consequence of insufficient blood flow or vascularization in relation to the energy consumption of a given tissue (Brahimi-Horn and Pouyssegur 2005). Under oxygen-insufficient conditions (low oxygen tension or hypoxia), instead of entering the TCA cycle and ETC in mitochondria, some of the glycolysis metabolite, pyruvate, may proceed to fermentation (Figure 11.3b). Although fermentation is less efficient in generating energy from glucose, under certain physiological conditions, such as sprinting, it may be used by a skeletal muscle cell to generate ATP and lactate even before the oxygen levels are depleted. This hypoxia-induced metabolism switch has been shown to be associated with an HIF (Brahimi-Horn et al. 2007; Kim and Dang 2006). Similarly, despite large numbers of mitochondria in the RPE indicative of the involvement of the TCA cycle in energy provision, fermentation also occurs in the RPE. As a result, concomitant with high oxygen consumption, the RPE also has a high lactate production even under physiological conditions (Coffe et al. 2006; Kaur et al. 2008; Miceli et al. 1990).

Local occlusive vascular diseases in the eye may also result in retinal hypoxia. Interestingly, in both DR and AMD, hypoxia has been shown to accelerate the progression of NV through an HIF-related pathway (Arjamaa and Nikinmaa 2006). It has been shown that in this pathway HIF serves as a transcription factor that controls the expression of many genes (HIF-inducible genes). Some of these genes regulate angiogenesis, such as the vascular endothelial growth factor (VEGF).

A novel hyperglycemic HIF pathway was proposed to explain hyperglycemic pathogenesis in the retina under hypoxic conditions (Figure 11.3b; also see Section 11.3.3.6) (Chiu and Taylor 2011). Like in aerobic respiration (Figure 11.3a), under hypoxic conditions, the four glycolysis-related pathways and the HIF pathway should be viewed as interrelated and independent mechanisms.

Simply speaking, the hyperglycemic pathogenesis consists of six pathways, including four glycolysis-related pathways, a mitochondria-derived ROS pathway, and an HIF pathway. The four glycolysis-related pathways are applicable in both normoxic and hypoxic conditions. The mitochondria-derived ROS pathway participates during normoxia and the HIF pathway dominates the hyperglycemic pathogenesis under hypoxia. Interestingly, recent data suggest that the HIF pathway may be also partially responsible for hyperglycemic pathogenesis in both diabetic and age-related retinopathy even under normoxia (Chang et al. 2014). In the following sections, we will discuss these six molecular mechanisms regarding how dietary hyperglycemia results in cellular dysfunctions that are associated with tissue damage and/or clinical manifestations of AMD and DR.

11.3.3.1 Hyperglycemic AGE Pathway

One of the major damages of the BRB is due to nonenzymatic modification of free amino groups of proteins, lipids, and DNA by aldehyde groups on sugars or sugar metabolites (such as dicarbonyls) (Stitt 2005). This reaction, called Maillard reaction, occurs naturally during aging in all tissues (Monnier et al. 1992). The initial unstable Schiff base slowly rearranges into an Amadori adduct, the first stable product formed during glycation of protein (Thorpe and Baynes 2003). These have half-lives of several months under physiological conditions (Lyons et al. 1991). The most well-known Amadori product is glycated hemoglobin A_{1c} (HbA_{1c}), which is used as an indicator for cumulative exposure of hemoglobin to elevated blood glucose (Glenn and Stitt 2009). Amadori adducts may undergo further oxidation, dehydration reactions, and crosslinking to form AGEs. Interestingly, these reactions are markedly accelerated during aging and even more so in diabetes, but the adducts formed during aging may differ (Brownlee 2005; Giardino et al. 1994; Glenn and

Stitt 2009; Queisser et al. 2010; Shinohara et al. 1998; Tessier et al. 1999). AGEs can come from many sources. A wide range of AGE precursor molecules give rise to a broad array of AGEs. The quantity and types of AGEs that are found at any time depend on rates of formation and rates of degradation. The most abundant AGE in human body is the N^{ε}-(carboxyl-methyl) lysine (CML) (Ikeda et al. 1996; Reddy et al. 1995).

Amino groups can also react with highly active glucose metabolites, including glyoxal (GO), methylglyoxal (MGO), 3-deoxyglucosone, and so on (Thorpe and Baynes 2003). These dicarbonyls can lead to very rapid AGE formation especially under circumstances of enhanced glycolytic activity (such as in hyperglycemia) (Lal et al. 1995; Thornalley et al. 1999; Thorpe and Baynes 2003). Interestingly, it was recently shown that in human aortic endothelial cells, hyperglycemia-induced ROS production increases the expression of RAGE and RAGE ligands, and this effect is mediated by ROS-induced MGO (Yao and Brownlee 2010). Furthermore, it is believed that these intracellular glucose-derived dicarbonyls are the major initiating molecules in the formation of both intracellular and extracellular AGEs (Degenhardt et al. 1998). Therefore, it is reasonable to anticipate that they constitute a more important source of AGEs in a highly energy-demanding tissue, such as retina, than other tissues.

11.3.3.1.1 Hyperglycemic AGE Pathway and DR

Clinical studies have shown that the levels of AGEs in serum (Dolhofer-Bliesener et al. 1996; Ono et al. 1998; Wagner et al. 2001), skin (Sell et al. 1992), and cornea (Sato et al. 2001) correlate with the onset or grade of DR. Importantly, AGEs are significantly increased in diabetic prepubescent children and adolescents with early or preproliferative retinopathy compared to both healthy and diabetic controls who are free from clinical signs of retinopathy (Chiarelli et al. 1999). While many of the studies measured nonspecific AGE moieties, others evaluated the associations between defined adducts, such as CML, pentosidine, or crossline (Sugiyama et al. 1998; Yamaguchi et al. 1998). There are also studies that reported no correlation between AGE levels and retinopathy in diabetic patients (Sugiyama et al. 1998; Wagner et al. 2001). The apparent inconsistency with other studies may be due to the variations in patient populations and/or the nonuniform assays for AGE quantification.

AGEs have a wide range of deleterious effects and play a role in initiation and progression of DR. In diabetic patients, AGEs and/or late Amadori products have been demonstrated to directly accumulate in retinal pericytes, vessels, neuroglia, and so on. Cross-linked AGEs are a significant feature of extracellular matrix dysfunction during diabetes progression (Gardiner et al. 2003; Hammes et al. 1994; 1999; Murata et al. 1997; Schalkwijk et al. 1999; Stitt et al. 1997).

In vivo, retinal pericytes are surrounded by a vascular basement membrane and lie outside the iBRB, and it is shown that retinal pericytes have a much lower replicative capacity than retinal microvascular endothelium (Sharma et al. 1985). Toxic AGEs accumulate in retinal pericytes in diabetic animal models (Chibber et al. 1997; Kalfa et al. 1995; Ruggiero-Lopez et al. 1997; Stitt et al. 1997). *In vitro*, pericytes grown on a "diabetic-like" AGE-modified basement membrane lead to dysfunction and apoptotic death (Stitt et al. 2004). Similarly, AGEs accumulation has been reported to have a detrimental influence on the cell function and survival ability of the retinal pericytes. This includes impaired phospholipid hydrolysis and phospholipid enzyme inhibition (Assero et al. 2001) or modification of the antioxidant enzymes catalase and superoxide dismutase (Paget et al. 1998). Studies also demonstrated that AGEs can induce osteoblastic differentiation, calcification (Yamagishi et al. 1999), and potent apoptotic death in pericytes (Yamagishi et al. 2002). These observations are consistent with the pathology of DR. For example, in diabetes, retinal endothelial cells, and pericytes undergo accelerated apoptosis, and this is related to the development of acellular capillaries and pericyte ghosts in the retinal microvasculature. These are preclinical signs of DR (Kern et al. 2000; Mizutani et al. 1996). In addition to direct biochemical effects, it appears that AGE-related toxicity in retinal pericytes acts in a receptor mediated fashion (Chibber et al. 1997). For example, a growing body of evidence indicates that AGEs–RAGE (receptor for AGEs) interaction-mediated oxidative stress generation plays an important role in DR (Yamagishi et al. 2008).

Exposure to AGEs results in several deleterious effects on the retinal vessels, including increasing vasopermeability, neovascularization, and evoking proinflammatory pathways, and so on. For example, *in vitro* and *in vivo* studies showed that exposure to AGEs causes significant upregulation of the VEGF (Lu et al. 1998; Stitt et al. 2000; Treins et al. 2001; Yamagishi et al. 2002), which can also be induced by a variety of stimuli, such as PKC (see Section 11.3.3.3) and HIF (see Section 11.3.3.6), to increase vascular permeability and induce DR-related neovascularization. Specifically, excessive permeability of the retinal microvasculature is related to iBRB dysfunction (Antonetti et al. 1999).

In nondiabetic rats, AGEs also compromise the retinal capillary unit leading to subtle but significant breakdown of the iBRB, with a concomitant increase in intracellular adhesion molecule-1 (Moore et al. 2003; Stitt et al. 2000). The increased amounts of adhesion molecules on the surface of retinal microvascular endothelial cells can activate proinflammatory pathways. In conjunction with an enhanced stickiness and reduced deformability of blood-borne leukocytes in the diabetic state, this can lead to a marked leukocyte adhesion to retinal vascular endothelium that precipitates capillary occlusion, vascular cell death, and finally DR (Kunt et al. 1998; Mamputu and Renier 2004; Miyamoto and Ogura 1999; Moore et al. 2003).

Interestingly, clinical observations indicate that development and progression of hyperglycemia-induced microvascular and macrovascular complications continues for many years after consistent improvement in HbA_{1c}. This is referred to as "hyperglycemic memory" (Brownlee 1992; Yamagishi et al. 2008). The persistence of accumulation of AGEs during periods of normal glucose homeostasis is considered to be the best explanation for this phenomenon.

The importance of AGEs in DR can also be seen from several novel therapeutics of DR. These include peroxisome proliferator-activated receptor agonist, blockade of the renin–angiotensin system with an angiotensin converting enzyme inhibitor or by using angiotensin II type 1 receptor blockers, and intravitreal anti-VEGF antibody administration (Simó and Hernández 2009), all of which have been at least indirectly related to AGEs (Yamagishi et al. 2008).

11.3.3.1.2 Hyperglycemic AGE Pathway and AMD

Among indicators of AMD are elevated levels of immunoreactive AGEs in Bruch's membrane and drusen (Farboud et al. 1999; Glenn and Stitt 2009; Hammes et al. 1999; Handa 1998; Handa et al. 1999; Hollyfield et al. 2003; Howes et al. 2004; Ishibashi et al. 1998; Schutt et al. 2003; Uchiki et al. 2011; Weikel et al. 2012; Yamada et al. 2006). In Bruch's membrane this leads to the progressive thickening and compromised permeability of the membrane (Moore et al. 1995; Okubo et al. 1999; 2000). Additional evidence of toxicity of AGEs is the finding that some of the components of drusen, such as lipids, tissue inhibitor of metalloproteinases 3, clusterin, serum albumin, apolipoprotein E, amyloid, and vitronectin (Hageman et al. 1999; Hollyfield et al. 2003; Mullins et al. 2000) are readily modified by AGEs and/or ALEs during aging (Hammes et al. 1996; Li and Dickson 1997; Schutt et al. 2003; Tabaton et al. 1997). As the accumulation of AGEs plays an important role in AMD pathogenesis, recent studies have tried to use the fluorescent and other spectroscopic properties of AGE adducts to develop noninvasive predictors for AMD (Birarda et al. 2013; Pawlak et al. 2008).

AGEs also induce upregulation of VEGF and platelet-derived growth factor-B (PDGF-B), both of which are important regulators in angiogenesis (Handa 1998; Lu et al. 1998; McFarlane et al. 2005). Prolonged exposure of RPE to AGEs or AGE-forming dicarbonyls induces changes in intracellular pH, maintenance of the choriocapillaris, and integrity of the RPE/photoreceptor complex. These dysfunctions may finally lead to apoptotic death in RPE (Stitt 2005).

As a part of cellular defense systems, some AGEs are transported through a receptor-mediated pathway to the lysosomal compartment for degradation. However, some AGEs escape degradation. AGEs are also substrates for degradation via the ubiquitin (Ub) proteasome pathway. Intracellular accumulation of highly reactive AGE adducts can markedly reduce degradative enzymatic activity (Kasper et al. 1999; Miyata et al. 1997; Queisser et al. 2010; Sebeková et al. 1998; Uchiki et al. 2011), that is, the lysosomal and Ub proteasomal degradation systems are also vulnerable to AGEs. This may lead to a reduction of intracellular proteolytic capacity and incomplete proteolysis of phagocytosed photoreceptor outer segments resulting in the accumulation of lipofuscin in the RPE (Boulton et al. 1989). Significantly, intracellular sequestration of these highly reactive adducts can markedly reduce degradative enzymatic activity in many types of epithelial cells (Kasper et al. 1999; Miyata et al. 1997; Sebeková et al. 1998; Stitt 2005).

Additional protective mechanisms involve a range of intracellular detoxifying enzymes against reactive dicarbonyls, such as GO and MGO (Figure 11.4). These detoxifying enzymes serve to limit advanced adduct formation. For example, a glutathione (GSH)-dependent glyoxalase complex has been found to serve as an effective detoxification system for GO and MGO (Kuhla et al. 2005). It is interesting to note that this enzyme's activity declines with aging and overexpression of this enzyme decreases the accumulation of MGO-derived AGEs in cells and elongates lifespan in *Caenorhabditis elegans* (Morcos et al. 2008; Shinohara et al. 1998). It has also been demonstrated that upregulation of glyoxalase-1 can reverse high-glucose mediated AGE formation over a short, 10-day period and prevent AGE-mediated cell abnormalities (Shinohara et al. 1998). Therefore, alterations in these enzymes during disease may result in AGE accumulation and pathogenic damage in cells and tissues (Miyata et al. 2001; Thornalley 1993; 2003).

In addition to the intracellular detoxifying enzymes, cells have several complex receptor systems that are responsible for removing senescent, glycation-modified molecules and/or degrading existing AGEs crosslinks from cells and tissues. Several AGE-binding molecules have been described, such as the RAGE (Schmidt et al. 1994), AGE-R1 (Li et al. 1996; Stitt et al. 1999), galectin-3 (Pugliese

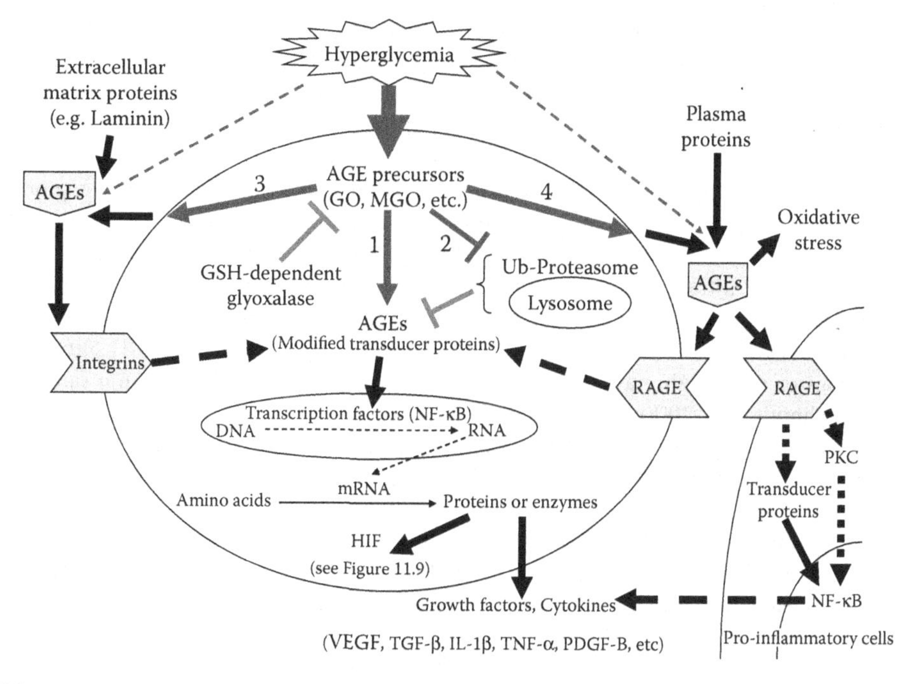

FIGURE 11.4 Hyperglycemic AGE pathway. The hyperglycemia-induced intracellular AGE precursors, such as MGO, induce pathological consequences in four routes, (1) direct intracellular glycation of proteins, including proteins involved in the regulation of gene transcription, such as NF-κB, (2) inhibiting enzymes responsible for protein degradation, such as proteasomal (including ubiquitin) and lysosomal systems, (3) the intracellular AGEs precursors can diffuse out of the cell and modify nearby cells (even the same cell itself), extracellular matrix, such as Bruch's membrane and choroidal capillary membranes, and (4) the intracellular AGEs precursors diffusing out of the cell to modify circulating proteins in the blood, which in turn activate RAGE on proinflammatory cells or CECs, thereby causing the production of inflammatory cytokines and/or growth factors.

et al. 2001; Stitt et al. 2005), CD36 (Ohgami et al. 2002), and the types I and II scavenger receptors (Horiuchi et al. 1996). These cell surface receptors interact with AGEs to maintain homeostatic function by clearing/detoxifying extracellular AGE-modified macromolecules from serum and the intercellular matrix. Among them, RAGE is the best characterized. It was first identified in endothelium and now is known to be present in multiple vascular, neural, and cardiac tissues (Neeper et al. 1992). The RAGE is a member of the immunoglobulin superfamily with a high affinity for several ligands, including AGEs, high mobility group-1 protein, amyloid-β peptide, and S100B/calgranulins, some of which are known components of drusen and Bruch's membrane deposits.

On the other hand, despite the protective role of AGE receptors, it is thought that many of the adverse effects caused by AGEs are mediated via AGE receptors and that these receptors play a critical role in AGE-related pathobiology associated with diabetes and aging disorders (Sano et al. 1999; Schmidt et al. 2000; Vlassara 2001). For example, the activation of the RAGE evokes downstream proinflammatory responses that could play a critical role in aging (Yan et al. 2007), such as skin aging (Lohwasser et al. 2006), and age-related diseases (Schmidt et al. 2000; Yan et al. 2007), such as Alzheimer's disease (Takeuchi and Yamagishi 2008), atherosclerosis (Ehlermann et al. 2006), dysfunction of cardiomyocytes (Gao et al. 2008), and retinal diseases (Stitt et al. 2005). The RAGE–ligand signals activate the wide range of pathophysiological responses linked to the downstream transcriptional activity of NF-κB (Figure 11.4), which induces proinflammatory cytokines and oxidative stress (Bierhaus et al. 2005; Pawlak et al. 2008).

In the context of the outer retina, studies have shown that RAGE is expressed on RPE and that RAGE levels are significantly increased in AMD (in postmortem tissue), especially on cells adjacent to drusen (Howes et al. 2004; Pawlak et al. 2008; Yamada et al. 2006). The activation of the RAGE axis in RPE cells upregulates the expression and secretion of VEGF (Glenn and Stitt 2009; Glenn et al. 2009; Ma et al. 2007; Yamada et al. 2006). This can elicit or propagate neovascularization. For example, exogenous AGE-albumin and S100B can activate RAGE and modulate proangiogenic VEGF expression in RPE (Justilien et al. 2007), and, with prolonged exposure, these ligands may lead to apoptosis (Howes et al. 2004). *In vitro*, in addition to RAGE (Ma et al. 2007), an increase of VEGF expression in RPE can also be modulated by another AGE receptor known as galectin-3 (McFarlane et al. 2005). Interestingly, the proteolytic fragment of RAGE, known as soluble RAGE, is elevated in the serum of elderly kidney disease patients and is associated with decreased glomerular filtration rate (Semba et al. 2009). The AGE-RAGE-NF-κB signal cascade in both RPE and photoreceptor cells has also been shown to contribute to the disease progression of early AMD and GA (Howes et al. 2004). Consistently, the suppression of RAGE signaling using peptide analogs or neutralizing antibodies can prevent key pathological events in a range of cells and tissues (Schmidt et al. 2000; Wautier and Schmidt 2004).

As summarized in Figure 11.4, the intracellular AGE precursors can damage cells by four routes described below. First, AGE accumulation in RPE can appear as free AGE adducts in the cytoplasm and as AGE-modified proteins in lipofuscin granules (Schutt et al. 2003). While some cytoplasm AGE-modified transducer proteins can affect the activity of downstream transcriptional factors, others are transported through a receptor-mediated transportation to the lysosomal compartment for degradation. However, because AGEs also compromise proteolytic capacity, the accumulation of lipofuscin in RPE reflects the effects of AGEs on both substrates and enzyme degradation systems (Stitt 2001; Uchiki et al. 2011). Indeed, incomplete proteolysis of phagocytosed photoreceptor outer segments is linked to the formation of lipofuscin in RPE (Boulton et al. 1989), and it has been shown that AGEs play an important role in the formation of age-related intracellular fluorophores and lipofuscin granules in postmitotic epithelial cells (Yin 1996).

A special case is that, when the detoxification enzymes *per se* become compromised, the situation may be exacerbated. For example, recent studies show that in microvascular endothelial cells of the retina, hyperglycemia-induced intracellular MGO reduces levels of the polyubiquitin receptor 19S, decreases the chymotrypsin-like activity of the proteasome, and causes polyubiquitinated proteins to accumulate in the cell. This may result in the decline of proteasomal activities over time

(Queisser et al. 2010). In addition, our recent work also showed that consuming high-GI diets causes accumulation of AGEs in RPE, and the AGE-modified intracellular proteins become resistant to the degradation by the Ub-dependent proteasome system (Uchiki et al. 2011), Furthermore, RPE grown on an AGE-modified substrate shows enhanced accumulation of lipofuscin that contributes to suppression of lysosomal enzymatic activity (Glenn and Stitt 2009; Glenn et al. 2009). The compromised lysosomal enzymatic activity could also account, at least partially, for the age-related RPE dysfunction resulting in the pathological accumulation of AGE crosslinks on Bruch's membrane, described below.

In addition to affecting RPE and Bruch's membrane, AGEs also occur at comparatively high levels in CNV membranes (Swamy-Mruthinti et al. 2002) where they may play a role in fibrous membrane formation by the induction of growth factors, such as transforming growth factor beta (TGF-β) and PDGF (Handa 1998; Rumble et al. 1997). For example, CML has been shown to promote CNV formation in cultured choroidal explants from aged rats via the stimulation of growth factors such as VEGF, tumor necrosis factor α (TNF-α), and PDGF-B (Kobayashi et al. 2007).

The intracellular AGEs precursors can diffuse out of the RPE cell and modify nearby RPE cells (even the same RPE cell itself) and extracellular matrix, such as Bruch's membrane and choroidal capillary membranes (Glenn and Stitt 2009; Glenn et al. 2009). In turn, these alterations may compromise cell-matrix signaling (e.g., integrin–laminin between RPE–Bruch's membrane) and cause physiological dysfunction (Aisenbrey et al. 2006; Charonis et al. 1990; Fang et al. 2009). Furthermore, dysfunction in the RPE can affect Bruch's membrane's function *per se*, and vice versa, and such dysfunction leaves the neural retina vulnerable because all metabolic exchange between the neural retina and choroidal plexus requires passage through the oBRB.

Intracellular AGE precursors can also diffuse out of the cell to modify circulating proteins in the blood, which can then bind to RAGE on proinflammatory cells or choroidal endothelial cells (CEC) to activate them, thereby causing the production of inflammatory cytokines and/or growth factors with associated vascular pathology (pathway #4 in Figure 11.4) (Abordo and Thornalley 1997; Doi et al. 1992; Kirstein et al. 1992; Li et al. 1996; Neeper et al. 1992; Schmidt et al. 1995; Skolnik et al. 1991; Smedsrod et al. 1997; Vlassara et al. 1988; 1995). Furthermore, by analogy with the angiogenesis-promoting abilities of AGEs in diabetic RNV (Hoffmann et al. 2002; Ishibashi 2000), AGEs have been hypothesized to be involved in the process of CNV formation. Indeed, studies have shown that AGEs accumulate significantly in the choriocapillaris during aging (Handa et al. 1998) and are highly expressed in CNV membranes (Hammes et al. 1999; Ishibashi et al. 1998). These AGE accumulations can stimulate CEC proliferation, matrix metalloproteinase 2 secretion, and VEGF upregulation, and are important promoters of CNV in exudative AMD *in vivo* (Hoffmann et al. 2002; Howes et al. 2004; Ma et al. 2007; Yamada et al. 2006). Together, these data indicate that the choriocapillaris is subject to damage from two different sources of AGEs, that is, one from cell-matrix communication and the other coming from the blood circulation.

11.3.3.1.3 Advanced Lipoxidation End Products in the Retina

Lipids are another important source of chemical modifications of proteins, especially in the lipid-rich and highly oxidative environments in the retina (Stitt et al. 2005). Lipid peroxidation products also form Maillard products called advanced lipoxidation end products (ALEs) (Onorato et al. 2000). It is not surprising that there are similarities between fatty acids and glucose (i.e., between ALEs and AGEs) in terms of age-related pathogenesis. Indeed, dyslipidemia, including hyperlipidemia, has been considered as a risk factor for AMD (Tan et al. 2007). The formation of ALEs through lipid peroxidation reactions may, at least partially, account for the underlying pathogenesis.

The outer retina is rich in polyunsaturated fatty acids (PUFAs), such as DHA (Bazan 1982; SanGiovanni and Chew 2005). PUFAs are highly susceptible to lipid peroxidation and this process yields lipid hydroperoxides, which in turn decompose into reactive aldehydes, such as acrolein,

4-hydroxynonenal, or malondialdehyde. Like reactive dicarbonyls derived from glucose, these reactive aldehydes can react with proteins to form stable ALE adducts (Januszewski et al. 2003).

ALEs add to the burden of protein modifications in the aging retina. For example, studies have shown that various ALEs can induce the proangiogenic growth factor expression by RPE *in vitro* (Glenn and Stitt 2009; Zhou et al. 2005).

Interestingly, studies indicate that higher intake of DHA and EPA reduces the risk for AMD (SanGiovanni and Chew 2005; SanGiovanni et al. 2008) and that the protective effect may be through modulating postprandial hyperlipidemia, which is a physiological consequence after consuming a high-GI diet (Anil 2007). Importantly, recent epidemiological observations also indicate that a diet high in DHA/EPA and low in GI offers a synergistic protection against AMD progression probably because the diet helps to eliminate deleterious effects from AGEs and ALEs (Chiu et al. 2009a; 2009b).

11.3.3.2 Hyperglycemic Polyol Pathway

Dietary hyperglycemia may manifest age-related or diabetic disorders through increases in the polyol pathway (Figure 11.5), which in turn lead to intracellular accumulation of sorbitol and oxidative stress. Flux through this pathway during hyperglycemia varies from 33% of total glucose used in the rabbit lens to 11% in human erythrocytes (Lee and Chung 1999). Therefore, the contribution of this pathway to age-related or diabetic disorders may be very much species, site, and tissue dependent (Brownlee 2001). The polyol pathway is primarily controlled by the enzyme aldose reductase (AR). Under euglycemia, AR can reduce toxic aldehydes in the cell to inactive alcohols, but when the glucose concentration in the cell becomes too high, AR also reduces glucose to sorbitol (a polyol or sugar alcohol), which is later oxidized to fructose. In the process of reducing high intracellular glucose to sorbitol, the AR consumes the cofactor NADPH (Lee and Chung 1999). However, as shown in Figure 11.5, NADPH is also the essential cofactor for regenerating a critical intracellular antioxidant, reduced glutathione (GSH). By competing NADPH with glutathione reductase and hence resulting in reduced amount of GSH, the polyol pathway increases susceptibility to intracellular oxidative stress. The accumulation of sorbitol also induces osmotic stress, and that has been linked to diabetic cataracts (Mulhern et al. 2007). Some studies also link this pathway to antioxidant taurine through an inhibitory effect on its Na^+-taurine cotransporter (TT) (Hansen 2001; Nakashima et al. 2005; Obrosova et al. 2001; Pop-Busui et al. 1999; Stevens et al. 1997a; 1997b; 1999).

In vascular smooth muscle cells isolated from rat aorta, AR was also found to affect PKC activation (see hyperglycemic PKC pathway for PKC activation) (Ramana et al. 2005). It was shown that inhibition of AR prevents membrane translocation (PKC-β2 and -δ) and phosphorylation (PKC-β1 and -ε) of multiple PKC enzymes by inhibiting high glucose-induced generation of diacylglycerol (DAG) from phospholipid hydrolysis.

11.3.3.2.1 Hyperglycemic Polyol Pathway and DR

In diabetes, the elevated expression of AR may impair antioxidant defense, which may render tissues susceptible to chronic diabetic complications. Thus, the increased expression of AR has been implicated as the critical link between chronic glucose toxicity and tissue damage (Burg and Kador 1988; Dent et al. 1991; Kasajima 2000; Nakashima et al. 2005; Shah et al. 1997; Stevens et al. 1997; Vinores et al. 1988). Although this pathway may play a minor role in retinopathies, there is also evidence linking AR activity with retinal capillary basement membrane thickening in galactosemic rats, suggesting a possible role in DR (Vinores et al. 1988). For example, electron microscopic immunocytochemical staining suggested that increased AR expression in retinal vascular endothelial cells and perivascular astrocytes is associated with hyperglycemia-related iBRB failure, which may finally lead to DR (Vinores et al. 1993a; 1993b).

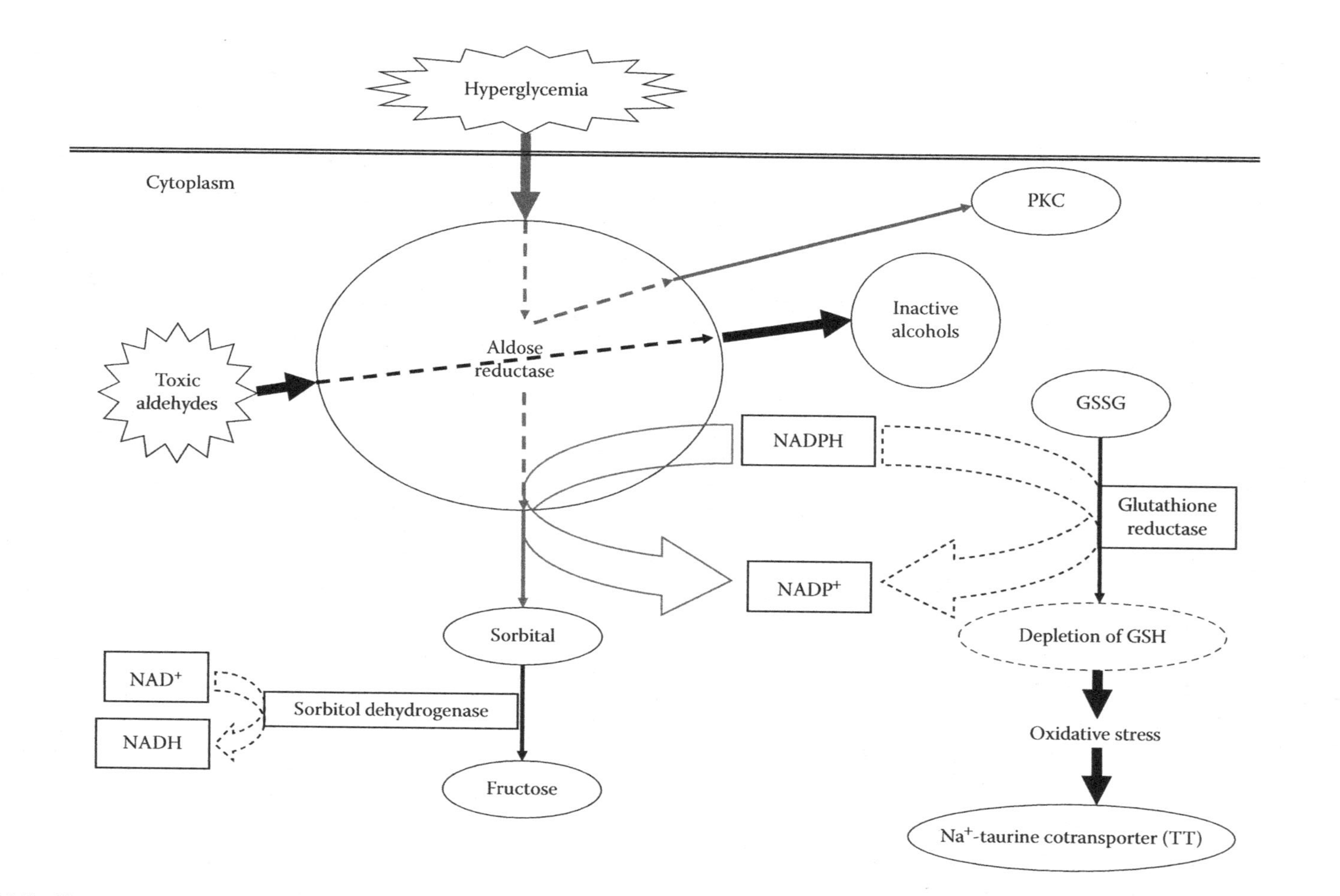

FIGURE 11.5 Hyperglycemic polyol pathway. Under hyperglycemia, AR reduces glucose to sorbitol (a polyol or sugar alcohol), which is later oxidized to fructose. In this process, the AR consumes cofactor NADPH. Therefore, the hyperglycemic polyol pathway consumes NADPH and hence results in the depletion of GSH. This increases intracellular oxidative stress.

11.3.3.2.2 Hyperglycemic Polyol Pathway and AMD

Human RPE cells contain two NADPH-dependent reductases, AR and aldehyde reductase with AR being the predominant reductase, because the levels of aldehyde reductase are insufficient to generate sugar alcohols (e.g., sorbitol) (Sato et al. 1993). In RPE cells, it is suggested that hyperglycemia upregulates AR gene expression, protein production, and activity (Henry et al. 2000), and that some hyperglycemia-related ultrastructural changes can be prevented by AR inhibitor, Sorbinil (Vinores and Campochiaro 1989). Furthermore, hyperglycemia also induces the loss of Na^{+}/K(+)-ATPase function in RPE cells, which affects the response to AR inhibitors and results in chronic accumulation of intracellular sorbitol (see Figure 11.5) (Crider et al. 1997).

The precise pathophysiological mechanism linking the polyol pathway to AMD remains uncertain, but depletion of the osmolyte and antioxidant taurine has been invoked (Obrosova et al. 2001; Pop-Busui et al. 1999; Stevens et al. 1997a; 1997b) through an inhibitory effect on its TT (Nakashima et al. 2005; Stevens et al. 1997a; 1997b; 1999). Taurine is an important organic osmolyte in mammalian cells, and, following osmotic cell swelling, taurine release via a volume-sensitive taurine efflux pathway is increased and the active taurine uptake via TT is decreased (Lambert 2004). It is found that in RPE cells the TT is regulated by oxidative stress and that overexpression of AR and hyperglycemia impair this response (Figure 11.5).

11.3.3.3 Hyperglycemic PKC Pathway

Hyperglycemia-induced PKC activation may lead to the visual loss associated with the BRB breakdown. For example, it has been shown that in RPE cells hyperglycemia induces PKC activation, which increases the expression of a variety of genes and further leads to a series of adverse effects. Since RPE forms the oBRB, the breakdown of the oBRB due to the disruption of the RPE tight junctions may lead to the development of AMD (Erickson et al. 2007). Conversely, the inhibition of PKC decreases the breakdown of the iBRB and prevents early changes in the diabetic retina (Bishara et al. 2002; Brownlee 2005; Ishii et al. 1996; Koya et al. 2000; Saishin et al. 2003).

PKC also affects the expression of gap junction proteins, connexins, which are critical for intercellular communication between RPE cells (Malfait et al. 2001). Many correlations between gap junctional intercellular communication and cellular processes, such as cellular growth control, cell differentiation, regulation of development, tissue homeostasis, and so on have been described (Goodenough et al. 1996).

As shown schematically in Figure 11.6, intracellular hyperglycemia induces synthesis of DAG, a critical activating cofactor for the isoforms of PKC, -β, -δ, and -α (DeRubertis and Craven 1994; Koya and King 1998; Koya et al. 1997; Xia et al. 1994). In turn, PKC activation activates transcriptional factors, such as NF-κB. This increases the expression of a variety of genes, which in turn give rise to physiological dysfunction. For example, in endothelial cells, hyperglycemia induces PKC-β activation, which inhibits the expression of endothelial nitric oxide synthase (eNOS) while increasing the expression of vasoconstrictor endothelin-1 (ET-1) (Ishii et al. 1996). This results in reduced blood flow. PKC-β activation also increases the expression of VEGF and plasminogen activator inhibitor-1 (PAI-1), leading to angiogenesis and vascular occlusion, respectively (Feener et al. 1996; Ishii et al. 1996; Koya et al. 1997; Kuboki et al. 2000; Studer et al. 1993). In the following two sections, we will focus on the effects of hyperglycemia-induced PKC activation on the VEGF, which is the major pharmaceutical target for DR and AMD (Abdallah and Fawzi 2009; Bressler 2009a; 2009b; Jardeleza and Miller 2009).

Hyperglycemia-induced PKC activation also increases the expression of TGF-β and contributes to capillary occlusion, probably through inhibition of nitric oxide (NO) production (Craven et al. 1997). Furthermore, hyperglycemia-induced PKC activation has also been implicated in the activation of membrane-associated NAD(P)H-dependent oxidase, which may increase the generation of ROS (Brownlee 2001). In addition to the DAG-related pathway, hyperglycemia may also activate the PKC pathway indirectly through ligation of AGE receptors (Portilla et al. 2000) (Figure 11.4),

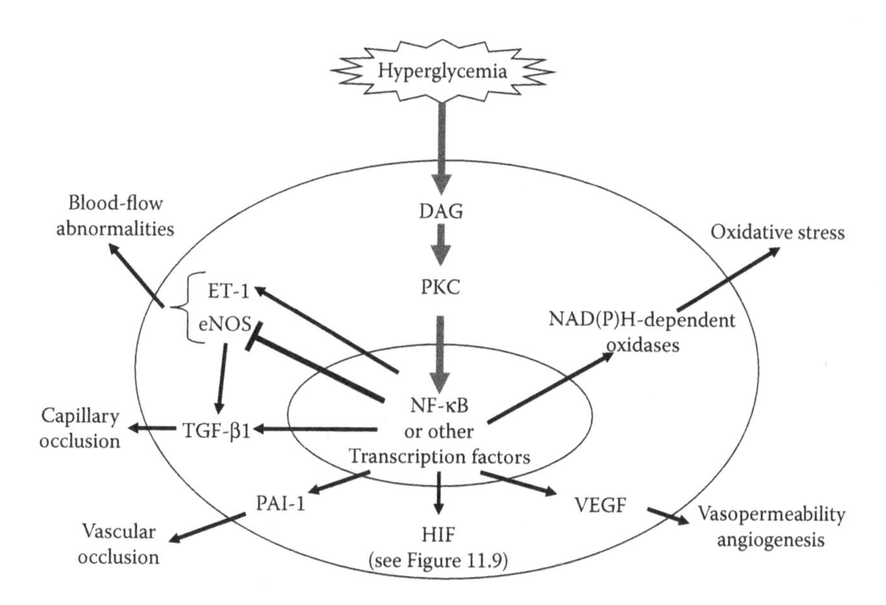

FIGURE 11.6 Hyperglycemic PKC pathway. The pathogenic consequences of hyperglycemic PKC through activating transcription factors for a wide range of proteins, including cytokines. Many transcription factors, such as NF-κB, are activated through hyperglycemia-induced PKC activation, resulting in oxidative stress, increased vasopermeability, angiogenesis, vascular occlusion, capillary occlusion, and abnormal blood flow.

increased flux of the polyol pathway (Keogh et al. 1997) (Figure 11.5), and increased flux of the hexosamine pathway (Goldberg et al. 2002) (Figure 11.7).

11.3.3.3.1 Hyperglycemic PKC Pathway and DR

VEGF, a potent endothelial cell mitogen and permeability factor, has been implicated as a cause of iBRB breakdown and angiogenesis in DR and other ischemic retinopathies (Aiello et al. 1994; 1997). In retinal endothelial cells and pericytes, high glucose causes activation of PKC-β and consequent expression of VEGF contributing to the progression of DR (Clarke and Dodson 2007; Enaida et al. 1999; Hata et al. 1999). It is also suggested that RPE cells may contribute to the pathogenesis of DR caused by hyperglycemia (Figure 11.6) and hypoxia (Figure 11.3b) through the PKC-mediated expression of VEGF (see Section 11.3.3.6) (Young et al. 2005).

11.3.3.3.2 Hyperglycemic PKC Pathway and AMD

In RPE cells, VEGF is expressed in response to mechanical stretch (Seko et al. 1999), hypoxia (Mousa et al. 1999) and high glucose (Sone et al. 1996), and may be mediated by PKC activation (Young et al. 2005). This is corroborated by the observation that inhibition of the PKC pathway using a mixture of ethanol extracts from herbal medicines inhibits high glucose or AGEs-induced VEGF expression in human RPE (Kim et al. 2007). Interestingly, it is well known that a number of cytokines and VEGF that are synthesized by RPE cells can exert autocrine function in addition to stimulating other cell types. Indeed, VEGF receptors are expressed on the surface of the RPE cell itself and the increased expression of VEGF in the RPE in maculae is involved in AMD (Kociok et al. 1998). It is also noted that VEGF expression and secretion by RPE under hyperglycemia and hypoxia are PKC-dependent, and the regulation appears to be more complicated than that in hyperglycemia alone (see Section 11.3.3.6) (Young et al. 2005).

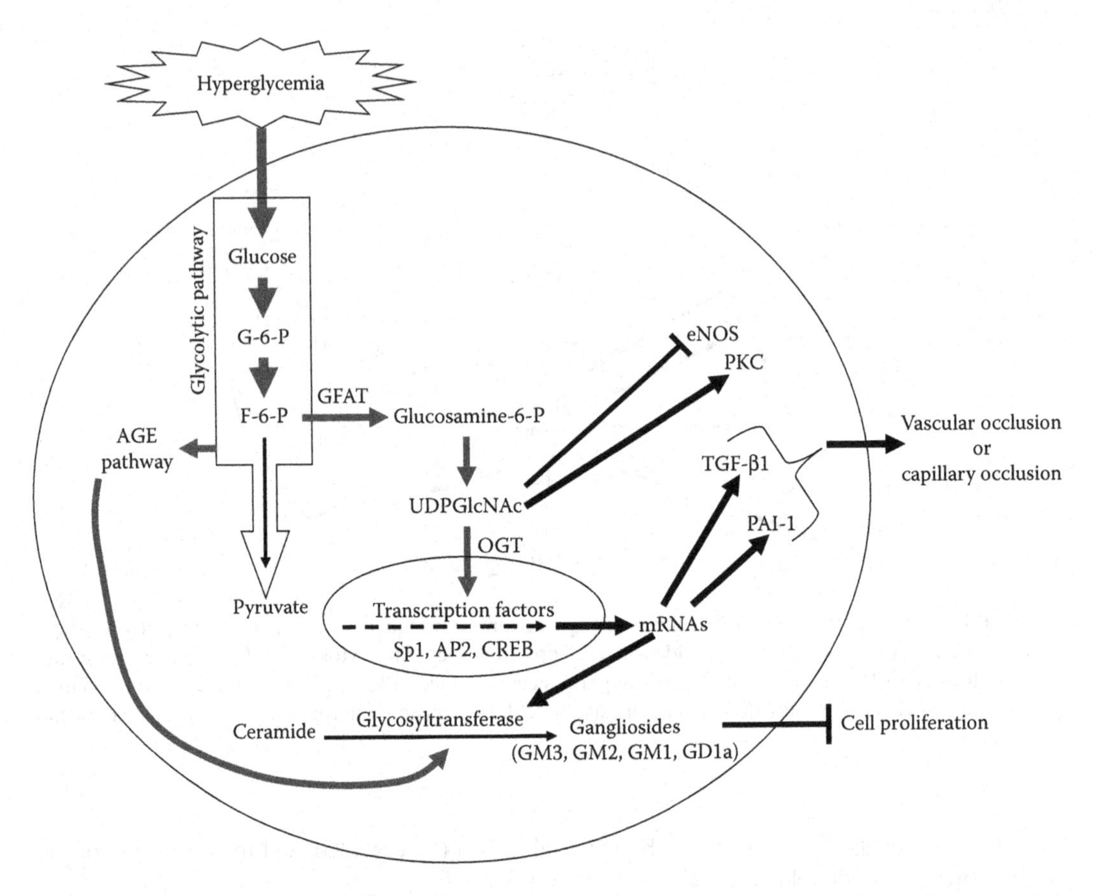

FIGURE 11.7 Hyperglycemic hexosamine pathway. The hyperglycemic hexosamine pathway starting from the glycolytic intermediate, F-6-P, which is converted by GFAT to glucosamine-6-P and eventually to UDPGlcNAc, an *O*-linked GlcNAc. Intracellular glycosylation by adding GlcNAc moieties to serine and threonine residues of proteins (e.g., transcription factors) is catalyzed by OGT. Increased glycosylation of transcription factors, such as Spl, AP2, and CREB, often at phosphorylation sites, increases the expression of cytokines and enzymes, including TGF- β1, PAI-1, and glycosyltransferase. In addition, AGEs can exert cellular effects by increasing a-series ganglioside levels to inhibit retinal pericyte cell proliferation. Other cytoplasmic proteins are also subject to dynamical modification by hyperglycemia-induced *O*-linked GlcNAc, such as the inhibition of eNOS activity by *O*-acetylglucosaminylation at the Akt site of the eNOS protein and activations of various PKC isoforms by glucosamine without membrane translocation.

11.3.3.4 Hyperglycemic Hexosamine Pathway

As shown schematically in Figure 11.7, glucose is metabolized through glycolysis, first being transformed into glucose-6 phosphate (G-6-P), then fructose-6 phosphate (F-6-P), and then on through the rest of the glycolytic pathway. However, when glucose concentration inside a cell is high, some of that F-6-P gets diverted into the hexosamine pathway in which glutamine:fructose-6 phosphate amidotransferase (GFAT) converts the F-6-P to glucosamine-6 phosphate and finally to uridine diphosphate *N*-acetyl glucosamine (UDPGlcNAc). Studies showed that the inhibition of GFAT blocks hyperglycemia-induced increases in the transcription of TGF-α, TGF-β1 (Kolm-Litty et al. 1998), and PAI-1 (Du et al. 2000). It is suggested that, in the hexosamine pathway, the hyperglycemia-induced increases in gene transcription may be through glycosylation of the transcription factor, Spl, by UDPGlcNAc (Brownlee 2001). Furthermore, the glycosylated form of Spl seems to be more transcriptionally active than the deglycosylated form (Kadonaga et al. 1988). However, because every RNA polymerase II transcription factor has been found to be *O*-acetylglucosaminylated (Hart 1997), it is possible that reciprocal modification by *O*-acetylglucosaminylation (*O*-GlcNAcylation) and phosphorylation of transcription factors other than Sp1 may function as a more generalized mechanism for regulating hyperglycemia-induced gene transcriptions in the hexosamine pathway (Brownlee 2001; Wang et al. 2007). Furthermore, Sp1, AP2, and CREB operate on the promoters of glycosyltransferase genes, which regulate the ganglioside biosynthetic pathway (see Section 11.3.3.4.1 for more details) (Zeng and Yu 2008).

Many other nuclear and cytoplasmic proteins are also subject to dynamic modification by *O*-linked *N*-acetyl-glucosamine (GlcNAc), and may show reciprocal modification by phosphorylation in a manner analogous to Sp1 (Hart 1997). For example, the eNOS activity can be inhibited by hyperglycemia-induced *O*-GlcNAcylation at the Akt site of the eNOS protein (Du et al. 2001). Additionally, various PKC isoforms (-βI and -δ) can be activated by glucosamine without membrane translocation (Goldberg et al. 2002).

11.3.3.4.1 Hyperglycemic Hexosamine Pathway and DR

Loss of retinal microvascular pericytes is etiologic for the early stages of DR. First, the increase flux of the hexosamine pathway increases gangliosides in retinal pericytes. This would result in the antiproliferative effect of glucosamine (Masson et al. 2005b). In addition, AGEs can increase a-series ganglioside (GM3, GM2, GM1, GD1a) levels, resulting in the inhibition of retinal pericyte cell proliferation. The possible mechanism could involve an increase in GM3 synthase activity (Figure 11.7) (Masson et al. 2005a).

Gangliosides play multiple functions including cellular recognition and adhesion as well as signaling. The expression of gangliosides is not only cell specific and developmentally regulated, but also closely related to the differentiation state of the cell (Yu et al. 2004). In general, ganglioside biosynthesis starts with the common precursor for acidic and nonacidic glycosphingolipids, ceramide (Figure 11.7). Ganglioside synthases are glycosyltransferases involved in the biosynthesis of glycoconjugates in the ganglioside biosynthetic pathway. The transcription of glycosyltransferases genes is subject to complex developmental and tissue-specific regulation. The promoters of glycosyltransferases genes are characteristic of house-keeping genes, including TATA-less and lacking a CCAAT box but containing GC-rich boxes. It has been shown that a set of cis-acting elements and transcription factors, including Sp1, AP2, and CREB, operate in the proximal promoters (Figure 11.7) (Zeng and Yu 2008). The hyperglycemia-induced transcription of glycosyltransferases may result in the increased synthesis of gangliosides, which in turn inhibits retinal pericyte cell proliferation and leads to the development of early DR (Masson et al. 2005a; 2005b).

11.3.3.4.2 Hyperglycemic Hexosamine Pathway and AMD

In fresh human donor macula-derived RPE, there are age-related decreases in the activity of *N*-acetyl-beta-glucosaminidase, an enzyme that is responsible for the degradation of GlcNAc. Since GlcNAc is the major carbohydrate monomer of the oligosaccharide chains of human rhodopsin, defects in its degradation may lead to the accumulation of undigested residual material in the RPE (Cingle et al. 1996). Indeed, GlcNAc is observed in drusen, RPE, Bruch's membrane, and photoreceptors in eyes with AMD (D'Souza et al. 2009). In keeping with Farkas' observation that drusen are derived from degenerating RPE cells containing abundant photoreceptor remnants (Farkas et al. 1971), this observation supports the hypothesis that the pathogenesis of drusen includes the hexosamine pathway.

11.3.3.5 Hyperglycemic Mitochondria-Derived ROS

There are four protein complexes in the mitochondrial ETC, including complexes I, II, III, and IV. Under euglycemic and normoxic conditions (left panel of Figure 11.3a), after pyruvate is metabolized through the TCA cycle, it generates electrons that are passed to coenzyme Q through complexes I and II, and then transferred to complex III, cytochrome-C (Cyt c), complex IV, and finally to molecular oxygen (O_2), which is then reduced to water. While electrons are transported from left to right as shown in the left panel of Figure 11.3a, some of the energy of those electrons is used to pump protons across the membrane at complexes I, III, and IV to generate a voltage potential across the mitochondrial membrane. The energy from this voltage gradient drives the synthesis of ATP by ATP synthase (Trumpower 1990; Wallace 1992). Regulation of the rate of ATP generation is achieved in part by uncoupling proteins (UCPs) that can dissipate the voltage gradient to generate heat.

However, under hyperglycemic normoxic conditions (right panel of Figure 11.3a), more glucose is oxidized. This pushes more electrons into the ETC. When the voltage gradient across the mitochondrial membrane increases to a critical threshold, transfer in complex III is blocked (Korshunov et al. 1997), causing the electrons to accumulate in coenzyme Q. This allows coenzyme Q to donate the electrons one at a time to O_2, thereby generating superoxide (O_2^-). The cell defends itself against this ROS using the mitochondrial isoform of superoxide dismutase (Mn-SOD). This enzyme dismutates O_2^- to hydrogen peroxide, which is then converted to H_2O and O_2 by catalase.

11.3.3.5.1 Hyperglycemic Mitochondria-Derived ROS and DR

Brownlee hypothesizes that the hyperglycemia-induced mitochondrial overproduction of ROS (i.e., the O_2^- described above) may activate poly(ADP-ribose) polymerase (PARP), a DNA repair enzyme that is only found in the nucleus and needs GAPDH as a cofactor (Sawa et al. 1997; Schmidtz 2001). By competing with glycolysis for GAPDH, the ROS-activated PARP impedes the glycolytic pathway and increases the level of all the glycolytic intermediates that are upstream of GAPDH (Figure 11.3a). This exacerbates the deleterious effects of the four glycolysis-associated pathways that are induced by hyperglycemia (Brownlee 2005). This unifying hypothesis of hyperglycemia-induced microvascular damage suggests that hyperglycemia-induced mitochondrial overproduction of ROS is the major culprit in the pathogenesis of DR (Brownlee 2001; 2005; Hammes 2005). In support of this theory, it has been shown that hyperglycemia increases superoxide production in mitochondria, and therapies that inhibit such superoxide production prevent the development of DR (Du et al. 2003; Kanwar et al. 2007).

Studies have shown that hyperglycemia-induced GAPDH nuclear translocation and accumulation participates in the development of various degenerative diseases. This is because nuclear translocation of GAPDH induces the formation of oxidative stress and production of proinflammatory stimuli, such as NO and cytokines that are associated with increased risk for DR (Chuang et al. 2005; Kanwar and Kowluru 2009). Translocation of GAPDH from the cytosol to the nucleus is a critical step in the induction of apoptosis in neuronal cells, such as Müller cells (Kusner et al. 2004). The mechanism underlying the movement of GAPDH from the cytosol to the nucleus under high glucose conditions involves the E3 Ub ligase siah-1, which facilitates hyperglycemia-induced GAPDH nuclear translocation via the formation of a complex with GAPDH (Figure 11.3a) (Yego and Mohr 2010).

Overproduction of ROS results in impaired antioxidant defense enzymes, oxidatively modified DNA, and nitrosylated proteins. Furthermore, the mitochondria become dysfunctional because the proapoptotic protein, Bax, translocates from the cytosol into the mitochondria. This results in Cyt c leaking out from the mitochondria. This is accompanied by increased retinal capillary cell apoptosis, and the formation of acellular capillaries and pericyte ghosts, early signs of DR (Kowluru 2005).

Studies suggest that diabetes-related endothelial injury in the retina may be due to glucose-induced cytokine release by other retinal cells (i.e., paracrine mediators), such as RPE and Müller cells, and not a direct effect of high glucose (Busik et al. 2008; Hammes 2005; Prow et al. 2008).

11.3.3.5.2 Hyperglycemic Mitochondria-Derived ROS and AMD

Age-related pathology, including AMD, has also been related to mitochondrial genomic instability. For example, an increased level of the mitochondrial superoxide dismutase (SOD2) (Figure 11.3a) has been shown to decrease the disruption of the mitochondrial transmembrane potential and the release of Cyt c, and thus to prevent apoptotic cell death in mouse RPE (Kasahara et al. 2005). Furthermore, it is suggested that in RPE mitochondria are the main target of oxidative injury, that the mitochondrial genome is a weak link in the antioxidant defenses, and that deficits in mitochondrial DNA repair pathways are important contributors to the pathogenesis of AMD (Cai et al. 2000; Jarrett et al. 2008). These data suggest that oxidative stress-induced mitochondrial genomic instability will result in loss of cell function and greater susceptibility to stress. This mitochondrial overproduction of ROS may play a significant role in AMD pathogenesis.

11.3.3.6 Hyperglycemic HIF Pathway

Cell respiration depends on the balance between glucose homeostasis and oxygen homeostasis. Cells may be rendered hypoxic because more oxygen is consumed in the ETC during hyperglycemia (Figure 11.3a). Therefore, hypoxia can be viewed as a frequently coincident event with hyperglycemia, even under physiological conditions. In addition, because vascular occlusion diseases, which often develop during the progression of DR or AMD, limit circulation and result in ischemia, they may also induce hypoxia.

It has been proposed that the increased cytosolic ratio of free NADH/NAD$^+$ caused by diabetes-related hyperglycemia mimics the effects of true hypoxia on vascular and neural function and plays an important role in the pathogenesis of diabetic complications, including DR (Nyengaard et al. 2004; Williamson et al. 1993). This is referred to as pseudohypoxia because tissue partial pressure oxygen is normal.

The aberrant stabilization of HIF-α proteins (HIF-1α and/or HIF-2α) (see HIF) under normoxic conditions is also termed pseudohypoxia. For example, dysfunction of TCA cycle enzymes causes pseudohypoxia, leading to the enhanced neovascularization and glycolysis that support cancer formation (Gottlieb and Tomlinson 2005). Pseudohypoxia can also result from von Hippel–Lindau (VHL) mutations (Kim and Kaelin 2004) because VHL mutations result in stabilization of HIF-α proteins (see Section 11.3.3.6). It has been proposed that identifying ways to prevent HIF-α stabilization under pseudohypoxia could lead to treatments for tumors (MacKenzie et al. 2007).

As discussed later in Section 11.3.4, hyperglycemia-induced proinflammatory cytokines, such as IL-1β and TNF-α, can result in the stabilization of HIF-1α under normoxic conditions (Figure 11.8a). This can also be considered pseudohypoxia.

Although some vertebrate species, such as fish, tolerate large variations in ambient oxygen tension during their normal life cycle, most mammals, including man, face serious problems if exposed, even for shorter periods of time, to low oxygen tension (Stecyk et al. 2004). The human retina is highly sensitive to the reduction in oxygen tension (Arjamaa and Nikinmaa 2006), but like the effects of hyperglycemia, the effects of hypoxia vary among retinal cell types (Young et al. 2005).

11.3.3.6.1 Hypoxia-Inducible Factor

HIF was first characterized from human hepatoma cells in which it influenced the transcription of the erythropoietin (Epo) gene (Semenza and Wang 1992). Roles for HIF in the etiologies of DR and AMD have also been proposed (Arjamaa and Nikinmaa 2006; Arjamaa et al. 2009). Stabilizing HIF is among the primary responses to low oxygen tension in cells. As HIF is found in a wide range of animal cells and tissues, and plays an indispensable role in cellular reactions, it can be regarded as a "master switch" of metabolism (Semenza 2000, 2003).

Some suggest that the oBRB, including RPE, is highly resistant to hypoxic damage (Kaur et al. 2008). We posit the novel hypothesis that the resistance to hypoxia is compromised when hypoxia coincides with hyperglycemia. Furthermore, the effects of hypoxia largely depend on the level of hyperglycemia.

With the objective of enhancing the understanding of hyperglycemia-related retinal pathology in both normoxia and hypoxia, in the following sections, we will explore relationships between the HIF pathway and the four glycolysis-associated pathways and the mitochondria-derived ROS pathway, which were described above.

HIF is a heterodimeric protein complex that is composed of two subunits, HIF-1α and HIF-1β (Wang et al. 1995). In contrast to the constitutively expressed HIF-1β subunit, HIF-α is an oxygen labile protein, which in the presence of O_2 is hydroxylated and then degraded (Cockman et al. 2000; Kamura et al. 2000; Lisztwan et al. 1999; Ohh et al. 2000; Tanimoto et al. 2000). HIF-1α becomes stabilized in response to hypoxia, dimerizes with HIF-1β, and binds to hypoxia response elements (HRE), thereby activating the expression of numerous target genes (HIF-inducible genes) (Park et al. 2006).

Although HIF is expressed under physiological conditions, the expression and degradation of the HIF protein are kept in balance (Figure 11.8). Under normoxic conditions (Figure 11.8a), there are

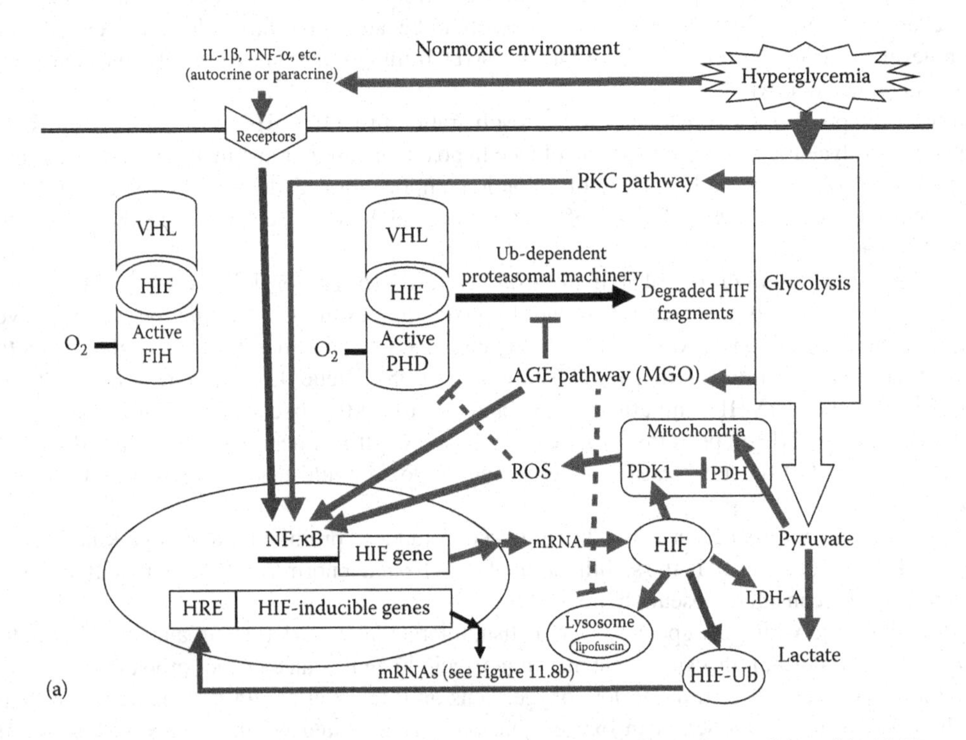

FIGURE 11.8 Hyperglycemic HIF pathway in both normoxic (a) and hypoxic conditions (b). (a) Normoxic, hyperglycemic HIF pathway. In normoxia, hyperglycemic PKC activation, AGEs formation, mitochondrial ROS, and proinflammatory cytokines (e.g., IL-1β and TNF-α) decrease the degradation (through impairing proteasomal system) and/or increase the expression of HIF (through activating NF-κB). The elevated cytoplasmic HIF proteins may switch glucose metabolism from aerobic respiration to fermentation giving rise to lactate accumulation (also see Figure 11.3a). The hyperglycemia-induced excess cytosolic HIF proteins may also lead to increased autophagy, while the lysosomal proteases are impaired by hyperglycemia. The combination of the two effects may also result in the accumulation of lysosomal lipofuscin. In addition, the excess cytosolic HIF proteins, such as an ubiquitinated form of HIF-1α induced by TNF-α, can also transactivate HIF-inducible genes (also see Figure 11.8b). However, under hypoxia the hyperglycemia-induced HIF protein is more stable. *(Continued)*

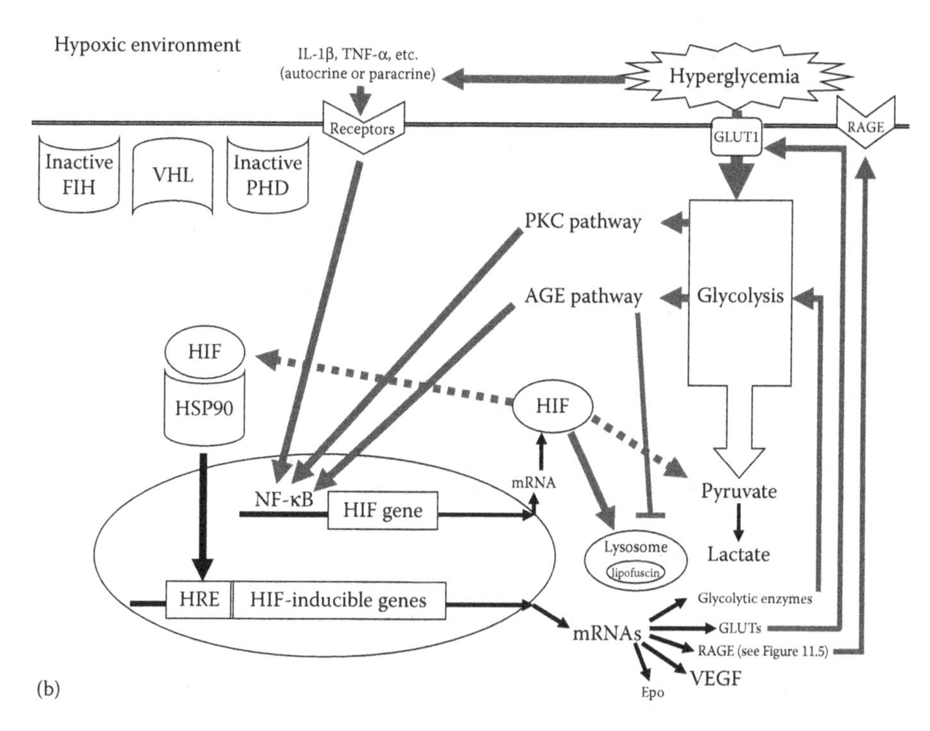

FIGURE 11.8 (Continued) (b) Hypoxic, hyperglycemic HIF pathway. In hypoxia, the transactivation activity of HIF is turned on because both oxygen sensors, PHD and FIH, become inactive. This eliminates proteasomal degradation of HIF proteins. The HIF proteins are further stabilized by hypoxia-induced HSP90 and bind to the HREs in the promoter or enhancer region of HIF-inducible genes to transactivate the transcriptions of the genes. The HIF pathway consists of many HIF-inducible genes, which encode a wide range of proteins, including RAGE, glycolytic enzymes, GLUTs, Epo, and VEGF. The hyperglycemic, hypoxic HIF pathway may be enhanced by hyperglycemic AGE formation and PKC activation, which can activate RAGE signaling cascades and increase HIF expression. Furthermore, in adaptation of lower efficiency of ATP generation from fermentation, the activation of GLUTs and glycolytic enzymes increase glucose uptake and upregulate the glycolysis pathway (also see Figure 11.3b). Therefore, in hyperglycemic, hypoxic conditions the HIF pathway may further deteriorate the four glycolysis-associated pathways and lactate accumulation in the cytoplasm. Furthermore, the hyperglycemia-induced excess cytosolic HIF proteins may also enhance autophage, while the lysosomal system is impaired by hyperglycemia. Together, they may also result in the accumulation of lysosomal lipofuscin. In addition, hyperglycemia-induced proinflammatory cytokines (e.g., IL-1β and TNF-α) can further enhance the HIF pathway.

two mechanisms that cells use to keep HIF inactive (Iyer and Leung 1998). The first mechanism is through the ubiquitin-dependent proteasomal degradation pathway. In this pathway, the conserved proline residues (402 and 564) of HIF are first hydroxylated by proline hydroxylase (PHD) enzymes. Next, the hydroxylated HIF interacts with a Ub-protein ligase, VHL protein (Iwai et al. 1999; Lisztwan et al. 1999) becomes ubiquitinated, and is degraded via the proteasomal pathway (Figure 11.8a) (Cockman et al. 2000; Kamura et al. 2000; Lisztwan et al. 1999; Ohh et al. 2000; Tanimoto et al. 2000). The degradation is dependent on the protein motifs found in the carboxyl terminus of HIF proteins, termed hypoxia-responsive domains (Huang et al. 1998). Thus, HIF is kept at a low level in the cytosol. In the second mechanism, HIF is prevented from binding to the HREs in the promoter or enhancer regions of HIF-inducible genes. Specifically, in normoxia, HIF binding to DNA is inhibited through asparagine hydroxylation by an oxygen-dependent factor inhibiting HIF

(FIH) (Figure 11.8a) (Lando et al. 2002; Lisy and Peet 2008; Mahon et al. 2001). In this situation, the transcription of HIF-inducible genes, such as VEGF, is limited.

Under hypoxia, both oxygen sensors, PHD and FIH, become inactive and unable to hydroxylate HIF-1α. The stabilized HIF binds to HIF-inducible genes (Figure 11.8b). In addition, hypoxia also induces the expression of heat shock proteins (HSPs). HSPs are molecular chaperones required for the stability and function of a number of conditionally activated and/or expressed protein kinases and transcription factors, such as HIF (Kaarniranta and Salminen 2009). For example, the ATP-dependent HSP90 can bind to the Per-Arnt-Sim (PAS) domain of HIF and increase its stability (Pearl et al. 2008). The PAS is situated in the amino terminal end of HIF and is involved in the formation and stabilization of HIF heterodimers (Park et al. 2006; Wang et al. 1995). Therefore, under hypoxia, the transcription activities of HIF-inducible genes are turned on by HIF. As noted earlier, these HIF-inducible genes are responsible for a wide range of hyperglycemic pathogenesis, such as VEGF-induced angiogenesis (Figures 11.3b and 11.8b).

The HIF system is also affected independently of O_2 (Dehne and Brüne 2009). Although oxygen seems to be the major determinant of PHD activity, the enzyme is also sensitive to cellular redox status, iron or metabolite homeostasis, and so on (Kaelin Jr. and Ratcliffe 2008). Among these effectors is nitric oxide (NO). NO is produced by activated macrophages and granulocytes during inflammation (Thomas et al. 2008). NO is synthesized from L-arginine by nitric oxide synthase (NOS). NOS from neurons (nNOS) and endothelium (eNOS) are constitutively expressed enzymes. Their activities are stimulated by increases in intracellular calcium (Kaur et al. 2008). Inducible NOS is calcium-independent, and NO generated from this isoform is known to mediate immune functions. Excess production of NO has been reported to increase blood flow and the permeability of the blood–brain barrier allowing substances to enter into the brain passively (Shukla et al. 1996; Thiel and Audus 2001). The modulation of NO availability by eNOS seems to be an important determinant in the maintenance of cerebral perfusion in hypoxic conditions. Vasodilatation occurring after hypoxic–ischemic episodes is mediated by eNOS (Bolanos and Almeida 1999), leading to increased blood flow. It has also been proposed that eNOS mediates VEGF-induced vascular hyperpermeability (Fukumura et al. 2001). NO, exogenously added or endogenously produced, stabilizes HIF protein and causes the transactivation of HIF under normoxia (Brune and Zhou 2007). It is suggested that hypoxia and NO use overlapping signaling pathways to stabilize HIF, because NO attenuates HIF ubiquitination in an *in vitro*-assay and decreases PHD activity (Brune and Zhou 2007). FIH activity is also inactivated by NO (Park et al. 2008). Besides, NO also increased PI3K-dependent HIF protein expression (Brune and Zhou 2007). Therefore, it is not surprising that NO, similar to hypoxia, can induce HIF-related responses.

In tumor cells, it has been shown that tumor suppressor gene and oncogene activity can also influence HIF activity and subsequent changes in glucose metabolism (Hammond and Giaccia 2005; Ramanathan et al. 2005; Semenza 2003).

11.3.3.6.2 Hyperglycemia and HIF

Accumulating evidence implies that there is an undescribed HIF-related mechanism that results in pathology under hyperglycemic, hypoxic conditions (Figure 11.8b). Hyperglycemia can enhance the activity of HIF through glycolysis-derived hyperglycemic AGE and PKC pathways (Figure 11.8b). First, hypoxia has been shown to result in the activation of NF-kB, which can bind to the HIF promoter in response to hypoxia (Belaiba et al. 2007; Bonello et al. 2007). As described previously, NF-κB can also be activated by hyperglycemia-induced AGE formation (Figure 11.4) and PKC activation (Figure 11.6). Thus, coincidental hyperglycemia and hypoxia lead to enhanced expression of HIF and HIF-inducible genes (Figure 11.8b). Indeed, it has been shown that when hyperglycemia coincides with hypoxia the secretion of VEGF is enhanced. This is partially mediated via activation of PKC (Young et al. 2005). Remarkably, PKC can also be activated through the hyperglycemic polyol pathway (see Section 11.3.3.2 and Figure 11.5) and the hyperglycemic hexosamine pathway (see Section 11.3.3.4 and Figure 11.7). Second, the hyperglycemic HIF pathway may amplify the deleterious effects of hyperglycemic AGE formation (Figure 11.4) by HIF-inducible RAGE expression (Figure 11.8b) (Pichiule et al. 2007).

Another example of the synergistic effect of hypoxia and hyperglycemia is on the lysosomal and proteasomal proteolysis systems. Autophagy is one of the cellular mechanisms that are responsible for proteolytic functions. It cooperates with the lysosomal and Ub proteasome pathway in protein clearance in response to cellular stress, such as hypoxia and disturbed energy balance (Korolchuk et al. 2009; Ryha¨nen et al. 2009; Salminen and Kaarniranta 2009). Interestingly, it has been shown that HIF can induce autophagy by preventing ATP depletion and by enhancing the elimination of damaged mitochondria (Bellot et al. 2009; Zhang et al. 2008a). However, hyperglycemia-induced glycating agents, such as MGO, impair both lysosomal and proteasomal functions (Kasper et al. 1999; Miyata et al. 1997; Queisser et al. 2010; Sebeková et al. 1998; Uchiki et al. 2011). Taken together, the higher input (increased autophagocytosis) than output (impaired proteolytic function) in proteolytic machinery may lead to the accumulation of intracellular lipofuscin and the formation of drusen, both of which are hallmarks of early AMD (Uchiki et al. 2011). This mechanistic proposal is corroborated by observations that in human AMD donor samples or in RPE cells, there are increased levels of autophagic markers, decreased lysosomal activity, increased exocytotic activity and the release of cytokines (Wang et al. 2009a). Interestingly, the exosomes released by the stressed RPE to remove damaged intracellular proteins are coated with complement and can bind a complement factor H (CFH), which has been identified as a major inflammatory factor in AMD pathogenesis (Edwards et al. 2005; Haines et al. 2005; Klein et al. 2005).

Even under normoxic conditions, hyperglycemia appears to be able to induce some effects of HIF. It has been shown that in RPE cells high concentrations of glucose enhance synthesis and accumulation of HIF (Xiao et al. 2006). As described earlier (Figures 11.4 and 11.6), AGEs and PKC can activate NF-kB. PKC can also be activated through the hyperglycemic polyol pathway (Figure 11.5) and hyperglycemic hexosamine pathway (Figure 11.7). This may cause the over expression of HIF (Figure 11.8a). The overexpressed HIF may be further stabilized by MGO, which has been shown to impair Ub proteasome function (Queisser et al. 2010). Elevated mitochondrial ROS can also enhance the expression of HIF through NF-kB signaling (Bonello et al. 2007; Decanini et al. 2007; Taylor 2008; van Uden et al. 2008; Wang et al. 2010) and stabilize HIF protein by inhibiting PHD (Yuan et al. 2008) (Figures 11.3a and 11.8a). Taken together, under hyperglycemic, normoxic conditions, the hyperglycemic AGE and PKC pathways may also result in excess cytosolic HIF proteins (Figure 11.8a), which can induce autophagy (Bellot et al. 2009; Zhang et al. 2008a) and, in conjunction with impaired proteolytic functions, lead to the accumulation of lysosomal lipofuscin.

Together, we propose that hyperglycemia can lead to HIF accumulation resulting in the formation of intracellular deposits and the expression of HIF-inducible genes under both hypoxic and normoxic conditions (Figures 11.8a and 11.8b) (see Section 11.3.4). However, studies have shown that under hypoxia, the hyperglycemia-induced HIF protein is more stable, and the expression of VEGF is increased (Xiao et al. 2006; Yao et al. 2003).

The effects of hypoxia can persist for some time after oxygen tension returns to a normoxic level, probably through mitochondrial ROS generation. For example, intermittent hypoxia, followed by reoxygenation, has been shown to potentiate the production of ROS, which may lead to HIF activation and accelerated aging and to the appearance of age-related diseases (Rapino et al. 2005; Yuan et al. 2008). In theory, this phenomenon may occur at the highly active retina during the transition from early to middle postprandial stage after ingesting a high-GI meal.

It has been known for long that, even under conditions of plentiful oxygen (normoxia), cancer cells switch from aerobic respiration to lactate fermentation (Warburg 1956). Studies have demonstrated that the phenomenon, including increased glucose uptake, upregulated glycolytic cascade and reduced aerobic respiration, increased lactate production, and acidosis of the microenvironment, is primarily due to the activation of HIF (Brahimi-Horn et al. 2007; Kim and Dang 2006). Actually, this phenomenon also occurs in nontumor cells under physiological conditions (Brahimi-Horn et al. 2007;

Kim and Dang 2006; Kim et al. 2006a; 2006b; Papandreou et al. 2006; Pouyssegur and Mechta-Grigoriou 2006). This may, at least partially, explain the physiological phenomenon of a high lactate production concomitant with high oxygen consumption in the RPE (Figures 11.3a and 11.8a) (Coffe et al. 2006; Kaur et al. 2008; Miceli et al. 1990). The possibility of using the lactate level in the RPE as a biomarker of hyperglycemic exposure or even a prognostic biomarker as well deserves further study.

The molecular mechanism for the HIF-dependent pyruvate metabolism switching has also been studied (Figure 11.8a). The increased metabolism of pyruvate to lactate is mainly a result of the activation of two HIF-dependent enzymes, mitochondrial pyruvate dehydrogenase kinase 1 (PDK1) and lactate dehydrogenase A (LDH-A). PDK1 inhibits the activity of pyruvate dehydrogenase (PDH), which is required in the TCA cycle (Kim et al. 2006a; 2006b; Papandreou et al. 2006; Pouyssegur and Mechta-Grigoriou 2006). LDH-A converts pyruvate into lactate (Koukourakis et al. 2005).

As the metabolism of glucose via pyruvate to lactate is less energy efficient, cells must increase glucose uptake and accelerate glycolysis to maintain the ATP level. It is remarkable that these adaptations are also mediated by the HIF pathway, which increases the expression of glucose transporters (GLUTs, e.g., GLUT-1) and upregulates glycolytic enzymes (e.g., LDH and aldolase protein levels) (Figures 11.3b and 11.8b) (Semenza 2003; Schofield and Ratcliffe 2004). Therefore, in hyperglycemic, hypoxic conditions HIF pathway may further potentiate the four glycolysis-associated pathways. The stabilization of HIF that occurs under conditions of hypoxia and sufficient glucose provides an additional explanation for synergistic effects of hypoxia and hyperglycemia compared with the effect from hypoxia alone (Vordermark et al. 2005).

Recently, the carbohydrate response element binding protein (ChREBP) was shown to be able to upregulate the transcription of HIF-1α and, therefore, downstream HIF-inducible gene expression in human renal mesangial cells exposed to normoxia and high glucose, and it is suggested that this phenomenon is tissue (cell type)-specific (Isoe et al. 2010). Carbohydrate response element binding protein (ChREBP) is a key regulator of glucose metabolism, which is activated in response to high glucose and upregulates more than 15 genes involved in the metabolic conversion of glucose to fat, such as the pyruvate kinase and lipogenesis enzyme genes, by binding to a carbohydrate response element (ChRE) of these genes (Uyeda et al. 2002). Through controlling the transcription of lipogenic enzyme genes in response to nutritional and hormonal inputs, ChREBP may play an important role in disease states, such as diabetes, obesity, and hypertension. Interestingly, our recent observations also suggest that ChREBP plays a role in the transcriptional upregulation of HIF-1α under hyperglycemic, nomoxic conditions in the RPE (Figure 11.9) (Chang et al. 2014). This ChREBP-mediated HIF-1α upregulation further transactivates VEGF, insulin-like growth factor 1 (IGF-1), glucose transporter 1 (GLUT-1), and many other HIF-inducible genes. This observation provides support for our hypothesis that the HIF pathway may also be responsible for pathogenesis under normoxia. Notably, unlike hypoxia, the normoxic hyperglycemia-induced, ChREBP-mediated HIF is regulated by increasing mRNA levels, and the phenomenon is cell-type specific, that is, we only observed the phenomenon in the RPE cells but not in either human lens epithelial cells (HLEC) or HeLa cells.

Interestingly, the normoxic hyperglycemia-induced, ChREBP-mediated HIF seems to be independent from glycolysis. It has been proposed that high glucose facilitates nuclear translocation of dephosphorylated ChREBP by protein phosphatase 2A (PP2A), which is upregulated by an intermediate, xylulose-5-P, in the pentose phosphate pathway (Haase 2010). Since the pentose phosphate pathway is an alternative to glycolysis and only activated in specific cell types, this may offer an explanation for the cell-type-specific glucose-induced ChREBP-mediated HIF activation under normoxia. Further deciphering this biochemical mechanism will advance our understanding of the underlying pathogenesis and enhance therapeutic options for metabolic retinal diseases, such as DR and AMD, preferably in the early stages of the diseases. Therefore, HIF is not only an HIF, but it can also be described as a "hyperglycemia-inducible factor." Through this mechanism, the hyperglycemic HIF pathway and its interactions with other hyperglycemic pathogenesis pathways, such as hyperglycemic AGE, PKC, polyol, and hexosamine pathways, can affect oxidative stress responses, inflammation, proteolytic mechanisms, and so on, all of which are involved in the pathogeneses of

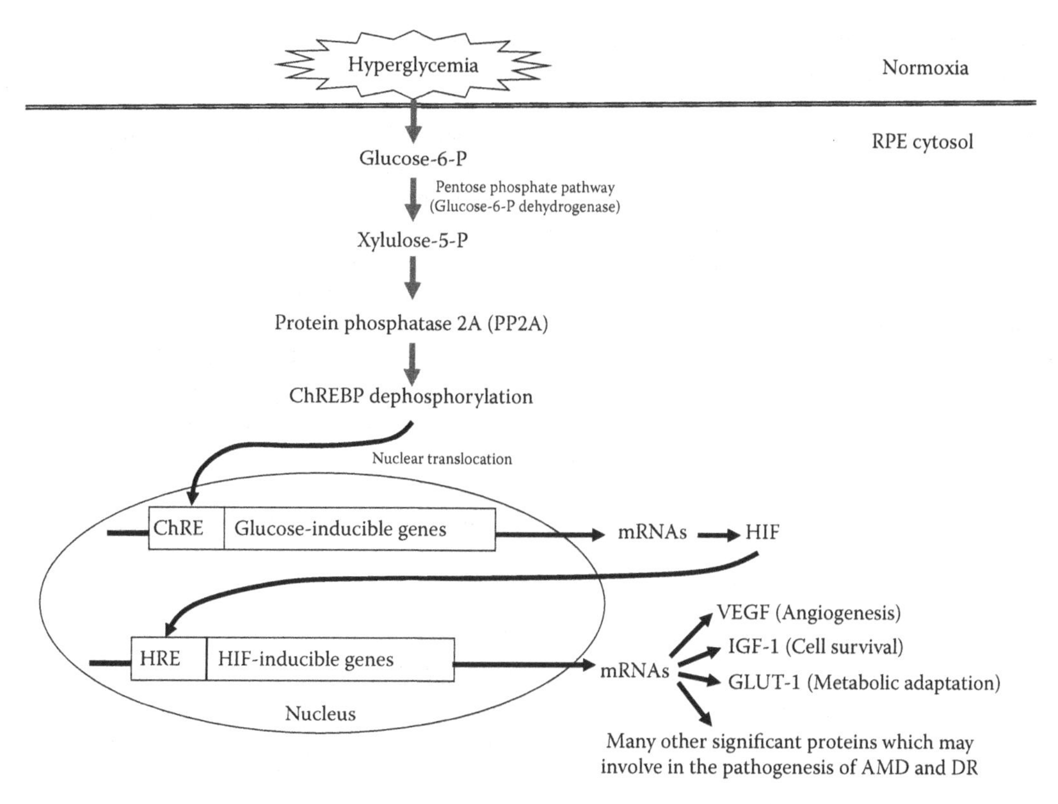

FIGURE 11.9 Normoxic, hyperglycemic ChREBP-mediated HIF pathway. Carbohydrate response element binding protein (ChREBP) upregulates the transcription of hypoxia-inducible factor (HIF)-1α and, therefore, downstream HIF-inducible gene expressions in human retinal pigment epithelial (RPE) cells exposed to normoxia and high glucose concentration.

DR and AMD. This wide range of HIF-mediated cellular effects may open new treatment indications, for example, for dry forms of AMD. Nevertheless, caution is advised because suppressing of HIF may be a double-edged sword. By serving as the major regulator in glucose metabolism, HIF is necessary for maintaining physiological homeostasis.

11.3.3.6.3 HIF and VEGF

From a clinical point of view, VEGF is one of the most important HIF-inducible genes (Figure 11.8b), because it induces postnatal neovascularization and angiogenesis seen after ischemic events in both DR and AMD patients (Lee et al. 2000). Although both hyperglycemia and hypoxia can induce the VEGF expression, it is remarkable that, while the hyperglycemia-induced VEGF expression is mediated by PKC (Figure 11.6), hypoxia mediates the VEGF expression by increased binding of the active HIF to the HRE of the VEGF promoter and by increasing the stability of the VEGF mRNA transcript through mitogen-activated protein kinase and Akt pathways, respectively (Figure 11.8b) (Suzuma et al. 2000). Importantly, it has been shown that exposure to hypoxia as well as AGEs causes additive VEGF expression by RPE cells (Lu et al. 1998).

The expression of HIF-inducible genes, including VEGF, can also be stimulated through HIF-independent mechanisms, such as the transcriptional coactivator peroxisome-proliferator-activated receptor-gamma coactivator-1alpha (PGC-1α). PGC-1α is a potent metabolic sensor and regulator induced by a lack of nutrients and oxygen. PGC-1α powerfully regulates the VEGF expression and angiogenesis in cultured muscle cells and skeletal muscle *in vivo* (Arany et al. 2008). Such observations may help explain why people with diabetes can have impaired new blood vessel growth in one tissue compartment (e.g., myocardium) and also exhibit hyperproliferative vascular disease in another (e.g., retina) (Thangarajah et al. 2010).

Anti-VEGF, such as Lucentis®, Avastin®, and Macugen®, has been used in clinics to treat exudative AMD (Bressler 2009a; 2009b) and is currently being evaluated for the treatment of proliferative DR and neovascular glaucoma (Rodriguez-Fontal et al. 2009). Recently, it has been shown that intravitreal ranibizumab (anti-VEGF therapy, trade name Lucentis) with the prompt or deferred laser is more effective through at least one year compared with the prompt laser alone for the treatment of DME involving the central macula (The Diabetic Retinopathy Clinical Research Network; Elman et al. 2010).

In addition to VEGF, recent studies have also explored the possibility of directly targeting HIF for a new therapeutic option for both DR and AMD, especially the neovascular types (Arjamaa and Nikinmaa 2006; Arjamaa et al. 2009; Wang et al. 2009b; Zhang et al. 2007).

Some studies suggested that the poor wound healing in diabetic patients is a result of compromised blood vessel formation in response to ischemia and that this impairment in neovascularization results from an MGO-induced defect in transactivation of HIF-1α, leading to the decreased expression of VEGF (Bento et al. 2010; Thangarajah et al. 2009; 2010). However, because ischemia is a phenomenon of lacking oxygen, glucose, and serum in the tissues (Osborne et al. 2004; Wood and Osborne 2001), it should be differentiated from the hypoxic, hyperglycemic conditions discussed here.

11.3.3.6.4 HIF and Erythropoietin

It was shown that Epo provides protection against apoptosis of photoreceptor cells in the rodent retina and this protection is through interfering with caspase-1 activation, a downstream event in the intracellular death cascade, but not through inhibiting initial events of the apoptosis cascade, such as activator protein-1 activation (Grimm et al. 2002; 2006; Junk et al. 2002). It has also been shown that Epo acts as a neuroprotective factor in diabetic neuropathy (Bianchi et al. 2004; Lipton 2004). However, although Epo overexpression is an early event in the retina of diabetic patients, at this stage, it is unrelated to a hypoxic stimulus (i.e., HIF-independent) (Forooghian et al. 2007; García-Ramírez et al. 2008). This is to say that, in the early stage of DR, HIF-independent Epo overexpression actually has beneficial rather than pathogenic actions. It appears that factors, apart from hypoxia, that could be responsible for Epo overexpression include hyperglycemia and inflammation (García-Ramírez et al. 2008; Sun and Zhang 2001; Watanabe et al. 2005).

However, Epo is also a potent retinal angiogenic factor independent of VEGF and, at least partially, responsible for retinal angiogenesis in proliferative DR, the late stage of the disease. This Epo expression is mainly stimulated by hypoxia (i.e., HIF-dependent) (Figure 11.8b) (Mowat et al. 2010; Watanabe et al. 2005).

Therefore, despite its neuroprotective effect, Epo administration may be hazardous for retinal diseases that involve retinal vasoproliferation (Bianchi et al. 2004; Lipton 2004). Conversely, Epo blockade may be hazardous for retinal diseases that involve apoptosis of retinal photoreceptors (Becerra and Amaral 2002; Watanabe et al. 2005). The clinical application of Epo needs further study.

11.3.4 Hyperglycemia Induces Inflammation and Apoptosis

Both DR and AMD have been characterized as chronic inflammatory diseases leading to cell death in the retina (Anderson et al. 2002; Hageman et al. 2001; Joussen et al. 2004; Mohr 2004). This is consistent with many molecular and epidemiological observations, reviewed above, that hyperglycemia results in the increased production of proinflammatory cytokines and apoptosis of the cells (Allen et al. 2005; Buyken et al. 2010; Node and Inoue 2009).

Caspases, a family of cysteine proteases, are known to be critically involved in both the activation of proinflammatory cytokines and the initiation and execution of apoptosis (Alnemri 1997; Alnemri et al. 1996). Caspase-1 is involved in the activation of inflammatory processes (Mariathasan et al. 2004). Two caspase pathways have been described by which cells undergo apoptosis. The extrinsic (receptor-mediated) pathway is triggered via cell surface receptors that are represented by TNF-α family receptors, leading to the activation of caspase-8 and caspase-3 proteolytic enzymes. The intrinsic (mitochondrial) pathway involves the mitochondrial Cyt c release and activation of the caspase-9, with the subsequent activation of caspase-3. The intrinsic pathway can be activated by agents that directly target the mitochondria, or indirectly via the extrinsic pathway through caspase-8-mediated cleavage of the inactive cytosolic protein BID. Once activated, BID translocates to the mitochondria where it stimulates Cyt c release (Fiers et al. 1999; Takahashi et al. 2004).

In Müller cells in the retina of streptozotocin-induced diabetic rats, hyperglycemia caused apoptosis that was associated with the activation of the caspase-3 and mitochondrial caspase-9 pathways (Xi et al. 2005). Recent studies also showed that inhibiting the activation of caspase-1, or former IL-1β converting enzyme that is responsible for the production of the proinflammatory cytokines IL-1β and IL-18, could be a potential new strategy to prevent the development of DR (Mohr 2004; Mohr et al. 2002; Vincent and Mohr 2007).

In the human RPE, the activation of caspase-8 pathway (i.e., extrinsic pathway), but not the mitochondrial caspase-9 pathway (i.e., intrinsic pathway) was shown to be involved in the 7-ketocholesterol (an oxidative stressor)-induced apoptosis (Luthra et al. 2006). However, in TNF-α-induced apoptosis in the human RPE cells, it was shown that the mitochondrial caspase-9 could be used to amplify the death signal mediated by caspase-8 (Yang et al. 2007).

As discussed in the four glycolysis-related pathways above, hyperglycemia can induce proinflammatory cytokines (e.g., Figure 11.4), such as IL-1β and TNF-α. Interestingly, IL-1β and TNF-α can prolong the activation of HIF-1α protein under conditions of inflammation via enhancing the translation of HIF-1α mRNA, further leading to the increased expression of HIF-inducible genes (Frede et al. 2005; 2007; Hellwig-Bürgel et al. 1999; Sandau et al. 2001; Zhou et al. 2003). Importantly, this can happen under both normoxic (Figure 11.8a) and hypoxic (Figure 11.8b) conditions (Yee Koh et al. 2008). This gives additional support to the idea that hyperglycemia is able to induce some effects of HIF (also see hyperglycemia and HIF).

11.4 SUMMARY AND CONCLUDING REMARKS

Diet is a major determinant of health. Just because carbohydrate is our major energy source, it is not unexpected that the metabolism of sugars plays a significant role in aging and disease. The GI reflects the kinetics of blood glucose concentrations after ingesting a meal irrespective of glucose tolerance or diabetes. Recent data from a wide range of epidemiological and molecular studies offer a strong support for the conclusion that dietary hyperglycemia is associated with risk for major metabolic disorders, including type 2 diabetes, CVD, and retinal diseases such as DR and AMD (Chiu et al. 2011; Uchiki et al. 2011). Therefore, it remains critical to elucidate the mechanisms of these relations and fully exploit the management of carbohydrate nutrition as a means to prevent the onset or progression of these diseases. Based on the research evidence, a low-GI diet should be recommended to those at a high risk of DR and AMD. In terms of identifying high risk populations, the development of susceptibility biomarkers, exposure biomarkers, and surrogate endpoints for a disease will be invaluable.

LIST OF ABBREVIATIONS

AGEs	advanced glycation end products
ALEs	advanced lipoxidation end products
AMD	age-related macular degeneration
AR	aldose reductase
AREDS	Age-Related Eye Disease Study
ATP	adenosine triphosphate
AUC	area under blood glucose curve and above the baseline blood glucose level

BDES	Beaver Dam Eye Study
BLDs	basal lamina deposits
BMES	Blue Mountains Eye Study
BRB	blood–retinal barrier
ChRE	carbohydrate response element
ChREBP	carbohydrate response element binding protein
CEC	choroidal endothelial cells
CHD	coronary heart disease
CI	confidence interval
CML	N^{ε}-(carboxyl-methyl) lysine
CNV	choroidal neovascularization
CVD	cardiovascular disease
Cyt c	cytochrome-C
DAG	diacylglycerol
DHA	docosahexaenoic acid
DME	diabetic macular edema
DR	diabetic retinopathy
eNOS	endothelial nitric oxide synthase
EPA	eicosapentaenoic acid
Epo	erythropoietin
ET-1	vasoconstrictor endothelin-1
ETC	electron transport chain
F-6-P	fructose-6-phosphate
FIH	factor inhibiting hypoxia-inducible factor
G-6-P	glucose-6-phosphate
GA	geographic atrophy
GA-3-P	glyceraldehyde-3-phosphate
GAPDH	glyceraldehyde-3 phosphate dehydrogenase
GFAT	glutamine:fructose-6 phosphate amidotransferase
GI	glycemic index
GL	glycemic load
Glucosamine-6-P	glucosamine-6-phosphate
GLUT-1	glucose transporter 1
GLUTs	glucose transporters
GO	glyoxal
GSH	glutathione
HbA_{1c}	hemoglobin A_{1c}
HDL	high-density lipoprotein
HIF	hypoxia-inducible factor
HLEC	human lens epithelial cell
HREs	hypoxia-responsive elements
HSP90	heat shock protein 90
HSPs	heat shock proteins
iBRB	inner blood–retinal barrier
IGF-1	insulin-like growth factor 1
IL	interleukin
LDH-A	lactate dehydrogenase A
LDL	low-density lipoprotein
MGO	methylglyoxal
Mn-SOD	mitochondrial isoform of superoxide dismutase
NF-κB	nuclear factor kappa B

NHANES	National Health and Nutrition Examination Surveys
NHS	Nurses' Health Study
nNOS	neurons nitric oxide synthase
NO	nitric oxide
NOS	nitric oxide synthase
NVP	Nutrition and Vision Project
oBRB	outer blood–retinal barrier
O-GlcNAcylation	*O*-acetylglucosaminylation
OGT	*O*-GlcNAc transferase
OR	odds ratio
PAI-1	plasminogen activator inhibitor-1
PARP	poly(ADP-ribose) polymerase
PAS	Per-Arnt-Sim
PDGF-B	platelet-derived growth factor-B
PDH	pyruvate dehydrogenase
PDK1	pyruvate dehydrogenase kinase 1
PGC-1α	peroxisome-proliferator-activated receptor-gamma coactivator-1alpha
PHD	praline hydroxylase
PKC	protein kinase C
PP2A	protein phosphatase 2A
PPAR	peroxisome proliferator-activated receptor
PUFAs	polyunsaturated fatty acids
RAGE	receptors for AGEs
RNV	retinal neovascularization
ROS	reactive oxygen species
RPE	retinal pigment epithelium
RR	relative risk
SDH	succinate dehydrogenase
SOD2	mitochondrial superoxide dismutase
TCA	tricarboxylic acid
TGF-β1	transforming growth factor-β1
TNF-α	tumor necrosis factor α
TT	Na^+-taurine cotransporter
Ub	ubiquitin
UCPs	uncoupling proteins
UDPGlcNAc	uridine diphosphate *N*-acetyl glucosamine
USDA	United States Department of Agriculture
VEGF	vascular endothelial growth factor
VHL	von Hippel–Lindau

ACKNOWLEDGMENTS

This work was supported, in part by grants from USDA contract 1950-510000-060-01A, NIH EY 013250, EY 021212, EY 021826, and Alcon, Johnson and Johnson Focused Giving.

REFERENCES

Abdallah, W. and A. A. Fawzi (2009). Anti-VEGF therapy in proliferative diabetic retinopathy. *Int Ophthalmol Clin.* **49**: 95–107.

Abordo, E. A. and P. J. Thornalley (1997). Synthesis and secretion of tumour necrosis factor-alpha by human monocytic THP-1 cells and chemotaxis induced by human serum albumin derivatives modified with methylglyoxal and glucose-derived advanced glycation endproducts. *Immunol Lett.* **58**: 139–147.

Age-Related Eye Disease Study Research Group (2001). A randomized, placebo-controlled, clinical trial of high-dose supplementation with vitamins C and E, beta carotene, and zinc for age-related macular degeneration and vision loss: AREDS report no. 8. *Arch Ophthalmol.* **119**(10): 1417–1436.

Age-Related Eye Disease Study Research Group (2005). Risk factors for the incidence of Advanced Age-Related Macular Degeneration in the Age-Related Eye Disease Study (AREDS) AREDS report no. 19. *Ophthalmology* **112**: 533–539.

Aiello, L. P., R. L. Avery, P. G. Arrigg, B. A. Keyt, H. D. Jampel, S. T. Shah et al. (1994). Vascular endothelial growth factor in ocular fluid of patients with diabetic retinopathy and other retinal disorders. *N. Engl. J. Med.* **331**: 1480–1487.

Aiello, L. P., S. E. Bursell, A. Clermont, E. Duh, H. Ishii, C. Takagi et al. (1997). Vascular endothelial growth factor-induced retinal permeability is mediated by protein kinase C in vivo and suppressed by an orally effective beta-isoform-selective inhibitor. *Diabetes* **46**: 1473–1480.

Aisenbrey, S., M. Zhang, D. Bacher, J. Yee, W. J. Brunken, and D. D. Hunter (2006). Retinal pigment epithelial cells synthesize laminins, including laminin 5, and adhere to them through alpha3- and alpha6-containing integrins. *Invest Ophthalmol Vis Sci.* **47**: 5537–5544.

Allen, D. A., M. M. Yaqoob, and S. M. Harwood (2005). Mechanisms of high glucose-induced apoptosis and its relationship to diabetic complications. *J Nutr Biochem.* **16**: 705–713.

Alnemri, E., D. J. Livingston, D. W. Nicholson, G. Salvesen, N. A. Thornberry, W. W. Wong, and J. Yuan (1996). Human ICE/CED-3 protease nomenclature (Letter). *Cell* **87**: 171.

Alnemri, E. S. (1997). Mammalian cell death proteases: A family of highly conserved aspartate specific cysteine proteases. *J Cell Biochem.* **64**: 33–42.

Anderson, D. H., R. F. Mullins, G. S. Hageman, and L. V. Johnson (2002). A role for local inflammation in the formation of drusen in the aging eye. *Am J Ophthalmol.* **134**: 411–431.

Anderson, D. H., M. J. Radeke, N. B. Gallo, E. A. Chapin, P. T. Johnson, C. R. Curletti et al. (2010). The pivotal role of the complement system in aging and age-related macular degeneration: Hypothesis re-visited. *Prog Retin Eye Res.* **29**(2): 95–112.

Anil, E. (2007). The impact of EPA and DHA on blood lipids and lipoprotein metabolism: Influence of apoE genotype. *Proc Nutr Soc.* **66**: 60–68.

Antonetti, D. A., A. J. Barber, L. A. Hollinger, E. B. Wolpert, and T. W. Gardner (1999). Vascular endothelial growth factor induces rapid phosphorylation of tight junction proteins occludin and zonula occluden 1. A potential mechanism for vascular permeability in diabetic retinopathy and tumors. *J Biol Chem.* **274**: 23463–23467.

Arany, Z., S. Y. Foo, Y. Ma, J. L. Ruas, A. Bommi-Reddy, G. Girnun et al. (2008). HIF-independent regulation of VEGF and angiogenesis by the transcriptional coactivator PGC-1alpha. *Nature* **451**: 1008–1012.

Arjamaa, O. and M. Nikinmaa (2006). Oxygen-dependent diseases in the retina: Role of hypoxia-inducible factors. *Exp Eye Res.* **83**: 473–483.

Arjamaa, O., M. Nikinmaa, A. Salminen, and K. Kaarniranta (2009). Regulatory role of HIF-1alpha in the pathogenesis of age-related macular degeneration (AMD). *Ageing Res Rev.* **8**: 349–358.

Assero, G., G. Lupo, C. D. Anfuso, N. Ragusa, and M. Alberghina (2001). High glucose and advanced glycation end products induce phospholipid hydrolysis and phospholipid enzyme inhibition in bovine retinal pericytes. *Biochim Biophys Acta.* **1533**: 128–140.

Balkau, B., M. Shipley, R. J. Jarrett, K. Pyörälä, M. Pyörälä, A. Forhan and E. Eschwège (1998). High blood glucose concentration is a risk factor for mortality in middle-aged nondiabetic men. 20-year follow-up in the Whitehall Study, the Paris Prospective Study, and the Helsinki Policemen Study. *Diabetes Care.* **21**: 360–367.

Bazan, N. G. (1982). Metabolism of phospholipids in the retina. *Vision Res.* **22**: 1539–1548.

Becerra, S. P. and J. Amaral (2002). Erythropoietin—An endogenous retinal survival factor. *N Engl J Med.* **347**: 1968–1970.

Beckman, K. B. and B. N. Ames (1998). The free radical theory of aging matures. *Physiol. Rev.* **78**: 547–581.

Belaiba, R. S., S. Bonello et al. (2007). Hypoxia up-regulates hypoxia-inducible factor-1 alpha transcription by involving phosphatidylinositol 3-kinase and nuclear factor kappaB in pulmonary artery smooth muscle cells. *Mol. Biol. Cell* **18**: 4691–4697.

Bellot, G., R. Garcia-Medina, P. Gounon, J. Chiche, D. Roux, J. Pouysségur, and N. M. Mazure (2009). Hypoxia-induced autophagy is mediated through hypoxia-inducible factor induction of BNIP3 and BNIP3L via their BH3 domains. *Mol. Cell. Biol.* **29**: 2570–2581.

Bento, C. F., R. Fernandes, P. Matafome, C. Sena, R. Seiça, and P. Pereira (2010). Methylglyoxal-induced imbalance in the ratio VEGF/Ang-2 secreted by retinal pigment epithelial cells leads to endothelial dysfunction. *Exp Physiol.* **95**: 955–970.

Bianchi, R., B. Buyukakilli, M. Brines, C. Savino, G. Cavaletti, and N. Oggioni (2004). Erythropoietin both protects from and reverses experimental diabetic neuropathy. *Proc Natl Acad Sci USA*. **101**: 823–828.

Bierhaus, A., P. M. Humpert, D. M. Stern, B. Arnold, and P. P. Nawroth (2005). Advanced glycation end product receptor-mediated cellular dysfunction. *Ann. N.Y. Acad. Sci*. **1043**: 676–680.

Birarda, G., E. A. Holman, S. K. W. Fu, P. Hua, F. G. Blankenberg et al. (2013). Synchrotron infrared imaging of advanced glycation end products (AGEs) in cardiac tissue from mice fed high glycemic diets. *Biomed Spectrosc Imaging*. **2**(4): 301–315.

Bishara, N. B., M. E. Dunlop, T. V. Murphy, I. A. Darby, M. A. Sharmini Rajanayagam, and M. A. Hill (2002). Matrix protein glycation impairs agonist-induced intracellular Ca2+ signaling in endothelial cells. *J Cell Physiol*. **193**: 80–92.

Bolanos, J. P. and A. Almeida (1999). Roles of nitric oxide in brain hypoxia-ischemia. *Biochim. Biophys. Acta*. **1411**: 415–436.

Bonello, S., C. Za¨hringer, R. S. BelAiba, T. Djordjevic, J. Hess, and C. Michiels et al. (2007). Reactive oxygen species activate the HIF-1alpha promoter via a functional NFkB site. *Arterioscler. Thromb. Vasc. Biol*. **27**: 755–761.

Boulton, M. and J. Marshall (1986). Effects of increasing numbers of phagocytic inclusions on human retinal pigment epithelial cells in culture: A model for aging. *Br J Ophthalmol*. **70**: 808–815.

Boulton, M., N. M. McKechnie, J. Breda, M. Bayly, and J. Marshall (1989). The formation of autofluorescent granules in cultured human RPE. *Invest Ophthalmol Vis Sci*. **30**: 82–89.

Boulton, M., P. Moriarty, J. Jarvis-Evans, and B. Marcyniuk (1994). Regional variation and age-related changes of lysosomal enzymes in the human retinal pigment epithelium. *Br J Ophthalmol*. **78**: 125–129.

Boulton, M., M. Rozanowska, B. Rozanowski, and T. Wess (2004). The photoreactivity of ocular lipofuscin. *Photochem Photobiol Sci*. **3**: 759–764.

Brahimi-Horn, M. C., J. Chiche, and J. Pouysségur (2007). Hypoxia signalling controls metabolic demand. *Curr Opin Cell Biol*. **19**: 223–229.

Brahimi-Horn, M. C. and J. Pouyssegur (2005). The hypoxia-inducible factor and tumor progression along the angiogenic pathway. *Int Rev Cytol*. **242**: 157–213.

Bressler, N. M. (2009a). Antiangiogenic approaches to age-related macular degeneration today. *Ophthalmology* **116**(10 Suppl): S15–S23.

Bressler, S. B. (2009b). Introduction: Understanding the role of angiogenesis and antiangiogenic agents in age-related macular degeneration. *Ophthalmology* **116**(10 Suppl): S1–S7.

Brownlee, M. (1992). Glycation products and the pathogenesis of diabetic complications. *Diabetes Care* **15**: 1835–1843.

Brownlee, M. (1995). Advanced protein glycosylation in diabetes and aging. *Annu Rev Med*. **46**: 223–234.

Brownlee, M. (2001). Biochemistry and molecular cell biology of diabetic complications. *Nature* **414**: 813–820.

Brownlee, M. (2005). The pathobiology of diabetic complications: A unifying mechanism. Diabetes **54**: 1615–1625.

Brune, B. and J. Zhou (2007). Nitric oxide and superoxide: Interference with hypoxic signaling. *Cardiovasc. Res*. **75**: 275–282.

Burg, M. B. and P. F. Kador (1988). Sorbitol, osmoregulation, and the complications of diabetes. *J Clin Invest*. **81**: 635–640.

Busik, J. V., S. Mohr, and M. B. Grant (2008). Hyperglycemia-induced reactive oxygen species toxicity to endothelial cells is dependent on paracrine mediators. *Diabetes* **57**: 1952–1965.

Buyken, A. E., V. Flood, M. Empson, E. Rochtchina, A. W. Barclay, J. Brand-Miller, and P. Mitchell (2010). Carbohydrate nutrition and inflammatory disease mortality in older adults. *Am J Clin Nutr*. **92**: 634–643.

Cai, J., K. C. Nelson, M. Wu, P. J. Sternberg, and D. P. Jones (2000). Oxidative damage and protection of the RPE. *Prog Retin Eye Res*. **19**: 205–221.

Chang, M. L., C. J. Chiu, F. Shang, and A. Taylor (2014). High glucose activates ChREBP-mediated HIF-1α and VEGF expression in human RPE Cells under normoxia. *Adv Exp Med Biol*. **801**: 609–621.

Charonis, A. S., L. A. Reger, J. E. Dege, K. Kouzi-Koliakos, L. T. Furcht, R. M. Wohlhueter, and E. C. Tsilibary (1990). Laminin alterations after in vitro nonenzymatic glycosylation. *Diabetes* **39**: 807–814.

Chen, X., S. S. Rong, Q. Xu, F. Y. Tang, Y. Liu, H. Gu et al. (2014). Diabetes mellitus and risk of age-related macular degeneration: A systematic review and meta-analysis. *PLoS One*. **9**(9): e108196.

Cherepanoff, S., P. G. McMenamin, M. C. Gillies, E. Kettle, and S. H. Sarks (2009). Bruch's membrane and choroidal macrophages in early and advanced age-related macular degeneration. *Br J Ophthalmol*. [Epub ahead of print].

Chiarelli, F., M. de Martino, A. Mezzetti, M. Catino, G. Morgese, F. Cuccurullo, and A. Verrotti (1999). Advanced glycation end products in children and adolescents with diabetes: Relation to glycemic control and early microvascular complications. *J Pediatr.* **134**: 486–491.

Chibber, R., P. A. Molinatti, N. Rosatto, B. Lambourne, and E. M. Kohner (1997). Toxic action of advanced glycation end products on cultured retinal capillary pericytes and endothelial cells: Relevance to diabetic retinopathy. *Diabetologia* **40**: 156–164.

Chiu, C. J., L. D. Hubbard, J. Armstrong, G. Rogers, P. F. Jacques, J. L. T. Chylack et al. (2006a). Dietary glycemic index and carbohydrate in relation to early age-related macular degeneration. *Am J Clin Nutr.* **83**(4): 880-886.

Chiu, C. J., R. Klein, R. C. Milton, G. Gensler, and A. Taylor (2009a). Does eating particular diets alter risk of age-related macular degeneration in users of the Age-Related Eye Disease Study supplements? *Br J Ophthalmol.* **93**(9): 1241–1246.

Chiu, C. J., S. Liu, W. C. Willett, T. M. S. Wolever, J. C. Brand-Miller, A. W. Barclay, and A. Taylor (2011). Informing food choices and health outcomes by use of the dietary glycemic index. *Nutrition Reviews* **69**: 231–242.

Chiu, C. J., R. C. Milton, G. Gensler, and A. Taylor (2006b). Dietary carbohydrate and glycemic index in relation to cortical and nuclear lens opacities in the Age-Related Eye Disease Study. *Am J Clin Nutr* **83**(5): 1177–1184.

Chiu, C. J., R. C. Milton, G. Gensler, and A. Taylor (2007a). Association between dietary glycemic index and age-related macular degeneration in nondiabetic participants in the Age-Related Eye Disease Study. *Am J Clin Nutr.* **86**(1): 180–188.

Chiu, C. J., R. C. Milton, R. Klein, G. Gensler, and A. Taylor (2007b). Dietary carbohydrate and progression of age-related macular degeneration, a prospective study from the Age-Related Eye Disease Study. *Am J Clin Nutr* **86**(4): 1210–1218.

Chiu, C. J., R. C. Milton, R. Klein, G. Gensler, and A. Taylor (2009b). Dietary compound score and risk of age-related macular degeneration in the Age-Related Eye Disease Study. *Ophthalmology.* **116**(5): 939–946.

Chiu, C. J., M. S. Morris, G. Rogers, P. F. Jacques, L. T. J. Chylack, W. Tung et al. (2005). Carbohydrate intake and glycemic index in relation to the odds of early cortical and nuclear lens opacities. *Am J Clin Nutr* **81**: 1411–1416.

Chiu, C. J., L. Robman, C. A. McCarty, B. N. Mukesh, A. Hodge, H. R. Taylor and A. Taylor (2010). Dietary carbohydrate in relation to cortical and nuclear lens opacities in the Melbourne Visual Impairment Project. *Invest Ophthalmol Vis Sci.* **51**: 2897–2905.

Chiu, C. J. and A. Taylor (2011b). Dietary hyperglycemia, glycemic index and metabolic retinal diseases. *Prog Retin Eye Res.* **30**(1): 18–53.

Chuang, D. M., C. Hough, and Senatorov, V (2005). Glyceraldehyde-3-phosphate dehydrogenase, apoptosis, and neurodegenerative diseases. *Annu Rev Pharmacol Toxicol* **45**: 269–290.

Cingle, K. A., R. S. Kalski, W. E. Bruner, C. M. O'Brien, P. Erhard, and R. E. Wyszynski (1996). Age-related changes of glycosidases in human retinal pigment epithelium. *Curr Eye Res.* **15**: 433–438.

Clarke, M. and P. M. Dodson (2007). PKC inhibition and diabetic microvascular complications. *Best Pract Res Clin Endocrinol Metab.* **21**: 573–586.

Cockman, M. E., N. Masson, D. R. Mole, P. Jaakkola, G. W. Chang, S. C. Clifford et al. (2000). Hypoxia inducible factoralpha binding and ubiquitylation by the von Hippel-Lindau tumor suppressor protein. *J. Biol. Chem.* **275**: 25733–25741.

Coffe, V., R. C. Carbajal, and R. Salceda (2006). Glucose metabolism in rat retinal pigment epithelium. *Neurochem Res.* **31**: 103–108.

Cohen, L. H. and W. K. Noell (1965). *Relationships between visual function and metabolism.* New York, Academic Press.

Craven, P. A., R. K. Studer, J. Felder, S. Phillips, and F. R. DeRubertis (1997). Nitric oxide inhibition of transforming growth factor-beta and collagen synthesis in mesangial cells. *Diabetes* **46**: 671–681.

Crider, J. Y., T. Yorio, N. A. Sharif, and B. W. Griffin (1997). The effects of elevated glucose on Na+/K(+)-ATPase of cultured bovine retinal pigment epithelial cells measured by a new nonradioactive rubidium uptake assay. *J Ocul Pharmacol Ther.* **13**: 337–352.

D'Souza, Y. B., C. J. Jones and R. E. Bonshek (2009). Comparison of lectin binding of drusen, RPE, Bruch's membrane, and photoreceptors. *Mol Vis.* **15**: 906–911.

D'Amico, D. J. (1994). Diseases of the retina. *N Engl J Med.* **331**: 95–106.

Decanini, A., C. L. Nordgaard, X. Feng, D. A. Ferrington, and T. W. Olsen (2007). Changes in select redox proteins of the retinal pigment epithelium in age-related macular degeneration. *Am. J. Ophthalmol.* **143**: 607–615.

Degenhardt, T. P., S. R. Thorpe, and J. W. Baynes (1998). Chemical modification of proteins by methylglyoxal. *Cell Mol Biol.* **44**: 1139–1145.

Dehne, N. and B. Brüne (2009). HIF-1 in the inflammatory microenvironment. *Exp Cell Res.* **315**: 1791–1797.

Delcourt, C., F. Michel, A. Colvez, A. Lacroux, M. Delage, M. H. Vernet, and POLA Study Group (2001). Association of cardiovascular disease and its risk factors with age-related macular degeneration: The POLA study. *Ophthalmic Epidemiol* **8**: 237–249.

Dent, M. T., S. E. Tebbs, A. M. Gonzalez, J. D. Ward, and R. M. Wilson (1991). Neutrophil aldose reductase activity and its association with established diabetic microvasulcar complications. *Diabet Med.* **8**: 439–442.

DeRubertis, F. R. and P. A. Craven (1994). Activation of protein kinase C in glomerular cells in diabetes: Mechanisms and potential links to the pathogenesis of diabetic glomerulopathy. *Diabetes* **43**: 1–8.

Diabetes Control and Complications Trial Research Group (1993a). Hypoglycemia in the diabetes control and complications trial. *Diabetes* **46**: 271–286.

The Diabetes Control and Complications Trial Research Group (1993b). The effect of intensive treatment of diabetes on the development and progression of long-term complications in insulin-dependent diabetes mellitus. *N Engl J Med.* **329**: 977–986.

The Diabetes Control and Complications Trial/Epidemiology of Diabetes Interventions and Complications Research Group (2000). Retinopathy and nephropathy in patients with type 1 diabetes four years after a trial of intensive therapy. *N Engl J Med.* **342**: 381–389.

The Diabetic Retinopathy Clinical Research Network, M. J. Elman, L. P. Aiello, R. W. Beck, N. M. Bressler, S. B. Bressler et al. (2010). Randomized trial evaluating ranibizumab plus prompt or deferred laser or triamcinolone plus prompt laser for diabetic macular edema. *Ophthalmology* **117**: 1064–1077.

Diederen, R. M., C. A. Starnes, B. A. Berkowitz, and B. S. Winkler (2006). Reexamining the hyperglycemic pseudohypoxia hypothesis of diabetic oculopathy. *Invest Ophthalmol Vis Sci.* **47**: 2726–2731.

Doi, T., H. Vlassara, M. Kirstein, Y. Yamada, G. E. Striker, and L. J. Striker (1992). Receptor-specific increase in extracellular matrix production in mouse mesangial cells by advanced glycosylation end products is mediated via platelet-derived growth factor. *Proc Natl Acad Sci USA.* **89**: 2873–2877.

Dolhofer-Bliesener, R., B. Lechner, and K. D. Gerbitz (1996). Possible significance of advanced glycation end products in serum in end-stage renal disease and in late complications of diabetes. *Eur J Clin Chem Clin Biochem.* **34**: 355–361.

Du, X. L., D. Edelstein, S. Dimmeler, Q. Ju, C. Sui, and M. Brownlee (2001). Hyperglycemia inhibits endothelial nitric oxide synthase activity by posttranslational modification at the Akt site. *J Clin Invest.* **108**: 1341–1348.

Du, X. L., D. Edelstein, L. Rossetti, I. G. Fantus, H. Goldberg, F. Ziyadeh et al. (2000). Hyperglycemia-induced mitochondrial superoxide overproduction activates the hexosamine pathway and induces plasminogen activator inhibitor-1 expression by increasing Sp1 glycosylation. *Proc Natl Acad Sci USA.* **97**: 12222–12226.

Du, Y., C. M. Miller, and T. S. Kern (2003). Hyperglycemia increases mitochondrial superoxide in retina and retinal cells. *Free Radic Biol Med.* **35**: 1491–1499.

Edwards, A. O., R. 3rd. Ritter, K. J. Abel, A. Manning, C. Panhuysen, and L. A. Farrer (2005). Complement factor H polymorphism and age-related macular degeneration. *Science* **308**: 421–424.

Ehlermann, P., K. Eggers, A. Bierhaus, P. Most, D. Weichenhan, J. Greten et al. (2006). Increased proinflammatory endothelial response to S100A8/A9 after preactivation through advanced glycation end products. *Cardiovasc Diabetol.* **5**: 6.

Enaida, H., Y. Kabuyama, Y. Oshima, T. Sakamoto, K. Kato, H. Kochi, and Y. Homma (1999). VEGF-dependent signaling in retinal microvascular endothelial cells. *Fukushima J Med Sci.* **45**: 77–91.

Engerman, R. L. and T. S. Kern (1986). Hyperglycemia as a cause of diabetic retinopathy. *Metabolism* **35**: 20–23.

Erickson, K. K., J. M. Sundstrom, and D. A. Antonetti (2007). Vascular permeability in ocular disease and the role of tight junctions. *Angiogenesis.* **10**: 103–117.

Eye Disease Case-Control Study Group (1992). Risk factors for neovascular age-related macular degeneration. *Arch. Ophthalmol.* **110**: 1701–1708.

Fang, I. M., C. H. Yang et al. (2009). Overexpression of integrin alpha6 and beta4 enhances adhesion and proliferation of human retinal pigment epithelial cells on layers of porcine Bruch's membrane. *Exp Eye Res.* **88**: 12–21.

Farboud, B., A. Aotaki-Keen et al. (1999). Development of a polyclonal antibody with broad epitope specificity for advanced glycation endproducts and localization of these epitopes in Bruch's membrane of the aging eye. *Mol Vis.* **5**: 11.

Farkas, T. G., V. Sylvester et al. (1971). The ultrastructure of drusen. *Am J Ophthalmol.* **71**: 1196–1205.

Feener, E. P., P. Xia et al. (1996). Role of protein kinase C in glucose- and angiotensin II-induced plasminogen activator inhibitor expression. *Contrib Nephrol.* **118**: 180–187.

Fiers, W., R. Beyaert et al. (1999). More than one way to die: Apoptosis, necrosis and reactive oxygen damage. *Oncogene* **18**: 7719–7730.

Fong, D. S., L. P. Aiello et al. (2004). Diabetic retinopathy. *Diabetes Care.* **27**: 2540–2553.

Forooghian, F., R. Razavi et al. (2007). Hypoxia-inducible factor expression in human RPE cells. *Br J Ophthalmol.* **91**: 1406–1410.

Foulds, W. S. (1990). The choroid circulation and retinal metabolism. Part 2: An overview. *Eye* **4**: 243–248.

Frank, R. N. (2004). Diabetic retinopathy. *N Engl J Med.* **350**: 48–58.

Fraser-Bell, S., J. Wu et al. (2008). Cardiovascular risk factors and age-related macular degeneration: The Los Angeles Latino Eye study. *Am J Ophthalmol* **145**: 308–316.

Frede, S., U. Berchner-Pfannschmidt et al. (2007). Regulation of hypoxia-inducible factors during inflammation. *Methods Enzymol.* **435**: 405–419.

Frede, S., P. Freitag et al. (2005). The proinflammatory cytokine interleukin 1beta and hypoxia cooperatively induce the expression of adrenomedullin in ovarian carcinoma cells through hypoxia inducible factor 1 activation. *Cancer Res.* **65**: 4690–4697.

Fukumura, D., L. Xu et al. (2001). Hypoxia and acidosis independently up-regulate vascular endothelial growth factor transcription in brain tumors in vivo. *Cancer Res.* **61**: 6020–6024.

Gao, Z. Q., C. Yang, Y. Y. Wang, P. Wang, H. Chen, X. D. Zhang et al. (2008). RAGE upregulation and nuclear factor-kappaB activation associated with ageing rat cardiomyocyte dysfunction. *Gen Physiol Biophys.* **27**: 152–158.

García-Ramírez, M., C. Hernández, and R. Simó (2008). Expression of erythropoietin and its receptor in the human retina: A comparative study of diabetic and nondiabetic subjects. *Diabetes Care.* **31**: 1189–1194.

Gardiner, T. A., H. R. Anderson, and A. W. Stitt (2003). Inhibition of advanced glycation end-products protects against retinal capillary basement membrane expansion during long-term diabetes. *J Pathol.* **201**: 328–333.

Giardino, I., D. Edelstein, and M. Brownlee (1994). Nonenzymatic glycosylation in vitro and in bovine endothelial cells alters basic fibroblast growth factor activity: A model for intracellular glycosylation in diabetes. *J Clin Invest.* **94**: 110–117.

Giugliano, D., A. Ceriello, and K. Esposito (2008). Glucose metabolism and hyperglycemia. *Am J Clin Nutr.* **87**: 217S–222S.

Glenn, J. V., H. Mahaffy, K. Wu, G. Smith, R. Nagai, D. A. Simpson et al. (2009). Advanced glycation end product (AGE) accumulation on Bruch's membrane: Links to age-related RPE dysfunction. *Investig. Ophthalmol. Vis. Sci.* **50**: 441–451.

Glenn, J. V. and A. W. Stitt (2009). The role of advanced glycation end products in retinal ageing and disease. *Biochim Biophys Acta.* **1790**: 1109–1116.

Goldberg, H. J., C. I. Whiteside, and I. G. Fantus (2002). The hexosamine pathway regulates the plasminogen activator inhibitor-1 gene promoter and Sp1 transcriptional activation through protein kinase C-beta I and -delta. *J Biol Chem.* **277**: 33833–33841.

Goldberg, J., G. Flowerdew, E. Smith, J. A. Brody, and M. O. M. Tso (1988). Factors associated with age-related macular degeneration. *Am. J.Epidemiol.* **128**(4633): 700–710.

Goodenough, D. A., J. A. Goliger, and D. L. Paul (1996). Connexins, connexons, and intercellular communication. Annu. Rev. Biochem. **65**: 475–502.

Gottlieb, E. and I. P. Tomlinson (2005). Mitochondrial tumour suppressors: A genetic and biochemical update. *Nat. Rev. Cancer.* **5**: 857–866.

Grimm, C., A. Wenzel, N. Acar, S. Keller, M. Seeliger, and M. Gassmann (2006). Hypoxic preconditioning and erythropoietin protect retinal neurons from degeneration. *Adv Exp Med Biol.* **588**: 119–131.

Grimm, C., A. Wenzel, M. Groszer, H. Mayser, M. Seeliger, M. Samardzija et al. (2002). HIF-1-induced erythropoietin in the hypoxic retina protects against light-induced retinal degeneration. *Nat Med.* **8**: 718–724.

Grune, T., T. Jung, K. Merker, and K. J. Davies (2004). Decreased proteolysis caused by protein aggregates, inclusion bodies, plaques, lipofuscin, ceroid, and "aggresomes" during oxidative stress, aging, and disease. Int J Biochem Cell Biol. **36**: 2519–2530.

Haase, V. H. (2010). The sweet side of HIF. *Kidney Int.* **78**: 10–13.

Hageman, G. S., P. J. Luthert, N. H. Victor Chong, L. V. Johnson, D. H. Anderson, and R. F. Mullins (2001). An integrated hypothesis that considers drusen as biomarkers of immune-mediated processes at the RPE-Bruch's membrane interface in aging and age-related macular degeneration. *Prog Retin Eye Res.* **20**: 705–732.

Hageman, G. S., R. F. Mullins, S. R. Russell, L. V. Johnson, and D. H. Anderson (1999). Vitronectin is a constituent of ocular drusen and the vitronectin gene is expressed in human retinal pigmented epithelial cells. *FASEB J.* **13**: 477–484.

Haines, J. L., M. A. Hauser, S. Schmidt, W. K. Scott, L. M. Olson, P. Gallins et al. (2005). Complement factor H variant increases the risk of age-related macular degeneration. *Science*. **308**: 419–421.

Hammes, H. P. (2005). Pericytes and the pathogenesis of diabetic retinopathy. *Horm Metab Res.* **37** (**Suppl 1**): 39–43.

Hammes, H. P., A. Alt, T. Niwa, J. T. Clausen, R. G. Bretzel, M. Brownlee, and E. D. Schleicher (1999). Differential accumulation of advanced glycation end products in the course of diabetic retinopathy. *Diabetologia*. **42**: 728–736.

Hammes, H. P., M. Brownlee, D. Edelstein, M. Saleck, S. Martin, and K. Federlin (1994). Aminoguanidine inhibits the development of accelerated diabetic retinopathy in the spontaneous hypertensive rat. *Diabetologia*. **37**: 32–35.

Hammes, H. P., X. Du, D. Edelstein, T. Taguchi, T. Matsumura, Q. Ju et al. (2003). Benfotiamine blocks three major pathways of hyperglycemic damage and prevents experimental diabetic retinopathy. *Nat Med.* **9**: 294–299.

Hammes, H. P., H. Hoerauf, A. Alt, E. Schleicher, J. T. Clausen, R. C. Bretzel, and H. Laqua (1999). N(epsilon)(carboxymethyl)lysin and the AGE receptor RAGE colocalize in age-related macular degeneration. *Invest Ophthalmol Vis Sci.* **40**: 1855–1859.

Hammes, H. P., A. Weiss, S. Hess, N. Araki, S. Horiuchi, M. Brownlee, and K. T. Preissner (1996). Modification of vitronectin by advanced glycation alters functional properties in vitro and in the diabetic retina. *Lab. Invest.* **75**: 325–338.

Hammond, E. M. and A. J. Giaccia (2005). The role of p53 in hypoxia-induced apoptosis. *Biochem Biophys Res Commun.* **331**: 718–725.

Handa, J. T. (1998). The advanced glycation endproduct pentosidine induces the expression of PDGF-B in human retinal pigment epithelial cells. *Exp. Eye Res.* **66**: 411–419.

Handa, J. T., A. Matsunaga, A. Aotaki-Keen, G. A. Lutty, and L. M. Hjelmeland (1998). Immunohistochemical evidence for deposition of advanced glycation endproducts (AGEs) in Bruch's membrane and choroid with age. *Invest Ophthalmol Vis Sci.* **39**: S370.

Handa, J. T., N. Verzijl, H. Matsunaga, A. Aotaki-Keen, G. A. Lutty, J. M. te Koppele et al. (1999). Increase in the advanced glycation end product pentosidine in Bruch's membrane with age. *Invest Ophthalmol Vis Sci.* **40**: 775–779.

Hansen, S. H. (2001). The role of taurine in diabetes and the development of diabetic complications. *Diabetes Metab Res Rev.* **17**: 330–346.

Harhaj, N. S. and D. A. Antonetti (2004). Regulation of tight junctions and loss of barrier function in pathophysiology. *Int J Biochem Cell Biol.* **36**: 1206–1237.

Hart, G. W. (1997). Dynamic O-linked glycosylation of nuclear and cytoskeletal proteins. *Annu. Rev. Biochem.* **66**: 315–335.

Hata, Y., S. L. Rook, and L. P. Aiello (1999). Basic fibroblast growth factor induces expression of VEGF receptor KDR through a protein kinase C and p44/p42 mitogen-activated protein kinase-dependent pathway. *Diabetes* **48**: 1145–1155.

Hellwig-Bürgel, T., K. Rutkowski, E. Metzen, J. Fandrey, and W. Jelkmann (1999). Interleukin-1beta and tumor necrosis factor-alpha stimulate DNA binding of hypoxia-inducible factor-1. *Blood* **94**: 1561–1567.

Henkind, P. (1981). Retinal blood vessels. Neovascularisation, collaterals, and shunts. *Trans Ophthalmol Soc N Z.* **33**: 46–50.

Henkind, P. and J. B. Walsh (1980). Retinal vascular anomalies. Pathogenesis, appearance, and history. *Trans Ophthalmol Soc U K.* **100**: 425–433.

Henry, D. N., R. N. Frank, S. R. Hootman, S. E. Rood, C. W. Heilig, and J. V. Busik (2000). Glucose-specific regulation of aldose reductase in human retinal pigment epithelial cells in vitro. *Invest Ophthalmol Vis Sci.* **41**: 1554–1560.

Hoffmann, S., U. Friedrichs, W. Eichler, A. Rosenthal, and P. Wiedemann (2002). Advanced glycation end products induce choroidal endothelial cell proliferation, matrix metalloproteinase-2 and VEGF upregulation in vitro. *Graefes Arch Clin Exp Ophthalmol.* **240**: 996–1002.

Hollyfield, J. G., R. G. Salomon, and J. W. Crabb (2003). Proteomic approaches to understanding age-related macular degeneration. *Adv. Exp Med. Biol.* **533**: 83–89.

Horiuchi, S., T. Higashi, K. Ikeda, T. Saishoji, Y. Jinnouchi, H. Sano et al. (1996). Advanced glycation end products and their recognition by macrophage and macrophage-derived cells. *Diabetes* **45 (Suppl 3)**: S73–S76.

Howes, K. A., Y. Liu, J. L. Dunaief, A. Milam, J. M. Frederick, A. Marks, and W. Baehr (2004). Receptor for advanced glycation end products and age-related macular degeneration. *Invest Ophthalmol Vis Sci.* **45**: 3713–3720.

Huang, L. E., J. Gu, M. Schau, and H. F. Bunn (1998). Regulation of hypoxia-inducible factor 1alpha is mediated by an O2-dependent degradation domain via the ubiquitin-proteasome pathway. *Proc Natl Acad Sci USA.* **95**(14): 7987–7992.

Hyman, L., A. P. Schachat, Q. He, and M. C. Leske (2000). Hypertension, cardiovascular disease, and age-related macular degeneration. Age-Related Macular Degeneration Risk Factors Study Group. *Arch Ophthalmol.* **118**: 351–358.

Ido, Y. and J. R. Williamson (1997). Hyperglycemic cytosolic reductive stress "pseudohypoxia": Implications for diabetic retinopathy. *Invest Ophthalmol Vis Sci.* **38**: 1467–1470.

Ikeda, K., T. Higashi, H. Sano, Y. Jinnouchi, M. Yoshida, T. Araki et al. (1996). N (epsilon)-(carboxymethyl) lysine protein adduct is a major immunological epitope in proteins modified with advanced glycation end products of the Maillard reaction. *Biochemistry.* **35**: 8075–8083.

Ishibashi, T. (2000). Cell biology of intraocular vascular diseases. *Jpn J Ophthalmol.* **44**: 323–324.

Ishibashi, T., T. Murata M. Hangai, R. Nagai, S. Horiuchi, P. F. Lopez et al. (1998). Advanced glycation end products in age related macular degeneration. *Arch. Ophthalmol.* **116**: 1629–1632.

Ishibashi, T., R. Patterson, Y. Ohnishi, H. Inomata, and S. J. Ryan (1986a). Formation of drusen in the human eye. *Am J Ophthalmol.* **101**: 342–353.

Ishibashi, T., N. Sorgente, R. Patterson, and S. J. Ryan (1986b). Pathogenesis of drusen in the primate. *Invest Ophthalmol Vis Sci.* **27**: 184–193.

Ishii, H., M. R. Jirousek, D. Koya, C. Takagi, P. Xia, A. Clermont (1996). Amelioration of vascular dysfunctions in diabetic rats by an oral PKC beta inhibitor. *Science* **272**: 728–731.

Isoe, T., Y. Makino, K. Mizumoto, H. Sakagami, Y. Fujita, J. Honjo et al. (2010). High glucose activates HIF-1-mediated signal transduction in glomerular mesangial cells through a carbohydrate response element binding protein. *Kidney Int.* **78**: 48–59.

Iwai, K., K. Yamanaka, T. Kamura, N. Minato, R. C. Conaway, J. W. Conaway et al. (1999). Identification of the von Hippel-Lindau tumor-suppressor protein as part of an active E3 ubiquitin ligase complex. *Proc. Nat. Acad. Sci., USA.* **96**: 12436–12441.

Iyer, N. V. and S. W. Leung (1998). The human hypoxia-inducible factor 1alpha gene: HIF1A structure and evolutionary conservation. *Genomics* **52**: 159–165.

Januszewski, A. S., N. L. Alderson, T. O. Metz, S. R. Thorpe, and J. W. Baynes (2003). Role of lipids in chemical modification of proteins and development of complications in diabetes. *Biochem. Soc. Trans.* **31**: 1413–1416.

Jardeleza, M. S. and J. W. Miller (2009). Review of anti-VEGF therapy in proliferative diabetic retinopathy. *Semin Ophthalmol.* **24**: 87–92.

Jarrett, S. G., H. Lin, B. J. Godley, and M. E. Boulton (2008). Mitochondrial DNA damage and its potential role in retinal degeneration. *Prog Retin Eye Res.* **27**: 596–607.

Jenkins, D. J. A., C. W. C. Kendall, L. S. A. Augustin, S. Franceschi, M. Hamidi, A. Marchie (2002). Glycemic index: Overview of implications in health and disease. *Am J Clin Nutr* **76 (suppl)**: 266S–273S.

Johnson, P. T., G. P. Lewis, K. C. Talaga, M. N. Brown, P. J. Kappel, S. K. Fisher et al. (2003). Drusen-associated degeneration in the retina. *Invest Ophthalmol Vis Sci.* **44**: 4481–4488.

Joussen, A. M., V. Poulaki, M. L. Le, K. Koizumi, C. Esser, and H. Janicki (2004). A central role for inflammation in the pathogenesis of diabetic retinopathy. *FASEB J* **18**: 1450–1452.

Junk, A. K., A. Mammis, S. I. Savitz, M. Singh, S. Roth, S. Malhotra et al. (2002). Erythropoietin administration protects retinal neurons from acute ischemia-reperfusion injury. *Proc Natl Acad Sci USA.* **99**: 10659–10664.

Justilien, V., J. J. Pang, K. Renganathan, X. Zhan, J. W. Crabb, S. R. Kim et al. (2007). SOD2 knockdown mouse model of early AMD. *Invest. Ophthalmol. Vis. Sci.* **48**: 4407–4420.

Kaarniranta, K. and A. Salminen (2009). Age-relatedmacular degeneration: Activation of innate immunity system via pattern recognition receptors. *J. Mol. Med.* **87**: 117–123.

Kadonaga, J. T., A. J. Courey, J. Ladika, and R. Tjian (1988). Distinct regions of Sp1 modulate DNA binding and transcriptional activation. *Science* **242**: 1566–1570.

Kaelin Jr., W. G. and P. J. Ratcliffe (2008). Oxygen sensing by metazoans: The central role of the HIF hydroxylase pathway. *Mol. Cell.* **30**: 393–402.

Kalfa, T. A., M. E. Gerritsen, E. C. Carlson, A. J. Binstock, and E. C. Tsilibary (1995). Altered proliferation of retinal microvascular cells on glycated matrix. *Invest Ophthalmol Vis Sci.* **36**: 2358–2367.

Kamura, T., S. Sato, K. Iwai, M. Czyzyk-Krzeska, R. C. Conaway, and J. W. Conaway (2000). Activation of HIF1alpha ubiquitination by a reconstituted von Hippel-Lindau (VHL) tumor suppressor complex. *Proc Natl Acad Sci USA* **97**(19): 10430–10435.

Kanwar, M., P. S. Chan, T. s. Kern, and R. A. Kowluru (2007). Oxidative damage in the retinal mitochondria of diabetic mice: Possible protection by superoxide dismutase. *Invest Ophthalmol Vis Sci.* **48**: 3805–3811.

Kanwar, M. and R. A. Kowluru (2009). Role of glyceraldehyde 3-phosphate dehydrogenase in the development and progression of diabetic retinopathy. *Diabetes* **58**: 227–234.

Kasahara, E., L. R. Lin, Y. S. Ho, and V. N. Reddy (2005). SOD2 protects against oxidation-induced apoptosis in mouse retinal pigment epithelium: Implications for age-related macular degeneration. *Invest Ophthalmol Vis Sci.* **46**: 3426–3434.

Kasajima, H. (2000). Enhanced in situ expression of aldose reductase in peripheral nerve and renal glomeruli in diabetic patients. *Virchows Arch.* **439**: 46–54.

Kasper, M., R. Schinzel, T. Niwa, G. Münch, M. Witt, H. Fehrenbach (1999). Experimental induction of AGEs in fetal L132 lung cells changes the level of intracellular cathepsin D. *Biochem. Biophys. Res. Commun.* **261**: 175–182.

Kaur, C., W. S. Foulds, and E. A. Ling (2008). Blood-retinal barrier in hypoxic ischaemic conditions: Basic concepts, clinical features and management. *Prog Retin Eye Res.* **27**: 622–647.

Kaushik, S., J. J. Wang, V. Flood, J. S. Tan, A. W. Barclay, T. Y. Wong et al. (2008). Dietary glycemic index and the risk of age-related macular degeneration. *Am J Clin Nutr.* **88**(4): 1104–1110.

Keogh, R. J., M. E. Dunlop, and R. G. Larkins (1997). Effect of inhibition of aldose reductase on glucose flux, diacylglycerol formation, protein kinase C, and phospholipase A2 activation. *Metabolism* **46**: 41–47.

Kern, T. S., J. Tang, M. Mizutani, R. Kowluru, R. Nagraj, and M. Lorenzi (2000). Response of capillary cell death to aminoguanidine predicts the development of retinopathy: Comparison of diabetes and galactosemia. *Invest Ophthalmol Vis Sci.* **41**: 3972–3978.

Kim, J. W. and C. V. Dang (2006). Cancer's molecular sweet tooth and the Warburg effect. *Cancer Res.* **66**: 8927–8930.

Kim, J. W., I. Tchernyshyov, G. L. Semenza, and C. V. Dang (2006). HIF-1-mediated expression of pyruvate dehydrogenase kinase: A metabolic switch required for cellular adaptation to hypoxia. *Cell Metab* **3**: 177–185.

Kim, W. Y. and W. G. Kaelin (2004). Role of VHL gene mutation in human cancer. *J. Clin. Oncol.* **22**: 4991–5004.

Kim, W. Y., M. Safran, M. R. Buckley, B. L. Ebert, J. Glickman, M. Bosenberg et al. (2006). Failure to prolyl hydroxylate hypoxia-inducible factor a phenocopies VHL inactivation in vivo. *EMBO J.* **25**: 4650–4662.

Kim, Y. S., D. H. Jung, N. H. Kim, Y. M. Lee, D. S. Jang, G. Y. Song, and J. S. Kim (2007). KIOM-79 inhibits high glucose or AGEs-induced VEGF expression in human retinal pigment epithelial cells. *J Ethnopharmacol.* **112**: 166–172.

Kirstein, M., C. Aston, R. Hintz, and H. Vlassara (1992). Receptor-specific induction of insulin-like growth factor I in human monocytes by advanced glycosylation end product-modified proteins. *J Clin Invest.* **90**: 439–446.

Klein, R., B. E. Klein, and S. C. Jeensen (1997). The relationship of cardiovascular disease and its risk factors to the 5-year incidence of age-related maculopathy. The Beaver Dam Eye study. *Ophthalmology* **104**: 1804–1812.

Klein, R., B. E. Klein, and S. E. Moss (1992). Diabetes, hyperglycemia, and age-related maculopathy. The Beaver Dam Eye Study. *Ophthalmology.* **99**: 1527–1534.

Klein, R., S. M. Meuer, M. D. Knudtson, S. K. Iyengar, and B. E. Klein (2008). The epidemiology of retinal reticular drusen. *Am J Ophthalmol* **145**: 317–326.

Klein, R. J., C. Zeiss, E. Y. Chew, J. Y. Tsai, R. S. Sackler, C. Haynes et al. (2005). Complement factor H polymorphism in age-related macular degeneration. *Science* **308**: 385–389.

Kobayashi, S., M. Nomura, T. Nishioka, M. Kikuchi, A. Ishihara, R. Nagai, and N. Hagino (2007). Overproduction of N(epsilon)-(carboxymethyl)lysine-induced neovascularization in cultured choroidal explant of aged rat. *Biol. Pharm. Bull.* **30**: 133–138.

Kociok, N., H. Heppekausen, U. Schraermeyer, P. Esser, G. Thumann, G. Gristanti, and K. Heimann (1998). The mRNA expression of cytokines and their receptors in cultured iris pigment epithelial cells: A comparison with retinal pigment epithelial cells. *Exp. Eye Res.* **67**: 237–250.

Kohner, E. M., S. J. Aldington, I. M. Stratton, S. E. Manley, R. R. Holman, D. R. Matthews, and R. C. Turner (1998). United Kingdom Prospective Diabetes Study, 30: Diabetic retinopathy at diagnosis of non-insulin-dependent diabetes mellitus and associated risk factors. *Arch Ophthalmol.* **116**: 297–303.

Kohner, E. M., I. M. Stratton, S. J. Aldington, R. R. Holman, D. R. Matthews, and UK Prospective Diabetes Study (UKPDS) Group. (2001). Relationship between the severity of retinopathy and progression to photocoagulation in patients with type 2 diabetes mellitus in the UKPDS (UKPDS 52). *Diabet Med.* **18**: 178–184.

Kolm-Litty, V., U. Sauer, A. Nerlich, R. Lehmann, and E. D. Schleicher (1998). High glucose-induced transforming growth factor beta1 production is mediated by the hexosamine pathway in porcine glomerular mesangial cells. *J. Clin. Invest.* **101**: 160–169.

Korolchuk, V. I., F. M. Menzies, and D. C. Rubinsztein (2009). Mechanisms of cross-talk between the ubiquitin-proteasome and autophagy-lysosome systems. *FEBS Lett.* [Epub ahead of print].

Korshunov, S. S., V. P. Skulachev, and A. A. Starkov (1997). High protonic potential actuates a mechanism of production of reactive oxygen species in mitochondria. *FEBS Lett.* **416**: 15–18.

Koukourakis, M. I., A. Giatromanolaki, C. Simopoulos, A. Polychronidis, and E. Sivridis (2005). Lactate dehydrogenase 5 (LDH5) relates to up-regulated hypoxia inducible factor pathway and metastasis in colorectal cancer. *Clin Exp Metastasis.* **22**: 25–30.

Kowluru, R. A. (2005). Diabetic retinopathy: Mitochondrial dysfunction and retinal capillary cell death. *Antioxid Redox Signal.* **7**: 1581–1587.

Koya, D., M. Haneda, H. Nakagawa, K. Isshiki, H. Sato, S. Maeda et al. (2000). Amelioration of accelerated diabetic mesangial expansion by treatment with a PKC beta inhibitor in diabetic db/db mice, a rodent model for type 2 diabetes. *FASEB J.* **14**: 439–447.

Koya, D., M. R. Jirousek, Y .W. Lin, H. Ishii, K. Kuboki, and G. L. King (1997). Characterization of protein kinase C beta isoform activation on the gene expression of transforming growth factor-beta, extracellular matrix components, and prostanoids in the glomeruli of diabetic rats. *J Clin Invest.* **100**: 115–126.

Koya, D. and G. L. King (1998). Protein kinase C activation and the development of diabetic complications. *Diabetes* **47**: 859–866.

Kuboki, K., Z. Y. Jiang, N. Takahara, S. W. Ha, M. Igarashi, T. Yamauchi et al. (2000). Regulation of endothelial constitutive nitric oxide synthase gene expression in endothelial cells and in vivo: A specific vascular action of insulin. *Circulation* **101**: 676–681.

Kuhla, B., H. J. Lüth, D. Haferburg, K. Boeck, T. Arendt, and G. Münch (2005). Methylglyoxal, glyoxal, and their detoxification in Alzheimer's disease. *Ann N Y Acad Sci.* **1043**: 211–216.

Kunt, T., T. Forst, O. Harzer, G. Buchert, A. Pfützner, M. Löbig et al. (1998). The influence of advanced glycation endproducts (AGE) on the expression of human endothelial adhesion molecules. *Exp Clin Endocrinol Diabetes* **106**: 183–188.

Kusner, L. L., V. P. Sarthy, and S. Mohr (2004). Nuclear translocation of glyceraldehyde-3-phosphate dehydrogenase: A role in high glucose-induced apoptosis in retinal Müller cells. *Invest Ophthalmol Vis Sci.* **45**: 1553–1561.

Lal, S., B. S. Szwergold, A. H. Taylor, W. C. Randall, F. Kappler, and K. Wells-Knecht (1995). Metabolism of fructose-3-phosphate in the diabetic rat lens. *Arch. Biochem. Biophys.* **318**(7269): 191–199.

Lambert, I. H. (2004). Regulation of the cellular content of the organic osmolyte taurine in mammalian cells. *Neurochem Res.* **29**(1): 27–63.

Lando, D., D. J. Peet, D. A. Whelan, J. J. Gorman, and M. L. Whitelaw (2002). Asparagine hydroxylation of the HIF transactivation domain a hypoxic switch. Science **295**: 858–861.

Lee, A. Y. and S. S. Chung (1999). Contributions of polyol pathway to oxidative stress in diabetic cataract. *FASEB J.* **13**: 23–30.

Lee, S. H., P. L. Wolf, R. Escudero, R. Deutsch, S. W. Jamieson, and P. A. Thistlethwaite (2000). Early expression of angiogenesis factors in acute myocardial ischemia and infarction. *N Engl J Med.* **342**: 626–633.

Leske, M. C., S. Y. Wu, A. Hennis, B. Nemesure, L. Yang, L. Hyman et al. (2006). Nine-year incidence of age-related macular degeneration in the Barbados Eye Studies. *Ophthalmology* **113**: 29–35.

Li, Y. M. and D. W. Dickson (1997). Enhanced binding of advanced glycation endproducts (AGE) by the ApoE4 isoform links the mechanism of plaque deposition in Alzheimer's disease. *Neurosci. Lett.* **226**: 155–158.

Li, Y. M., T. Mitsuhashi, D. Wojciechowicz, N. Shimizu, J. Li, A. Stitt et al. (1996). Molecular identity and cellular distribution of advanced glycation endproduct receptors: Relationship of p60 to OST-48 and p90 to 80K-H membrane proteins. *Proc Natl Acad Sci USA*. **93**: 11047–11052.

Lipton, S. A. (2004). Erythropoietin for neurologic protection and diabetic neuropathy. *N Engl J Med.* **350**: 2516–2517.

Lisy, K. and D. J. Peet (2008). Turn me on: Regulating HIF transcriptional activity. *Cell Death Differ* **15**: 642–649.

Lisztwan, J., G. Imbert, C. Wirbelauer, M. Gstaiger, and W. Krek (1999). The von Hippel-Lindau tumor suppressor protein is a component of an E3 ubiquitin-protein ligase activity. *Genes Dev.* **13**(14): 1822–1833.

Lohwasser, C., D. Neureiter, B. Weigle, T. Kirchner, and D. Schuppan (2006). The receptor for advanced glycation end products is highly expressed in the skin and upregulated by advanced glycation end products and tumor necrosis factor-alpha. *J. Invest. Dermatol.* **126**: 291–299.

Lorenzi, M. and C. Gerhardinger (2001). Early cellular and microvascular changes induced by diabetes in the retina. *Diabetologia.* **44**: 791–804.

Louie, J. L., R. J. Kapphahn, and D. A. Ferrington (2002). Proteasome function and protein oxidation in the aged retina. *Exp Eye Res.* **75**: 271–284.

Lu, M., M. Kuroki, S. Amano, M. Tolentino, K. Keough, I. Kim et al. (1998). Advanced glycation end products increase retinal vascular endothelial growth factor expression. *J Clin Invest.* **101**: 1219–1224.

Ludwig, D. S. (2002). The glycemic index: Physiological mechanisms relating to obesity, diabetes, and cardiovascular disease. *JAMA*. **287**: 2414–2423.

Luthra, S., B. Fardin, J. Dong, D. Hertzog, S. Kamjoo, S. Gebremariam et al. (2006). Activation of caspase-8 and caspase-12 pathways by 7-ketocholesterol in human retinal pigment epithelial cells. *Invest Ophthalmol Vis Sci.* **47**: 5569–5575.

Lyons, T. J., G. Silvestri, J. A. Dunn, D. G. Dyer, and J. W. Baynes (1991). Role of glycation in modification of lens crystallins in diabetic and nondiabetic senile cataracts. *Diabetes* **40**: 1010–1015.

Ma, W., S. E. Lee, J. Guo, W. Qu, B. I. Hudson, A. M. Schmidt, and G. R. Barile (2007). RAGE ligand upregulation of VEGF secretion in ARPE-19 cells. *Invest Ophthalmol Vis Sci.* **48**: 1355–1361.

MacKenzie, E. D., M. A. Selak, D. A. Tennant, L. J. Payne, S. Crosby, C. M. Frederiksen et al. (2007). Cell-permeating alpha-ketoglutarate derivatives alleviate pseudohypoxia in succinate dehydrogenase-deficient cells. *Mol Cell Biol.* **27**: 3282–3289.

Madsen-Bouterse, S. A. and R. A. Kowluru (2008). Oxidative stress and diabetic retinopathy: Pathophysiological mechanisms and treatment perspectives. *Rev Endocr Metab Disord* **9**: 315–327.

Maeda, A., J. W. Crabb, and K. Palczewski (2005). Microsomal glutathione S-transferase 1 in the retinal pigment epithelium: Protection against oxidative stress and a potential role in aging. *Biochemistry.* **44**: 480–489.

Mahon, P. C., K. Hirota, and G. L. Semenza (2001). FIH-1, a novel protein that interacts with HIF-1alpha and VHL to mediate repression of HIF-1 transcriptional activity. *Genes Dev.* **15**: 2675–2686.

Malfait, M., P. Gomez, T. A. Van Veen, J. B. Parys, H. De Smedt, J. Vereecke, and B. Himpens (2001). Effects of hyperglycemia and protein kinase C on connexin43 expression in cultured rat retinal pigment epithelial cells. *J Membr Biol.* **181**: 31–40.

Mamputu, J. C. and G. Renier (2004). Advanced glycation end-products increase monocyte adhesion to retinal endothelial cells through vascular endothelial growth factor-induced ICAM-1 expression: Inhibitory effect of antioxidants. *J Leukoc Biol.* **75**: 1062–1069.

Mariathasan, S., K. Newton, D. Monack, D. Vucic, D. French, W. Lee et al. (2004). Differential activation of the inflammasome by caspase-1 adaptors ASC and Ipaf. *Nature* **430**: 213–218.

Masson, E., L. Troncy, D. Ruggiero, N. Wiernsperger, M. Lagarde, and S. El Bawab (2005a). a-Series gangliosides mediate the effects of advanced glycation end products on pericyte and mesangial cell proliferation: A common mediator for retinal and renal microangiopathy? *Diabetes.* **54**: 220–227.

Masson, E., N. Wiernsperger, M. Lagarde, and S. El Bawab (2005b). Involvement of gangliosides in glucosamine-induced proliferation decrease of retinal pericytes. *Glycobiology.* **15**: 585–591.

McFarlane, S., J. V. Glenn, and A. M. Lichanska (2005). Characterisation of the advanced glycation endproduct receptor complex in the retinal pigment epithelium. *Br J Ophthalmol.* **89**: 107–112.

Miceli, M. V., D. A. Newsome, and G. W. Schriver (1990). Glucose uptake, hexose monophosphate shunt activity, and oxygen consumption in cultured human retinal pigment epithelial cells. *Invest Ophthalmol Vis Sci.* **31**: 277–283.

Mitchell, P. and J. J. Wang (1999). Diabetes, fasting blood glucose and age-related maculopathy: The Blue Mountains Eye Study. *Aust N Z J Ophthalmol.* **27**: 197–199.

Miyamoto, K. and Y. Ogura (1999). Pathogenetic potential of leukocytes in diabetic retinopathy. *Semin Ophthalmol.* **14**: 233–239.

Miyata, S., B. F. Liu, H. Shoda, T. Ohara, H. Yamada, K. Suzuki, and M. Kasuga (1997). Accumulation of pyrraline-modified albumin in phagocytes due to reduced degradation by lysosomal enzymes. *J. Biol. Chem.* **272**: 4037–4042.

Miyata, T., C. van Ypersele de Strihou, T. Imasawa, A. Yoshino, Y. Ueda, H. Ogura et al. (2001). Glyoxalase I deficiency is associated with an unusual level of advanced glycation end products in a hemodialysis patient. *Kidney Int.* **60**: 2351–2359.

Mizutani, M., T. S. Kern, and M. Lorenzi (1996). Accelerated death of retinal microvascular cells in human and experimental diabetic retinopathy. *J Clin Invest.* **97**: 2883–2890.

Mohr, S. (2004). Potential new strategies to prevent the development of diabetic retinopathy. *Expert Opin Investig Drugs.* **13**: 189–198.

Mohr, S., X. Xi, J. Tang, and T. S. Kern (2002). Caspase activation in retinas of diabetic and galactosemic mice and diabetic patients.. Diabetes **51**: 1172–1179.

Monnier, V. M., D. R. Sell, R. H. Nagaraj, S. Miyata, S. Grandhee, P. Odetti, and S. Ibrahim (1992). Maillard reaction-mediated molecular damage to extracellular matrix and other tissue proteins in diabetes, aging, and uremia. Diabetes. **41 (Suppl 2)**: 36–41.

Moore, D. J. and G. M. Clover (2001). The effect of age on the macromolecular permeability of human Bruch's membrane. *Invest Ophthalmol Vis Sci.* **42**: 2970-2975.

Moore, D. J., A. A. Hussain, and J. Marshall (1995). Age-related variation in the hydraulic conductivity of Bruch's membrane. *Invest. Ophthalmol. Vis. Sci.* **36**: 1290–1297.

Moore, T. C., J. E. Moore, Y. Kaji, N. Frizzell, T. Usui, V. Poulaki et al. (2003). The role of advanced glycation end products in retinal microvascular leukostasis. *Invest Ophthalmol Vis Sci.* **44**: 4457–4464.

Morcos, M., X. Du, F. Pfisterer, H. Hutter, A. A. Sayed, P. Thornalley et al. (2008). Glyoxalase-1 prevents mitochondrial protein modification and enhances lifespan in Caenorhabditis elegans. *Aging Cell.* **7**: 260–269.

Mousa, S. A., W. Lorelli, and P. A. Campochiaro (1999). Role of hypoxia and extracellular matrix-integrin binding in the modulation of angiogenic growth factors secretion by retinal pigmented epithelial cells. *J. Cell. Biochem.* **74**: 135–143.

Mowat, F. M., U. F. Luhmann, A. J. Smith, C. Lange, Y. Duran, S. Harten et al. (2010). HIF-1alpha and HIF-2alpha are differentially activated in distinct cell populations in retinal ischaemia. *PLoS One.* **5**: e11103.

Mulder, D. J., M. Bieze, R. Graaff, A. Smit, and A. Hooymans (2010). Skin autofluorescence is elevated in neovascular age-related macular degeneration. Br J Ophthalmol. **94**: 622–625.

Mulhern, M. L., C. J. Madson, P. F. Kador, J. Randazzo, and T. Shinohara (2007). Cellular osmolytes reduce lens epithelial cell death and alleviate cataract formation in galactosemic rats. *Mol Vis.* **13**: 1397–1405.

Mullins, R. F., S. R. Russell, D. H. Anderson, and G. S. Hageman (2000). Drusen associated with aging and age-related macular degeneration contain proteins common to extracellular deposits associated with atherosclerosis, elastosis, amyloidosis, and dense deposit disease. *Faseb J.* **14**(7): 835–846.

Murata, T., R. Nagai, T. Ishibashi, H. Inomuta, K. Ikeda, and S. Horiuchi (1997). The relationship between accumulation of advanced glycation end products and expression of vascular endothelial growth factor in human diabetic retinas. *Diabetologia.* **40**: 764–769.

Nakashima, E., R. Pop-Busui, R. Towns, T. P. Thomas, Y. Hosaka, J. Nakamura et al. (2005). Regulation of the human taurine transporter by oxidative stress in retinal pigment epithelial cells stably transformed to overexpress aldose reductase. *Antioxid Redox Signal.* **7**: 1530–1542.

Neeper, M., A. M. Schmidt, J. Brett, S. D. Yan, F. Wang, Y. C. Pan et al. (1992). Cloning and expression of a cell surface receptor for advanced glycosylation end products of proteins. *J Biol Chem.* **267**: 14998–15004.

Nishikawa, T. and E. Araki (2008). Investigation of a novel mechanism of diabetic complications: Impacts of mitochondrial reactive oxygen species. *Rinsho Byori.* **56**: 712–719.

Nishikawa, T., D. Edelstein, X. L. Du, S. Yamagishi, T. Matsumura, Y. Kaneda et al. (2000). Normalizing mitochondrial superoxide production blocks three pathways of hyperglycaemic damage. *Nature.* **404**: 787–790.

Node, K. and T. Inouc (2009). Postprandial hyperglycemia as an etiological factor in vascular failure. *Cardiovasc Diabetol.* **8**: 23.

Nyengaard, J. R., Y. Ido, C. Kilo, and J. R. Williamson (2004). Interactions between hyperglycemia and hypoxia: Implications for diabetic retinopathy. *Diabetes* **53**: 2931–2938.

Obrosova, I. G., L. Fathallah, and M. J. Stevens (2001). Taurine counteracts oxidative stress and nerve growth factor deficit in early experimental diabetic neuropathy. *Exp Neurol.* **172**: 211–219.

Ohgami, N., R. Nagai, M. Ikemoto, H. Arai, A. Miyazaki, H. Hakamata et al. (2002). CD36, serves as a receptor for advanced glycation endproducts (AGE). *J Diabetes Complications*. **16**: 56–59.

Ohh, M., C. W. Park, M. Ivan, M. A. Hoffman, T. Y. Kim, L. E. Huang et al. (2000). Ubiquitination of hypoxia-inducible factor requires direct binding to the beta-domain of the von Hippel-Lindau protein. *Nature Cell Biol.* **2**: 423–427.

Okubo, A., R. H. J. Rosa, C. V. Bunce, R. A. Alexander, J. T. Fan, A. C. Bird, and P. J. Luthert (1999). The relationships of age changes in retinal pigment epithelium and Bruch's membrane. *Invest. Ophthalmol. Vis. Sci.* **40**: 443–449.

Okubo, A., M. Sameshima, K. Unoki, F. Uehara, and A. C. Bird (2000). Ultrastructural changes associated with accumulation of inclusion bodies in rat retinal pigment epithelium. *Invest. Ophthalmol. Vis. Sci.* **41**: 4305–4312.

Ola, M. S., D. A. Berkich, Y. Xu, M. T. King, T. W. Gardner, I. Simpson, and K. F. LaNoue (2006). Analysis of glucose metabolism in diabetic rat retinas. *Am J Physiol Endocrinol Metab.* **290**: E1057–E1067.

Ono, Y., S. Aoki, K. Ohnishi, T. Yasuda, K. Kawano, and Y. Tsukada (1998). Increased serum levels of advanced glycation end-products and diabetic complications. *Diabetes Res Clin Pract.* **41**: 131–137.

Onorato, J. M., A. J. Jenkins, S. R. Thorpe, and J. W. Baynes (2000). Pyridoxamine, an inhibitor of advanced glycation reactions, also inhibits advanced lipoxidation reactions. Mechanism of action of pyridoxamine. *J Biol Chem.* **275**: 21177–21184.

Osborne, N. N., R. J. Casson, J. P. Wood, G. Chidlow, M. Graham, and J. Melena (2004). Retinal ischemia: Mechanisms of damage and potential therapeutic strategies. *Prog Retin Eye Res.* **23**: 91–147.

Paget, C., M. Lecomte, D. Ruggiero, N. Wiernsperger, and M. Lagarde (1998). Modification of enzymatic antioxidants in retinal microvascular cells by glucose or advanced glycation end products. *Free Radic Biol Med.* **25**: 121–129.

Papandreou, I., R. A. Cairns, L. Fontana, A. L. Lim, and N. C. Denko (2006). HIF-1 mediates adaptation to hypoxia by actively downregulating mitochondrial oxygen consumption. *Cell Metab.* **3**: 187–197.

Park, E. J., D. Kong, R. Fisher, J. Cardellina, R. H. Shoemaker, and G. Melillo (2006). Targeting the PAS-A domain of HIF-1alpha for development of small molecule inhibitors of HIF-1. *Cell Cycle.* **5**: 1847–1853.

Park, Y. K., D. R. Ahn, M. Oh, T. Lee, E. G. Yang, M. Son, and H. Park (2008). Nitric oxide donor, (+/−)-S-nitroso-N-acetylpenicillamine, stabilizes transactive hypoxia-inducible factor-1alpha by inhibiting von Hippel–Lindau recruitment and asparagine hydroxylation. *Mol. Pharmacol.* **74** 236–245.

Pascuzzo, G. J., J. E. Johnson, and E. L. Pautler (1980). Glucose transport in isolated mammalian pigment epithelium. *Exp. Eye Res.* **30**: 53–58.

Pawlak, A. M., J. V. Glenn, J. R. Beattie, J. J. McGarvey, and A. W. Stitt (2008). Advanced glycation as a basis for understanding retinal aging and noninvasive risk prediction. *Ann N Y Acad Sci.* **1126**: 59–65.

Pearl, L. H., C. Prodromou, and P. Workman (2008). The Hsp90 molecular chaperone: An open and shut case for treatment. *Biochem. J.* **410**: 439–453.

Pichiule, P., J. C. Chavez, L. Beyer, and M. J. Stevens (2007). Hypoxia-inducible factor-1 mediates neuronal expression of the receptor for advanced glycation end products following hypoxia/ischemia. *J Biol Chem.* **282**: 36330–36340.

Pop-Busui, R., C. Van Huysen et al. (1999). Attenuation of nerve vascular and functional deficits by taurine in the streptozotocin-diabetic rat. *Diabetes* **47**: A229.

Portilla, D., G. Dai, J. M. Peters, F. J. Gonzalez, M. D. Crew, and A. D. Proia (2000). Etomoxir -induced PPARalpha-modulated enzymes protect during acute renal failure. *Am J Physiol Renal Physiol.* **278**: F667–F675.

Pouyssegur, J. and F. Mechta-Grigoriou (2006). Redox regulation of the hypoxia-inducible factor. *Biol Chem.* **387**: 1337–1346.

Prow, T. W., I. Bhutto, R. Grebe, K. Uno, C. Merges, D. S. McLeod, and G. A. Lutty (2008). Nanoparticle-delivered biosensor for reactive oxygen species in diabetes. *Vision Res.* **48**: 478–485.

Pugliese, G., F. Pricci, C. Iacobini, G. Leto, L. Amadio, P. Barsotti et al. (2001). Accelerated diabetic glomerulopathy in galectin-3/AGE receptor 3 knockout mice. *FASEB J.* **15**: 2471–2479.

Queisser, M. A., D. Yao, S. Geisler, H. P. Hammes, G. Lochnit, E. D. Schleicher et al. (2010). Hyperglycemia impairs proteasome function by methylglyoxal. *Diabetes.* **59**: 670–678.

Rakoczy, P. E., M. Baines, C. J. Kennedy, and I. J. Constable (1996). Correlation between autofluorescent debris accumulation and the presence of partially processed forms of cathepsin D in cultured retinal pigment epithelial cells challenged with rod outer segments. *Exp. Eye Res.* **63**: 159–167.

Ramana, K. V., B. Friedrich, R. Tammali, M. B. West, A. Bhatnagar, and S. K. Srivastava (2005). Requirement of aldose reductase for the hyperglycemic activation of protein kinase C and formation of diacylglycerol in vascular smooth muscle cells. *Diabetes* **54**: 818–829.

Ramanathan, A., C. Wang, and S. L. Schreiber (2005). Perturbational profiling of a cell-line model of tumorigenesis by using metabolic measurements. *Proc Natl Acad Sci USA* **102**: 5992–5997.

Rapino, C., G. Bianchi, C. Di Giulio, L. Centurione, M. Cacchio, A. Antonucci, and A. Cataldi (2005). HIF-1alpha cytoplasmic accumulation is associated with cell death in old rat cerebral cortex exposed to intermittent hypoxia. *Aging Cell.* **4**: 177–185.

Reddy, S., J. Bichler, K. J. Wells-Knecht, S. R. Thorpe, and J. W. Baynes (1995). N epsilon-(carboxymethyl) lysine is a dominant advanced glycation end product (AGE) antigen in tissue proteins. *Biochemistry.* **34**(7513): 10872–10878.

Rodriguez-Fontal, M., V. Alfaro, J. B. Kerrison, and E. P. Jablon (2009). Ranibizumab for diabetic retinopathy. *Curr Diabetes Rev.* **5**: 47–51.

Ruggiero-Lopez, D., N. Rellier, M. Lecomte, M. Lagarde, and N. Wiernsperger (1997). Growth modulation of retinal microvascular cells by early and advanced glycation products. *Diabetes Res Clin Pract.* **34**: 135–142.

Rumble, J. R., M. E. Cooper, T. Soulis, A. Cox, L. Wu, S. Youssef et al. (1997). Vascular hypertrophy in experimental diabetes. Role of advanced glycation end products. *J. Clin. Invest.* **99**: 1016–1027.

Ryhänen, T., J. M. Hyttinen, J. Kopitz, K. Rilla, E. Kuusisto, E. Mannermaa et al. (2009). Crosstalk between Hsp70 molecular chaperone, lysosomes and proteasomes in autophagy-mediated proteolysis in human retinal pigment epithelial cells. *J. Cell. Mol. Med.* **13**: 3616–3631.

Saishin, Y., Y. Saishin, K. Takahashi, M. Melia, S. A.Vinores, and P. A. Campochiaro (2003). Inhibition of protein kinase C decreases prostaglandin-induced breakdown of the blood-retinal barrier. *J Cell Physiol.* **195**: 210–219.

Salminen, A. and K. Kaarniranta (2009). Regulation of the aging process by autophagy. *Trends Mol Med.* **15**: 217–224.

Sandau, K. B., J. Zhou, T. Kietzmann, and B. Brune (2001). Regulation of the hypoxia-inducible factor 1alpha by the inflammatory mediators nitric oxide and tumor necrosis factor-alpha in contrast to desferroxamine and phenylarsine oxide. *J. Biol. Chem.* **276**: 39805–39811.

SanGiovanni, J. P. and E. Y. Chew (2005). The role of omega-3 long-chain polyunsaturated fatty acids in health and disease of the retina. *Prog Retin Eye Res.* **24**: 87–138.

SanGiovanni, J. P., E. Y. Chew, E. Agrón, T. E. Clemons, G. Gensler et al. (2008). The relationship of dietary omega-3 long-chain polyunsaturated fatty acid intake with incident age-related macular degeneration: AREDS report no. 23. *Arch Ophthalmol.* **126**: 1274–1279.

Sano, H., R. Nagai, K. Matsumoto, and S. Horiuchi (1999). Receptors for proteins modified by advanced glycation endproducts (AGE)—their functional role in atherosclerosis. *Mech Ageing Dev.* **107**: 333–346.

Sarks, S. H., J. J. Arnold, M. C. Killingsworth, and J. P. Sarks (1999). Early drusen formation in the normal and aging eye and their relation to age related maculopathy: A clinicopathological study. *Br J Ophthalmol.* **83**: 358–368.

Sato, E., F. Mori, S. Igarashi, T. Abiko, M. Takeda, S. Ishiko, and A. Yoshida (2001). Corneal advanced glycation end products increase in patients with proliferative diabetic retinopathy. *Diabetes Care* **24**: 479–482.

Sato, S., L. R. Lin, V. N. Reddy, and P. F. Kador (1993). Aldose reductase in human retinal pigment epithelial cells. *Exp Eye Res.* **57**: 235–241.

Sawa, A., A. A. Khan, L. D. Hester, and S. H. Snyder (1997). Glyceraldehyde-3-phosphate dehydrogenase: Nuclear translocation participates in neuronal and nonneuronal cell death. *Proc Natl Acad Sci USA.* **94**: 11669–11674.

Schalkwijk, C. G., N. Ligtvoet, H. Twaalfhoven, A. Jager, H. G. Blaauwgeers, R. O. Schlingemann et al. (1999). Amadori albumin in type 1 diabetic patients: Correlation with markers of endothelial function, association with diabetic nephropathy, and localization in retinal capillaries. *Diabetes.* **48**: 2446–2453.

Schmidt, A. M., O. Hori, J. Brett, S. D. Yan, J. L. Wautier, and D. Stern (1994). Cellular receptors for advanced glycation end products. Implications for induction of oxidant stress and cellular dysfunction in the pathogenesis of vascular lesions. *Arterioscler Thromb.* **14**: 1521–1528.

Schmidt, A. M., O. Hori, J. X. Chen, J. F. Li, J. Crandall, J. Zhang et al. (1995). Advanced glycation endproducts interacting with their endothelial receptor induce expression of vascular cell adhesion molecule-1 (VCAM-1) in cultured human endothelial cells and in mice: A potential mechanism for the accelerated vasculopathy of diabetes. *J Clin Invest.* **96**: 1395–1403.

Schmidt, A. M., S. D. Yan, S. F. Yan, and D. M. Stern (2000). The biology of the receptor for advanced glycation end products and its ligands. *Biochim Biophys Acta.* **1498**: 99–111.

Schmidtz, H. D. (2001). Reversible nuclear translocation of glyceraldehyde-3-phosphate dehydrogenase upon serum depletion. *Eur J Cell Biol.* **80**: 419–427.

Schofield, C. J. and P. J. Ratcliffe (2004). Oxygen sensing by HIF hydroxylases. *Nat Rev Mol Cell Biol.* **5**: 343–354.

Schutt, F., M. Bergmann, F. G. Holz, and J. Kopitz (2003). Proteins modified by malondialdehyde, 4-hydroxynonenal, or advanced glycation end products in lipofuscin of human retinal pigment epithelium. *Invest Ophthalmol Vis Sci.* **44**: 3663–3668.

Sebeková, K., R. Schinzel, H. Ling, A. Simm, G. Xiang, M. Gekle et al. (1998). Advanced glycated albumin impairs protein degradation in the kidney proximal tubules cell line LLC-PK1. *Cell. Mol. Biol.* **44**: 1051–1060.

Seko, Y., Y. Seko, H. Fujikura, J. Pang, T. Tokoro, and H. Shimokawa (1999.). Induction of vascular endothelial growth factor after application of mechanical stress to retinal pigment epithelium of the rat in vitro. *Invest. Ophthalmol. Vis. Sci.* **40**: 3287–3291.

Sell, D. R., A. Lapolla, P. Odetti, J. Fogarty, and V. M. Monnier (1992). Pentosidine formation in skin correlates with severity of complications in individuals with long-standing IDDM. *Diabetes* **41**: 1286–1292.

Semba, R. D., L. Ferrucci, J. C. Fink, K. Sun, J. Beck, M. Dalal et al. (2009). Advanced glycation end products and their circulating receptors and level of kidney function in older community-dwelling women. *Am J Kidney Dis.* **53**: 51–58.

Semenza, G. L. (2000). HIF-1 and human disease: One highly involved factor. *Genes Dev.* **14**: 1983–1991.

Semenza, G. L. (2003). Targeting HIF-1 for cancer therapy. *Nat. Rev. Cancer.* **3**: 721–732.

Semenza, G. L. and G. L. Wang (1992). A nuclear factor induced by hypoxia via de novo protein synthesis binds to the human erythropoietin gene enhancer at a site required for transcriptional activation. *Mol. Cell. Biol.* **12**: 5447–5454.

Shah, V. O., R. I. Dorin, Y. Sun, M. Braun, and P. G. Zager (1997). Aldose reductase gene expression is increased in diabetic nephropathy. *J Clin Endocrinol Metab.* **82**: 2294–2298.

Sharma, N. K., T. A. Gardiner, and D. B. Archer (1985). A morphologic and autoradiographic study of cell death and regeneration in the retinal microvasculature of normal and diabetic rats. *Am J Ophthalmol.* **100**: 51–60.

Shinohara, M., P. J. Thornalley, I. Giardino, P. Beisswenger, S. R. Thorpe, J. Onorato, and M. Brownlee (1998). Overexpression of glyoxalase-I in bovine endothelial cells inhibits intracellular advanced glycation end-product formation and prevents hyperglycemia-induced increases in macromolecular endocytosis. *J Clin Invest.* **101**: 1142–1147.

Shukla, A., M. Dikshit, and R. C. Srimal (1996). Nitric oxide-dependent blood–brain barrier permeability alteration in the rat brain. *Experientia* **52**: 136–140.

Simó, R. and C. Hernández (2009). Advances in the medical treatment of diabetic retinopathy. *Diabetes Care* **32**: 1556–1562.

Singh, A. and J. M. Stewart (2009). Pathophysiology of diabetic macular edema. *Int Ophthalmol Clin.* **49**: 1–11.

Skolnik, E. Y., Z. Yang, Z. Makita, S. Radoff, M. Kirstein, and H. Vlassara (1991). Human and rat mesangial cell receptors for glucose-modified proteins: Potential role in kidney tissue remodelling and diabetic nephropathy. *J Exp Med.* **174**: 931–939.

Smedsrod, B., J. Melkko, N. Araki, H. Sano, and S. Horiuchi (1997). Advanced glycation end products are eliminated by scavenger-receptor-mediated endocytosis in hepatic sinusoidal kupffer and endothelial cells. *Biochem J.* **322**: 567–573.

Smith, R. T., J. K. Chan, M. Busuoic, V. Sivagnanavel, A. C. Bird, and N. V. Chong (2006). Autofluorescence characteristics of early, atrophic, and high-risk fellow eyes in age-related macular degeneration. *Invest Ophthalmol Vis Sci.* **47**: 5495–5504.

Smith, W., J. Assink, R. Klein, P. Mitchell, C. C. Klaver, B. E. Klein et al. (2001). Risk factors for age-related macular degeneration: Pooled findings from three continents. *Ophthalmology.* **108**: 697–704.

Sone, H., Y. Kawakami, Y. Okuda, S. Kondo, M. Hanatani, H. Suzuki, and K. Yamashita (1996). Vascular endothelial growth factor is induced by long-term high glucose concentration and upregulated by acute glucose deprivation in cultured bovine retinal pigmented epithelial cells. *Biochem. Biophys. Res. Commun.* **221**: 193–198.

Stecyk, J. A., K. O. Stensløkken, A. P. Farrell, and G. E. Nilsson (2004). Maintained cardiac pumping in anoxic Crucian carp. *Science* **306**: 77.

Stevens, M. J., E. L. Feldman, T. P. Thomas, and D. A. Greene (1997a). The pathogenesis of diabetic neuropathy. Clinical Management of Diabetic Neuropathy. A. Veves and P. M. C. Conn. Totowa, NJ, Humana Press: 13–47.

Stevens, M. J., Y. Hosaka, J. A. Masterson, S. M. Jones, T. P. Thomas, and D. D. Larkin (1999). Downregulation of the human taurine transporter by glucose in cultured retinal pigment epithelial cells. *Am J Physiol.* **277**: E760–E771.

Stevens, M. J., D. Larkin, Y. Hosaka, C. Porcellati, T. P. Thomas, J. M. Masterson et al. (1997b). Suppression of endogenous osmoregulatory genes in human retinal pigment epithelial cells transfected to overpress aldose reductase. *Diabetologia.* **40**: A491.

Stitt, A. W. (2001). Advanced glycation: An important pathological event in diabetic and age related ocular disease. *Br J Ophthalmol* **85**(6): 746–753.

Stitt, A. W. (2005). The maillard reaction in eye diseases. *Ann. N.Y. Acad. Sci.* **1043**: 582–597.

Stitt, A. W., T. Bhaduri, C. B. McMullen, T. A. Gardiner, and D. B. Archer (2000). Advanced glycation end products induce blood-retinal barrier dysfunction in normoglycemic rats. *Mol Cell Biol Res Commun.* **3**: 380–388.

Stitt, A. W., C. He, and H. Vlassara (1999). Characterization of the advanced glycation end-product receptor complex in human vascular endothelial cells. *Biochem Biophys Res Commun.* **256**: 549–556.

Stitt, A. W., S. J. Hughes, P. Canning, O. Lynch, O. Cox, N. Frizzell et al. (2004). Substrates modified by advanced glycation end-products cause dysfunction and death in retinal pericytes by reducing survival signals mediated by platelet-derived growth factor. *Diabetologia.* **47**: 1735–1746.

Stitt, A. W., Y. M. Li, T. A. Gardiner, R. Bucala, D. B. Archer, and H. Vlassara (1997). Advanced glycation end products (AGEs) co-localize with AGE receptors in the retinal vasculature of diabetic and of AGE-infused rats. *Am J Pathol.* **150**: 523–531.

Stitt, A. W., C. McGoldrick, A. Rice-McCaldin, D. R. McCance, J. V. Glenn, D. K. Hsu et al. (2005). Impaired retinal angiogenesis in diabetes: Role of advanced glycation end products and galectin-3. *Diabetes.* **54**: 785–794.

Strauss, O. (2005). The retinal pigment epithelium in visual function. *Physiol. Rev.* **85**: 845–881.

Studer, R. K., P. A. Craven, and F. R. Derubertis (1993). Role for protein kinase C in the mediation of increased fibronectin accumulation by mesangial cells grown in high-glucose medium. *Diabetes* **42**: 118–126.

Sugiyama, S., T. Miyata, Y. Ueda, H. Tanaka, K. Maeda, S. Kawashima et al. (1998). Plasma levels of pentosidine in diabetic patients: An advanced glycation end product. *J Am Soc Nephrol.* **9**: 1681–1688.

Sun, X. M. and Y. X. Zhang (2001). Effects of glucose on growth, metabolism and EPO expression in recombinant CHO cell cultures. *Sheng Wu Gong Cheng Xue Bao* **17**: 698–702.

Suzuma, K., K. Naruse, I. Suzuma, N. Takahara, K. Ueki, L. P. Aiello, and G. L. King (2000). Vascular endothelial growth factor induces expression of connective tissue growth factor via KDR, Flt1, and phosphatidylinositol 3-kinase-akt-dependent pathways in retinal vascular cells. *J. Biol. Chem.* **275**: 40725–40731.

Swamy-Mruthinti, S., K. C. Miriam, S. K. Kumar, J. Biswas, S. Ramakrishnan, R. H. Nagaraj, and K. N. Sulochana (2002). Immunolocalization and quantification of advanced glycation end products in retinal neovascular membranes and serum: A possible role in ocular neovascularization. *Curr. Eye Res.* **25**: 139–145.

Szweda, P. A., M. Camouse, K. C. Lundberg, T. D. Oberley, and L. I. Szweda (2003). Aging, lipofuscin formation, and free radical-mediated inhibition of cellular proteolytic systems. *Ageing Res Rev.* **2**: 383–405.

Tabaton, M., G. Perry, M. Smith, M. Vitek, G. Angelini, D. Dapino et al. (1997). Is amyloid beta-protein glycated in Alzheimer's disease? *Neuroreport.* **8**: 907–909.

Takahashi, A., A. Masuda, M. Sun, V. E. Centonze, and B. Herman (2004). Oxidative stress-induced apoptosis is associated with alterations in mitochondrial caspase activity and Bcl-2-dependent alterations in mitochondrial pH (pHm). *Brain Res Bull.* **62**: 497–504.

Takeuchi, M. and S. Yamagishi (2008). Possible involvement of advanced glycation endproducts (AGEs) in the pathogenesis of Alzheimer's disease. *Curr. Pharm. Des.* **14**: 973–978.

Tan, J. S., P. Mitchell, W. Smith, and J. J. Wang (2007). Cardiovascular risk factors and the long-term incidence of age-related macular degeneration: The Blue Mountains Eye Study. *Ophthalmology.* **114**: 1143–1150.

Tanimoto, K., Y. Makino, T. Pereira, and L. Poellinger (2000). Mechanism of regulation of the hypoxia-inducible factor 1alpha by the von Hippel-Lindau tumor suppressor protein. *EMBO J.* **19**: 4298–4309.

Taylor, C. T. (2008). Interdependent roles for hypoxia inducible factor and nuclear factor-kB in hypoxic inflammation. *J. Physiol.* **586**: 4055–4059.

Terman, A., B. Gustafsson, and U. T. Brunk (2007). Autophagy, organelles and ageing. *J Pathol.* **211**: 134–143.

Tessier, F., M. Obrenovich, and V. M. Monnier (1999). Structure and mechanism of formation of human lens fluorophore LM-1. Relationship to vesperlysine A and the advanced maillard reaction in aging, diabetes, and cataractogenesis. *J Biol Chem.* **274**: 20796–20804.

Thangarajah, H., I. N. Vial, R. H. Grogan, D. Yao, Y. Shi et al. (2010). HIF-1alpha dysfunction in diabetes. *Cell Cycle* **9**: 75–79.

Thangarajah, H., D. Yao, E. I. Chang, Y. Shi, L. Jazayeri, I. N. Vial et al. (2009). The molecular basis for impaired hypoxia-induced VEGF expression in diabetic tissues. *Proc Natl Acad Sci USA.* **106**: 13505–13510.

Thiel, V. E. and K. L. Audus (2001). Nitric oxide and blood–brain barrier integrity. *Antioxid. Redox Signal.* **3**: 273–278.

Thomas, D. D., L. A. Ridnour, J. S. Isenberg, W. Flores-Santana, C. H. Switzer et al. (2008). The chemical biology of nitric oxide: Implications in cellular signaling. *Free Radic. Biol. Med.* **45**: 18–31.

Thornalley, P. J. (1993). The glyoxalase system in health and disease. *Mol Aspects Med.* **14**: 287–371.

Thornalley, P. J. (2003). Protecting the genome: Defence against nucleotide glycation and emerging role of glyoxalase I overexpression in multidrug resistance in cancer chemotherapy. *Biochem Soc Trans.* **31(Pt 6)**: 1372–1377.

Thornalley, P. J., A. Langborg, and H. S. Minhas (1999). Formation of glyoxal, methylglyoxal and 3-deoxyglucosone in the glycation of proteins by glucose. *Biochem J.* **344** (**Pt 1**): 109–116.

Thorpe, S. R. and J. W. Baynes (2003). Maillard reaction products in tissue proteins: New products and new perspectives. *Amino Acids* **25**: 275–281.

To, C. H., K. K. Cheung, S. H. Chiu, H. M. Lai, and K.S. Lung (1998). The saturation characteristics of glucose transport in bovine retinal pigment epithelium. *Yan Ke Xue Bao.* **14**: 126–129.

Tomany, S. C., J. J. Wang, R. van Leeuwen, R. Klein, P. Mitchell, J. R. Vingerling et al. (2004). Risk factors for incident age-related macular degeneration: Pooled findings from 3 continents. *Ophthalmology.* **111**: 1280–1287.

Topouzis, F., E. Anastasopoulos, C. Augood, G. C Bentham, U. Chakravarthy, P.T. de Jong et al. (2009). Association of diabetes with age-related macular degeneration in the EUREYE study. *Br J Ophthalmol.* **93**: 1037–1041.

Treins, C., S. Giorgetti-Peraldi, J. Murdaca, and E. Van Obberghen (2001). Regulation of vascular endothelial growth factor expression by advanced glycation end products. *J Biol Chem.* **276**: 43836–43841.

Trumpower, B. L. (1990). The protonmotive Q cycle: Energy transduction by coupling of proton translocation to electron transfer by the cytochrome bc1 complex. *J Biol Chem.* **265**: 11409–11412.

Uchiki, T., K. A. Weikel, W. Jiao, F. Shang, A. Caceres, D. Pawlak, and A. Taylor (2011). Glycation-altered proteolysis as a pathobiologic mechanism that links dietary glycemic index, aging, and age-related disease (in nondiabetics). *Aging Cell.* [Epub ahead of print].

UK Prospective Diabetes Study (UKPDS) Group (1991). UK Prospective Diabetes Study (UKPDS). VIII. Study design, progress and performance. *Diabetologia.* **34**: 877–890.

UK Prospective Diabetes Study Group (1998). Effect of intensive blood-glucose control with metformin on complications in overweight patients with type 2 diabetes (UKPDS 34). *Lancet* **352**: 854–865.

Uyeda, K., H. Yamashita, and T. Kawaguchi (2002). Carbohydrate responsive element-binding protein (ChREBP): A key regulator of glucose metabolism and fat storage. Biochem Pharmacol. **63**: 2075–2080.

van Uden, P., N. S. Kenneth, and S. Rocha (2008). Regulation of hypoxia-inducible factor-1alpha by NF-kappaB. *Biochem. J.* **412**: 477–484.

Vilchis, C. and R. Salceda (1996). Characterization of [3H] deoxy-D-glucose uptake in retina and retinal pigment epithelium of normal and diabetic rats. *Neurochem. Int.* **28**: 213–219.

Vincent, J. A. and S. Mohr (2007). Inhibition of caspase-1/interleukin-1beta signaling prevents degeneration of retinal capillaries in diabetes and galactosemia. *Diabetes* **56**: 224–230.

Vinores, S. A. and P. A. Campochiaro (1989). Prevention or moderation of some ultrastructural changes in the RPE and retina of galactosemic rats by aldose reductase inhibition. *Exp Eye Res.* **49**: 495–510.

Vinores, S. A., P. A. Campochiaro, E. H. Williams, E. E. May, W. R. Green, and R. Sorenson (1988). Aldose reductase expression in human diabetic retina and retinal pigment epithelium. *Diabetes.* **37**: 1658–1664.

Vinores, S. A., E. Van Niel, J. L. Swerdloff, and P. A. Campochiaro (1993a). Electron microscopic immunocytochemical demonstration of blood-retinal barrier breakdown in human diabetics and its association with aldose reductase in retinal vascular endothelium and retinal pigment epithelium. *Histochem J.* **25**: 648–663.

Vinores, S. A., E. Van Niel, J. L. Swerdloff, and P. A. Campochiaro (1993b). Electron microscopic immunocytochemical evidence for the mechanism of blood-retinal barrier breakdown in galactosemic rats and its association with aldose reductase expression and inhibition. *Exp. Eye. Res.* **57**: 723–735.

Vlassara, H. (2001). The AGE-receptor in the pathogenesis of diabetic complications. *Diabetes Metab Res Rev.* **17**: 436–443.

Vlassara, H., M. Brownlee, K. R. Manogue, C. A. Dinarello, and A. Pasagian (1988). Cachectin/TNF and IL-1 induced by glucose-modified proteins: Role in normal tissue remodeling. *Science* **240**: 1546–1548.

Vlassara, H., Y. M. Li, F. Imani, D. Wojciechowicz, Z. Yang, F. T. Liu, and A. Cerami (1995). Identification of galectin-3 as a high-affinity binding protein for advanced glycation end products (AGE): A new member of the AGE-receptor complex. *Mol Med.* **1**: 634–646.

Vordermark, D., P. Kraft, A. Katzer, T. Bolling, J. Willner, and M. Flentje (2005). Glucose requirement for hypoxic accumulation of hypoxia-inducible factor-1a (HIF-1a). *Cancer Lett.* **230**: 122–133.

Wagner, Z., I. Wittmann, I. Mazák, R. Schinzel, A. Heidland, R. Kientsch-Engel, and J. Nagy (2001). N(epsilon)-(carboxymethyl)lysine levels in patients with type 2 diabetes: Role of renal function. *Am J Kidney Dis.* **38**: 785–791.

Wallace, D. C. (1992). Diseases of the mitochondrial DNA (Review). *Annu Rev Biochem.* **61**: 1175–1212.

Wang, A. L., T. J. Lukas, M. Yuan, N. Du, M. O. Tso, and A. H. Neufeld (2009a). Autophagy and exosomes in the aged retinal pigment epithelium: Possible relevance to drusen formation and age-related macular degeneration. *PLoS One* **24**: e4160.

Wang, D., D. Malo, and S. Hekimi (2010). Elevated mitochondrial reactive oxygen species generation affects the immune response via hypoxia-inducible factor-1alpha in long-lived Mclk1+/- mouse mutants. *J Immunol.* **184**: 582–590.

Wang, G. L., B. H. Jiang, E. A. Rue, and G. L. Semenza (1995). Hypoxia-inducible factor 1 is a basic-helix-loop-helix-PAS heterodimer regulated by cellular O2 tension. *Proc Natl Acad Sci USA.* **92**: 5510–5514.

Wang, X., G. Wang, and Y. Wang (2009b). Intravitreous vascular endothelial growth factor and hypoxia-inducible factor 1a in patients with proliferative diabetic retinopathy. *Am J Ophthalmol.* **148**: 883–889.

Wang, Z., A. Pandey, and G. W. Hart (2007). Dynamic interplay between O-linked N-acetylglucosaminylation and glycogen synthase kinase-3-dependent phosphorylation. *Mol Cell Proteomics.* **6**: 1365–1379.

Warburg, O. (1956). On the origin of cancer cells. *Science* **123**: 309–314.

Watanabe, D., K. Suzuma, S. Matsui, M. Kurimoto, J. Kiryu, M. Kita, and H. Takagi (2005). Erythropoietin as a retinal angiogenic factor in proliferative diabetic retinopathy. N Engl J Med. **353**: 782–792.

Wautier, J. L. and A. M. Schmidt (2004). Protein glycation: A firm link to endothelial cell dysfunction. Circ. Res. **95**: 233–238.

Weikel, K. A., P. Fitzgerald, F. Shang, M. A. Caceres, Q. Bian, J. T. Handa, and A. Taylor (2012). "Natural history of age-related retinal lesions that precede AMD in mice fed high or low glycemic index diets. *Invest Ophthalmol Vis Sci.* **53**(2): 622–632.

Williams, R., M. Airey, H. Baxter, J. Forrester, T. Kennedy-Martin, and A. Girach (2004). Epidemiology of diabetic retinopathy and macular oedema: A systematic review. *Eye* **18**: 963–983.

Williamson, J. R., K. Chang, M. Frangos, K. S. Hasan, Y. Ido, T. Kawamura, and R. G. Tilton (1993). Hyperglycemic pseudohypoxia and diabetic complications. *Diabetes* **42**: 801–813.

Wilson, T. M., R. Strang, J. Wallace, P. W. Horton, and N. F. Johnson (1973). The measurement of the choroidal blood flow in the rabbit using Krypton-85. *Exp Eye Res.* **16**: 421–425.

Wood, J. P. and N. N. Osborne (2001). The influence of zinc on caspase-3 and DNA breakdown in cultured human retinal pigment epithelial cells. *Arch Ophthalmol.* **119**: 81–88.

Xi, X., L. Gao, D. A. Hatala, D. G. Smith, M. C. Codispoti, B. Gong, and J. Z. Zhang (2005). Chronically elevated glucose-induced apoptosis is mediated by inactivation of Akt in cultured Müller cells. *Biochem Biophys Res Commun.* **326**: 548–553.

Xia, P., T. Inoguchi, T. S. Kern, R. L. Engerman, P. J. Oates, and G. L. King (1994). Characterization of the mechanism for the chronic activation of diacylglycerol-protein kinase C pathway in diabetes and hypergalactosemia. *Diabetes* **43**: 1122–1129.

Xiao, Q., S. Zeng, S. Ling, and M. Lv (2006). Up-regulation of HIF-1alpha and VEGF expression by elevated glucose concentration and hypoxia in cultured human retinal pigment epithelial cells. *J Huazhong Univ Sci Technolog Med Sci.* **26**: 463–465.

Yamada, Y., K. Ishibashi, I. A. Bhutto, J. Tian, G. A. Lutty, and J. T. Handa (2006). The expression of advanced glycation endproduct receptors in rpe cells associated with basal deposits in human maculas. *Exp Eye Res.* **82**: 840–848.

Yamagishi, S., S. Amano, Y. Inagaki, T. Okamoto, K. Koga, N. Sasaki, and Z. Makita (2002). Advanced glycation end products-induced apoptosis and overexpression of vascular endothelial growth factor in bovine retinal pericytes. *Biochem Biophys Res Commun.* **290**: 973–978.

Yamagishi, S., H. Fujimori, H. Yonekura, N. Tanaka, and H. Yamamoto (1999). Advanced glycation endproducts accelerate calcification in microvascular pericytes. *Biochem Biophys Res Commun.* **258**: 353–357.

Yamagishi, S., S. Ueda, T. Matsui, K. Nakamura, and S. Okuda (2008). Role of advanced glycation end products (AGEs) and oxidative stress in diabetic retinopathy. *Curr Pharm Des.* **14**: 962–968.

Yamaguchi, M., N. Nakamura, K. Nakano, Y. Kitagawa, H. Shigeta, G. Hasegawa, and M. Kondo (1998). Immunochemical quantification of crossline as a fluorescent advanced glycation endproduct in erythrocyte membrane proteins from diabetic patients with or without retinopathy. *Diabet Med.* **15**: 458–462.

Yan, S. F., V. D'Agati, A. M. Schmidt, and R. Ramasamy (2007). Receptor for advanced glycation endproducts (RAGE): A formidable force in the pathogenesis of the cardiovascular complications of diabetes & aging. *Curr. Mol. Med.* **7**: 699–710.

Yang, P., J. J. Peairs, R. Tano, N. Zhang, J. Tyrell, and G. J. Jaffe (2007). Caspase-8-mediated apoptosis in human RPE cells. *Invest Ophthalmol Vis Sci.* **48**: 3341–3349.

Yao, D. and M. Brownlee (2010). Hyperglycemia-induced reactive oxygen species increase expression of the receptor for advanced glycation end products (RAGE) and RAGE ligands. *Diabetes* **59**: 249–255.

Yao, Y., M. Guan, X. Q. Zhao, and Y. F. Huang (2003). Downregulation of the pigment epithelium derived factor by hypoxia and elevated glucose concentration in cultured human retinal pigment epithelial cells [Article in Chinese]. *Zhonghua Yi Xue Za Zhi.* **83**: 1989–1992.

Yee Koh, M., T. R. Spivak-Kroizman, and G. Powis (2008). HIF-1 regulation: Not so easy come, easy go. *Trends Biochem Sci.* **33**: 526–534.

Yego, E. C. and S. Mohr (2010). siah-1 Protein is necessary for high glucose-induced glyceraldehyde-3-phosphate dehydrogenase nuclear accumulation and cell death in Muller cells. *J Biol Chem.* **285**: 3181–3190.

Yin, D. (1996). Biochemical basis of lipofuscin, ceroid, and age pigment-like fluorophores. *Free Radic Biol Med.* **21**: 871–888.

Young, R. W. and D. Bok (1969). Participation of the retinal pigment epithelium in the rod outer segment renewal process. *J. Cell Biol.* **42**: 392–403.

Young, T. A., H. Wang, S. Munk, D. S. Hammoudi, D. S. Young, M. S. Mandelcorn, and C. I. Whiteside (2005). Vascular endothelial growth factor expression and secretion by retinal pigment epithelial cells in high glucose and hypoxia is protein kinase C-dependent. *Exp Eye Res.* **80**: 651–662.

Yu, R. K., E. Bieberich, T. Xia and G. Zeng (2004). Regulation of ganglioside biosynthesis in the nervous system. *J Lipid Res.* **45**: 783–793.

Yuan, G., J. Nanduri, S. Khan, G. L. Semenza, and N. R. Prabhakar (2008). Induction of HIF-1alpha expression by intermittent hypoxia: Involvement of NADPH oxidase, Ca2+ signaling, prolyl hydroxylases, and mTOR. *J. Cell. Physiol.* **217**: 674–685.

Zadunaisky, J. A. and K. J. Degnan (1976). Passage of sugars and urea across the isolated retina pigment epithelium of the frog. *Exp. Eye Res.* **23**: 191–196.

Zeng, G. and R. K. Yu (2008). Cloning and transcriptional regulation of genes responsible for synthesis of gangliosides. *Curr Drug Targets.* **9**: 317–324.

Zhang, H., M. Bosch-Marce, L. A. Shimoda, Y.S Tan, J. H. Baek, J. B. Wesley, and G. L. Semenza (2008a). Mitochondrial autophagy is an HIF-1-dependent adaptive metabolic response to hypoxia. *J. Biol. Chem.* **283**: 10892–10903.

Zhang, P., Y. Wang, Y. Hui, D. Hu, H. Wang, J. Zhou, and H. Du (2007). Inhibition of VEGF expression by targeting HIF-1 alpha with small interference RNA in human RPE cells. *Ophthalmologica* **221**: 411–417.

Zhang, X., J. Zhou, A. F. Fernandes, J. R. Sparrow, P. Pereira, A. Taylor, and F. Shang (2008b). The proteasome: A target of oxidative damage in cultured human retina pigment epithelial cells. *Invest Ophthalmol Vis Sci.* **49**: 3622–3630.

Zhou, J., B. Cai, Y. P. Jang, S. Pachydaki, A. M. Schmidt, and J. R. Sparrow (2005). Mechanisms for the induction of HNE- MDA- and AGE-adducts, RAGE and VEGF in retinal pigment epithelial cells. *Exp Eye Res.* **80**: 567–580.

Zhou, J., T. Schmid, and B. Brune (2003). Tumor necrosis factor-alpha causes accumulation of a ubiquitinated form of hypoxia inducible factor-1alpha through a nuclear factor-kappaB-dependent pathway. *Mol. Biol. Cell.* **14**: 2216–2225.

12 Glycemic Index Use on Food Labels

Informed Food Choice or Misuse?

Alan W. Barclay

CONTENTS

12.1 INTRODUCTION

Rates of overweight/obesity, type 2 diabetes, and their sequelae are increasing around the globe in both developed and developing nations (International Diabetes Federation 2011; WHO 2003).

Carbohydrates (sugars, maltodextrins, starches, and fiber) in foods and drinks are associated with the risk of developing these conditions (Hauner et al. 2012). Nutrition Information/Facts are provided either voluntarily or are mandated on the labels of packaged foods in developed and developing nations, and are regulated by government agencies (Food Standards Australia New Zealand 2013). In some nations, the only requirement is information on total carbohydrates per 100 g/mL of food, whereas in others, sugars (total) and dietary fiber are also included. In addition, in most nations, ingredient lists are mandated on the labels of most packaged foods and these incorporate the names of common carbohydrate-containing ingredients. Consumers are able to utilize this information about the amount and quality of the carbohydrate in a food or beverage to make informed food purchasing decisions at the point of sale to assist with the prevention and management of overweight/obesity and their sequelae.

There is a rapidly growing body of evidence that low glycemic index (GI) or glycemic load (GL) diets assist with weight loss (Thomas et al. 2007), weight maintenance (Larsen et al. 2010), and chronic disease prevention (Barclay et al. 2008; Livesey et al. 2013) and management (Thomas and Elliott 2009). However, few nations regulate the use of GI or GL information in food and drink Nutrition Information/Facts panels, or associated nutrition claims (Food Standards Australia New Zealand 2013). In addition, it is not possible for the average consumer to estimate the GI or GL of a food or beverage from information provided in the Nutrition Information/Facts panel or ingredient list. The reader is referred to Chapter 3 for the methodology of measuring the GI of foods and for a detailed explanation of how this is done.

To help consumers manage their weight and reduce their risk of chronic disease, provision of information about GI and/or GL on the labels of foods and drinks is warranted if regulated effectively. Like all nutrition information and associated claims, care must be taken to ensure that consumers are able to utilize the information provided to make all-round healthy choices.

12.2 STANDARDIZED MEASUREMENT OF THE GLYCEMIC INDEX

Variability of GI values is often cited as a barrier to recommending the use of the GI (U.S. Department of Health and Human Services and U.S. Department of Agriculture 2005). Over the past 14 years, there have been two interlaboratory studies comparing the results of GI testing laboratories around the globe (Wolever et al. 2003, 2008). Results from the first interlaboratory study (Wolever et al. 2003) were used in the development of the world's first standard for measuring the GI of foods, Australian Standard Glycemic Index of Foods AS 4694-2007, and results from the second interlaboratory study (Wolever et al. 2008) were used in the development of the first international standard for measuring the GI of foods (ISO 26642:2010 Food products—Determination of the GI and recommendation for food classification (International Organization for Standardization 2010)). These two standards have addressed most of the issues identified in the two interlaboratory studies, helping to decrease the variability of GI values.

It is important to consider the fact that all nutrition information on the labels of foods or in nutrient composition databases is subject to variation. This is due to a number of factors including the inherent variability of foods due to changes in soil, environment, cultivar, processing, storage, etc., and limitations of the particular test method for the specific nutrient. For this reason, variations in nutrient values of ±20% are considered acceptable by most food regulatory agencies (Food Standards Australia New Zealand 2013).

12.3 FOOD PURCHASING DECISION MAKING

The availability of healthy low GI foods and drinks for purchase is often cited as a barrier to recommending the use of the GI (U.S. Department of Health and Human Services and U.S. Department of Agriculture 2005). Even when they are available, easy identification of healthy low GI choices amongst the many thousands of food choices available within an average supermarket is another potential barrier.

It has been estimated that at least 50% of food purchasing decisions are made at the point of sale (Mayer et al. 1989), so having information about the GI on the labels of foods would most likely facilitate its use by consumers, especially if the information was displayed prominently on the label as a nutrition content claim, or as part of a front-of-pack labeling scheme or endorsement program.

Indeed, there is evidence in Australia and New Zealand that low GI claims on foods, particularly those endorsed using the GI symbol (see Section 12.7), increase sales of specific foods and beverages.

12.4 POTENTIAL MISUSE

In the observational studies and clinical trials that make up the body of evidence that supports the consumption of low GI foods and meals (Barclay et al. 2008), the foods are with a few notable exceptions (see below) naturally low GI and moderate in carbohydrate, and overall the diets are moderate carbohydrate (44% of energy from carbohydrates on average; range 37–53%).

Around the globe, most foods and drinks are no longer naturally low GI due to cultivation of high-GI crops and modern food processing/manufacturing techniques. From a food technology perspective, however, there are potentially many ways to formulate processed foods to make them low GI (see Chapter 13). Ways of achieving this include adding relatively large amounts of fat, protein, certain added sugars (e.g., fructose), and/or specific dietary fiber fractions (e.g., beta glucans). It is of course also possible to lower the GL of a food or beverage by simply reducing the amount of carbohydrate it contains. These highly processed foods may indeed end up having a low GI and/or GL, but they may not be all-round healthy choices due to their high energy density, type of fat and sugars used, and/or lack of micronutrients.

Some foods that are low GI and have a long tradition of use from a culinary perspective are still discretionary foods that should be consumed in moderation, or perhaps limited to special occasions only. Examples include chocolate and chocolate bars, many high fat cakes, corn chips, ice cream, and jelly/jello (gelatin dessert) (Atkinson et al. 2008).

Many health professionals who do not support the use of the GI use these discretionary foods as examples as to why it is not an ideal tool for rating the nutritional quality of foods and beverages. However, no food or beverage should be judged solely on a single nutrient or nutritional attribute, just as no diet should be judged on a specific food or meal. The commercial focus on reducing fat in the United States and many other parts of the developed world in the 1980s and 1990s did not necessarily improve the overall nutritional profile of the food supply, for example, so this potential for misuse is by no means unique to the GI or GL.

From a regulatory perspective, it is relatively easy to prevent the use of low GI/GL claims on the labels of foods or in promotional material for discretionary foods and beverages. Nutrient profiling models can be mandated within food standards (Food Standards Australia New Zealand 2013) that only allow low GI/GL claims on foods that meet a range of predefined nutrient criteria. This will help identify foods and beverages suitable for frequent consumption as specified in dietary guidelines set by government agencies (see Section 12.6).

12.5 BARRIERS

There are a number of potential barriers to using the GI or GL on the label of foods including the availability of GI testing laboratories that are able to accurately and reliably measure the GI of local foods or beverages, the actual cost of testing, and interpretation of GI and GL values published in international tables.

Most countries have their own set of databases that contain information about the nutrient content of major foods and beverages consumed by the majority of people within that nation at a particular point in time. Also, most nations require packaged foods to carry nutrition information that usually includes as a minimum the amount of energy (kilocalories (kcal) or kilojoules (kJ)), protein (g), fat (g), carbohydrate (g) and sodium (mg)/salt (g) per 100 g/100 mL and/or per serve, in particular if the food or beverage is making a nutrition, health, or related claim (Food Standards Australia New Zealand 2013).

Relatively few nations regulate the use of GI or GL information in food and beverage Nutrition Information/Facts panels, or associated nutrition claims, however (Food Standards Australia New Zealand 2013), with the exceptions being Australia, New Zealand, Singapore, and South Africa. Unfortunately, as mentioned above, it is not possible to estimate the GI or GL of a food or beverage from information provided in the Nutrition Information/Facts panel or ingredient list. It is therefore necessary for the GI of each food or beverage to be measured directly, and these data in turn can be used to calculate the GL, that is, GI × amount of carbohydrate in the food per portion.

To measure the GI of foods directly, laboratories need to be established in each major region of the world, if not every country. At present, there are only a small number of commercial GI test laboratories located in Australia and New Zealand, Canada, Singapore, and the United Kingdom, and in addition, a number of universities throughout the world conduct GI testing for research purposes on an ad hoc basis.

Furthermore, to obtain acceptably accurate and reliable results, laboratories need to at the very least follow the procedures outlined in ISO 26642:2010. To ensure that laboratories are interpreting and implementing the procedures outlined in ISO 26642:2010, a global GI testing accreditation program is being piloted by Australia's Glycemic Index Foundation (GI Foundation), and it is anticipated that it will be rolled out globally from 2016 onward.

In the meantime, both consumer advice and research must utilize GI test result data published online (e.g., the University of Sydney's http:www.glycemicindex.com) or in the most recent version of the international tables of GI and GL values (Atkinson et al. 2008). While it is arguably appropriate to utilize GI test results from the international tables on the labels of minimally processed core foods such as fruits, vegetables, plain milks, natural yoghurts, and legumes, it may not always be appropriate to use GI values for highly processed foods from another nation because ingredients and manufacturing processes vary widely around the globe depending on a nation's food supply and cultural preferences. Kellogg's Special K™, for example, has different formulations in Australia/New Zealand, the United Kingdom, and the United States, so GI test values from Australian samples are most likely not going to be the same as those for products manufactured in the United Kingdom or the United States.

One of the more significant barriers to utilizing the GI on food labels is the relatively high cost of GI testing. For example, in Australia, it costs between $3,000 and $10,000 for each food or beverage tested due primarily to the expenses related to recruiting 10 or more volunteers for a minimum of 4 sessions (3 glucose standard and 1 or more test foods), whereas it costs around $500–600 for all of the other components required in the mandatory nutrition information panel. While this cost may appear relatively small compared to the amount of money spent on the promotion of foods by large food companies, it may in fact be prohibitive for small food companies. Some nations such as Singapore subsidize the cost of GI testing through government health initiatives.

Whenever a food or beverage is significantly reformulated (if the macronutrient composition [% fat, protein, carbohydrate, fiber] has changed by more than 1.5% point, the product is considered to have been reformulated), it must be retested, adding an additional cost burden to food industry.

Finally, both consumer research and market experience indicate that low GI claims are valued the most by consumers. If a food or beverage has a medium or high GI, manufacturers generally prefer not to inform consumers; however, many will reformulate foods with the intention of lowering the GI if possible.

12.6 FOOD STANDARDS CODES

Three nations have specific regulations for GI within their food standards code: Australia, New Zealand, and South Africa, and two of these (Australia and New Zealand) mention GL.

12.6.1 South Africa

South Africa was the first nation globally to officially allow GI claims on the labels of food. Developed in 2002, South Africa's REGULATIONS RELATING TO LABELLING AND ADVERTISING OF FOODSTUFFS No. R. 1055 (Capetown Government 2002) define the GI:

> Glycemic index (GI) means the blood glucose responses of carbohydrate foods and is defined as the incremental area under the blood glucose response curve of a 50 g carbohydrate portion of a test food expressed as a percentage of the response to the same amount of carbohydrate from pure glucose taken by the same subject.

Glycemic index category claims

> The glycemic index category claim shall, if used, be the category as determined according to the method described in Annexure 10 and does not include any method whereby a glycemic index value

is calculated to determine its category and may only be used for foodstuffs with a total glycemic carbohydrate content of 40% or more of the total energy value of the foodstuff; and may, if used, only be indicated as low, intermediate or high Glycemic index or low, intermediate or high GI, in the table with nutritional information or when used as part of a logo, provided the Glycemic index category corresponds with the conditions described hereunder:

Gi Category Claim	Condition
Low GI	GI value: 0 to 55
Intermediate GI	GI value: 56 to 69
High GI	GI value: 70 and more

12.6.2 Australia and New Zealand

In 2013, a new standard (1.2.7) for nutrition, health, and related claims was gazetted in Food Standards Australia New Zealand's (FSANZ) Food Standards Code (Food Standards Australia New Zealand 2013). Similar to the South African regulations, it defines GI:

> glycemic index (GI) means the property of the carbohydrates in different foods, specifically the blood glucose raising ability of the digestible carbohydrates in a given food.

It proscribes the use of AS 4694-2007:

> A method for determining glycaemic index of carbohydrates in foods is described in the Standards Australia Australian Standard Glycemic index of foods (AS 4694-007). In particular, glycaemic index testing is carried out by the determination of glycaemic (blood glucose) responses in human volunteers (in-vivo testing).
>
> The objective of AS 4694-2007 is to establish the recognised scientific method as the standard method for the determination of glycaemic index (GI) in foods.

and lists it as a nutrition content claim with special conditions:

Glycemic index		(a) the food meets the NPSC,[a] unless the food is a food standardized by Part 2.9 of the [Food Standards] Code; and (b) the claim or the nutrition information panel under Standard 1.2.8 includes the numerical value of the glycemic index of the food.
	Low	The numerical value of the glycemic index of the food is 55 or below.
	Medium	The numerical value of the glycemic index of the food is at least 56 and not exceeding 69.
	High	The numerical value of the glycemic index of the food is 70 or above.

[a] The NPSC, or Nutrient Profile Scoring Criterion, is a complex algorithm that takes into account the food group (three broad categories of beverages; fats, oils and spreads; and all other foods), energy density, saturated fat, total sugars, sodium, protein, fiber, fruits, vegetables, nuts, and legume content of the food or beverage (Food Standards Australia New Zealand 2014). Its intention is to ensure that higher level nutrition claims are able to be made on healthy foods and beverages only.

Standard 1.2.7 also lists GL as a permitted nutrition content claim on Australian and New Zealand foods and beverages. Like GI claims, foods and drinks must meet FSANZ NPSC before they are eligible to make GL claims. Unlike GI, low, medium, or high GL are not defined within Standard 1.2.7; however, so in theory manufacturers can claim that a food has low GL regardless of its value. However, in practice, all claims on food labels must be evidence based and food authorities within Australia and New Zealand are able to ask manufacturers to substantiate claims that a food has a low GL. Guidelines as to what constitute a low GL food or beverage have been published (Brand-Miller et al. 2003).

12.7 FRONT-OF-PACK LABELING SCHEMES

As well as including nutrition information like GI values in Nutrition Facts/Nutrition Information Panels, there is growing interest globally in the development of front-of-pack labeling (FoPL) schemes to assist consumers with healthy food purchasing decisions (Lichtenstein et al. 2014).

In Australia and New Zealand, the Health Star Rating (http://www.healthstarrating.gov.au) is a new voluntary FoPL scheme that rates packaged foods of 5 stars—with 5 of 5 stars being the highest rated and 0.5 of 5 stars being the lowest (Figure 12.1). The star rating is calculated using a complex formula that takes into account the amount of energy (kJ), saturated fat, total sugars, sodium, fiber, protein, and the percent of fruits, vegetables, nuts, and legumes in 100 g/100 mL of a food or beverage. In addition to the star rating, the amount of energy, saturated fat, total sugars, sodium, and fiber may also be provided (optionally) on the front of pack, with an optional statement as to whether the food is high or low in that particular nutrient.

Similarly, in the United Kingdom, there is a voluntary FoPL scheme for packaged foods that is a color coded version of the daily intake guide for energy, plus fat, saturated fat, sugars, and salt in 100 g/100 mL of a food or beverage (U.K. Department of Health and Foods Standards Agency 2014); see Figure 12.2. The energy content can appear by itself, or with the other four nutrients. For any particular nutrient, a color rating can be incorporated, grading the food from low (green) to high (red), for that particular nutrient.

Both these systems are useful guides for the general population to help improve packaged food choices. They do not include any nutrition information that will help consumers gauge the effect of a food or beverage on blood glucose concentration, however.

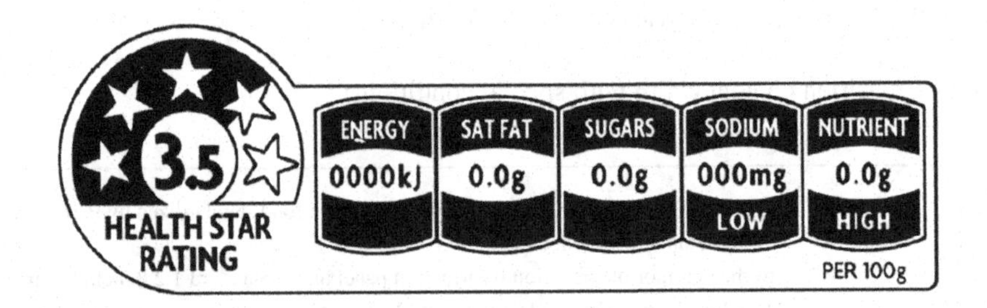

FIGURE 12.1 Australia's Health Star Rating System.

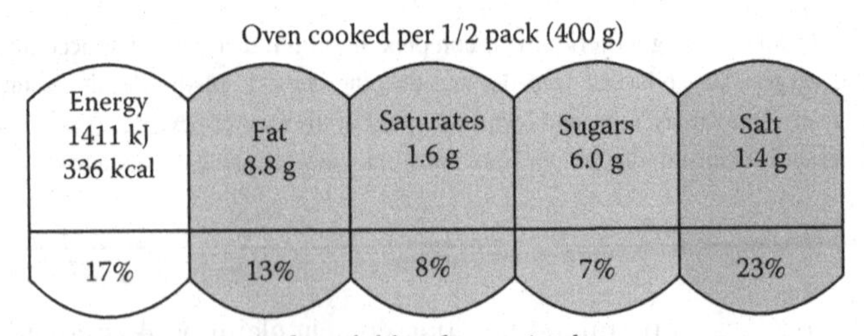

FIGURE 12.2 The United Kingdom's FoPL System.

Around the globe, there are at present two FoPL schemes that specifically focus on the GI of food: Australia's Glycemic Index Symbol Program and the GI Foundation of South Africa's endorsement program. In addition, Singapore's Health Promotion Board has a version of their healthier choice logo that includes a statement that the food has a low GI. Finally, Canada commenced the investigation of a GI-based food-endorsement scheme in 2015.

12.8 THE GLYCEMIC INDEX SYMBOL PROGRAM

The GI Symbol (http:www.gisymbol.com) is an FoPL scheme that also includes the requirement to include a GI value in the Nutrition Facts/Nutrition Information Panel (Figure 12.3). It was registered as a Certification Trademark (CTM) in Australia-New Zealand, North America, the EU, and Asian nations between 2002 and 2015.

To utilize the CTM (GI Symbol), foods must be low GI according to ISO 26642:2010 (International Organization for Standardization 2010) and also meet stringent nutrient criteria for kilojoules/kilocalories, carbohydrate, saturated fat, sodium, and in certain foods fiber and calcium (Glycemic Index Foundation 2015). Nutrient criteria are in line with international dietary guidelines (National Health and Medical Research Council 2013). As an example, the criteria for breads and crisp breads can be found in Table 12.1.

Food modeling by the Glycemic Index Foundation has demonstrated that the GI Symbol Programs Product Eligibility and Nutrient Criteria correlate very strongly with FSANZ NPSC.

The GI Symbol was launched in Australia in 2002 (Glycemic Index Foundation 2014) with a total of 5 foods carrying the GI Symbol and this increased to over 150 foods by 2013 (Glycemic Index

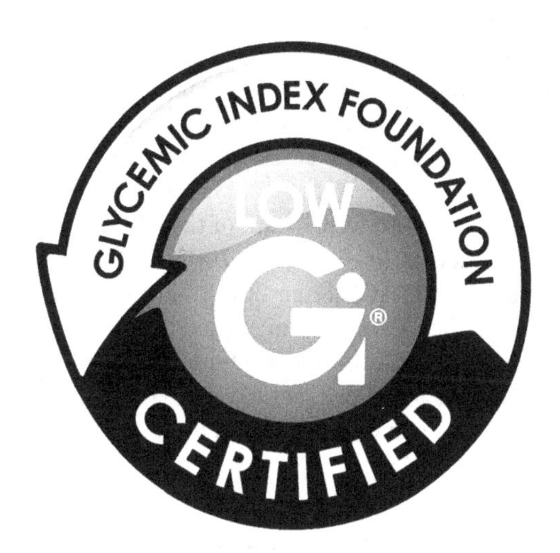

FIGURE 12.3 Australia's GI Symbol.

TABLE 12.1
Example GI Symbol Program Nutrient Criteria for Breads and Crisp Breads

Nutrient	Criterion
Carbohydrate	Contains at least 10 g per serve but no more than 45 g per serve
Fat	≤15 g/100 g, provided that saturated fat is ≤5 g/100 g
Dietary fiber	3 g/100 g or more
Sodium	450 mg /100 g or less

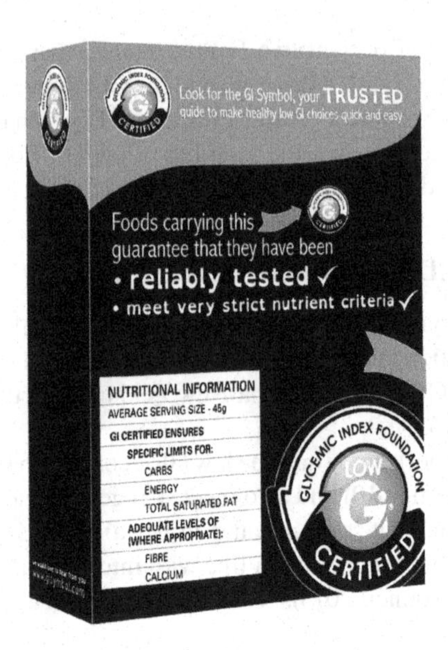

FIGURE 12.4 Example of food packaging carrying Australia's GI Symbol.

Foundation 2014) (Figure 12.4). In 2015, food companies paid a license fee of between AUD 3,000 and 50,000 per annum per stock keeping unit to use the GI Symbol.

Prior to the launch of the GI symbol, market research was conducted in Australia by Newspoll (Newspoll Market Research 2002), and then annually until 2007, and then again in 2012 (ACNielsen 2012) investigating consumer awareness and understanding. Survey participants were 490–1,502 main grocery buyers representative of the Australian adult (aged 18+ years) population and living in the five mainland capital cities (Adelaide, Brisbane, Melbourne, Perth, and Sydney) of Australia.

In 2002, 28% of respondents ($n = 490$) were aware of the GI (Newspoll Market Research 2002). This increased to 86% of respondents ($n = 458$) by 2005, and has remained approximately the same from that point in time onward (ACNielsen 2012). Awareness of the GI Symbol was 2% at baseline (Newspoll Market Research 2002), and increased to 37% by 2012 ($n = 1502$) (ACNielsen 2012). Most (94%) consumers who were aware of the GI looked for the GI Symbol when shopping (ACNielsen 2012). The majority (80%) believe that the GI Symbol indicates that foods that carry it are "healthy, wholesome and a good choice," "scientifically tested," and "provide sustained energy/glucose release" (ACNielsen 2012).

12.9 OTHER GLYCEMIC INDEX FRONT-OF-PACK LABELING SCHEMES

GI Foundation of South Africa's (GIFSA) endorsement program (http://www.gifoundation.com/) was developed shortly after Australia's GI Symbol program and was officially recognized as an endorsement program by the Director General of Health Republic of South Africa in 2011.

According to the company's website,

> Endorsed products bear the GIFSA endorsement logo and are lower in fat, have a GI rating and reduced sodium. The logo appears on selected products that comply with strict specifications and are available in most supermarkets. The GIFSA logo indicates that the endorsed food is healthy, has a lower fat content and is suitable for diabetics.
>
> **Glycemic Index Foundation**
> *GIFSA & Diabetes SA Food Endorsement Logos, 2011*

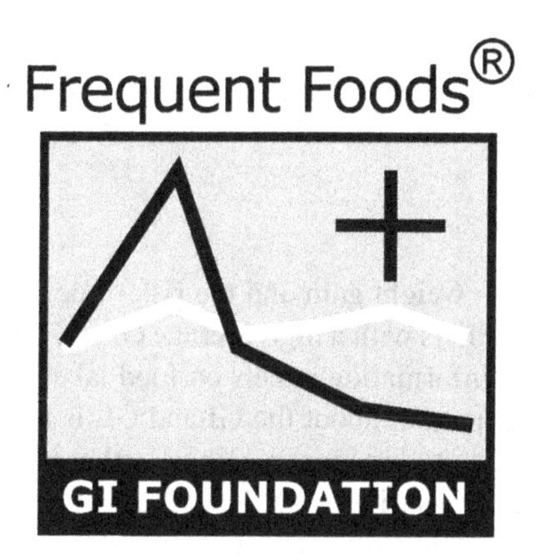

FIGURE 12.5 Example of GI Foundation South Africa's endorsement logo.

There are a number of GIFSA endorsement logos that differentiate "frequent foods" that are color coded green and are low GI and very low fat, from "Best after/with exercise" that are color coded red and are high GI (Figure 12.5). Around 200 foods and beverages were listed as endorsed on GIFSA's website in mid-2015.

Unfortunately, no consumer research information is made publically available by GIFSA.

The Singapore government's Health Promotion Board developed a Healthier Choice Symbol (HCS) Program and made it publically available in late 2009 (Singapore Government Health Promotion Board 2013). One variant incorporates a nutrition content claim alerting potential consumers to the fact that the food or beverage is "low GI."

The nutrient profiling system that underlies the HCS is similar to that of Australia's GI Symbol Program. Products carrying the HCS are generally lower in total fat, saturated fat, sodium, and sugar. Some are also higher in dietary fiber and calcium compared to similar products within the same food category. There are over 60 food categories, and each one has a separate set of nutritional criteria to adhere to. For example, breads displaying the HCS contain no trans fat, less sodium (450 mg/100 g), and more dietary fiber (3 g per 100 g) compared to the regular bread.

Foods claiming to have a low GI must fulfill the following criteria:

> At least 80% of the macronutrients within a food product must be contributed by carbohydrates, or be a special purpose food formulated for people with diabetes.
>
> AND
>
> Must have a GI value (according to ISO 26642:2010) of less than 55.
>
> The low GI logo is only applicable to food products in the HCS cereal category (e.g., mixed rice, noodles, buns, cakes, etc.) and as such must meet all the HCS nutrient guidelines as specified in the cereal category.
>
> **Singapore Government Health Promotion Board**
> *Healthier Choice Symbol Programme, 2013*

While no market research data are available for the low GI version of the HCS per se, for the program as a whole, 7 in 10 Singaporeans were found to be aware of the HCS and 69% had used the symbol to assist them in making healthier food choices.

Finally, in June 2015, the Canadian Diabetes Association (CDA) announced at the Diabetes and Nutrition Study Group of the European Association for the study of Diabetes meeting in Toronto, that it was investigating the development of an FoPL scheme similar to Australia's GI Symbol

Program, which would inform consumers about the GI of carbohydrate-containing foods and beverages. CDA are working with Health Canada on the development of the new FoPL scheme, and the latter have given it in principle approval (Canadian Diabetes Association 2015).

12.10 CONCLUSIONS

Carbohydrates are associated with weight gain and the risk of developing certain chronic diseases like type 2 diabetes. In particular, diets with a high average GI and GL are associated with increased risk. Around the globe, nutrition information panels on food labels provide information about carbohydrates, but provision of information about the GI and GL is relatively uncommon, making its use in food purchasing decisions limited in most nations. Furthermore, just because a food or beverage has a low GI or GL does not necessarily mean that it is an all-round healthy choice—no nutrient or property of a food should be used in isolation to make food purchasing decisions.

To facilitate the process of accurate GI labeling on foods, GI test laboratories that utilize ISO 26642:2010 need to be established in each major region of the world to measure the local food supply. Testing foods locally will help reduce one of the other barriers to GI testing—cost. To prevent misuse of low GI claims on discretionary foods and beverages that are energy dense but nutrient poor, nutrient profiling models need to be developed and included in government food standards.

Australia, New Zealand, and South Africa have all incorporated provisions for GI labeling in their food standards codes, and two of the three (Australia and South Africa) plus Singapore have developed endorsement programs that are FoPL schemes, which are underpinned with nutrient profiling models, to again limit the claims to healthier food choices within their respective food supplies. Canada is currently investigating the development of a GI labeling scheme.

The GI Symbol program is the Australian FoPL tool that helps people identify healthier low GI foods when shopping. Awareness of both the GI and the GI Symbol increased rapidly on introduction of the tool into the Australian food environment, helping people make healthy low GI choices easy choices. This program can be used as a basis for the development of similar programs in other parts of the world.

REFERENCES

ACNielsen. 2012. Online Omnibus 1207 (GI Symbol Omnibus). Glycemic Index Foundation.

Atkinson, F.S., Foster-Powell, K., & Brand-Miller, J.C. 2008. International tables of glycemic index and glycemic load values: 2008. *Diabetes Care*, 31(12), 2281–2283.

Barclay, A.W., Petocz, P., McMillan-Price, J., Flood, V.M., Prvan, T., Mitchell, P., & Brand-Miller, J.C. 2008. Glycemic index, glycemic load, and chronic disease risk—a meta-analysis of observational studies. *Am. J. Clin. Nutr.*, 87(3), 627–637.

Brand-Miller, J.C., Holt, S.H., & Petocz, P. 2003. Reply to R Mendosa. *Am. J. Clin. Nutr.*, 77(4), 994–995.

Canadian Diabetes Association. 2015. *Diabetes and Nutrition Study Group of the European Association for the Study of Diabetes.* Toronto, Canada.

Capetown Government. 2002. R 1055 of 08 August 2002 Foodstuffs, Cosmetics and Disinfectants Act, 1972 (Act no. 54 of 1972) Regulations Relating to Labelling and Advertising of Foodstuffs. South Africa. http://www.capetown.gov.za/en/CityHealth/Documents/Legislation/Regulations%20-%20Relating%20to%20the%20Labelling%20and%20Advertising%20of%20Foodstuffs%20-%20R%201055%20of%202002%20-%20DRAFT.pdf. (Accessed June 17, 2016.)

Food Standards Australia New Zealand. 2013. *Australia New Zealand Food Standards Code*, Commonwealth of Australia, Canberra, Australia.

Food Standards Australia New Zealand. 2014. *Nutrient Profiling Scoring Calculator for Standard 1.2.7, Australia.* http://www.foodstandards.gov.au/industry/labelling/pages/nutrientprofilingcalculator/Default.aspx. (Accessed June 17, 2016.)

Glycemic Index Foundation. 2011. GIFSA & Diabetes SA Food Endorsement Logos. http://www.gifoundation.com. (Accessed June 17, 2016.)

Glycemic Index Foundation. 2014. GI Symbol Program. http://www.gisymbol.com/. (Accessed June 17, 2016.)

Glycemic Index Foundation. 2015. Product Eligibility and Nutrient Criteria. http://www.gisymbol.com/cms/wp-content/uploads/2013/09/GI-Foundation-Product-Eligibility-and-Nutrient-Criteria-November-2015.pdf. (Accessed June 17, 2016.)

Hauner, H., Bechthold, A., Boeing, H., Bronstrup, A., Buyken, A., Leschik-Bonnet, E., Linseisen, J., Schulze, M., Strohm, D., & Wolfram, G. 2012. Evidence-based guideline of the German Nutrition Society: carbohydrate intake and prevention of nutrition-related diseases. *Ann. Nutr. Metab.*, 60(Suppl 1), 1–58.

International Diabetes Federation. 2011. *IDF Diabetes Atlas*, 5th edition.

International Organization for Standardization. 2010. Food products—Determination of the glycaemic index (GI) and recommendation for food classification: ISO 26642.

Larsen, T.M., Dalskov, S.M., van Baak, M., Jebb, S.A., Papadaki, A., Pfeiffer, A.F., Martinez, J.A., Handjieva-Darlenska, T., Kunesova, M., Pihlsgard, M., Stender, S., Holst, C., Saris, W.H., & Astrup, A. 2010. Diets with high or low protein content and glycemic index for weight-loss maintenance. *N. Engl. J. Med.*, 363(22), 2102–2113.

Lichtenstein, A.H., Carson, J.S., Johnson, R.K., Kris-Etherton, P.M., Pappas, A., Rupp, L., Stitzel, K.F., Vafiadis, D.K., & Fulgoni, V.L., III. 2014. Food-intake patterns assessed by using front-of-pack labeling program criteria associated with better diet quality and lower cardiometabolic risk. *Am. J. Clin. Nutr.*, 99(3), 454–462.

Livesey, G., Taylor, R., Livesey, H., & Liu, S. 2013. Is there a dose-response relation of dietary glycemic load to risk of type 2 diabetes? Meta-analysis of prospective cohort studies. *Am. J. Clin. Nutr.*, 97(3), 584–596.

Mayer, J., Dubbert, P., & Elder, J. 1989. Promoting nutrition at the point of choice: A review. *Health Edu. Q.*, 16(1), 31–43.

National Health and Medical Research Council. Australian Dietary Guidelines. 2013. Health and Medical Research Council, Canberra, Australia.

Newspoll Market Research. 2002. Omnibus Study.

Singapore Government Health Promotion Board. 2013. *Healthier Choice Symbol Programme.* Singapore. http://www.hpb.gov.sg/HOPPortal/health-article/2780. (Accessed June 17, 2016.)

Thomas, D., & Elliott, E.J. 2009. Low glycaemic index, or low glycaemic load, diets for diabetes mellitus. *Cochrane Database Syst. Rev.* 1, CD006296.

Thomas, D.E., Elliott, E.J., & Baur, L. 2007. Low glycaemic index or low glycaemic load diets for overweight and obesity. *Cochrane Database Syst. Rev.* 3, CD005105.

U.K. Department of Health and Foods Standards Agency. 2014. Guide to creating a front of pack (FoP) nutrition label for pre-packed products sold through retail outlets. https://www.gov.uk/government/uploads/system/uploads/attachment_data/file/300886/2902158_FoP_Nutrition_2014.pdf. (Accessed June 17, 2016.)

U.S. Department of Health and Human Services and U.S. Department of Agriculture. 2005. *Dietary Guidelines for Americans, 2005*, 6th ed. Government Printing Office, Washington, D.C.

WHO. 2003. *Diet, Nutrition and the Prevention of Chronic Diseases.* World Health Organization, Geneva, Switzerland, Technical Report Series No. 916.

Wolever, T.M., Brand-Miller, J.C., Abernethy, J., Astrup, A., Atkinson, F., Axelsen, M., Bjorck, I., Brighenti, F., Brown, R., Brynes, A., Casiraghi, M.C., Cazaubiel, M., Dahlqvist, L., Delport, E., Denyer, G.S., Erba, D., Frost, G., Granfeldt, Y., Hampton, S., Hart, V.A., Hatonen, K.A., Henry, C.J., Hertzler, S., Hull, S., Jerling, J., Johnston, K.L., Lightowler, H., Mann, N., Morgan, L., Panlasigui, L.N., Pelkman, C., Perry, T., Pfeiffer, A.F., Pieters, M., Ramdath, D.D., Ramsingh, R.T., Robert, S.D., Robinson, C., Sarkkinen, E., Scazzina, F., Sison, D.C., Sloth, B., Staniforth, J., Tapola, N., Valsta, L.M., Verkooijen, I., Weickert, M.O., Weseler, A.R., Wilkie, P., & Zhang, J. 2008. Measuring the glycemic index of foods: Interlaboratory study. *Am. J. Clin. Nutr.*, 87(1), 247S–257S.

Wolever, T.M., Vorster, H.H., Bjorck, I., Brand-Miller, J., Brighenti, F., Mann, J.I., Ramdath, D.D., Granfeldt, Y., Holt, S., Perry, T.L., Venter, C., & Xiaomei, W. 2003. Determination of the glycaemic index of foods: Interlaboratory study. *Eur. J. Clin. Nutr.*, 57(3), 475–482.

13 Creating Food Products with a Lower Glycemic Index

Sophie Vinoy, Aurélie Lesdéma, Gautier Cesbron-Lavau, Aurélie Goux, and Alexandra Meynier

CONTENTS

13.1 INTRODUCTION TO THE DIVERSITY OF CHO-RICH FOODS AND THE GLYCEMIC INDEX

According to international nutrition guidelines, carbohydrates (CHOs) should represent 45%–55% of the daily energy intake (EI), 10%–15% being simple CHOs or sugars, and the remainder being starches and oligosaccharides (FAO/WHO 1998; World Health Organization 2015).

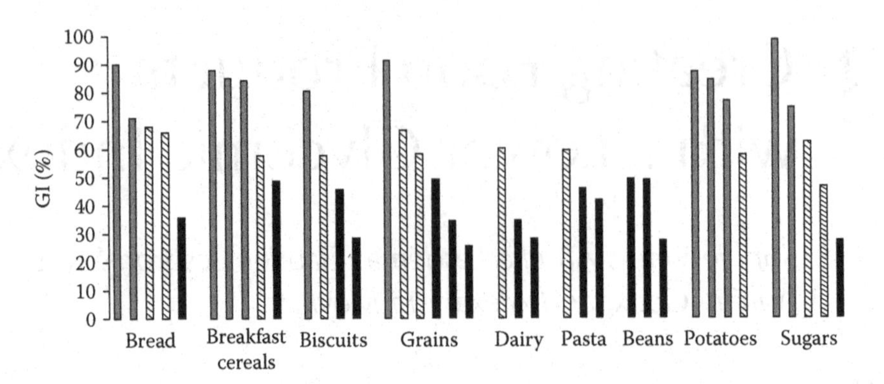

FIGURE 13.1 Example of the wide range of GI values of CHO-rich foods. (Data from Foster-Powell K, Holt SHA, and Brand-Miller JC. International table of glycemic index and glycemic load values: 2002. *American Journal of Clinical Nutrition* 76 no. 1, 2002: 5–56. With Permission.) Glucose is used as the reference. ■ GI ≤ 55; □ 55 < GI ≤ 70; ■ GI > 70.

Nearly 80% of the food consumed in developed countries is processed by the food industry, and it clearly has a significant influence on the way people eat and we must be aware of the essential role it plays in the diet (Dwyer and Ouyang 2000). Nevertheless, the glycemic index (GI) values of CHO-rich foods vary widely, even within a same food category (Atkinson et al. 2008; Foster-Powell et al. 2002) (Figure 13.1).

Postprandial glycemia, as well as the related phenomena of insulinemia and lipemia, have been implicated in the etiology of chronic metabolic diseases such as type-2 diabetes mellitus (T2DM) and cardiovascular disease. Globally, low GI diets have been shown to promote the management and prevention of metabolic disease (Ajala et al. 2013; Livesey et al. 2008; Maki and Phillips 2015), although some of the effects of a low GI diet on disease prevention have been less convincing (Blaak et al. 2012; Goff et al. 2013). One potential explanation, is the different ways foods and diets modulate the GI or the glycemic response (Russell et al. 2013). Indeed, these metabolic parameters are the result of different digestive and/or metabolic regulatory processes that interact with decreasing peripheral blood glucose (Vinoy et al. 2013). Two examples illustrate this by showing the different ways in which a food may result in a lower glycemic response. First, two different studies reported a low glycemic response to starchy foods that provided the same amount of available CHOs, but with different mechanisms (Nazare et al. 2010; Schenk et al. 2003). In the first study, the authors showed that this low glycemic response of a bran cereal was due to a rapid rate of appearance of the ingested CHOs and rapid uptake by tissues. In this case, insulin secretion was enhanced compared to the glycemic response (Schenk et al. 2003). The glycemic peak was much lower and the baseline glucose concentration level was reached earlier than the control product (corn flakes) that did not result in an exacerbated insulin response. In the second study, two biscuits that differed by their slowly digestible starch (SDS) content were compared. The low glycemic response was due to a slow rate of appearance of the ingested CHOs and slow tissue uptake with moderate insulin secretion (Nazare et al. 2010). The second example involves modification of the type of simple CHOs. Additionally, several short-term studies have replaced sucrose with fructose. In this case, there is an immediate effect in reducing the GI of foods, but the beneficial effect of fructose when eaten in high quantities is still a topic of debate because of its potential effect on metabolic complications such as dyslipidemia (Laville and Nazare 2009; Sanchez-Lozada et al. 2008).

The aim of this chapter is to discuss the technological details of CHO-rich foods in combination with their digestive and metabolic fates. The type of CHOs and their digestibility, the quantity of CHOs and their interactions with other macronutrients such as lipids, proteins, and fiber will be taken into account, as they can dramatically modify the postmeal response. The focus will be on solid foods to evaluate the impact of food processing. Sweetened beverages will also be addressed when food processing is not relevant or when no other information is available. Pharmaceutical compounds such as acidity inhibitors or acarbose will not be discussed here as they are not directly related to food or food processing.

13.2 DIFFERENT WAYS TO REDUCE THE GI OF FOODS

This section will discuss the impact of food characteristics, including macronutrients, food processing, and the physical properties of foods, on the fate of CHO in foods. The different ways that food can decrease the GI during the digestive and postabsorptive phases are shown in Figure 13.2 and each relevant step is described, from the buccal phase to colonic impact, including digestion in the small intestine. All ingredients or food components that can interfere with CHO digestibility and or metabolism will be discussed. However, only those foods that impact the GI or the glycemic response will be included, while ingredients that may decrease the glycemic load by decreasing the quantity of available CHO will not be discussed. The detailed digestibility processes will include the major metabolic and physiological mechanisms involved in glucose regulation.

13.2.1 The Buccal Phase: Salivary Amylase and Chewing Modification

The buccal phase refers to digestion that takes place in the mouth. While it is the first and shortest step in digestion, it is still important. Oral digestion involves two simultaneous processes. The first process is the mechanical disruption of ingested food by chewing. During mastication, ingested food is comminuted and lubricated with saliva to form a bolus that is safe and easy to swallow (Chen 2009). Lubrication of foods also initiates the digestion of starches and lipids by enzymes that are present in saliva (amylase and lipase).

Several studies have shown a direct influence of oral digestion parameters on starch hydrolysis (Bornhorst and Singh 2012; Hoebler et al. 1998; Pedersen et al. 2002) and described the influence

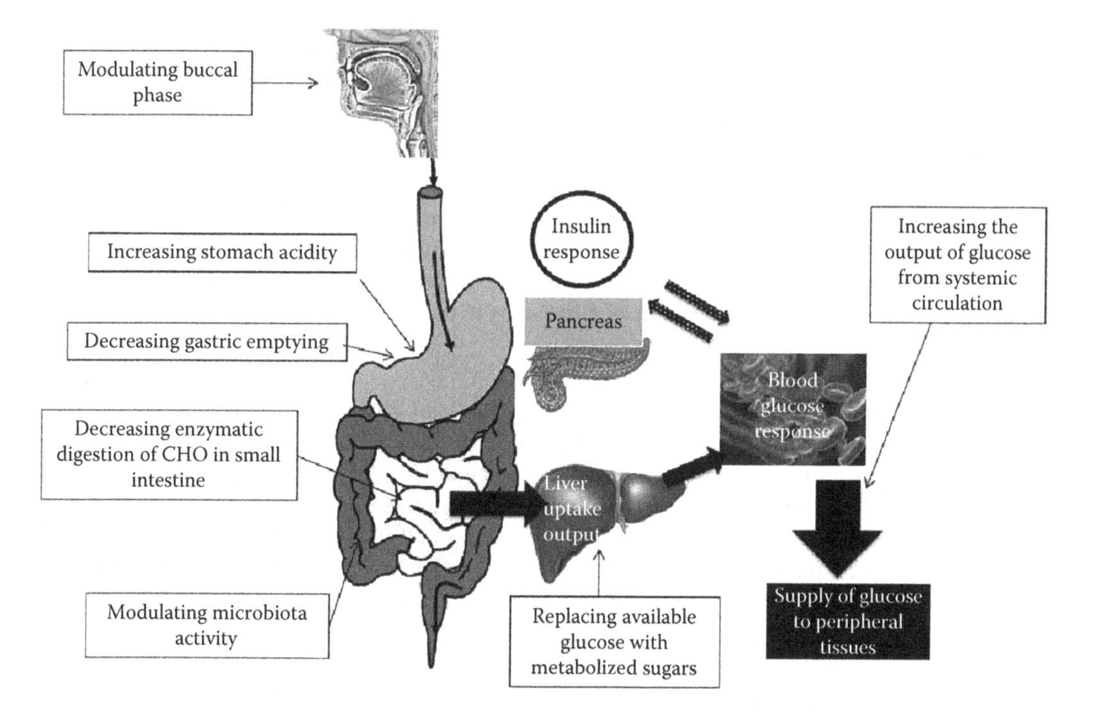

FIGURE 13.2 The different ways that food can decrease the GI during the digestive and postabsorptive phases.

of several of these parameters (hardness, toughness, cohesiveness, moisture content, fat content, macronutrient content, etc.) on chewing and lubrication of foods (Bourne 2004; Flynn 2012; Foster et al. 2006; Gaviao and Bilt 2004; Pereira et al. 2007; Steele et al. 2015). However, few studies have explored the effects of oral digestion on food GI. Read et al. (1986) showed that chewing increased the area under the curve (AUC) of the glycemic response over 2.5 h following rice intake by 184% compared to unchewed food. These results were corroborated by Ranawana et al. (2014), who found that chewing 30 times instead of 15 times increased the GI of a rice meal from 68 ± 3 to 88 ± 10.

While the buccal phase, and especially mastication and salivary amylases, is important to the overall digestion process (Fried et al. 1987; Lebenthal 1987; Rosenblum et al. 1988), not enough studies have been performed to fully understand how this phase impacts the GI of different foods.

13.2.2 Decreasing Gastric Emptying

13.2.2.1 Effect of Organic Acids

In 1995, it was observed that sourdough breads induced low glycemic responses. This phenomenon was attributed to the presence of organic acids formed during sourdough fermentation (Liljeberg et al. 1995). In addition, organic acids such as acetic and propionic acids have been shown to lower the GI and insulin response when added to white bread meals in healthy subjects. Administering high doses of vinegar (between 18 and 28 g of vinegar containing 6% acetic acid) significantly reduced the GI of the meal by about 30% (Darwiche et al. 2001; Liljeberg and Bjorck 1998; Ostman et al. 2005). In a more recent study, the addition of 20 g of vinegar containing 6% acetic acid to a high-GI CHO-rich meal significantly decreased the glycemic response by 42% and the insulin response by 33% in type-2 diabetic patients (Liatis et al. 2010). Interestingly, adding vinegar had no effect on the low GI meal. However, in another study that administered 28 mmol of acetic acid along with a milk rice meal, no decrease in the glucose response was observed (Mettler et al. 2009). It is possible that the increase in glycemia after ingestion of the milk rice meal without acetic acid was not exacerbated enough to detect any decrease induced by the addition of acetic acid, as some rice varieties already have a low GI value. Acetic acid is thought to decrease postprandial glucose and insulin responses by slowing down the gastric emptying phase (Darwiche et al. 2001; Liljeberg and Bjorck 1998). However, this effect was not detected in a study by Hlebowicz et al. (2008) that involved bread dipped in 28 g of vinegar (with 5% acetic acid) for a portion equivalent to 50 g of available CHO.

In all of these studies, the tested doses ranged from 18 to 28 g of vinegar (equivalent of around 2 to 3 tablespoons), providing around 1.1 to 1.7 g of acetic acid. The highest quantities of acetic acid tested decreased the glycemic responses in high-GI meals but had no effect on low GI meals. The mechanism of action is unclear, although delayed gastric emptying is the most likely candidate. Not enough data are available regarding other organic acids to draw any conclusion.

13.2.2.2 Effect of Lipids

Since the 1980s, many researchers have studied the effects of CHO and fat content on plasma substrates and postprandial insulin profiles. The results from these studies showed that adding large amounts of fat (from 37 to 50 g) to a CHO-rich meal decreased the postprandial glycemic response (Collier et al. 1984; Gannon et al. 1993). The primary mechanism identified in these studies was slower gastric emptying resulting in delayed CHO absorption (Cecil et al. 1999; Cunningham and Read 1989). However, the effect on the insulin response is controversial with, as an example, one study demonstrating that adding fat to a CHO-rich meal can potentially exacerbate the insulin response (Gannon et al. 1993).

A very sophisticated study using the stable isotope method evaluated the impact of adding fat (2, 15, or 40 g of fat) to a pasta meal including 75 g of CHO (Normand et al. 2001). Adding 15 g of fat decreased the glycemic response by 24% over the 3 h postprandial period. The effect on the rate of appearance of exogenous CHO was significantly lower when 40 g of fat were added, compared to

TABLE 13.1
Impact of Three Quantities of Fat on GI and II

Extruded Cereal	1.5 g Fat/100 g Cereal (3% of Total Energy Content)	6 g Fat/100 g Cereal (12% of Total Energy Content)	10 g Fat/100 g Cereal (21% of Total Energy Content)
GI (%)	77 ± 11	73 ± 10	70 ± 12
II (%)	77 ± 6	79 ± 8	71 ± 7

Note: GI: Glycemic index, using glucose solution as the reference, II: Insulin index.
There was no significant difference in GI or II regardless of the fat content (1.5, 6, or 10 g fat/100 g cereal).

low (2 g) and medium (15 g) amounts of added fat (Normand et al. 2001). The insulin response was not affected by the addition of fat, meaning it did not decrease in parallel with the glucose response. These results were confirmed in a study of 13 European breakfasts, which showed that 3–42 g of dietary fat, either present intrinsically in the test food or added to the meal as butter or cheese, were strongly inversely correlated to the GI of the meal (Flint et al. 2004). In addition, a few studies have evaluated the effect of intrinsic fat in cereal products. Inverse correlations were found between fat content and GI, as well as correlations with some other food parameters including the amount of SDS in 26 cereal products (Englyst et al. 2003) and 24 plain biscuits (Garsetti et al. 2005). Fat content did not correlate with the insulin response. A recent study confirmed the inverse effect of fat (from 1 to 18 g) on the GI of 190 cereal products (Meynier et al. 2015). The originality of this study was that it investigated the interactions between food characteristics and GI. Fat had a major effect on the GI when the tested food contained a small amount of fiber and SDS. In contrast, the ability of fat to affect the GI was dramatically decreased in products with large amounts of either SDS or fiber.

A prospective study evaluated the effect of three quantities of fat on the GI of a cereal product (Vinoy 2006). A high-GI product obtained by extrusion that contained 1.5 g fat/100 g portion had a measured GI of 77 ± 11. Additional fat was added to the formula during processing to yield 6 and 10 g fat/100 g portion. There was no significant decrease in the GI values of the cereal containing the highest doses of fat compared to low fat extruded cereal, although the GI was reduced by 4 and 7 points by including 6 and 10g of fat in the product, respectively. The impact of the three quantities of fat on GI and insulin index (II) are shown in Table 13.1 (Vinoy 2006).

Another aspect that has been addressed is the lipid quality that may have a greater influence on the insulin response than the GI in both healthy subjects and patients with type-2 diabetes. For example, butter has been shown to induce an exacerbated insulin response compared to olive oil (Lardinois et al. 1987; Rasmussen et al. 1996). However, this effect has not been confirmed by more recent studies (Burdge et al. 2006; Cortes et al. 2006; Shah et al. 2007; Thomsen et al. 2003).

In conclusion, there is a significant negative correlation between the fat content of a meal and the GI or the postmeal glycemic response. Consuming a meal with a medium to high fat content (15–40 g) significantly decreases the glycemic response. However, a lower fat content may have less of an impact on the GI, especially if other food components such as fiber or SDS interfere with its effect. Furthermore, fat did not decrease the insulin response in any of the aforementioned studies.

13.2.2.3 Effect of Soluble Viscous Dietary Fiber

This section will focus on the types of fiber that may interfere with gastric emptying. Resistant starch (RS) will not be discussed as it has not been shown to modulate gastric emptying. Dietary fiber is a general term for a chemically heterogeneous group of compounds with various chemical structures, molecular weights, and different physicochemical properties, such as water solubility, viscosity, cation exchange properties, organic acid absorption, and water-holding capacity (Eastwood and Morris 1992), and it has several interesting health benefits (Russell et al. 2013). Among the different fiber classifications the traditional system is based on water solubility and divides fibers into soluble (pectins, gums, mucilages) and insoluble (cellulose, hemicelluloses, lignin) types (Raninen et al. 2011; Slavin et al. 2009). (For a more detailed discussion on fiber, the reader is referred to Chapter 1.) This section will focus on fibers that have a direct effect on gastric emptying. Among them, studies where fibers were used in addition to, instead of as a replacement for, available CHOs will be specifically discussed.

Soluble viscous fibers play a significant role in managing postprandial glucose and insulin concentrations via the formation of viscous gels, thereby reducing gastric emptying (Darwiche et al. 2003; Marciani et al. 2001; Sanaka et al. 2007) and decreasing the rate of subsequent glucose absorption (Dikeman et al. 2006). Soluble fiber may also alter intestinal motility, decrease the diffusion rate of starch digestion products and reduce accessibility to α-amylase (Leclere et al. 1994). The most commonly used soluble viscous fibers are guar gum, glucomannan, xanthan gum, psyllium, pectin, alginate, arabinoxylan, and β-glucan concentrates and various combinations of these fibers (Granfeldt et al. 2008; Juvonen et al. 2011; Lu et al. 2000; Nilsson et al. 2008a, b; Rokka et al. 2013; Russell et al. 2013; Scazzina et al. 2013). Studies have shown that 4 g or more of soluble β-glucan can significantly reduce postprandial glucose and insulin responses in healthy individuals (Granfeldt et al. 2008; Juvonen et al. 2011). Moreover, the addition of wheat soluble arabinoxylan extract to a bread meal significantly lowered the postprandial glucose and insulin responses in healthy individuals in a dose-dependent manner; the glycemic response was reduced by 20% and 41% and insulin response by 17% and 33% in meals containing 6 and 12 g of arabinoxylan, respectively (Lu et al. 2000). In addition, Nilsson et al. (2008b) tested six types of fiber derived from wheat, barley, and rye and eaten either as kernels or incorporated in bread. The soluble fiber content ranged from 2 to 6 g/portion, while the total fiber content ranged from 4 to 14 g/portion. The breads containing rye and barley kernels, which had the highest fiber content (4 and 3 g of soluble fiber/portion, respectively), decreased the GI significantly (27% and 51%, respectively) compared to the standard white bread. Surprisingly, adding 6 g of soluble fiber from barley extract to white bread did not decrease the GI compared to standard white bread. The apparent lack of effect from this barley fiber-enriched bread was determined based on the shape of the curve over the 2 postprandial hours; the incremental AUC (iAUC) between 0 and 60 min clearly showed a significant decrease in the glycemic peak, but this was followed by a net prolonged maintenance in the later postprandial phase (60–120 min). In this study, the wheat and oat kernels (2 and 2.5 g of soluble fiber, respectively) did not reach statistically significant decrease in the GI and glycemic peak compared to standard white bread (Nilsson et al. 2008b), even though the GI decreased by 15% and 21%, respectively.

Our data showed that there is a clear dose response relationship between the amount of guar gum, a type of viscous soluble fiber, in biscuits and *in vitro* viscosity, gastric emptying and GI (Vinoy et al. 2011). This experiment was performed using three different biscuits made with 4, 9, or 13 g per portion of guar gum, with a total consumed weight of 80, 82, or 86 g, respectively. The amount of total fiber in each biscuit was 9, 14, or 18 g per portion, respectively. The glycemic peak was almost completely suppressed by the biscuit with the highest guar gum content, and the insulin demand was dramatically decreased (Table 13.2, Vinoy et al. 2011). This biscuit had the highest *in vitro* viscosity

TABLE 13.2
Impact of Three Quantities of Viscous Soluble Fiber (Guar Gum) on GI and II

Plain Biscuit (Portion Size)	4 g Fiber/Portion (80 g)	9 g Fiber/Portion (82 g)	13 g Fiber/Portion (86 g)
GI (%)	49 ± 6	25 ± 3*	17 ± 3*
II (%)	49 ± 4	17 ± 3*	10 ± 2*

Note: GI: Glycemic index, using glucose solution as the reference, II: Insulin index.
*Indicates a significant difference compared to the biscuit with 4 g fiber/portion; $p < .05$.

and induced the slowest gastric emptying. The GI was decreased by 49% and 65%, respectively, when 5 and 9 g of additional guar gum were added to a low-GI biscuit already containing 4 g of guar gum.

In conclusion, viscous soluble fibers have clearly been shown to actively decrease GI and the insulin response. Based on the data reported above, adding at least 4 g of these fibers per portion is effective in reducing GI. This has been demonstrated primarily with β-glucans. Furthermore, fibers behave differently in the digestive tract, especially in terms of developing viscosity in the gastric phase. This viscosity may depend on the origin of the fiber and potentially on the process that occurs during food manufacturing. This last parameter needs to be evaluated case by case.

13.2.3 Decreasing the Enzymatic Digestion of CHO in the Small Intestine

13.2.3.1 Molecular Conformation of Available CHO and Starch

Common food starch is derived from cereals (e.g., wheat, maize, rice, barley, and buckwheat), tubers (e.g., potatoes and cassava), and legumes (e.g., peas, lentils, kidney beans, and mung beans). Starch is a semicrystalline material produced by plants that forms roughly spherical granules in plant tissues. The sizes and shapes of the granules depend on their botanical origin, as well as the relative amounts of amylose (polymer made of α-1,4-linked glucose units) and amylopectin (polymer with a branched structure that has α-1,6-linked glucose units at the branch point and α-1,4 links in the linear regions). Native starch granules are slowly degraded by salivary and pancreatic amylases. All mechanical processes that cause fissures on the surface of granules increase their susceptibility to digestive enzymes. The rate and extent of starch digestion is influenced by its botanical origin, as this determines the amylose:amylopectin ratio and the structure of the starch granule (Miao et al. 2013).

13.2.3.1.1 Reducing the Starch Gelatinization during Processing

Another important factor in addition to starch structure is food processing, which determines the extent of starch gelatinization and the integrity of the particle size and plant cell wall (Colonna et al. 1992; Heaton et al. 1988). The structure of the starch granule undergoes dramatic changes when it is heated in the presence of water (Bornhorst and Paul Singh 2014; Lang 2004). As the temperature increases, hydrogen bonds between the starch chains are disrupted, and water is absorbed by the starch granule. This leads to swelling of the granule, which is followed by amylose leaching. The starch dissolves progressively, gradually increasing the viscosity of the solution. Gelatinization leads to the formation of a starch paste (Figure 13.3).

To monitor the rate and extent of starch digestibility or the intestinal absorption of starch-derived glucose, Englyst et al. (1992, 1999) developed the *Slowly Digestible Starch (SDS) method* to quantify nutritionally important starch fractions *in vitro*. This method mimics the human digestive system.

It was shown that there is a clear relationship between SDS, the gelatinization stage of starch in 23 cereal products, and their GI values (Englyst et al. 2003). Cereal products with the highest SDS had the lowest degree of starch gelatinization and led to the lowest GI and II values (Englyst et al. 2003). Increased amounts of SDS (within a range of 2%–41% of SDS/available starch) significantly decreased GI values. The impact on the insulin response was lower, decreasing the response by 10%. In addition, several studies have identified a clear link between the SDS content of starchy foods and the GI or glycemic response (Englyst et al. 1996, 1999; Garsetti et al. 2005; Nazare et al. 2010; Vinoy et al. 2013, 2015). Two groups have studied the dynamic metabolic fate of glucose using the stable isotope labeling method (Nazare et al. 2010; Vinoy et al. 2013). In both of these studies, cereal products with a high SDS content (50% and 35% SDS/available starch) induced a slower rate of appearance of CHO from the products during the postprandial period, leading to a reduction of the glycemic response by 33% and 30%, respectively, compared to a cereal product low in SDS (2% SDS/available starch) (Nazare et al. 2010; Vinoy et al. 2013). The effect on the insulin response is less clear, as Nazare et al. observed no significant difference in overweight subjects, whereas Vinoy et al. reported a 27% decrease in normal weight subjects after a high SDS meal compared to a low

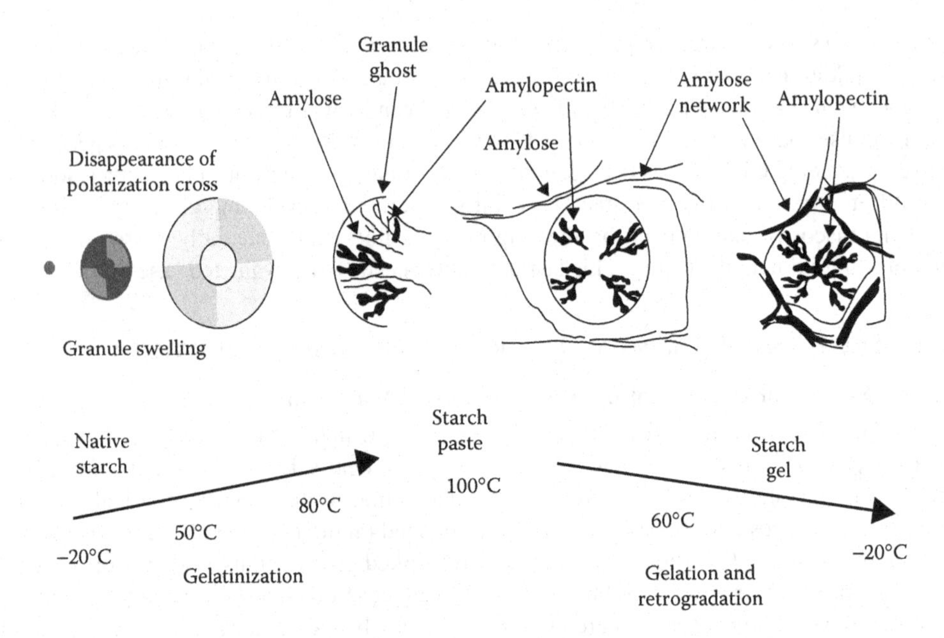

FIGURE 13.3 Influence of hydrothermic processing on physical starch characteristics. (Adapted from Bornet F. Technological treatments of cereals. Repercussions on the physiological properties of starch. *Carbohydrates Polymers* 21 no. 2–3, 1993: 195–203. With permission.)

SDS meal. Very recently, the impact of high SDS products on rate of appearance of CHO has been confirmed (Peronnet et al. 2015). Postprandial glycemic and insulin response were also decreased after the high SDS meal compared to the low SDS one.

The hydrothermic parameters used to process starchy foods (temperature, moisture content, cooking time, and pressure) dramatically modify the degree of starch gelatinization (Table 13.3). The moisture content in particular is a critical parameter. The combination of high moisture with high temperatures (baking or drum-drying) or high pressure and shearing (as in extrusion cooking process) leads to completely gelatinized starch and high-GI and II values (Englyst et al. 2003). In contrast, in other foods such as barley porridge, parboiled rice, biscuits, and pasta, the lower degree of gelatinization or limited starch swelling, which is mainly determined by a limited moisture level, cooking time, and temperature, maintains the SDS content and moderates the glycemic response (Garsetti et al. 2005; Holm et al. 1992; Wolever et al. 1986).

The SDS content is dramatically modified in three cereal products that are processed differently: plain biscuit, bread making, baking-extrusion (Figure 13.4; Cartier, pers. comm.). The SDS content is better maintained in the plain biscuit as the moisture is low during processing with a low dough hydration, no high pressure, and a controlled baking time.

In addition, interactions between starch and different components of the food product formula during processing can influence starch forms that are slowly digested or not digested at all. The two most important forms of starch interactions are starch–protein interactions and the formation of starch–lipid complexes (see Section 13.2.3.2). A good example of starch–protein interactions is cooked pasta. Each starch granule is encapsulated by a protein matrix and after 11 min of cooking in boiling water, the starch is completely gelatinized (Colonna et al. 1990). Preincubation of pasta with protease *in vitro* enhanced starch α-amylase hydrolysis (Colonna et al. 1990). The protein network limits starch swelling, thereby providing a structural explanation for the slow digestion of the starch in pasta and its reduced GI.

We recently analyzed a database of 190 cereal products to evaluate the relationship between the nutritional composition and the digestibility of CHOs in food products and the metabolic responses that they induce (including GI and II). The model describing the glycemic response showed that

TABLE 13.3
Hydrothermal Conditions of Manufacturing Processes for Various Types of Cereal Products

Manufacturing Process	Food Type	Hydrothermal Parameters: Dough Core Temperature (°C)	Dough Hydration Level (%)	Baking Time (min)	Pressure (bar)	Starch Digestibility (SDS[a] in %)	GI[b] (%)
Biscuit and bread products	Biscuits	100–130	15–30	5–15	1	Moderate to slow (14%–50%)	30–80
	Bakery products Sandwich loaf	100–120	40	20	1	Rapid (3%–9%)	60–90
	Crackers	100–130	25–35	2–3	1	Moderate (8%–17%)	50–65
Baking extrusion	Extruded cereals	120–180	14–30	5	50–200	Rapid (2%–10%)	75–95

Source: Calculated from data in:

(a) Bornet F. Technological treatments of cereals. Repercussions on the physiological properties of starch. *Carbohydrates Polymers* 21 no. 2–3 (1993): 195–203.

(b) Foster-Powell K, Holt SHA, and Brand-Miller JC. International table of glycemic index and glycemic load values: 2002. *American Journal of Clinical Nutrition* 76 no. 1 (2002): 5–56.

(c) Garsetti M, Vinoy S, Lang V et al. The glycemic and insulinemic index of plain sweet biscuits: relationships to in vitro starch digestibility. *Journal of the American College of Nutrition* 24 no. 6 (2005): 441–47.

[a] SDS: slowly digestible starch fraction determined *in vitro* using the Englyst method and expressed as a percent of the quantity of available starch.

[b] GI: Glycemic index.

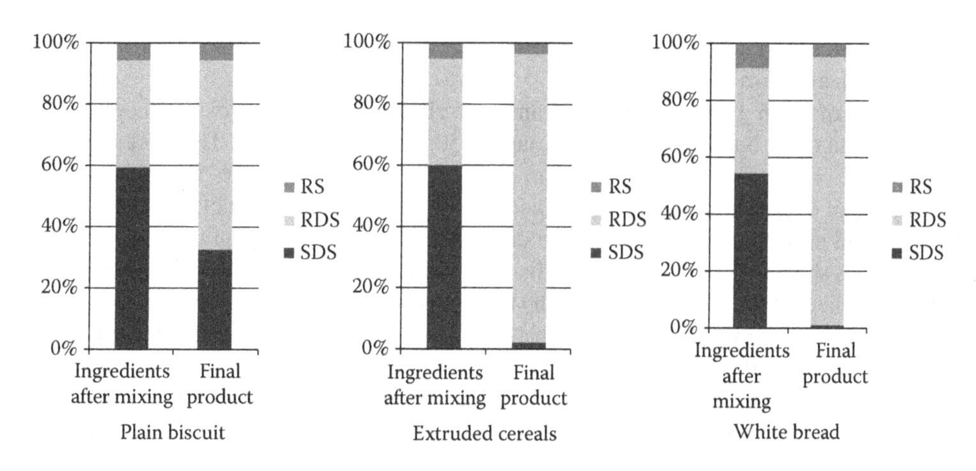

FIGURE 13.4 Percent of each starch fraction compared to the total starch content of three different cereal products during food processing (Cartier, pers. comm.). Slowly digestible starch (SDS), rapidly digestible starch (RDS), and resistant starch (RS) as a percent of total starch.

SDS, rapidly digestible starch (RDS), fat, fibers, and interactions between these components significantly explained GI by 53% and delta peak (difference between baseline and the highest value) of glycemia by 60%. SDS was one of the major contributors of GI (Meynier et al. 2015).

In conclusion, preserving the native structure of starch and thus the maintenance of a high SDS content (around 35% to 40% of the total available starch) can effectively reduce the GI and II of starchy foods. Using grains that contain specific starch structures may help to protect these starches from gelatinization. Indeed, food processing is the major modulator of starch gelatinization and thus of SDS content. Recent studies have provided insights into how to modify starch to decrease its susceptibility to gelatinization during food processing.

13.2.3.1.2 Ratio of Amylose/Amylopectin

Starch is mainly composed of 60% to 90% amylopectin and 10% to 30% amylose. There are high-amylose starches that contain up to 70% of amylose, as well as high-amylopectin (100%) varieties, which are called waxy starches. Cereal and tuber contain a wide range of amylose:amylopectin ratios (rice, wheat, barley, maize, and potatoes can be rich in amylose or waxy, depending on the variety) (Copeland et al. 2009; Fredriksson et al. 1998).

Many studies have explored the effect of amylose and amylopectin on GI. The amount of amylose or amylopectin has a significant influence on the overall rate of starch digestion. Several studies have shown that amylose-rich diets elicited a lower insulin response (Akerberg et al. 1998; Amelsvoort and Weststrate 1992; Behall et al. 1988, 1989; Behall and Howe 1995). For example, a 27% decrease in the total insulin AUC was recorded after consumption of a meal with a 45:55 amylose:amylopectin ratio compared to a meal with a 0:100 amylose:amylopectin ratio (Amelsvoort and Weststrate 1992).

Grandfeldt et al. (1994) demonstrated that an increased amylose content (33% to 42%) corresponded to a 75 ± 5% to 56 ± 2% reduction in the hydrolysis index of barley flours. A similar trend was detected in the GI values, which decreased slightly from 65 ± 9 to 55 ± 6. Zhang et al. (2006b) reported that there was no correlation between amylose content and SDS in native starch. This indicates that amylose alone is not a suitable predictor of GI, and that some other factors play a role. However, it has been reported that for similar amylose contents (26.7%–27%), the digestibility and GI of three rice cultivars with different physicochemical properties differed (61 ± 9, 72 ± 10, and 91 ± 12) (Panlasigui et al. 1991). In addition, the fine structures of both amylose and amylopectin may significantly affect overall starch digestion (Syahariza et al. 2013).

The structure of amylopectin plays an important role in delaying enzyme-mediated starch digestion. Indeed, rice cultivars containing amylopectin with longer chains (DP > 33) are digested more slowly than those containing amylopectin with short or medium chains (DP < 13 and 13 < DP < 33, respectively) (Benmoussa et al. 2007).

The number of α-1,6 glycosidic bonds in amylopectin may also play a role, as they are digested more slowly than α-1,4 bonds (French and Knapp 1950; Zihua et al. 2007). The more branches that an amylopectin chain has (and therefore, the greater the number of α-1,6 glycosidic bonds), the slower the rate of digestion (Singh et al. 2010; Zhang et al. 2006b; Zihua et al. 2007).

Amylose and amylopectin appear to have different effects depending on the state of the starch and its origin, as shown by seemingly contradictory findings for amylopectin. In one study, SDS was positively correlated with starch chain length (Benmoussa et al. 2007), whereas in a second study, shorter chains appeared to be more favorable to slow digestion in native and gelatinized starch (Zhang et al. 2006b). Fully gelatinized amylose seems to favor slow digestion, as its ability to form complexes with lipids when heated and its fast retrogradation rate make the starch harder to digest. However, in native starch (especially cereal starches), amylopectin is crucial in maintaining starch crystallinity, which is responsible for its slow digestion properties (Zhang et al. 2006a, b).

To summarize, the amylose:amylopectin ratio cannot fully explain GI values. The impact of the variations in amylose or amylopectin fine structures as well as the botanical origin of starches affects GI values as strongly as the amylose:amylopectin ratio itself. Further research is needed to elucidate this topic.

13.2.3.1.3 Synthesized or Modified CHOs

Synthesized or modified CHOs may represent an additional means of decreasing the rate of digestibility and consequent GI of food products. Several groups of investigators in the past few years have studied modified starches from corn, rice, potato, and tapioca aiming to limit their gelatinization and/or slow down their rate of digestion (Kittisuban et al. 2014; Lin et al. 2014). There are two main challenges in developing these modified starches: to avoid producing RS instead of SDS and to develop modified slow starches that resist food processing methods. Severijnen et al. (2007) modified a high-amylose starch high in RS by heating it in distilled water or a clinical sterile liquid to modify its functional properties. The SDS content increased threefold to 33.1 ± 2.4 g/100 g of powder when heated at 130°C. When rats were fed 2 g of available CHO/kg from this modified starch in water, they exhibited a 75% reduction in postprandial glycemia over the 45 first min compared to rats that were fed maltodextrin.

Another potential strategy is to use CHOs such as isomaltulose or trehalose. The GI of isomaltulose is 32 ± 3 (Atkinson et al. 2008), and ingested isomaltulose is completely absorbed regardless of the food matrix (Lina et al. 2002). *In vitro* studies have shown that isomaltulose and trehalose are hydrolyzed slowly (Lina et al. 2002); however, these results have not been confirmed *in vivo*. Ingestion of a solution containing 50 g of isomaltulose lead to a 36% lower glycemic response compared to ingestion of a solution containing 50 g of sucrose (Holub et al. 2010). In subjects with impaired glucose tolerance (IGT), the glycemic response to ingestion of a solution containing 75 g CHO-equivalents of isomaltulose was reduced by 43% compared to ingestion of the same amount of sucrose (Can et al. 2012). On the other hand, trehalose showed less convincing results. In two studies performed in healthy subjects and subjects with IGT, ingesting a solution containing 75 g CHO-equivalents of trehalose did not modify the postprandial glycemic response and only led to a reduced peak in the glycemic response (33% in subjects with IGT and about 15% in healthy subjects) when consumed alone compared to a sucrose solution (Can et al. 2009, 2012). These effects were confirmed when a trehalose solution was consumed in combination with a mixed lunch. Obese subjects who consumed a beverage containing 75 g of trehalose exhibited a significantly lower glycemic response (20%) compared to that elicited by glucose (Maki et al. 2009). In all of these studies, the insulin responses were also reduced. Therefore, consuming 50–75 g of isomaltulose or trehalose instead of sucrose or glucose leads to a 15%–36% reduction in the glycemic response. However, all these studies tested CHOs dissolved in a beverage; therefore, the impact of food processing on solid foods containing these CHOs remains to be investigated.

13.2.3.2 Formation of Starch–Lipid Complexes during Food Processing

Amylose forms complexes with amphiphilic or hydrophobic ligands, and most notably lipids. Complexed amylose, which is often referred to as *V-amylose*, loses its linear structure, folding to take on a helical structure (Lopez et al. 2012). This new conformation induces changes in its chemical and physical properties. Specifically, starch retrogradation is delayed (Chung et al. 1978), swelling is reduced (Ahmadi-Abhari et al. 2013a), and most importantly, the digestibility of the starch is decreased. This mechanism applies to lipids that interact with amylose to form complexes. These complexes form during processing when the right conditions are met, that is, heat, chain length, pressure, and lipid type (Tufvesson et al. 2003a, b).

Several *in vitro* studies have reported a significant decrease in starch digestibility after formation of an amylose-lipid complex (Ahmadi-Abhari et al. 2013b; Crowe et al. 2000; Guraya et al. 1997; Seneviratne and Biliaderis 1991). The decrease in *in vitro* starch digestibility reportedly ranged from 12% (Crowe et al. 2000) to up to 33% (Guraya et al. 1997).

Despite registering a substantially reduced digestion *in vitro*, Holm et al. (1983) reported that, in an *in vivo* rat model, lipid-complexed amylose was not digested slower than regular amylose. These observations suggest that amylose-lipid complexes decrease the enzyme-mediated digestion of starch *in vitro*, although more research is needed to confirm the relevance of these results on the GI of starches *in vivo*. Human studies are especially needed to draw reliable conclusions.

13.2.3.3 Compounds That Partially Inhibit Enzyme Activity

Starch digestion and absorption rely on the activity of several enzymes and transporters. Therefore, the glycemic response could be modulated by inhibiting the activity of the enzymes implicated in CHO digestion, such as α-amylase or amyloglucosidase. Another potential strategy would be inhibiting glucose transport in the bloodstream.

TABLE 13.4
Evaluation of Polyphenol Content and GI of Four Potato Species

Potato Species	Polyphenol Content (mg GAE /100 g DW)	GI
Purple Majesty	234 ± 28	77 ± 9
Red-Y38	190 ± 15	78 ± 14
Yukon Gold	108 ± 39	81 ± 16
Snowden	82 ± 1	93 ± 17

The values are expressed as the mean ± SEM.
GAE: Gallic acid equivalents; GI: Glycemic index; DW: Dry weight.

Dietary polyphenols are compounds originating from plants. Polyphenols display a wide range of chemical structures and are found in abundant quantities in fruits, vegetables, spices, chocolate, tea, coffee, wine, cereals, and other foods (Manach et al. 2005). Several early studies reported a significant inverse correlation between the phenolic content of food products and their glycemic response or GI. In 1984, Thompson et al. showed that the polyphenol content of foods is inversely correlated with their GI in both healthy and diabetic subjects. In this study, the amount of polyphenol ingested in the fruits and vegetables studied ranged between 8.0 ± 0.0 and 363.6 ± 2.2 mg. The GI values for these products were between 21 ± 7 and 111 ± 8 in healthy subjects and between 20 ± 8 and 123 ± 5 in diabetic patients (Thompson et al. 1984). The GI values observed in both the healthy and diabetic subjects correlated with the polyphenol intake, with r values of −0.58 to −0.69 ($p < 0.05$–0.01), respectively. Interestingly, this correlation was stronger with large polymeric polyphenols (condensed tannins) compared to the total polyphenol content. Recently, Ramdath et al. (2014) investigated the GI of four colored potato species (Purple Majesty, Red-Y38, Yukon Gold, and Snowden), using glucose solution as reference. These potatoes differed in terms of both polyphenol content and GI values (Table 13.4).

The measured GI values demonstrated a strong inverse correlation to the total polyphenol content ($r = -0.825$, $p < .05$). Finally, Coe et al. (2013) evaluated the impact of consuming a solution containing two different doses of baobab (a type of fruit) compared to white bread on the subsequent glycemic response. Both extracts provided 534 mg of gallic acid equivalents (GAE) (Low Dose [LD] test) and 1067 mg GAE (High Dose [HD] test), respectively. The three test products provided 50 g of available CHOs. Adding the two baobab extracts reduced the glycemic response by 19% (as measured by the LD test) and 23% (as measured by the HD test) compared to the control. Despite the large difference in polyphenol content between the two extracts, there was no difference in the glycemic response induced by their consumption.

Many *in vitro* studies have investigated the potential mechanism of action of polyphenols on the glycemic response. Flavonoids and phenolic acids are potent inhibitors of the activity of both α-amylase and α-glucosidase (Hanhineva et al. 2010; McDougall et al. 2005; Mkandawire et al. 2013). The potency of these compounds depends on their chemical structure (Barrett et al. 2013; Narita and Inouye 2009; Sirichai et al. 2009) and the quantity in the extract (Mkandawire et al. 2013).

Another potential strategy for modulating the glycemic response would be altering glucose uptake by tissues. Indeed, several *in vitro* studies have shown that polyphenols can modulate glucose transporter activity (Hanhineva et al. 2010; Johnston et al. 2005; Wang et al. 2013). However, this has not yet been confirmed *in vivo*.

Therefore, ingesting polyphenols along with food can reduce the GI of these food products. This effect appears to be dose dependent; however, only few intervention studies have been performed, and the mechanism of action is still unclear.

13.2.4 Replacing Available Glucose with Metabolized Sugars

13.2.4.1 Fructose

Fructose is a naturally abundant monosaccharide. The availability of fructose increased substantially in the 1960s when it became economically possible to produce high-fructose syrups from corn starch and other starches. These high-fructose syrups are now used to sweeten soft drinks, fruit drinks, baked goods, jams, syrups, and candies (Bantle 2006). Based on the United States Department of Agriculture Nationwide Food Consumption records, the average daily fructose intake in the United States in 1977–1978 was 37 g (Park and Yetley 1993). Based on more recent data from the National Health and Nutrition Examination Survey 1999–2004 study, the average fructose intake has increased to an estimated 49 g/day (Marriott et al. 2009). Although fructose and glucose have the same chemical formula ($C_6H_{12}O_6$), they are metabolized very differently due to the almost complete hepatic extraction and rapid hepatic conversion of fructose into glucose, glycogen, lactate, and fat (Tappy and Le 2010). Food products in which the main CHO is fructose or lactose elicit a low GI (Lang 2004; Wolever et al. 1994) and as reported by Foster-Powell et al. (2002) fructose eaten alone induces a very low GI (19 ± 2) compared to a glucose solution.

According to Bantle (2006), the consumption of fructose by both healthy and diabetic subjects produces a smaller postprandial rise in plasma glucose and serum insulin than other common CHOs. The same group compared the effect of isocaloric high fructose (20% of energy derived from fructose) and high starch diets (less than 3% of energy derived from fructose) in individuals with type-1 and type-2 diabetes (Bantle et al. 1992). Both diets were composed of common foods, including some cereal products. Substituting dietary fructose for other CHOs resulted in a 13% reduction in mean plasma glucose. Several other studies have confirmed these findings, and the lower glycemic response to fructose has also been observed in healthy and diabetic subjects in studies of solid foods (see Table 13.5).

Based on these studies, consuming foods that contain 25 to 50 g fructose as a replacement of available glucose leads to a decrease in the glycemic response of at least 30% in the acute phase, which is not systematically linked to lower insulin secretion.

13.2.4.2 Polyols

Polyols such as erythritol, xylitol, sorbitol, mannitol, isomalt, lactitol, maltitol, and polyglycitol are hydrogenated CHOs. These sugar-free sweeteners, also called sugar alcohols, are used as sugar replacements in foods such as confectionery, bakery, and dairy products. Among other potential health benefits, polyols are poorly digested and induce low glycemic and insulin responses. These properties are due to the interference of the alcohol group that replaces the carbonyl group and the occurrence of saccharide bonds other than the α-1,4 and α-1,6 bonds that are present in available CHOs. In clinical trials evaluating the impact of polyols on the glycemic response, a confounding factor is the quantity of CHO tested. In several studies, polyols have been used as 1:1 replacements for sugar. This replacement resulted in a decrease in the available CHO content of the tested products. Table 13.6 summarizes the effects of maltitol on glucose and insulin responses in healthy and diabetic subjects.

In both studies, the total quantity of sugar was replaced with maltitol, so the quantity of available CHOs was not equivalent in the maltitol tested food compared to the control one (Respondek et al. 2014; Rizkalla et al. 2002). Indeed, according to Livesey (2003), maltitol absorbability is only 45%, based on the consensus of energy values proposed by several authorities. Only one study, which tested muffins and bread, adapted the quantity of available CHO administered to the subjects (Quilez et al. 2007). The foods tested in this study provided an equivalent to 50 g of available CHOs in bread, the control muffin, and the muffin containing maltitol. The muffins containing maltitol induced lower glucose and insulin AUCs compared to the control muffin (20% for glucose, NS, and 30% for insulin, $p = .03$) and bread (48% for glucose, $p = .03$; 37% insulin, $p = .01$).

TABLE 13.5
Studies of Glucose and Insulin Responses When Fructose is Used as Sugar Replacement

Author	Delay	Food Form	Carbohydrates (g)	Fructose (g)	Subjects	Glycemic Response and GI for Fructose	Insulin Response
Bantle et al.1983	Acute (4 h)	Glucose meal, fructose meal, sucrose meal, potato meal, wheat meal	84 of total carbohydrates for each meal	42.00	10 healthy men	Smaller mean peak increment (38%), and mean iAUC than glucose (77%)	NS
					12 type-I diabetic subjects	NS	not studied
					10 type 2 diabetic subjects	Smaller mean peak increment (38%), and mean iAUC than glucose (46%)	NS
Wolever et al. 1985	Acute (3 h)	White bread, Oats 1/2 Oats plus 1/2 White bread 1/2 Oats plus Sucrose 1/2 Oats plus Fructose 1/2 Oats plus Glucose 1/2 Oats plus Lactose	50 of available carbohydrates	25.00	6 diabetic volunteers (2 men and 4 women)	AUC for fructose and lactose were significantly less than that for oats plus bread (32% and 17% less) Lactose and fructose had GIs significantly below that of bread reference (69 ± 10 and 35 ± 12, respectively)	not studied
Bantle et al.1992	Long term (28 d)	High fructose diet (20% of energy from fructose) crystalline fructose in baked goods, sweeten beverages, breakfast cereals	261 of available carbohydrates	88.00	6 type-I and 12 type 2 diabetic subjects	13% reduction with fructose diet after 28 days	NS
		High starch diet (<3% of energy from fructose), bread, potatoes, wheat or corn flour and oats	261 of available carbohydrates	5.00			
Lee and Wolever 1998	Acute (2 h)	Meals with 0–100 g of available carbohydrates from bread, glucose, sucrose, and fructose with 500 ml of either tea or water	0–100 of available carbohydrates	25 and 50	8 healthy subjects	Lower AUC after fructose than all the other carbohydrates at 25 and 50 g (89% and 86% reduction respectively for these doses compared to glucose) The GI value of fructose, 16 ± 4 was lower than bread (100) with no difference with any of the other sugars	Fructose induced a lower insulin response (85%) than bread and glucose at 50 g

Note: AUC: Area under the curve; iAUC: Incremental area under the curve; NS: Not significant; GI: Glycemic index.

TABLE 13.6
Effects of Maltitol on Glycemic and Insulin Responses in Healthy and Diabetic Subjects

Author	Delay	Food Form	Glucose and Polyol Content	Equivalent Quantity of Available Carbohydrates (Yes/No)	Subjects	Glycemic Response and GI for Polyols	Insulin Response
Rizkalla et al. 2002	Acute (3 h)	Lycasin syrup: hydrogenated starch hydrolysate 50%–55% maltitol, 5%–8% sorbitol, and 35%–40% hydrogenated oligosaccharides	50 g Lycasin vs. 50 g glucose	NO	6 healthy and 6 type 2 diabetic subjects	The GI was 47 ± 10% in healthy and 25 ± 6% in type 2 diabetic subjects Lower plasma glucose response with Lycasin between 60 and 180 min in type 2 diabetic subjects only (approximately 30%)	The insulin response was 23 ± 4% in healthy and 39 ± 14% in type 2 diabetic subjects Lower plasma insulin response with Lycasin between 15 and 90 min for healthy and at 90 min for type 2 diabetic subjects
Quilez et al. 2007	Acute (2 h)	Low calorie muffins	22% of maltitol in the low calorie muffin (49.2 g of total CHO) vs. plain muffin (48 g of total CHO) and bread (56.5 g of total CHO) food portions equivalent to 50 g of available carbohydrate	YES	14 healthy volunteers	Low calorie muffin GI = 37 ± 3% and plain muffin = 46 ± 8% Lower glucose AUC maltitol muffin compared to bread (48%) but NS compared to plain muffin (20%)	Lower insulin AUC maltitol muffin compared to bread (37%) and compared to plain muffin (30%)
Respondek et al. 2014	Acute (2 h)	Chocolate dairy dessert	35 g of maltitol in replacement of 35 g of D-glucose	NO	18 healthy subjects	45% reduction in glucose $AUC_{(0-120\ min)}$	38% reduction in insulin $AUC_{(0-120\ min)}$

Note: GI: glycemic index.

In conclusion, several studies that tested polyols as a sugar replacement observed a decrease in the glycemic response, due to a reduced quantity of available CHO and potentially a modified quality of sugars. However, the impact of the qualities of the sugars cannot be clearly evaluated because of the concomitant reduction in the quantity of available CHO. Thus, there is not enough data to clearly elucidate the effect of polyols on the GI. To address this question, specific studies should be designed to evaluate control and polyol-enriched products that provide the same amount of available CHO. These experiments should also test individual polyols.

13.2.5 Effect of Prebiotic Fibers

Fibers are nondigestible CHOs composed of three or more monomers. Fibers can have a direct effect on the GI by delaying gastric emptying, as discussed in Section 13.2.2.3. Moreover, as fibers are nondigestible, they are intact when they reach the colon, where they are metabolized by the microbiota. They can therefore modify both the activity and the composition of gut microbiota. Several studies have demonstrated that consuming barley kernel-based bread or wheat bread enriched with barley fibers in the evening has a beneficial effect on metabolism the following morning. Nilsson et al. (2008b) showed that meals including barley kernel-based bread and bread enriched with barley fibers providing 9 and 13 g of total dietary fibers (TDF) per serving, respectively, elicited a lower postprandial glycemia iAUC (−53% and −20%, respectively) compared to a meal including white wheat bread that contained 4 g of TDF per serving. The authors also observed an improvement in glucose tolerance at the subsequent breakfast. In this study, the glucose response was inversely correlated to colonic fermentation ($r = -0.25$; $p < .05$) that suggests that microbiota activity plays a role in these beneficial effects, most likely through the secretion of short chain fatty acids (SCFAs). Moreover, barley β-glucans appeared to be less efficient in decreasing the glycemic response compared to intrinsic fibers from barley kernels.

In addition to these short term effects, several studies have implicated the gut microbiota in longer-term regulation of postprandial glycemia in healthy individuals and patients with T2DM (Cani et al. 2009; Garcia et al. 2007; Lu et al. 2004; Parnell and Reimer 2009). Consuming 15 to 21 g/day of inulin, oligofructose, or arabinoxylanes for at least 6 weeks significantly decreased postprandial glycemia following the ingestion of a standardized breakfast meal or after an Oral Glucose Tolerance Test.

In conclusion, consuming between 9 and 13 g of prebiotic fibers indirectly reduces postprandial glycemia in the short term (about 12 h) through the production of SCFA. However, these studies did not provide sufficient information on the food matrix and fiber interactions to draw any further conclusions.

13.2.6 Increasing Glucose Output from Systemic Circulation by Increasing Insulin Secretion

13.2.6.1 Increasing Protein Quantity

The glycemic response to CHO-rich foods can be influenced by various factors in addition to the CHO content (Liljeberg Elmstahl and Bjorck 2001). Therefore, it is important to consider the food complexity and more specifically the influence of the combination of proteins and CHOs when studying the glycemic response. Plasma glucose concentration is the main regulator of insulin secretion. In addition to glucose, some dietary proteins and amino acids have an insulinotropic effect (Azzout-Marniche et al. 2014). Proteins are also strong stimulators of glucagon-like peptide-1 (GLP-1) (Raben et al. 2003). After ingesting a meal, intestinal hormones such as gastrointestinal-inhibitory peptide (GIP) and GLP-1 promote insulin secretion (Shrayyef and Gerich 2010).

Several studies have investigated the effect of milk and, more particularly, the whey protein fraction of milk on postprandial insulinemia. Three studies showed that the ingestion of 16–18 g of protein in a liquid food form, significantly reduced the glucose response and increased the insulin response (Frid et al. 2005; Gunnerud et al. 2012a; Liljeberg Elmstahl and Bjorck 2001) (Table 13.7).

TABLE 13.7
The Impact of Protein Combined with a CHO-Rich Meal on the Postprandial Metabolic Response

Author	Delay	Food Form	Carbohydrates (g)	Protein (g)	Subjects	Glycemic Response	Insulin Response
Frid et al. 2005	4 h after breakfast and 3 h after lunch	Breakfast: white wheat bread with or without whey powder in water	44.7 available carbohydrates	18.2 of whey protein	14 type 2 diabetic subjects	NS	The addition of whey increases the insulin response after both meals (18%–68% for breakfast and 49%–57% for lunch)
		Lunch: 52.2 g instant potato powder dissolved in water and 50 g of meatballs without whey powder in water	45.9 total carbohydrates of which 35.6 from potatoes			Reduced glycemia (around 20%) when whey proteins were introduced in the meal only after lunch	
Liljeberg Elmstahl and Bjorck 2001	2 h	High-GI bread and Low-GI spaghetti with or without 200 ml of milk	39.8 of total carbohydrates (30 from bread or spaghetti)	–	10 healthy subjects	NS for glucose $AUC_{0\text{–}95\ min}$	Increase $AUC_{0\text{–}95\ min}$ for the spaghetti (+300%)
		High-GI bread and Low-GI spaghetti with or without 400 ml of milk	49.6 of total carbohydrates (30 from bread or spaghetti)			NS for glucose $AUC_{0\text{–}95\ min}$	Increase $AUC_{0\text{–}95\ min}$ for both the spaghetti (+300%) and the bread (+65%)
Gunnerud et al. 2012a	2 h	White wheat bread (WWB)	25 of available carbohydrates	3.7	9 healthy subjects	$iAUC_{0\text{–}120\ min}$ is lower after all the drinks than after WWB (from 44%–64% reduction)	$iAUC_{0\text{–}120\ min}$ is increased only after whey (+58%)
		Whey drink		16.2			
		Casein drink		16.8			
		Bovine milk		16.8			
		Human milk		3.5			

Note: GI: Glycemic index, NS: Not significant, iAUC: Incremental area under the curve.

The interactions between CHO and proteins have also been studied in processed foods. In an analysis of 23 products (mean protein content 6.2 ± 2.9 g, range from 3 to 10 g/portion, providing 50 g of available CHOs) that excluded available CHO parameters, a 59% change in the GI was observed in response to the combined effects of the fat, protein, and nonstarch polysaccharide content. However, of these parameters, only the fat content was significant (Englyst et al. 2003). On the other hand, the protein content was strongly linked to an exacerbated insulin response (Englyst et al. 2003). More recently, a model derived from a database including 190 cereal products (mean protein content 6 ± 2 g/portion, range from 2 to 22 g/portion, providing 50 g of available CHOs) showed that SDS, RDS, fat, fibers, and interactions between these components account for 53% of the GI of a product (Meynier et al. 2015). Thus, these two studies have shown that the protein content of CHO-rich foods (mean content of around 6 g/portion) does not have a significant effect on the GI (Englyst et al. 2003). However, adding a greater range of high protein foods to a meal (14 breakfasts, mean protein content 15 ± 7 g, range from 5 to 28 g/portion) had a major effect on the GI (Flint et al. 2004). Indeed, in this study, the GI was inversely correlated to the amount of protein. The study by Flint et al. (2004) used a higher proportion of foods with protein content between 12 and 28 g (64%) than in the studies performed by Englyst et al. (2003) and Meynier et al. (2015), where 74% and 71% of the products, respectively, contained less than 6 g of protein. These doses are comparable to the milk protein study, in which an effect was observed with doses between 16 and 18 g.

In conclusion, proteins can reduce the glycemic response (from 20% to 64%) by stimulating the insulin response (from 50% to 300%) with a dose of at least 15 g/portion in a cereal product. Therefore, the ratio of protein:available CHO could have a significant effect on GI, although it entails an increase in insulin demand.

13.2.6.2 Effect of Amino Acids on Insulin Secretion

Dietary protein and amino acids regulate glucose homeostasis directly, by modulating blood glucose concentration, or indirectly, by modulating insulin secretion. Numerous studies have described the specific insulinotropic properties of amino acids such as arginine, leucine, alanine, and phenylalanine (Azzout-Marniche et al. 2014; Liu et al. 2008; Manders et al. 2012; Salehi et al. 2012). Most of these studies used liquid food forms. For instance, Gunnerud et al. (2012b) investigated the effects of premeal protein drinks (PMPD) and amino acids on glycemic, insulinemic, and incretin (GIP, GLP-1) responses at a subsequent meal. These drinks contained whey or soy protein either alone, with five added amino acids (4.5 g of amino acids in the drink) or with six added amino acids (5.2 g of amino acids in the drink). The amino acids used were isoleucine, leucine, lysine, threonine, and valine or these five amino acids plus arginine. All of the whey- or soy-based PMPD contained 50 g of available CHOs and 22–23 g of protein. The three whey-based PMPD meals, but not the soy-based PMPD meals, displayed lower GIs (73 ± 11 for whey, 53 ± 8 for whey + five amino acids, 60 ± 6 for whey + six amino acids) compared to the reference meal (GI = 100). In addition, a combination of whey and five amino acids (leucine, isoleucine, valine, lysine, and threonine; 4.5–7.4 g of amino acids) induced a reduced glycemic response (around 50%) and a higher insulin response (31%–50%) compared to the reference meal (Gunnerud et al. 2012b; Nilsson et al. 2007).

In conclusion, adding specific amino acids to liquid foods could lower the GI and glucose response beyond the global effect of protein content. The observed reduction in glycemia could be due to stimulation of the early phase of insulin secretion. Unfortunately, the lack of studies using solid food forms prevents us from drawing any conclusions regarding the interactions between food processing, food matrices, and amino acids. The quality of amino acids is also a determining factor, but the relative efficacy of different amino acid mixes remains to be investigated. As for the insulinotropic potential of amino acids, several studies have reported that a mixture containing a protein hydrolysate and free leucine has the greatest potential (Russell et al. 2013; van Loon et al. 2000a, b).

13.2.7 Summary of the Effects of Food Components on the GI

Decreasing the GI of processed foods is one of the major challenges faced by the food industry. In this chapter, we have discussed a variety of strategies that can be used to decrease the GI of foods that involve a very wide range of ingredients and food processing methods.

The interactions between food processing methods and ingredients can be neutral, but other interactions have a positive or negative effect on GI values. For instance, the physical characteristics of food (such as softness, cohesiveness, or toughness) have no clear influence on GI. Starch–lipid complexes, on the other hand have a potentially positive effect on GI (i.e., by decreasing the GI), and starch gelatinization has a demonstrable negative impact on GI.

Thus, controlling food processing and food composition is crucial for producing low GI CHO-rich foods (Table 13.8).

13.2.7.1 Validated Components That Decrease the GI

As reviewed here, some food components clearly decrease the GI (Table 13.8). The data show that viscous soluble fibers, SDS, lipids, and fructose significantly decrease the GI or glycemic response without exacerbating the insulin demand. The studies reviewed here reported a minimum decrease in the GI of around 30% compared to reference products with less or without active components. Some components also induced a decreased insulin response, which is an additional benefit in combination with the reduced GI. Viscous soluble fibers have the most significant effect on the insulin response, while SDS and fructose showed a less marked, but still positive, effect. On the other hand, lipids exhibited either no effect or a detrimental effect on the insulin response. In contrast, some types of protein dramatically exacerbate the insulin response, which results in a decrease in the GI. This increase in the insulin response stimulates blood glucose uptake by peripheral tissues.

Other food components may affect the GI, but there are either not enough data to clearly quantify the extend of the effect, or the effect is too limited to be effective. For example, organic acids, particularly acetic acid, strongly decrease the GI of high-GI foods only. Isomaltulose consistently decreases GI, whereas the reported effects of trehalose are contradictory. Modified or synthesized starches may also be useful candidates for decreasing the GI. As this effect depends directly on the structure of starch, a general recommendation cannot be made for all starches. Instead, each molecule needs to be investigated individually to determine its effect on the GI and postprandial metabolism, and to evaluate any potential side effects. Several other promising molecules, including modified starches, have been investigated, but the results are too preliminary to draw any conclusions (Kittisuban et al. 2014).

13.2.7.2 Food Components That Could Potentially Decrease the GI

In this chapter, several candidates for decreasing the GI of processed foods have been discussed. Polyphenols, the amylose:amylopectin ratio, polyols, and prebiotic fibers are promising candidates, although the results are still inconclusive (Table 13.8). Some studies, such as those investigating the amylose:amylopectin ratio and polyols, have too many confounding factors to allow us to draw any conclusions. For polyphenols and prebiotic fibers, there is not enough evidence to support a decrease in the GI. The buccal phase has been studied as well; however, there are too many complex interactions between the physical characteristics of foods, buccal enzymes, and mastication to merit further investigation of this topic.

Polyphenols have a wide range of chemical structures that lead to different effects on CHO digestion. However, the lack of characterization of the tested foods and sparse data regarding their effects do not allow us to draw any conclusions about their effect on the GI.

The amylose:amylopectin ratio has been studied for several years. Unfortunately, the different behavior of these two molecules during food processing dramatically increases the complexity of their potential beneficial effects. Thus, it is difficult to draw any conclusions regarding their effect on the GI. The formation of amylose:lipid complexes during food processing has been reported

TABLE 13.8
Summary of the Effect of Food Components on the GI and the II and Their Longer Term Health Impact

Component	Origin	Effect on GI	Effect on II	Mechanism Involved	Long-Term Health Impact
Texture	Food processing and composition	?	?	Buccal phase	No direct impact
Organic acids	Ingredient	+/0	0	Gastric emptying delay	Unknown
Lipids	Ingredient	++	0/-	Gastric emptying delay	High quantities linked to the development of metabolic disease
Viscous soluble fibers	Ingredient	+++	++	Gastric emptying delay	Prevent the development of metabolic disease
Slowly digestible starch	Preserved during processing (from flour)	+++	+	Small intestine digestion	Starch is the basis of daily CHO intake. By extrapolation, if this type of starch decreases the GI, it can be linked to the prevention of metabolic disease
Amylose:amylopectin	Structure of starch (from flour)	?	?	Small intestine digestion	
Synthesized or modified CHO*	Ingredient	++/0	+/0	Small intestine digestion	Unknown; will depend on the individual synthesized or modified starch
Starch–lipid complexes	Created during food processing	?	?	Small intestine digestion	Unknown
Polyphenols	Ingredients	?	?	Small intestine digestion	Potential health interest in preventing metabolic disease (antioxidant capacity) (Warning on high doses)
Prebiotic fibers	Ingredient	?	?	Microbiota activity	Prevent the development of metabolic disease (Warning on gastrointestinal discomfort)
Fructose	Ingredient	+++	+	Metabolized in the liver	Safety dose Associated with the development of metabolic disease, like sugars
Polyols	Ingredient	?	?		Transitory intestinal disorders; unknown long-term effects
Proteins	Ingredient	++	--	Stimulation of blood glucose output	Exacerbated insulin secretion is deleterious in the long term

Note: GI: Glycemic index; II: Insulin index.+: proven effect to decrease GI or II; 0: no effect on GI or II; -: proven effect to increase GI or II; ? not enough data to conclude on GI or II decrease; *: selected examples include isomaltulose and trehalose.

in vitro only. Thus, it is not possible to draw any conclusions regarding the potentially slower rate of starch digestion when complexed with lipids and the consequent effect on GI. Polyols are usually used as a sugar replacement by the food industry, and the quantity of available CHOs is not adjusted. It is therefore difficult to draw any conclusions regarding the effect of polyol use due to the confounding factors of the quantity and quality of available CHOs.

Fibers clearly decrease the GI and the II when they delay gastric emptying. Fibers exert an additional beneficial effect on the GI by modulating microbiota activity. This effect is detectable during a second meal, as glucose tolerance is improved a few hours after fiber consumption, resulting in a decrease in the GI of the next meal. Unfortunately, few data are available regarding this phenomenon.

13.3 LONG-TERM HEALTH IMPACT OF COMPONENTS THAT DECREASE THE GI

Several ingredients can influence the GI and the II. Decreasing the GI is associated with the prevention of metabolic disease (Blaak et al. 2012; Maki and Phillips 2015). However, some components that decrease GI efficiently have also been linked to the development of metabolic disease. In this section, this apparent contradiction will be discussed. In addition, some strategies for decreasing the GI may be relevant at an individual level, but considering the scale of food industry, implementing such changes would dramatically increase the exposure of consumers to these components.

13.3.1 Health Implications of Food Components Known to Decrease the GI

Viscous soluble fibers have been associated with a wide range of beneficial health effects, and particularly with the prevention of metabolic disease (Russell et al. 2013). SDS is an abundant component of raw flours derived from cereals and beans. During food processing, however, a portion of these SDSs is modified to become more rapidly digestible. Controlling food processing conditions could prevent this modification, resulting in the maintenance of a high level of SDS in processed starchy foods. Starch is a mandatory part of daily EI, as CHOs should represent between 45% and 55% of daily calorie consumption (FAO/WHO 1998). According to dietary recommendations, sugar intake should be limited to 10% of the total daily intake, and around 40% of the total daily EI should be provided by starch, which means around 200 g of starch per day for a diet providing 2000 kcal/day (World Health Organization 2015). Thus, preserving a high level of SDS in starchy products is beneficial for overall health.

Fat is directly related to high energy diets and is associated with the development of obesity because of its high energy density (Perez-Escamilla et al. 2012; Pourshahidi et al. 2014; Rolls et al. 2005). In addition, high fat diets have been associated with deleterious health effects including cardiovascular complications (Lottenberg et al. 2012; Ortega and Fernandez-Real 2013; Schwab et al. 2014). Furthermore, the addition of a large amount of lipids (40 g) to a starchy meal initially delays exogenous glucose absorption but leads to secondary glycemia later. Moreover, it is associated with high triglyceride concentration, a higher insulin:glucose ratio and decreased inhibition of endogenous glucose production, which imply insulin resistance (Normand et al. 2001). Thus, there may be some interest to use lipids to decrease the GI, if they are included in the diet in a way that does not modify the energy density of the overall diet. Additionally, food products with a low GI that is induced only by modifying the fat content should be included cautiously in a balanced diet.

Several studies have identified a deleterious effect of fructose consumption on glucose metabolism and insulin sensitivity, leading to metabolic complications such as dyslipidemia (Laville and Nazare 2009). A high fructose diet increased glucose and insulin responses to a sucrose load (Hallfrisch et al. 1983), increased fasting glycemia (Liu et al. 2006), and led to hepatic insulin resistance in healthy men (Faeh et al. 2005). However, there is no evidence that fructose intake in moderate doses is directly related to these adverse metabolic effects (Chiavaroli et al. 2015; Le et al. 2009; van Buul et al. 2014). The deleterious effects are only observed in high doses of fructose (≥25% of the total daily energy intake, corresponding to around 125 g/day) (Stanhope and Havel 2008), but not in lower doses (40–50 g/day when taken instead of starch or sucrose) (Jayalath et al. 2014; Rizkalla 2010). However, according to general diet recommendations, all sugars, including fructose, should account for only 10% of the daily EI (World Health Organization 2015). Therefore, fructose is not recommended as a promising candidate for decreasing the GI of CHO-rich foods produced by the food industry.

Organic acids, such as acetic acid, which is present in vinegar, induce a moderate decrease in the GI. Even though there is no obvious risk involved in slightly increasing the consumption of organic acids, further studies are needed to develop a clear recommendation for their use in decreasing the GI of processed foods.

Increasing the protein content of processed foods exacerbates the insulin response, leading to a corresponding decrease in the GI. This overstimulation of the pancreas contradicts recommendations for preventing T2DM (Grill and Bjorklund 2001; Russell et al. 2013; Weickert et al. 2011). The elevation of blood glucose during the postprandial period, in combination with an exacerbated insulin secretion, leads to transitory deleterious metabolic and hormonal states and oxidative stress. These negative effects involve the liver, pancreas, and skeletal muscles, and have an impact on lipid metabolism and inflammatory parameters in healthy subjects, and the effects are exacerbated in individuals with IGT (Blaak et al. 2012; Weickert et al. 2011). Interestingly, the exacerbated insulin response is not necessarily induced by all types of amino acids (Hattersley et al. 2014; Nilsson et al. 2007). Thus, further investigation of the amino acid composition of proteins may be more promising.

13.3.2 Health Implications of Potential Candidates for Decreasing the GI

For some components that have been studied for their impact on GI—polyphenols, the amylose:amylopectin ratio, polyols, and prebiotic fibers—there is no clear conclusion on their effect. Amylose and amylopectin are natural starch structures, and starch is a mandatory component of the daily EI, as CHOs should represent between 45% and 55% of the daily energy consumption (FAO/WHO 1998).

Two members of this list—polyols and prebiotic fibers—are partially or totally indigestible. Despite the potential health benefits, increasing fiber intake can lead to undesirable side effects such as gas, bloating, abdominal distension, and increased stool frequency (Grabitske and Slavin 2009). These effects are primarily due to two phenomena. The first is the fermentation of these fibers by the gut microbiota, which leads to the production of gases in the colon (Nyman 2002). This can induce bloating, distention, borborygmi, and flatulence. The second is the osmotic effect of an increased amount of water in the colon (Grabitske and Slavin 2009), which can lead to increased stool frequency and diarrhea. Generally, these gastrointestinal symptoms increase with increasing doses of fiber (Bonnema et al. 2010). However, the gastrointestinal tolerance may increase with regular fiber intake. Indeed, it is thought that the digestive tract can adapt to increased fiber intake over time. However, not enough information is currently available to confirm this hypothesis (Bonnema et al. 2010).

In a study of 59 healthy volunteers, Koutsou et al. (1996) showed that different polyols induce gastrointestinal symptoms with differing degrees of severity. Ingesting 40 g of lactitol in milk chocolate induced a significant increase in the frequency and severity of gastrointestinal symptoms compared to a standard sucrose-containing chocolate. This increase in symptoms was also observed when the study participants consumed 40 g of isomalt, although the effects were mild. Finally, 40 g of maltitol induced fewer symptoms than isomalt, and there was a significant decrease in all of the symptoms when the dose was decreased to 30 g. A recent study by Respondek et al. (2014) showed that ingesting 35 g of maltitol in a chocolate dairy dessert induced higher discomfort than the control, although the effects were considered to be mild. Precautions should be taken when using polyols as sugar replacements, as mild side effects are observed in response to doses that are similar to or even lower than the dose needed to have a beneficial effect on the GI.

Polyphenols have many health benefits (Tapiero et al. 2002); however, some adverse effects have also been linked to polyphenol intake. Some polyphenols, such as quercetin or caffeic acid, may be carcinogenic when consumed in high doses (Catterall et al. 2000; Hagiwara et al. 1991).

However, these effects are only observed with high levels of polyphenol intake. Some polyphenols, when consumed in excess, develop pro-oxidant properties (Awad et al. 2002; Lecci et al. 2014). Isoflavones are a family of polyphenols that have a specific estrogen-like activity due to their structure. This can have positive and negative effects on consumer health, especially by affecting fertility and the development of some types of cancers (Ososki and Kennelly 2003). Finally, polyphenols may also have antinutritional effects. For example, consuming tea can inhibit the absorption of nonheme iron, which can lead to iron depletion in the case of individuals with diagnosed anemia or at risk of anemia who consume large amounts of tea (Temme and Van Hoydonck 2002; Wierzejska 2014). However, in light of the current understanding of polyphenol side effects, it is not possible to define an upper limit for safe consumption of polyphenols.

These effects should be considered when designing food products, and appropriate doses should be determined taking into account the potential global intake of these compounds to avoid excessive intake.

13.3.3 Relevance of Component Combinations to Optimize GI Decrease

The available data show that some components can decrease the GI without affecting the II. In this chapter, the impact of these food components on the palatability of food products has not been directly addressed. However, it is generally acknowledged that fiber (especially viscous soluble fiber), which is one of the best candidates for decreasing the GI, can decrease the palatability of solid food. On the other hand, some food processing methods do not provide an adequate SDS content in the final food products, as these processing conditions require high dough hydration or high pressure. Therefore, combining some compounds may have better effects on the GI and improve the acceptability of these food products to consumers.

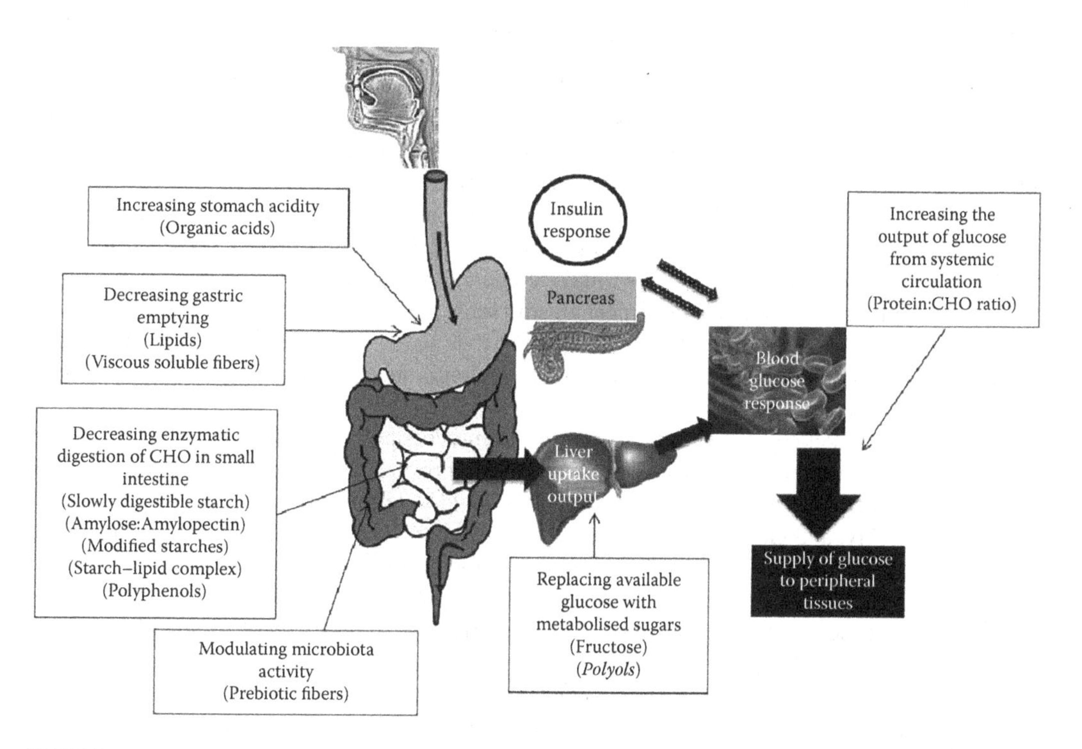

FIGURE 13.5 Description of how food components may decrease the GI during the digestive and postabsorptive phases.

To evaluate the effectiveness of a mixture of active components in decreasing the GI, it is important to consider the mechanism by which these components act (Figure 13.5). Obviously, the health impact of these items needs to be considered as well. There are two approaches to producing foods with reduced GIs: either by emphasizing one mechanism of action or incorporating complementary mechanisms of action. Very few studies have evaluated the impact of components alone or in combination within a specific food matrix. Thus, our discussion of this strategy will be based on hypotheses and studies in which statistical analyses were performed on combined components.

13.3.3.1 Combination of Components to Reinforce One Mechanism

Reinforcing a single mechanism for decreasing the GI seems easily achievable, in theory, especially with regard to decreasing gastric emptying or promoting the enzymatic digestion of CHO in the small intestine (Zhang et al. 2015). For example, combining viscous soluble fibers and a moderate amount of fat could be an appropriate approach for delaying gastric emptying. Recent work has shown that fiber and moderate amounts of fat combine to decrease the GI, based on data from 190 processed cereal foods (Meynier et al. 2015). However, the quantities of each component required to produce this effect and the magnitude of the effect on the GI require further investigation. To date, there is no clear consensus on this topic.

Starch digestion could be modulated by modifying the starch structure in complementary ways. For example, the food processing methods could be controlled to maintain native SDS levels, as well as including some synthesized or modified starches. However, there are currently no data available regarding this strategy, and each combination would need to be studied on a case-by-case basis.

Another promising approach that requires further investigation is the combination of favorable starch structures (either SDS or modified starch) with polyphenols to decrease the GI (Peng et al. 2015). However, polyphenols can have a negative effect on flavor; therefore, each combination should be tested for its effects on metabolism and product palatability.

13.3.3.2 Combination of Components with Complementary Mechanisms

The combination of multiple mechanisms of action leads to more potential ways to decrease the GI without exacerbating insulin demand. A recent study proposed several combinations of food components that could be used to slow down small intestine digestion of starch and lower the GI by additional mechanisms (Zhang et al. 2015). The combinations discussed included mixing SDS with proteins, polyphenols, or fat. Based on a statistical analysis of cereal products, SDS, fat, and fiber are the three most important components linked to decreasing the GI of solid foods (Meynier et al. 2015). Combining two complementary mechanisms such as gastric emptying and small intestine digestion could limit the amount of each component that needs to be added to the food formula. However, further research is needed to identify the optimal ratio for combining these components to decrease the GI.

Additional combinations that take into account food processing constraints should also be tested, such as slowing gastric emptying with viscous soluble fibers and/or fat and the use of metabolized sugars such as fructose or isomaltulose. Other factors could be tested, such as processing feasibility, product palatability, and GI impact. Furthermore, it is important to remember that the effects and feasibility of these combinations may be related to the food matrix as well.

Other suggested approaches combine polyols with prebiotic fibers. The main purpose of this combination is to decrease the gastrointestinal side effects of these components while reducing the glycemic response. For example, maltitol may cause gastrointestinal symptoms by increasing osmotic pressure, and some fibers, such as cellulose or partially hydrolyzed guar gum, could reduce this pressure due to their ability to form gels and delay gastric emptying (Nakamura et al. 2007; Oku et al. 2008). Similar approaches should be explored before drawing any conclusions regarding their efficacy.

Since the food matrix is often a complex structure, the concept of using complementary components to decrease the GI presents new possibilities that may be more feasible for food design.

13.4 CONCLUSION

The GI of processed foods can be decreased using several already validated ways and/or promising solutions that are still under investigation. The health impact of the components is an important consideration in identifying the best candidates. Fiber and SDS can decrease the GI effectively and are associated with long-term health benefits. They can be combined in complex food matrices with limited amounts of fat or fructose to reinforce their activity, if needed. Polyphenols, specifically modified or synthesized CHOs, and organic acids also have promising effects and should be investigated further.

In all cases, the low GIs of these improved foods should be validated in clinical trials where the appropriate procedures used to measure the GI are fully respected (Brouns et al. 2005; FAO/WHO 1998; International Standard Organisation 2010). Indeed, it is very difficult to calculate a valid GI from a formula. Interactions between ingredients during processing can induce reactions that interfere with CHO digestibility, for example, the formation of starch–lipid complexes. In addition, interactions between components within the gut could modify CHO degradation and absorption; for example, polyphenols could affect CHO digestion by acting at the enzyme level. Therefore, combining components to decrease the GI of food products and promote long-term health benefits is a promising area of research for optimizing the production of low GI foods and improving consumer health.

Some components, such as fiber (Jannie et al. 2014) and organic acids (Partanen and Mroz 1999) may decrease palatability while polyphenols may increase astringency (King-Thom et al. 1998). Therefore, it is an important challenge to formulate foods enriched with these components that maintain an acceptable level of taste for consumers.

Finally, after finding ways to decrease the GI, the second challenge for food industry is to guarantee that all batches of a same product remain low GI all throughout their shelf life. Specific quality controls must be planned by each company to provide this guarantee to consumers.

REFERENCES

Ahmadi-Abhari S, Woortman AJJ, Hamer RJ, Oudhuis AACM, and Loos K. Influence of lysophosphatidylcholine on the gelation of diluted wheat starch suspensions. *Carbohydrate Polymers* 93 no. 1 (2013a): 224–31.

Ahmadi-Abhari S, Woortman AJJ, Oudhuis AACM, Hamer RJ, and Loos K. The influence of amylose-LPC complex formation on the susceptibility of wheat starch to amylase. *Carbohydrate Polymers* 97 no. 2 (2013b): 436–40.

Ajala O, English P, and Pinkney J. Systematic review and meta-analysis of different dietary approaches to the management of type 2 diabetes. *American Journal of Clinical Nutrition* 97 no. 3 (2013): 505–16.

Akerberg A, Liljeberg H, and Bjorck I. Effects of amylose/amylopectin ratio and baking conditions on resistant starch formation and glycaemic indices. *Journal of Cereal Science* 28 no. 1 (1998): 71–80.

Amelsvoort JMM, and Weststrate JA. Amylose-amylopectin ratio in a meal affects postprandial variables in male volunteers. *American Journal of Clinical Nutrition* 55 no. 3 (1992): 712–18.

Atkinson FS, Foster-Powell K, and Brand-Miller JC. International tables of glycemic index and glycemic load values: 2008. *Diabetes Care* 31 no. 12 (2008): 2281–83.

Awad HM, Boersma MG, Boeren S, van der Woude H, and van Zanden J. Identification of o-quinone/quinone methide metabolites of quercetin in a cellular in vitro system. *FEBS Letters* 520 no. 1–3 (2002): 30.

Azzout-Marniche D, Gaudichon C, and Tome D. Dietary protein and blood glucose control. *Current Opinion in Clinical Nutrition and Metabolic Care* 17 no. 4 (2014): 349–54.

Bantle JP, Laine DC, Castle GW, Thomas JW, and Hoogwerf BJ. Postprandial glucose and insulin responses to meals containing different carbohydrates in normal and diabetic subjects. *New England Journal of Medicine* 309 no. 1 (1983): 7–12.

Bantle JP, Swanson JE, Thomas W, and Laine DC. Metabolic effects of dietary fructose in diabetic subjects. *Diabetes Care* 15 no. 11 (1992): 1468–76.

Bantle JP. Is fructose the optimal low glycemic index sweetener? *Nestlé Nutrition Workshop Series Clinical & Performance Programme* 11 (2006): 83–91.

Barrett A, Ndou T, Hughey CA, Straut C, and Howell A. Inhibition of alpha-amylase and glucoamylase by tannins extracted from cocoa, pomegranates, cranberries, and grapes. *Journal of Agricultural and Food Chemistry* 61 no. 7 (2013): 1477–86.

Behall KM, and Howe JC. Effect of long-term consumption of amylose vs amylopectin starch on metabolic variables in human subjects. *American Journal of Clinical Nutrition* 61 no. 2 (1995): 334–40.

Behall KM, Scholfield DJ, and Canary J. Effect of starch structure on glucose and insulin responses in adults. *American Journal of Clinical Nutrition* 47 no. 3 (1988): 428–32.

Behall KM, Scholfield DJ, Yuhaniak I, and Canary J. Diets containing high amylose vs amylopectin starch: Effects on metabolic variables in human subjects. *American Journal of Clinical Nutrition* 49 no. 2 (1989): 337–44.

Benmoussa M, Moldenhauer KAK, and Hamaker BR. Rice amylopectin fine structure variability affects starch digestion properties. *Journal of Agricultural and Food Chemistry* 55 no. 4 (2007): 1475–79.

Blaak EE, Antoine JM, Benton D, Bjorck I, and Bozzetto L. Impact of postprandial glycaemia on health and prevention of disease. *Obesity Reviews* 13 no. 10 (2012): 923–84.

Bonnema AL, Kolberg LW, Thomas W, and Slavin JL. Gastrointestinal tolerance of chicory inulin products. *Journal of the American Dietetic Association* 110 no. 6 (2010): 865–68.

Bornet F. Technological treatments of cereals. Repercussions on the physiological properties of starch. *Carbohydrates Polymers* 21 no. 2–3 (1993): 195–203.

Bornhorst GM, and Paul Singh R. Bolus formation and disintegration during digestion of food carbohydrates. *Comprehensive Reviews in Food Science and Food Safety* 11 no. 2 (2012): 101–18.

Bornhorst GM, and Paul Singh R. Gastric digestion in vivo and in vitro: How the structural aspects of food influence the digestion process. *Annual Review of Food Science and Technology* 5 (2014): 111–32.

Bourne M. Relation between texture and mastication. *Journal of Texture Studies* 35 no. 2 (2004): 125–43.

Brouns F, Bjorck I, Frayn KN, Gibbs AL, and Lang V. Glycaemic index methodology. *Nutrition Research Reviews* 18 no. 1 (2005): 145–71.

Burdge GC, Powell J, and Calder PC. Lack of effect of meal fatty acid composition on postprandial lipid, glucose and insulin responses in men and women aged 50–65 years consuming their habitual diets. *British Journal of Nutrition* 96 no. 3 (2006): 489–500.

Can JGP, IJzerman TH, Loon LJC, Brouns F, and Blaak EE. Reduced glycaemic and insulinaemic responses following trehalose ingestion: Implications for postprandial substrate use. *British Journal of Nutrition* 102 no. 10 (2009): 1395–99.

Can JGP, Loon LJC, Brouns F, and Blaak EE. Reduced glycaemic and insulinaemic responses following trehalose and isomaltulose ingestion: Implications for postprandial substrate use in impaired glucose-tolerant subjects. *British Journal of Nutrition* 108 no. 7 (2012): 1210–17.

Cani PD, Lecourt E, Dewulf EM, Sohet FM, and Pachikian BD. Gut microbiota fermentation of prebiotics increases satietogenic and incretin gut peptide production with consequences for appetite sensation and glucose response after a meal. *American Journal of Clinical Nutrition* 90 no. 5 (2009): 1236–43.

Catterall F, Souquet JM, Cheynier V, Clifford MN, and Ioannides C. Modulation of the mutagenicity of food carcinogens by oligomeric and polymeric procyanidins isolated from grape seeds: Synergistic genotoxicity with N-nitrosopyrrolidine. *Journal of the Science of Food and Agriculture* 80 no. 1 (2000): 91–101.

Cecil JE, Francis J, and Read NW. Comparison of the effects of a high-fat and high-carbohydrate soup delivered orally and intragastrically on gastric emptying, appetite, and eating behaviour. *Physiology & Behavior* 67 no. 2 (1999): 299–306.

Chen J. Food oral processing—a review. *Food Hydrocolloids* 23 no. 1 (2009): 1–25.

Chiavaroli L, Ha V, de Souza RJ, Kendall CWC, and Sievenpiper JL. Overstated associations between fructose and nonalcoholic fatty liver disease. *Journal of Pediatric Gastroenterology and Nutrition* 60 no. 4 (2015): e35.

Chung OK, Pomeranz Y, and Finney KF. Wheat flour lipids in breadmaking. *Cereal Chemistry* 55 (1978): 598–618.

Coe SA, Clegg M, Armengol M, and Ryan L. The polyphenol-rich baobab fruit (Adansonia digitata L.) reduces starch digestion and glycemic response in humans. *Nutrition Research* 33 no. 11 (2013): 888–96.

Collier G, McLean A, and O'Dea K. Effect of co-ingestion of fat on the metabolic responses to slowly and rapidly absorbed carbohydrates. *Diabetologia* 26 no. 1 (1984): 50–54.

Colonna P, Barry JL, Cloarec D, Bornet F, and Gouilloud S. Enzymic susceptibility of starch from pasta. *Journal of Cereal Science* 11 no. 1 (1990): 59–70.

Colonna P, Leloup V, and Buleon A. Limiting factors of starch hydrolysis. *European Journal of Clinical Nutrition* 46 Suppl. 2 (1992): S17–S32.

Copeland L, Blazek J, Salman H, and Tang MC. Form and functionality of starch. *Food Hydrocolloids* 23 no. 6 (2009): 1527–34.

Cortes B, Nunez I, Cofan M, Gilabert R, and Perez-Heras A. Acute effects of high-fat meals enriched with walnuts or olive oil on postprandial endothelial function. *Journal of the American College of Cardiology* 48 no. 8 (2006): 1666–71.

Crowe TC, Seligman SA, and Copeland L. Inhibition of enzymic digestion of amylose by free fatty acids in vitro contributes to resistant starch formation. *Journal of Nutrition* 130 no. 8S (2000): 2006–08.

Cunningham KM, and Read NW. The effect of incorporating fat into different components of a meal on gastric emptying and postprandial blood glucose and insulin responses. *British Journal of Nutrition* 61 no. 2 (1989): 285–90.

Darwiche G, Ostman EM, Liljeberg HG, Kallinen N, and Bjorgell O. Measurements of the gastric emptying rate by use of ultrasonography: Studies in humans using bread with added sodium propionate. *American Journal of Clinical Nutrition* 74 no. 2 (2001): 254–58.

Darwiche G, Bjorgell O, and Almer LO. The addition of locust bean gum but not water delayed the gastric emptying rate of a nutrient semisolid meal in healthy subjects. *BMC Gastroenterology* 3 (2003): 12.

Dikeman CL, Murphy MR, and Fahey GC, Jr. Dietary fibers affect viscosity of solutions and simulated human gastric and small intestinal digesta. *Journal of Nutrition* 136 no. 4 (2006): 913–19.

Dwyer JT, and Ouyang CM. What can industry do to facilitate dietary and behavioural changes?. *British Journal of Nutrition* 83 Suppl. 1 (2000): S173–S180.

Eastwood MA, and Morris ER. Physical properties of dietary fiber that influence physiological function: A model for polymers along the gastrointestinal tract. *American Journal of Clinical Nutrition* 55 no. 2 (1992): 436–42.

Englyst HN, Kingman SM, and Cummings JH. Classification and measurement of nutritionally important starch fractions. *European Journal of Clinical Nutrition* 46 Suppl. 2 (1992): S33–S50.

Englyst HN, Veenstra J, and Hudson GJ. Measurement of rapidly available glucose (RAG) in plant foods: A potential in vitro predictor of the glycaemic response. *British Journal of Nutrition* 75 no. 3 (1996): 327–37.

Englyst KN, Englyst HN, Hudson GJ, Cole TJ, and Cummings JH. Rapidly available glucose in foods: An in vitro measurement that reflects the glycemic response. *American Journal of Clinical Nutrition* 69 no. 3 (1999): 448–54.

Englyst KN, Vinoy S, Englyst HN, and Lang V. Glycaemic index of cereal products explained by their content of rapidly and slowly available glucose. *British Journal of Nutrition* 89 no. 3 (2003): 329–40.

Faeh D, Minehira K, Schwarz JM, Periasamy R, and Park S. Effect of fructose overfeeding and fish oil administration on hepatic de novo lipogenesis and insulin sensitivity in healthy men. *Diabetes* 54 no. 7 (2005): 1907–13.

FAO/WHO. Carbohydrates in human nutrition. Report of a Joint FAO/WHO Expert Consultation. *FAO Food and Nutrition Paper* 66 (1998): 1–140.

Flint A, Moller BK, Raben A, Pedersen D, and Tetens I. The use of glycaemic index tables to predict glycaemic index of composite breakfast meals. *British Journal of Nutrition* 91 no. 6 (2004): 979–89.

Flynn CS. 2012. The particle size distribution of solid foods after human mastication: A thesis presented in partial fulfilment of the requirements for the degree of Doctor of Philosophy in Food Technology at Massey University, Auckland, New Zealand. PhD

Foster KD, Woda A, and Peyron MA. Effect of texture of plastic and elastic model foods on the parameters of mastication. *Journal of Neurophysiology* 95 no. 6 (2006): 3469–79.

Foster-Powell K, Holt SHA, and Brand-Miller JC. International table of glycemic index and glycemic load values: 2002. *American Journal of Clinical Nutrition* 76 no. 1 (2002): 5–56.

Fredriksson H, Salomonsson L, Andersson R, and Salomonsson AC. Effects of protein and starch characteristics on the baking properties of wheat cultivated by different strategies with organic fertilizers and urea. *Acta Agriculturae Scandinavica. Section B, Soil and Plant Science* 48 no. 1 (1998): 49–57.

French D, and Knapp DW. The maltase of Clostridium acetobutylicum: Its specificity range and mode of action. *The Journal of Biological Chemistry* 187 no. 2 (1950): 463–71.

Frid AH, Nilsson M, Holst JJ, and Bjorck IME. Effect of whey on blood glucose and insulin responses to composite breakfast and lunch meals in type 2 diabetic subjects. *American Journal of Clinical Nutrition* 82 no. 1 (2005): 69–75.

Fried M, Abramson S, and Meyer JH. Passage of salivary amylase through the stomach in humans. *Digestive Diseases and Sciences* 32 no. 10 (1987): 1097–103.

Gannon MC, Nuttall FQ, Westphal SA, and Seaquist ER. The effect of fat and CHO on plasma glucose, insulin, C-peptide, and triglycerides in normal male subjects. *Journal of the American College of Nutrition* 12 no. 1 (1993): 36–41.

Garcia AL, Otto B, Reich SC, Weickert MO, and Steiniger J. Arabinoxylan consumption decreases postprandial serum glucose, serum insulin and plasma total ghrelin response in subjects with impaired glucose tolerance. *European Journal of Clinical Nutrition* 61 no. 3 (2007): 334–41.

Garsetti M, Vinoy S, Lang V, Holt S, and Loyer S. The glycemic and insulinemic index of plain sweet biscuits: Relationships to in vitro starch digestibility. *Journal of the American College of Nutrition* 24 no. 6 (2005): 441–47.

Gaviao MBD, and Bilt AVd. Salivary secretion and chewing: Stimulatory effects from artificial and natural foods. *Journal of Applied Oral Science: Revista FOB* 12 no. 2 (2004): 159–63.

Goff LM, Cowland DE, Hooper L, and Frost GS. Low glycaemic index diets and blood lipids: A systematic review and meta-analysis of randomised controlled trials. *Nutrition, Metabolism and Cardiovascular Diseases* 23 no. 1 (2013): 1–10.

Grabitske HA, and Slavin JL. Gastrointestinal effects of low-digestible carbohydrates. *Critical Reviews In Food Science And Nutrition* 49 no. 4 (2009):327–60.

Granfeldt Y, Liljeberg H, Drews A, Newman R, and Bjoerk I. Glucose and insulin responses to barley products: Influence of food structure and amylose-amylopectin ratio. *American Journal of Clinical Nutrition* 59 no. 5 (1994): 1075–82.

Granfeldt Y, Nyberg L, and Bjorck I. Muesli with 4 g oat beta-glucans lowers glucose and insulin responses after a bread meal in healthy subjects. *European Journal of Clinical Nutrition* 62 no. 5 (2008): 600–07.

Grill V, and Bjorklund A. Overstimulation and beta-cell function. *Diabetes* 50 Suppl. 1 (2001): S122–S124.

Gunnerud U, Holst JJ, Ostman E, and Bjorck I. The glycemic, insulinemic and plasma amino acid responses to equi-carbohydrate milk meals, a pilot-study of bovine and human milk. *Nutrition Journal* 11 (2012a): 83.

Gunnerud UJ, Heinzle C, Holst JJ, Ostman EM, and Bjorck IME. Effects of pre-meal drinks with protein and amino acids on glycemic and metabolic responses at a subsequent composite meal. *Plos One* 7 no. 9 (2012b): e44731.

Guraya HS, Kadan RS, and Champagne ET. Effect of rice starch–lipid complexes on in vitro digestibility, complexing index, and viscosity. *Cereal Chemistry* 74 no. 5 (1997): 561–65.

Hagiwara A, Hirose M, Takahashi S, Ogawa K, and Shirai T. Forestomach and kidney carcinogenicity of caffeic acid in F344 rats and C57BL/6N × C3H/HeN F1 mice. *Cancer Research* 51 no. 20 (1991): 5655–60.

Hallfrisch J, Ellwood KC, Michaelis OE, Reiser S, and O'Dorisio TM. Effects of dietary fructose on plasma glucose and hormone responses in normal and hyperinsulinemic men. *Journal of Nutrition* 113 no. 9 (1983): 1819–26.

Hanhineva K, Torronen R, Bondia-Pons I, Pekkinen J, and Kolehmainen M. Impact of dietary polyphenols on carbohydrate metabolism. *International Journal of Molecular Sciences* 11 no. 4 (2010): 1365–402.

Hattersley JG, Pfeiffer AFH, Roden M, Petzke KJ, and Hoffmann D. Modulation of amino acid metabolic signatures by supplemented isoenergetic diets differing in protein and cereal fiber content. *Journal of Clinical Endocrinology and Metabolism* 99 no. 12 (2014): E2599–E2609.

Heaton KW, Marcus SN, Emmett PM, and Bolton CH. Particle size of wheat, maize, and oat test meals: Effects on plasma glucose and insulin responses and on the rate of starch digestion in vitro. *American Journal of Clinical Nutrition* 47 no. 4 (1988): 675–82.

Hlebowicz J, Darwiche G, Bjorgell O, and Almer LO. Effect of muesli with 4 g oat beta-glucan on postprandial blood glucose, gastric emptying and satiety in healthy subjects: A randomized crossover trial. *Journal of the American College of Nutrition* 27 no. 4 (2008): 470–75.

Hoebler C, Karinthi A, Devaux MF, Guillon F, and Gallant DJG. Physical and chemical transformations of cereal food during oral digestion in human subjects. *British Journal of Nutrition* 80 no. 5 (1998): 429–36.

Holm J, Bjoerck I, Ostrowska S, Eliasson AC, and Asp NG. Digestibility of amylose-lipid complexes in-vitro and in-vivo. *Starch/Staerke* 35 no. 9 (1983): 294–97.

Holm J, Koellreutter B, and Wursch P. Influence of sterilization, drying and oat bran enrichment of pasta on glucose and insulin responses in healthy subjects and on the rate and extent of in vitro starch digestion. *European Journal of Clinical Nutrition* 46 no. 9 (1992): 629–40.

Holub I, Gostner A, Theis S, Nosek L, and Kudlich T. Novel findings on the metabolic effects of the low glycaemic carbohydrate isomaltulose (Palatinose). *British Journal of Nutrition* 103 no. 12 (2010): 1730–37.

International Standard Organisation. Food products - Determination of the glycaemic index (GI) and recommendation for food classification. ISO/FDIS 26642. (2010).

Jannie Yi FY, Smeele RJM, Harington KD, Loon FM, and Wanders AJ. The effects of functional fiber on postprandial glycemia, energy intake, satiety, palatability and gastrointestinal wellbeing: A randomized crossover trial. *Nutrition Journal* 13 (2014): 9.

Jayalath VH, Sievenpiper JL, de Souza RJ, Ha V, and Mirrahimi A. Total fructose intake and risk of hypertension: A systematic review and meta-analysis of prospective cohorts. *Journal of the American College of Nutrition* 33 no. 4 (2014): 328–39.

Johnston K, Sharp P, Clifford M, and Morgan L. Dietary polyphenols decrease glucose uptake by human intestinal Caco-2 cells. *FEBS Letters* 579 no. 7 (2005): 1653–57.

Juvonen KR, Salmenkallio-Marttila M, Lyly M, Liukkonen KH, and Lahteenmaki L. Semisolid meal enriched in oat bran decreases plasma glucose and insulin levels, but does not change gastrointestinal peptide responses or short-term appetite in healthy subjects. *Nutrition, Metabolism and Cardiovascular Diseases* 21 no. 9 (2011): 748–56.

King-Thom C, Tit YW, Cheng I, Yao-Wen H, and Yuan L. Tannins and human health: A review. *Critical Reviews In Food Science And Nutrition* 38 no. 6 (1998):421–64.

Kittisuban P, Lee BH, Suphantharika M, and Hamaker BR. Slow glucose release property of enzyme-synthesized highly branched maltodextrins differs among starch sources. *Carbohydrate Polymers* 107 (2014): 182–91.

Koutsou GA, Storey DM, Lee A, Zumbe A, and Flourie B. Dose-related gastrointestinal response to the ingestion of either isomalt, lactitol or maltitol in milk chocolate. *European Journal of Clinical Nutrition* 50 no. 1 (1996): 17–21.

Lang V. Development of a range of industrialised cereal-based foodstuffs, high in slowly digestible starch. In *Starch in Food: Structure, Function and Applications:* Eliasson AC, ed., 477–504. Cambridge: Woodhead Publishing (2004).

Lardinois CK, Starich GH, Mazzaferri EL, and DeLett A. Polyunsaturated fatty acids augment insulin secretion. *Journal of the American College of Nutrition* 6 no. 6 (1987): 507–15.

Laville M, and Nazare JA. Diabetes, insulin resistance and sugars. *Obesity Reviews* 10 Suppl. 1 (2009): 24–33.

Le KA, Ith M, Kreis R, Faeh D, and Bortolotti M. Fructose overconsumption causes dyslipidemia and ectopic lipid deposition in healthy subjects with and without a family history of type 2 diabetes. *American Journal of Clinical Nutrition* 89 no. 6 (2009): 1760–65.

Lebenthal E. Role of salivary amylase in gastric and intestinal digestion of starch. *Digestive Diseases and Sciences* 32 no. 10 (1987): 1155–57.

Lecci RM, Logrieco A, and Leone A. Pro-oxidative action of polyphenols as action mechanism for their pro-apoptotic activity. *Anti-Cancer Agents in Medicinal Chemistry* 14 no. 10 (2014): 1363–75.

Leclere CJ, Champ M, Boillot J, Guille G, and Lecannu G. Role of viscous guar gums in lowering the glycemic response after a solid meal. *American Journal of Clinical Nutrition* 59 no. 4 (1994): 914–21.

Lee BM, and Wolever TM. Effect of glucose, sucrose and fructose on plasma glucose and insulin responses in normal humans: Comparison with white bread. *European Journal of Clinical Nutrition* 52 no. 12 (1998): 924–28.

Liatis S, Grammatikou S, Poulia KA, Perrea D, and Makrilakis K. Vinegar reduces postprandial hyperglycaemia in patients with type II diabetes when added to a high, but not to a low, glycaemic index meal. *European Journal of Clinical Nutrition* 64 no. 7 (2010): 727–32.

Liljeberg Elmstahl H, and Bjorck I. Milk as a supplement to mixed meals may elevate postprandial insulinaemia. *European Journal of Clinical Nutrition* 55 no. 11 (2001): 994–99.

Liljeberg H, and Bjorck I. Delayed gastric emptying rate may explain improved glycaemia in healthy subjects to a starchy meal with added vinegar. *European Journal of Clinical Nutrition* 52 no. 5 (1998): 368–71.

Liljeberg HG, Lonner CH, and Bjorck IM. Sourdough fermentation or addition of organic acids or corresponding salts to bread improves nutritional properties of starch in healthy humans. *Journal of Nutrition* 125 no. 6 (1995): 1503–11.

Lin AH-M, Zihua A, Quezada-Calvillo R, Nichols BL, and Chi-Tien L. Branch pattern of starch internal structure influences the glucogenesis by mucosal Nt-maltase-glucoamylase. *Carbohydrate Polymers* 111 (2014): 33–40.

Lina BAR, Jonker D, and Kozianowski G. Isomaltulose (Palatinose): A review of biological and toxicological studies. *Food and Chemical Toxicology* 40 no. 10 (2002):1375–81.

Liu J, Grundy SM, Wang W, Smith SC, and Vega GL, Jr. Ethnic-specific criteria for the metabolic syndrome: Evidence from China. *Diabetes Care* 29 no. 6 (2006): 1414–16.

Liu Z, Jeppesen PB, Gregersen S, Chen X, and Hermansen K. Dose- and glucose-dependent effects of amino acids on insulin secretion from isolated mouse islets and clonal INS-1E beta-cells. *The Review of Diabetic Studies: RDS* 5 no. 4 (2008): 232–44.

Livesey G. Health potential of polyols as sugar replacers, with emphasis on low glycaemic properties. *Nutrition Research Reviews* 16 no. 2 (2003): 163–91.

Livesey G, Taylor R, Hulshof T, and Howlett J. Glycemic response and health—a systematic review and meta-analysis: Relations between dietary glycemic properties and health outcomes. *American Journal of Clinical Nutrition* 87 no. 1 (2008): 258S–68S.

Lopez CA, Vries AH, and Marrink SJ. Amylose folding under the influence of lipids. *Carbohydrate Research* 364 (2012): 1–7.

Lottenberg AM, Afonso MdS, Lavrador MSF, Machado RM, and Nakandakare ER. The role of dietary fatty acids in the pathology of metabolic syndrome. *Journal of Nutritional Biochemistry* 23 no. 9 (2012): 1027–40.

Lu ZX, Walker KZ, Muir JG, Mascara T, and O'Dea K. Arabinoxylan fiber, a byproduct of wheat flour processing, reduces the postprandial glucose response in normoglycemic subjects. *American Journal of Clinical Nutrition* 71 no. 5 (2000): 1123–28.

Lu ZX, Walker KZ, Muir JG, and O'Dea K. Arabinoxylan fibre improves metabolic control in people with Type II diabetes. *European Journal of Clinical Nutrition* 58 no. 4 (2004): 621–28.

Maki KC, Kanter M, Rains TM, Hess SP, and Geohas J. Acute effects of low insulinemic sweeteners on post-prandial insulin and glucose concentrations in obese men. *International Journal of Food Sciences and Nutrition* 60 Suppl. 3 (2009): 48–55.

Maki KC, and Phillips AK. Dietary substitutions for refined carbohydrate that show promise for reducing risk of type 2 diabetes in men and women. *Journal of Nutrition* 145 no. 1 (2015): 159S–63S.

Manach C, Williamson G, Morand C, Scalbert A, and Remesy C. Bioavailability and bioefficacy of polyphenols in humans I. Review of 97 bioavailability studies. *American Journal of Clinical Nutrition* 81 no. 1, Suppl. (2005):230S–42S.

Manders RJ, Little JP, Forbes SC, and Candow DG. Insulinotropic and muscle protein synthetic effects of branched-chain amino acids: Potential therapy for type 2 diabetes and sarcopenia. *Nutrients* 4 no. 11 (2012): 1664–78.

Marciani L, Gowland PA, Spiller RC, Manoj P, and Moore RJ. Effect of meal viscosity and nutrients on satiety, intragastric dilution, and emptying assessed by MRI. *American Journal of Physiology. Gastrointestinal and Liver Physiology* 280 no. 6 (2001): G1227–G1233.

Marriott BP, Cole N, and Lee E. National estimates of dietary fructose intake increased from 1977 to 2004 in the United States. *Journal of Nutrition* 139 no. 6 (2009): 1228S–35S.

McDougall GJ, Shpiro F, Dobson P, Smith P, and Blake A. Different polyphenolic components of soft fruits inhibit alpha-amylase and alpha-glucosidase. *Journal of Agricultural and Food Chemistry* 53 no. 7 (2005): 2760–66.

Mettler S, Schwarz I, and Colombani PC. Additive postprandial blood glucose-attenuating and satiety-enhancing effect of cinnamon and acetic acid. *Nutrition Research* 29 no. 10 (2009): 723–27.

Meynier A, Goux A, Atkinson FS, Brack O, and Vinoy S. Postprandial glycemic response: How is it influenced by characteristics of cereal products?. *British Journal of Nutrition* 113 no. 12 (2015): 1931–39.

Miao M, Jiang B, Cui SW, Zhang T, and Jin Z. Slowly digestible starch-a review. *Critical Reviews in Food Science and Nutrition* 55 no. 12 (2015): 1642–57.

Mkandawire NL, Kaufman RC, Bean SR, Weller CL, and Jackson DS. Effects of sorghum (Sorghum bicolor (L.) Moench) tannins on alpha-amylase activity and in vitro digestibility of starch in raw and processed flours. *Journal of Agricultural and Food Chemistry* 61 no. 18 (2013): 4448–54.

Nakamura S, Hongo R, Moji K, and Oku T. Suppressive effect of partially hydrolyzed guar gum on transitory diarrhea induced by ingestion of maltitol and lactitol in healthy humans. *European Journal of Clinical Nutrition* 61 no. 9 (2007): 1086–93.

Narita Y, and Inouye K. Kinetic analysis and mechanism on the inhibition of chlorogenic acid and its components against porcine pancreas alpha-amylase isozymes I and II. *Journal of Agricultural and Food Chemistry* 57 no. 19 (2009): 9218–25.

Nazare JA, Rougemont Ad, Normand S, Sauvinet V, and Sothier M. Effect of postprandial modulation of glucose availability: Short- and long-term analysis. *British Journal of Nutrition* 103 no. 10 (2010): 1461–70.

Nilsson A, Ostman E, Preston T, and Bjorck I. Effects of GI vs content of cereal fibre of the evening meal on glucose tolerance at a subsequent standardized breakfast. *European Journal of Clinical Nutrition* 62 no. 6 (2008a): 712–20.

Nilsson AC, Ostman EM, Granfeldt Y, and Bjorck IME. Effect of cereal test breakfasts differing in glycemic index and content of indigestible carbohydrates on daylong glucose tolerance in healthy subjects. *American Journal of Clinical Nutrition* 87 no. 3 (2008b): 645–54.

Nilsson M, Holst JJ, and Bjorck IME. Metabolic effects of amino acid mixtures and whey protein in healthy subjects: Studies using glucose-equivalent drinks. *American Journal of Clinical Nutrition* 85 no. 4 (2007): 996–1004.

Normand S, Khalfallah Y, Louche-Pelissier C, Pachiaudi C, and Antoine JM. Influence of dietary fat on post-prandial glucose metabolism (exogenous and endogenous) using intrinsically 13C-enriched durum wheat. *British Journal of Nutrition* 86 no. 1 (2001): 3–11.

Nyman M. Fermentation and bulking capacity of indigestible carbohydrates: The case of inulin and oligofructose. *British Journal of Nutrition* 87 Suppl. 2 (2002): S163–S168.

Oku T, Hongo R, and Nakamura S. Suppressive effect of cellulose on osmotic diarrhea caused by maltitol in healthy female subjects. *Journal of Nutritional Science and Vitaminology* 54 no. 4 (2008): 309–14.

Ortega FJ, and Fernandez-Real JM. Inflammation in adipose tissue and fatty acid anabolism: When enough is enough!. *Hormone and Metabolic Research* 45 no. 13 (2013): 1009–19.

Ososki AL, and Kennelly EJ. Phytoestrogens: A review of the present state of research. *Phytotherapy Research* 17 no. 8 (2003): 845–69.

Ostman E, Granfeldt Y, Persson L, and Bjorck I. Vinegar supplementation lowers glucose and insulin responses and increases satiety after a bread meal in healthy subjects. *European Journal of Clinical Nutrition* 59 no. 9 (2005): 983–88.

Panlasigui LN, Thompson LU, Juliano BO, Perez CM, and Yiu SH. Rice varieties with similar amylose content differ in starch digestibility and glycemic response in humans. *American Journal of Clinical Nutrition* 54 no. 5 (1991): 871–77.

Park YK, and Yetley EA. Intakes and food sources of fructose in the United States. *American Journal of Clinical Nutrition* 58 Suppl. 5 (1993): 737S–47S.

Parnell JA, and Reimer RA. Weight loss during oligofructose supplementation is associated with decreased ghrelin and increased peptide YY in overweight and obese adults. *American Journal of Clinical Nutrition* 89 no. 6 (2009): 1751–59.

Partanen KH, and Mroz Z. Organic acids for performance enhancement in pig diets. *Nutrition Research Reviews* 12 no. 1 (1999): 117–45.

Pedersen AM, Bardow A, Jensen SB, and Nauntofte B. Saliva and gastrointestinal functions of taste, mastication, swallowing and digestion. *Oral Diseases* 8 no. 3 (2002): 117–29.

Peng S, Xue L, Leng X, Yang R, and Zhang G. Slow digestion property of octenyl succinic anhydride modified waxy maize starch in the presence of tea polyphenols. *Journal of Agricultural and Food Chemistry* 63 no. 10 (2015): 2820–29.

Pereira LJ, Gaviao MBD, Engelen L, and Van der Bilt A. Mastication and swallowing: Influence of fluid addition to foods. *Journal of Applied Oral Science: Revista FOB* 15 no. 1 (2007): 55–60.

Perez-Escamilla R, Obbagy JE, Altman JM, Essery EV, and McGrane MM. Dietary energy density and body weight in adults and children: A systematic review. *Journal of the Academy of Nutrition and Dietetics* 112 no. 5 (2012): 671–84.

Peronnet F, Meynier A, Sauvinet V, Normand S, and Bourdon E. Plasma glucose kinetics and response of insulin and GIP following a cereal breakfast in female subjects: Effect of starch digestibility. *European Journal of Clinical Nutrition* 69 no. 6 (2015): 740–45.

Pourshahidi LK, Kerr MA, McCaffrey TA, and Livingstone MB. Influencing and modifying children's energy intake: The role of portion size and energy density. *Proceedings of the Nutrition Society* 73 no. 3 (2014): 397–406.

Quilez J, Bullo M, and Salas-Salvado J. Improved postprandial response and feeling of satiety after consumption of low-calorie muffins with maltitol and high-amylose corn starch. *Journal of Food Science* 72 no. 6 (2007): S407–S411.

Raben A, Agerholm-Larsen L, Flint A, Holst JJ, and Astrup A. Meals with similar energy densities but rich in protein, fat, carbohydrate, or alcohol have different effects on energy expenditure and substrate metabolism but not on appetite and energy intake. *American Journal of Clinical Nutrition* 77 no. 1 (2003): 91–100.

Ramdath Dd, Padhi E, Hawke A, Theva S, and Tsaoa R. The glycemic index of pigmented potatoes is related to their polyphenol content. *Food & Function* 5 no. 5 (2014): 909–15.

Ranawana V, Leow MKS, and Henry CJK. Mastication effects on the glycaemic index: Impact on variability and practical implications. *European Journal of Clinical Nutrition* 68 no. 1 (2014): 137–39.

Raninen K, Lappi J, Mykkanen H, and Poutanen K. Dietary fiber type reflects physiological functionality: Comparison of grain fiber, inulin, and polydextrose. *Nutrition Reviews* 69 no. 1 (2011): 9–21.

Rasmussen O, Lauszus FF, Christiansen C, Thomsen C, and Hermansen K. Differential effects of saturated and monounsaturated fat on blood glucose and insulin responses in subjects with non-insulin-dependent diabetes mellitus. *American Journal of Clinical Nutrition* 63 no. 2 (1996): 249–53.

Read NW, Welch IM, Austen CJ, Barnish C, and Bartlett CE. Swallowing food without chewing: A simple way to reduce postprandial glycaemia. *British Journal of Nutrition* 55 no. 1 (1986): 43–47.

Respondek F, Hilpipre C, Chauveau P, Cazaubiel M, and Gendre D. Digestive tolerance and postprandial glycaemic and insulinaemic responses after consumption of dairy desserts containing maltitol and fructo-oligosaccharides in adults. *European Journal of Clinical Nutrition* 68 no. 5 (2014): 575–80.

Rizkalla SW, Luo J, Wils D, Bruzzo F, and Slama G. Glycaemic and insulinaemic responses to a new hydrogenated starch hydrolysate in healthy and type 2 diabetic subjects. *Diabetes & Metabolism* 28 no. 5 (2002): 385–90.

Rizkalla SW. Health implications of fructose consumption: A review of recent data. *Nutrition & Metabolism* 7 (2010): 82.

Rokka S, Ketoja E, Jarvenpaa E, and Tahvonen R. The glycaemic and C-peptide responses of foods rich in dietary fibre from oat, buckwheat and lingonberry. *International Journal of Food Sciences and Nutrition* 64 no. 5 (2013): 528–34.

Rolls BJ, Drewnowski A, and Ledikwe JH. Changing the energy density of the diet as a strategy for weight management. *Journal of the American Dietetic Association* 105 (2005): 98–103.

Rosenblum JL, Irwin CL, and Alpers DH. Starch and glucose oligosaccharides protect salivary-type amylase activity at acid pH. *American Journal of Physiology* 254 no. 5,I (1988): G775–G780.

Russell WR, Baka A, Bjorck I, Delzenne N, and Gao D. Impact of diet composition on blood glucose regulation. *Critical Reviews in Food Science and Nutrition* 56 no. 4 (2016): 541–90.

Salehi A, Gunnerud U, Muhammed SJ, Ostman E, and Holst JJ. The insulinogenic effect of whey protein is partially mediated by a direct effect of amino acids and GIP on beta-cells. *Nutrition & Metabolism* 9 no. 1 (2012): 48.

Sanaka M, Yamamoto T, Anjiki H, Nagasawa K, and Kuyama Y. Effects of agar and pectin on gastric emptying and post-prandial glycaemic profiles in healthy human volunteers. *Clinical and Experimental Pharmacology and Physiology* 34 no. 11 (2007): 1151–55.

Sanchez-Lozada LG, Le M, Segal M, and Johnson RJ. How safe is fructose for persons with or without diabetes?. *American Journal of Clinical Nutrition* 88 no. 5 (2008): 1189–90.

Scazzina F, Siebenhandl-Ehn S, and Pellegrini N. The effect of dietary fibre on reducing the glycaemic index of bread. *British Journal of Nutrition* 109 no. 7 (2013): 1163–74.

Schenk S, Davidson CJ, Zderic TW, Byerley LO, and Coyle EF. Different glycemic indexes of breakfast cereals are not due to glucose entry into blood but to glucose removal by tissue. *American Journal of Clinical Nutrition* 78 no. 4 (2003): 742–48.

Schwab U, Lauritzen L, Tholstrup T, Haldorssoni T, and Riserus U. Effect of the amount and type of dietary fat on cardiometabolic risk factors and risk of developing type 2 diabetes, cardiovascular diseases, and cancer: A systematic review. *Food & Nutrition Research* 58 (2014).

Seneviratne HD, and Biliaderis CG. Action of alpha-amylases on amylose-lipid complex superstructures. *Journal of Cereal Science* 13 no. 2 (1991): 129–43.

Severijnen C, Abrahamse E, Beek EMBuco A, and Heijning BJM. Sterilization in a liquid of a specific starch makes it slowly digestible in vitro and low glycemic in rats. *Journal of Nutrition* 137 no. 10 (2007): 2202–07.

Shah M, Adams-Huet B, and Garg A. Effect of high-carbohydrate or high-cis-monounsaturated fat diets on blood pressure: A meta-analysis of intervention trials. *American Journal of Clinical Nutrition* 85 no. 5 (2007): 1251–56.

Shrayyef MZ, and Gerich JE. Normal glucose homeostasis. In *Principles of Diabetes Mellitus*, L Poretsky, ed., 19–35. New York: Springer (2010).

Singh J, Dartois A, and Kaur L. Starch digestibility in food matrix: A review. *Trends in Food Science & Technology* 21 no. 4 (2010): 168–80.

Sirichai A, Praew C, Haruthai T, and Sirintorn Y. A series of cinnamic acid derivatives and their inhibitory activity on intestinal alpha-glucosidase. *Journal of Enzyme Inhibition and Medicinal Chemistry* 24 no. 5 (2009): 1194–200.

Slavin JL, Savarino V, Paredes-Diaz A, and Fotopoulos G. A review of the role of soluble fiber in health with specific reference to wheat dextrin. *Journal of International Medical Research* 37 no. 1 (2009): 1–17.

Stanhope KL, and Havel PJ. Endocrine and metabolic effects of consuming beverages sweetened with fructose, glucose, sucrose, or high-fructose corn syrup. *American Journal of Clinical Nutrition* 88 no. 6 (2008): 1733S–37S.

Steele CM, Alsanei WA, Ayanikalath S, Barbon CEA, and Chen J. The influence of food texture and liquid consistency modification on swallowing physiology and function: A systematic review. *Dysphagia* 30 no. 1 (2015): 2–26.

Syahariza ZA, Sar S, Hasjim J, Tizzotti MJ, and Gilbert RG. The importance of amylose and amylopectin fine structures for starch digestibility in cooked rice grains. *Food Chemistry* 136 no. 2 (2013): 742–49.

Tapiero H, Tew KD, Nguyen Ba G, and Mathe G. Polyphenols: Do they play a role in the prevention of human pathologies?. *Biomedicine & Pharmacotherapy* 56 no. 4 (2002): 200–07.

Tappy L, and Le KA. Metabolic effects of fructose and the worldwide increase in obesity. *Physiological Reviews* 90 no. 1 (2010): 23–46.

Temme EHM, and Van Hoydonck PGA. Tea consumption and iron status. *European Journal of Clinical Nutrition* 56 no. 5 (2002): 379–86.

Thompson LU, Yoon JH, Jenkins DJA, Wolever TMS, and Jenkins AL. Relationship between polyphenol intake and blood glucose response of normal and diabetic individuals. *American Journal of Clinical Nutrition* 39 no. 5 (1984): 745–51.

Thomsen C, Storm H, Holst JJ, and Hermansen K. Differential effects of saturated and monounsaturated fats on postprandial lipemia and glucagon-like peptide 1 responses in patients with type 2 diabetes. *American Journal of Clinical Nutrition* 77 no. 3 (2003): 605–11.

Tufvesson F, Wahlgren M, and Eliasson AC. Formation of amylose-lipid complexes and effects of temperature treatment. Part 1. Monoglycerides. *Starch/Staerke* 55 no. 2 (2003a): 61–71.

Tufvesson F, Wahlgren M, and Eliasson AC. Formation of amylose-lipid complexes and effects of temperature treatment. Part 2. Fatty acids. *Starch/Staerke* 55 no. 3–4 (2003b): 138–49.

van Buul VJ, Tappy L, and Brouns FJPH. Misconceptions about fructose-containing sugars and their role in the obesity epidemic. *Nutrition Research Reviews* 27 no. 1 (2014): 119–30.

van Loon LJ, Kruijshoop M, Verhagen H, Saris WH, and Wagenmakers AJ. Ingestion of protein hydrolysate and amino acid-carbohydrate mixtures increases postexercise plasma insulin responses in men. *Journal of Nutrition* 130 no. 10 (2000a): 2508–13.

van Loon LJ, Saris WH, Verhagen H, and Wagenmakers AJ. Plasma insulin responses after ingestion of different amino acid or protein mixtures with carbohydrate. *American Journal of Clinical Nutrition* 72 no. 1 (2000b): 96–105.

Vinoy S. Influence of low GI cereal food on postprandial metabolism. Eurostarch final meeting, Gröningen, the Netherlands, April 28, 2006.

Vinoy S, Arlotti A, Meynier A, and Fuzellier G. How to reduce glycaemic response in processed foods: Mechanisms of action. *Annals of Nutrition and Metabolism* 58 Suppl. 3 (2011): 362.

Vinoy S, Normand S, Meynier A, Sothier M, and Louche-Pelissier C. Cereal processing influences postprandial glucose metabolism as well as the GI effect. *Journal of the American College of Nutrition* 32 no. 2 (2013): 79–91.

Vinoy S, Meynier A, Conrad M, and Goux A. Authorised EU health claim for slowly digestible starch. In *Foods, Nutrients and Food Ingredients with Authorised EU Health Claims: Volume 2, 1st Edition*, M Sadler, ed., 49–74. Cambridge: Woodhead Publishing (2015).

Wang M, Gao XJ, Zhao WW, Zhao WJ, and Jiang CH. Opposite effects of genistein on the regulation of insulin-mediated glucose homeostasis in adipose tissue. *British Journal of Pharmacology* 170 no. 2 (2013): 328–40.

Weickert MO, Roden M, Isken F, Hoffmann D, and Nowotny P. Effects of supplemented isoenergetic diets differing in cereal fiber and protein content on insulin sensitivity in overweight humans. *American Journal of Clinical Nutrition* 94 no. 2 (2011): 459–71.

Wierzejska R. Tea and health—a review of the current state of knowledge. *Przeglad Epidemiologiczny* 68 no. 3 (2014): 501–99.

Wolever TM, Jenkins DJ, Kalmusky J, Giordano C, and Giudici S. Glycemic response to pasta: Effect of surface area, degree of cooking, and protein enrichment. *Diabetes Care* 9 no. 4 (1986): 401–04.

Wolever TM, Nguyen PM, Chiasson JL, Hunt JA, and Josse RG. Determinants of diet glycemic index calculated retrospectively from diet records of 342 individuals with non-insulin-dependent diabetes mellitus. *American Journal of Clinical Nutrition* 59 no. 6 (1994): 1265–69.

Wolever TMS, Wong GS, Kenshole A , Josse RG, and Thompson LU. Lactose in the diabetic diet: A comparison with other carbohydrates. *Nutrition Research* 5 no. 12 (1985): 1335–45.

Zhang G, Ao Z, and Hamaker BR. Slow digestion property of native cereal starches. *Biomacromolecules* 7 no. 11 (2006a): 3252–58.

Zhang G, Hasek LY, Lee BH, and Hamaker BR. Gut feedback mechanisms and food intake: A physiological approach to slow carbohydrate bioavailability. *Food & Function* 6 no. 4 (2015): 1072–89.

Zhang G, Venkatachalam M, and Hamaker BR. Structural basis for the slow digestion property of native cereal starches. *Biomacromolecules* 7 no. 11 (2006b): 3259–66.

Zihua A, Simsek S, Genyi Z, Mahesh V, and Reuhs BL. Starch with a slow digestion property produced by altering its chain length, branch density, and crystalline structure. *Journal of Agricultural and Food Chemistry* 55 no. 11 (2007): 4540–47.

Appendix A: Glycemic Index of Some Commonly Consumed Foods

The following table includes glycemic index (GI) values of some commonly consumed foods taken from two sources (Foster-Powell et al., 2002; Atkinson et al., 2008). It is not intended to be a complete or sole source of information on GI of foods.

The reader is advised to refer to the above two sources and the University of Sydney's GI webpage (http://www.glycemicindex.com) to obtain information on specific foods, branded foods or foods less commonly consumed. Owing to possible differences in formulations between brands and/or countries, only foods where at least two types have been tested and no brand names were mentioned are shown below.

The GI values are reported either as a single value, if based on one study or as mean ± standard error of the mean (SEM), if based on a number of studies.

TABLE A.1
GI of Some Commonly Consumed Foods

Bakery Products	**GI Value**
Croissant[a]	67
Crumpet[a]	69
Doughnut[a]	76
Sponge cake, plain[a]	46 ± 6
Muffin, blueberry[a]	59
Pastry[a]	59 ± 6
Scones plain, made from packet mix[a]	92 ± 8
Waffles[a]	76
Pancakes from shake mix[a]	67 ± 5
Beverages	
Cordial, orange, reconstituted[a]	66 ± 8
Smoothie, raspberry[a]	33 ± 9
Soft drink/soda[b]	59 ± 3
Breads	
Bagel, white[a]	72
Chapatti[b]	52 ± 4
Corn tortilla[b]	45 ± 4
French baguette, plain[a]	95 ± 15
Gluten-free bread[a]	76 ± 5
Lebanese bread[a]	75 ± 9
Rye bread[a]	50 ± 4
Specialty grain bread[b]	53 ± 2
Unleavened wheat bread[b]	70 ± 5
Wheat roti[b]	62 ± 3
White pita bread[a]	57
White-wheat bread[b,c]	75 ± 2
Whole wheat/whole meal bread[b]	74 ± 2

(Continued)

TABLE A.1 (*Continued*)
GI of Some Commonly Consumed Foods

Food	GI
Breakfast Cereals	
All-bran (mean of four studies)[a,d]	42 ± 5
Cornflakes[b]	81 ± 6
Grapenuts (mean of two studies)[a,d]	71 ± 4
Instant oat porridge[b]	79 ± 3
Millet porridge[b]	67 ± 5
Muesli[b]	57 ± 2
Oat bran (mean of two studies)[a,d]	55 ± 5
Porridge, rolled oats[b]	55 ± 2
Puff wheat (mean of two studies)[a,d]	74 ± 7
Rice bubbles (mean of three studies)[a,d]	87 ± 4
Rice porridge/congee[b]	78 ± 9
Shredded wheat (mean of two studies)[a,d]	75 ± 8
Weetabix (mean of seven studies)[a,d]	70 ± 2
Wheat flake biscuits[b]	69 ± 2
Cereal Grains	
Amaranth (popped, eaten with milk and non-nutritive sweetener)[a]	97 ± 19
Barley[b]	28 ± 2
Buckwheat (mean of three studies)[a]	54 ± 4
Cornmeal (mean of two studies)[a]	69 ± 1
Couscous[be]	65 ± 4
Cracked wheat (bulgur or bourghul, mean of four studies)[a]	48 ± 2
Maize, flour made into chapatti[a]	59
Maize meal porridge[a]	109
Millet, boiled[a]	71 ± 10
Millet flour porridge[a]	107
Pearl barley (mean of five studies)[a]	25 ± 1
Semolina (mean of two studies)[a]	55 ± 1
Wheat, whole kernels (mean of four studies)[a]	41 ± 3
Cookies/Crackers[d]	
Arrowroot (mean of three studies)[a,d]	65 ± 2
Digestives (mean of three studies)[a,d]	59 ± 2
Rice cakes (mean of three studies)[a,d]	78 ± 9
Rye crispbread (mean of four studies)[a,d]	64 ± 2
Water cracker (mean of two studies)[a,d]	71 ± 8
Dairy Products and Alternatives	
Milk, full fat[b]	39 ± 3
Milk, skim[b]	37 ± 4
Ice cream[b]	51 ± 3
Yoghurt, fruit[b]	41 ± 2
Soy milk[b]	34 ± 4
Rice milk[b]	86 ± 7
Fruit and Fruit Products	
Apple, raw[b,e]	36 ± 2
Apple juice[b]	41 ± 2
Apricots, raw[a]	57

(*Continued*)

TABLE A.1 (*Continued*)
GI of Some Commonly Consumed Foods

Apricots, canned in light syrup[a]	64
Apricots, dried (mean of two studies)[a]	31 ± 1
Banana, raw[b,e]	51 ± 3
Dates, raw[b]	42 ± 4
Grapefruit, raw[a]	25
Grapefruit juice[a]	48
Grapes (mean of two studies)[a]	46 ± 3
Cherries, raw[a]	22
Kiwi (mean of two studies)[a]	53 ± 6
Orange, raw[b,e]	43 ± 3
Orange juice[b]	50 ± 2
Peaches, raw (mean of two studies)[a]	42 ± 14
Pears, raw (mean of four studies)[a]	48 ± 2
Pineapple, raw[b]	59 ± 8
Plum, raw (mean of two studies)[a]	39 ± 15
Prunes[a]	29 ± 4
Mango, raw[b,e]	51 ± 5
Watermelon, raw[b]	76 ± 4
Peaches, canned[b,e]	43 ± 5
Raisins[a]	64 ± 11
Strawberry jam/jelly[b]	49 ± 3
Sultanas[a]	56 ± 11
Legumes and Nuts	
Baked beans (mean of two studies)[a]	48 ± 8
Beans, dried, boiled (mean of two studies)[a]	29 ± 9
Black-eyed beans and peas (mean of two studies)[a]	42 ± 9
Butter beans (mean of two studies)[a]	51 ± 3
Cashew nuts, salted[a]	22 ± 5
Chickpeas[b]	28 ± 9
Haricot and navy beans (mean of five studies)[a]	38 ± 6
Kidney beans[b]	24 ± 4
Lentils[b]	32 ± 5
Marrowfat peas[a]	39 ± 8
Peanuts (mean of three studies)[a]	14 ± 8
Peas, dried, boiled[a]	22
Soybeans[b]	16 ± 1
Sweet corn[b]	52 ± 5
Pasta	
Fettucine, egg (mean of three studies)[a]	40 ± 8
Linguine, thick (mean of four studies)[a]	52 ± 3
Linguine, thin (mean of two studies)[a]	46 ± 3
Mung bean noodles (mean of two studies)[a]	33 ± 7
Spaghetti, white[b]	49 ± 2
Spaghetti, whole meal[b]	48 ± 5
Noodles	
Rice noodles[b,e]	53 ± 7
Udon noodles[b]	55 ± 7

(*Continued*)

TABLE A.1 (*Continued*)
GI of Some Commonly Consumed Foods

Rice	
White rice, boiled[b,c]	73 ± 4
Brown rice, boiled[b]	68 ± 4
Snack Foods	
Chocolate[b]	40 ± 3
Corn chips (mean of three studies)[a]	63 ± 10
Jelly beans (mean of two studies)[a]	78 ± 2
Popcorn[b]	65 ± 5
Potato crisps[b]	56 ± 3
Rice crackers/crisps[b]	87 ± 2
Sugars	
Fructose[b]	15 ± 4
Sucrose[b]	65 ± 4
Glucose[b]	103 ± 3
Honey[b]	61 ± 3
Vegetables	
Beetroot[a]	64 ± 6
Broad beans[a]	79 ± 16
Carrots, boiled[b]	39 ± 4
Green peas (mean of three studies)[a]	48 ± 5
Plantain/green banana[b]	55 ± 6
Potato, boiled[b]	78 ± 4
Potato, french fries[b]	63 ± 5
Potato, instant mash[b]	87 ± 3
Pumpkin, boiled[b]	64 ± 7
Sweet corn (mean of six studies)[a]	54 ± 4
Sweet potato, boiled[b]	63 ± 6
Taro, boiled[b]	53 ± 2
Vegetable soup[b]	48 ± 5
Yam (mean of three studies)[a]	37 ± 8

[a] Data from Foster-Power, K. et al., *Am. J. Clin. Nutr.*, 76, 5–56, 2002. Data are means ± SEM.
[b] Data from Atkinson, F.S. et al., *Diabetes Care*, 31, 2281–2283, 2008. Derived from multiple studies by different laboratories.
[c] Low-GI varieties were also identified.
[d] Owing to possible differences in formulations between brands and/or countries, reported foods are only those that, at least two types, have been tested and no brand names are mentioned.
[e] Average of all available data.

REFERENCES

Atkinson, F.S., Foster-Powell, K., and Brand-Miller, J.C. (2008). International tables of glycemic index and glycemic load values: 2008. *Diabetes Care*, 31, 2281–2283.

Foster-Powell, K., Holt, S.H., and Brand-Miller, J.C. (2002). International table of glycemic index and glycemic load values: 2002. *Am. J. Clin. Nutr.*, 76, 5–56.

Index

Note: Page numbers followed by f and t refer to figures and tables, respectively.

G

H

I

K

L

M

N

O

V

W